First Responder Mental Health

Michael L. Bourke
Vincent B. Van Hasselt • Sam J. Buser
Editors

First Responder Mental Health

A Clinician's Guide

Springer

Editors
Michael L. Bourke
Michael Bourke, Ph.D., PLLC
Springfield, VA, USA

Vincent B. Van Hasselt
College of Psychology
Nova Southeastern University
Davie, FL, USA

Sam J. Buser
Houston Fire Department (Retired)
Houston, TX, USA

ISBN 978-3-031-38148-5 ISBN 978-3-031-38149-2 (eBook)
https://doi.org/10.1007/978-3-031-38149-2

This Springer imprint is published by the registered company Springer Nature Switzerland AG
The registered company address is: Gewerbestrasse 11, 6330 Cham, Switzerland

Paper in this product is recyclable.

Editors
Michael L. Bourke
Michael Bourke, Ph.D., PLLC
Springfield, VA, USA

Vincent B. Van Hasselt
College of Psychology
Nova Southeastern University
Davie, FL, USA

Sam J. Buser
Houston Fire Department (Retired)
Houston, TX, USA

ISBN 978-3-031-38148-5 ISBN 978-3-031-38149-2 (eBook)
https://doi.org/10.1007/978-3-031-38149-2

This Springer imprint is published by the registered company Springer Nature Switzerland AG
The registered company address is: Gewerbestrasse 11, 6330 Cham, Switzerland

Paper in this product is recyclable.

Michael L. Bourke
Vincent B. Van Hasselt • Sam J. Buser
Editors

First Responder Mental Health

A Clinician's Guide

Springer

Overview and Introduction

This book was inspired by our more than 100 collective years of experience in nearly every first responder setting: local, county, and federal law enforcement; fire services; EMS; state and federal corrections; emergency communications; and the military. The fact we have not simply worked as psychologists in these fields but also have served on the front lines has given us a unique perspective on the issue of first responder wellness. We saw this book as an opportunity to contribute to other clinicians who may practice in these settings, as well as those who are considering whether to work with one or more first responder populations.

While each profession has unique characteristics, and each possesses a subculture all its own, there are commonalities that wind their way among the groups described herein. Working with the darker sides of humanity and being regularly exposed to disasters and other critical incidents can take their toll on any first responder, and wellness should be a goal no matter which uniform one wears. For this volume, we invited some of the leading experts in the field to share their perspectives on important issues that almost inevitably arise when clinicians work with first responders.

Part I, Mental Health of First Responders, contains descriptions of psychological issues that arise in public safety settings. Miller discusses stress and coping in law enforcement officers, describes effective interventions, and identifies issues relevant to psychotherapy with this population. Buser tackles similar issues in the fire services, including obstacles to seeking mental health care and common mental health issues faced by firefighters. He also offers tips for clinicians who want to work with either professional or volunteer firefighters and/or EMS personnel. The next chapter, by Lowe et al., deals with an oft-neglected group of first responders – correctional workers. The authors discuss occupational stressors that can emerge behind the prison walls; they then provide a conceptual framework for prevention and intervention efforts. Next, Plombon and her colleagues discuss subtypes of crime scene investigators and distinguish stressors particular to this profession. Finally, Beamer et al. address emergency communications operators (dispatchers), a group that is arguably the "first" among first responders yet may be the least likely to receive appropriate psychological assistance.

In Part II, Assessment and Prevention, Mangan provides an overview of psychological evaluations in public safety settings. He includes a discussion on two of the most common evaluations requested in the field: pre-employment psychological evaluations and fitness for duty evaluations.

Presley and colleagues then discuss Behavioral Health Training and peer support programs. In the following chapter, Bourke distinguishes secondary traumatic stress from vicarious trauma and posttraumatic stress, and offers insights for working with first responders who experience stressors secondarily (e.g., online). Lebeaut et al. then provide a similar inquiry into wellness, focusing on resilience and mindfulness. They offer pragmatic guidelines for large-scale as well as client-specific program implementation. The section ends with a multi-part chapter by Mitchell and Everly on Critical Incident Stress Management (CISM). In the first half, they introduce key concepts and describe the history and development of CISM, and in the second they describe specific applications, such as Rest, Information and Transition Services (RITS), Crisis Management Briefing (CMB), Defusing, and Critical Incident Stress Debriefing (CISD).

Part III, Treatment Strategies, begins with Martin's chapter on cognitive-behavioral approaches when working with public safety personnel, including variations of CBT that may be used with this population. Cipriano and colleagues then discuss the development of Eye Movement Desensitization Reprocessing (EMDR) from the inception of the process in the late 1980s to present-day applications in law enforcement settings. In the next chapter, Cox et al. use several case studies to illustrate how exposure treatments were effectively applied to public safety personnel, and they highlight the potential utility of the embedded behavioral health perspective. Next, Gralnik and Rey describe pharmacological interventions; in this extremely comprehensive chapter, several useful tables are offered for quick reference. In the following chapter, Beidel et al. introduce an innovative and promising treatment modality – virtual reality treatment – and provide the reader with an understanding of how the procedure could be incorporated into clinical work with first responders. The part wraps up with Eickleberry's discussion of how motivational interviewing can be used with first responders; she also provides helpful vignettes as examples of how the techniques can show up in clinical work.

Those who provide clinical services in public safety settings will be familiar with what we call Special Topics – these categories are found in Part IV of this book. They include the role of the chaplaincy by Braswell and Beamer, followed by chapters by Pepper and Cnapich on the mental health of retired first responders, and on Employee Assistance Programs by Couwels. Suicide prevention and intervention, a growing and concerning problem, is addressed by Ammendola and colleagues. Last, the issue of trauma and PTSD is tackled by Zegel et al.

Part V is titled Advocacy, and here we placed Garmezy's chapter on working with families of first responders, Massey's description of the role of administrators in the public safety arena, and McGrew et al.'s perspective on look at mental health issues among female first responders. These are followed by Belsches and Blackmon's in-depth look at first responders of color and Buser's examination of veterans who work in the public safety arena. The last chapter, by Chan and Dryden, is an in-depth discussion of legal issues that pertain to the first responder community.

We should note that some chapters include hypothetical interactions with first responders. These "quotes" are merely exemplars, and are not excerpts from any specific conversation. Most of these statements are a paraphrased amalgam of remarks made by multiple first responders; they are provided merely to provide a summary of how first responders tend to view a particular issue, or to illustrate how a technique might be used in clinical practice.

It goes without saying that first responders today are adapting to a rapidly changing world and facing crises never before experienced, from political and social unrest to pandemics to an exponential rise in online criminality. To date there has been no more appropriate time to focus on finding answers to the question, "How do we protect the protectors?" Caring for first responders is noble work; if you are serving (or intend to serve) any of the first responders in our extensive family of public safety professionals, you have our sincere thanks. We are confident you will find it as professionally and personally rewarding as we have.

Springfield, VA, USA — Michael L. Bourke
Davie, FL, USA — Vincent B. Van Hasselt
Houston, TX, USA — Sam J. Buser

Contents

Part III Treatment Strategies

Part IV Special Topics

Part V Advocacy

Contributors

Ron Acierno University of Texas Health Science Center, Houston, TX, USA

Faillace Department of Psychiatry and Ralph H. Johnson VA Medical Center, Charleston, SC, USA

Ennio Ammendola The Ohio State University Wexner Medical Center, Columbus, OH, USA

Justin Baker The Ohio State University Wexner Medical Center, Columbus, OH, USA

Rick Baker Responder Support Services, Asheville, NC, USA

Angela T. Beamer College of Psychology, Nova Southeastern University, Fort Lauderdale, FL, USA

Deborah C. Beidel Department of Psychology, University of Central Florida, Orlando, FL, USA

Leah J. Belsches Houston Fire Department, Houston, TX, USA

Garry W. Blackmon Houston Fire Department, Houston, TX, USA

Jessica R. Blalock College of Psychology, Nova Southeastern University, Fort Lauderdale, FL, USA

Michael L. Bourke Michael Bourke, Ph.D., PLLC, Springfield, VA, USA

United States Marshals Service Behavioral Analysis Unit (Retired), Arlington, VA, USA

Clint A. Bowers Department of Psychology, University of Central Florida, Orlando, FL, USA

Richard Braswell Broward Sheriff's Office (Retired), Fort Lauderdale, FL, USA

Teresa Bryant , Town of Jupiter, FL, USA

Keiser University, West, FL, USA

Sam J. Buser Houston Fire Department (Retired), Houston, TX, USA

Leonard N. Chan Houston Fire Department, Houston, TX, USA

Robert J. Cipriano Jr Fort Lauderdale Police Department, Fort Lauderdale, FL, USA

Emily M. Cnapich College of Psychology, Nova Southeastern University, Fort Lauderdale, FL, USA

Judy Couwels Broward Sheriff's Office, Fort Lauderdale, FL, USA

Keith Cox , Asheville, NC, USA

Responder Support Services, Asheville, NC, USA

Caitlin N. Dryden Bucks County District Attorney's Office, Doylestown, PA, USA

Lori L. Eickleberry Motivational Institute for Behavioral Health, Fort Lauderdale, FL, USA

Institute for Life Renovation, LLC, Fort Lauderdale, FL, USA

College of Psychology, Nova Southeastern University, Davie, FL, USA

David Englert Uniformed Services University of the Health Sciences (USUHS), FL, USA

George S. Everly Jr School of Public Health, Johns Hopkins University, Baltimore, MD, USA

International Critical Incident Stress Foundation, Ellicott City, MD, USA

Elizabeth Anderson Fletcher Department of Decision and Information Sciences, University of Houston, Houston, TX, USA

Lisa Berg Garmezy Independent Practice, Houston, TX, USA

Leonard M. Gralnik Department of Psychiatry and Behavioral Health, Herbert Wertheim College of Medicine, Florida International University, Miami, FL, USA

Caroline Haskamp College of Psychology, Nova Southeastern University, Fort Lauderdale, FL, USA

Nathanial A. Healy Department of Psychology, University of Houston, Houston, TX, USA

Crystal Joudry Responder Support Services, Asheville, NC, USA

Katherine Kuhlman Kuhlman Psychology and Counseling, Scottsdale, AZ, USA

Antoine Lebeaut Department of Psychology, University of Houston, Houston, TX, USA

Samuel J. Leonard Department of Psychology, University of Houston, Houston, TX, USA

Krystal Lowe Saint Mary's University, Halifax, NS, Canada

Philip R. Magaletta ICF, Columbia, MD, USA

Federal Bureau of Prisons (Retired), Columbia, MD, USA

Brian Mangan Law Enforcement Psychological & Counseling Associates, Inc., Medley, FL, USA

Colleen E. Martin Cincinnati VA Medical Center, Cincinnati, OH, USA

Larry L. Massey Jr Abraham S. Fischler College of Education, School of Criminal Justice, Nova Southeastern University, Fort Lauderdale, FL, USA

Shelby J. McGrew University of Houston, Houston, TX, USA

Laurence Miller Miller Psychological Associates, Boca Raton, FL, USA

Jeffrey T. Mitchell International Critical Incident Stress Foundation, Ellicott City, MD, USA

Department of Emergency Health Services, University of Maryland, Baltimore, MD, USA

Marc Patry Saint Mary's University, Halifax, NS, Canada

Jordana Pepper Federal Bureau of Prisons, Lompoc, CA, USA

Brittany Plombon College of Psychology, Nova Southeastern University, Fort Lauderdale, FL, USA

Hannah Pressley College of Psychology, Nova Southeastern University, Fort Lauderdale, FL, USA

Jose A. Rey Department of Pharmacy Practice, College of Pharmacy, Nova Southeastern University, Fort Lauderdale, FL, USA

Samantha Rodriguez College of Psychology, Nova Southeastern University, Fort Lauderdale, FL, USA

Carrington Slaughter University of Houston, Houston, TX, USA

Kathryn D. Sunderman Department of Psychology, University of Central Florida, Orlando, FL, USA

Edwin Szeto The Ohio State University Wexner Medical Center, Columbus, OH, USA

Tara D. Thomas Broward Sheriff's Office, Fort Lauderdale, FL, USA

Jana Tran National Aeronautics and Space Administration, Houston, TX, USA

Eleni Travers Federal Bureau of Prisons, Ayer, MA, USA

Vincent B. Van Hasselt College of Psychology, Nova Southeastern University, Davie, FL, USA

Anka A. Vujanovic University of Houston, Houston, TX, USA

Sherri L. White Broward Sheriff's Office, Fort Lauderdale, FL, USA

Ashley T. Winch Department of Psychology, University of Central Florida, Orlando, FL, USA

Maya Zegel Department of Psychology, University of Houston, Houston, TX, USA

Part I
Mental Health of First Responders

Psychological Stress Syndromes and Treatment Strategies for Law Enforcement Personnel

Laurence Miller

Stress and Coping in Law Enforcement Professionals

Police officers regularly deal with the most violent, impulsive, and predatory members of society, sometimes putting their lives on the line and handling traumatic crises that most of us view from the sanitized distance of pages and screens. In addition to the daily grind and critical incidents, officers are frequently the targets of criticism and complaints by citizens, the media, the judicial system, opportunistic politicians, hostile attorneys, "do-gooder" clinicians and social service workers, and their own administrators and law enforcement agencies. In some cases, police work stress may bleed over into personal lives, leading to family distress and dissolution (Blau, 1994; Borum & Philpot, 1993; Miller, 1995, 1998, 2000, 2006c, 2007b, 2009b, 2011; Woody, 2006).

While police officers generally carry out their sworn duties and responsibilities with competence and dedication, the stress load may sometimes be too much to handle, and every officer has their breaking point. For some, it may come in the form of a particularly dramatic event, such as a gruesome accident or homicide, a vicious crime against a child, a close personal brush with death, the killing or wounding of a partner, the mistaken shooting of an innocent civilian, or an especially grisly accident or crime scene (Henry, 2004; Miller, 2006a, 2007a).

For other officers, there may be no single major trauma; however, the identified mental breakdown occurs under the cumulative weight of a number of more moderate stresses over the course of the officer's career. In either case, an officer may feel that the department does not support them and that there is nowhere else to vent their frustration and distress. Consequently, the officer bottles up their feelings, becomes surly with coworkers and civilians, and grows hypersensitive to small annoyances on and off the job. As their isolation and feelings of alienation grow,

L. Miller (✉)
Miller Psychological Associates, Boca Raton, FL, USA

M. L. Bourke et al. (eds.), *First Responder Mental Health*,
https://doi.org/10.1007/978-3-031-38149-2_1

health and home life begin to deteriorate, work becomes a burden, and the officer may ultimately feel that he is going "squirrelly" (McCafferty et al., 1992; Russell & Beigel, 1990).

Most police officers deal with both routine and exceptional stresses by using a variety of situationally adaptive coping and defense mechanisms, such as repression, displacement, isolation of feelings, humor, or just clamming up and toughing it out. Officers develop an insular "cop culture" centering around *The Job*. Part of this closed-society credo is based on the shared belief that no civilian or outsider could possibly understand what police officers go through on a day-to-day basis (Anderson et al., 1995; Blau, 1994; Miller, 2006b; Woody, 2005).

According to one estimate (Sewell et al., 1988), after a traumatically stressful incident, such as an officer-involved shooting, approximately one-third of officers have minimal or no problems, another third have moderate problems, and the final third have severe problems affecting the officer, their family, and the department. It is still unclear whether police work produces an inordinate number of stress disabilities compared to other professions (Curran, 2003; Henry, 2004). And, in my experience, the overwhelming majority of officers recover spontaneously or experience minimal psychological sequelae from critical incidents, unless their actions are contested and subject to adverse investigation or other proceedings, which occur in use of force or deadly force cases (Miller, 2006a, b, 2015a, 2019, 2020, in press). In such cases, officers may experience significant emotional reactions, which include a heightened sense of danger, flashbacks, intrusive imagery and thoughts, anger, guilt, sleep disturbances, withdrawal, depression, and other stress symptoms; in rare cases, this may result in PTSD-like symptoms (Miller, 2015c, 2020, in press).

In some instances, the untreated after-effects of a traumatic incident may persist for months or years in the form of anger, hostility, irritability, conflicts with authority, fatigue, impaired concentration, loss of self-confidence, or increased indulgence in food or substances. Many of these long-term effects interfere with work performance and threaten the stability of personal relationships. Ultimately, they may be responsible for early retirement, burnout, or, in rare cases, suicide (Cummings, 1996; Miller, 2005a, 2006a; Regehr & Bober, 2004).

In other cases, the delayed or prolonged stress reaction manifests itself in the form of somatic symptoms such as headaches, chronic musculoskeletal pain syndromes, stomachaches, heart palpitations, or breathing disturbances. Typically, physical symptoms are easier to justify as a cause of stress-related disability than "mental problems" for police officers, first responders, military personnel, and others who are invested in their sense of toughness and resilience (Benedikt & Kolb, 1986; McFarlane et al., 1994; Miller, 1995, 2008a, 2013a, b; Regehr & Bober, 2004; Toch, 2002; Woody, 2005).

Extreme critical incidents aside, officers often overlook the cumulative effect of more ordinary stressors, such as long overtime hours during disasters, dealing with child victims, attempting resuscitation on a victim who dies, or working a fatal accident scene where the officer knows the victim. Failure to resolve these issues may lead to a variety of maladaptive response patterns. Some officers begin to overreact to perceived or imagined threats, while others ignore clear danger signals.

Some cops retire prematurely, while others become discipline problems or show increased absenteeism, impaired work performance, stress disorders, substance abuse, or a host of other personal problems that can interfere with functioning at home and on the job (Miller, 2011; Solomon, 1988, 1990, 1995; Solomon & Horn, 1986).

Special pressures are experienced by higher-ranking officers or those attached to special units, such as hostage negotiation, undercover work, or homicide and sex crimes detectives, especially those who are involved in the investigation of particularly brutal crimes, such as multiple murders, serial killings, or child sexual abuse (Miller, 2005b, 2006d, 2009a, 2013a, b; Sewell, 1993, 1994). The normally expected societal protective role of the police officer becomes heightened at the same time as their responsibilities as public servants who protect individual rights become compounded by the pressures to solve the crime.

A murder or child sex crime investigation forces an officer to confront stressors directly related to their projected role and image of showing unflagging strength in the face of adversity and frustration, responding competently and dispassionately to crises, and placing the needs and demands of the public above personal feelings. Moreover, the sheer magnitude and shock effect of many mass-homicide scenes (e.g., school shootings) or the violence and sadism associated with many sex crimes, sometimes involving children, often exceed the defense mechanisms and coping capacities of even the most seasoned and hard-boiled investigator. Revulsion may be tinged with rage when fellow officers have been killed or injured, or when the offender is known, but the existing evidence is insufficient to support an arrest or conviction. The cumulative effect of fatigue compounds the problem, which may lead to case errors, deteriorating work quality, and the wearing down of the investigator's normal defenses, rendering them even more vulnerable to stress and burnout (Miller, 2009a; Sewell, 1993, 1994).

Interventions with Police Officers in Distress

To avoid overly clinical-sounding connotations, mental health intervention services with emergency service and crisis personnel have often been contextualized in more neutral terminology as *debriefing, stress management, or psychological first aid* (Anderson et al., 1995; Belles & Norvell, 1990; Everly & Lating, 2022; Miller, 1999, 2008b; Mitchell & Bray, 1990). Where spontaneous recovery does not fully occur, incident-specific, one-time interventions will be most appropriate for handling the effects of an isolated overwhelmingly traumatic event on otherwise normal, well-functioning personnel. Where posttraumatic sequelae persist, or where the psychological problems relate to a longer-term pattern of maladaptive functioning under relatively routine stresses, more extensive individual psychotherapeutic approaches are called for (Everly & Lating, 2022; Miller, 1995, 1998, 2003, 2006b).

Critical Incident Stress Debriefing

Although the stress debriefing approach has grown out of the general field of crisis intervention, and is an important element of all therapeutic work with traumatized individuals, *critical incident stress debriefing* (CISD) was organizationally formalized for law enforcement and first-responder services by Jeff Mitchell and his colleagues (Mitchell, 1983, 1988, 1991; Mitchell & Bray, 1990; Mitchell & Everly, 1996). Despite some recent controversies (see Everly & Lating, 2022, for a review), CISD is now implemented in public safety departments throughout the United States, Britain, Europe, Australia, and other parts of the world (Dyregrov, 1989; Everly & Lating, 2022, Miller, 1999). CISD is often subsumed under the broader umbrella category of *critical incident stress management* (CISM), which includes a range of preventive and crisis intervention strategies, such as one-on-one defusings, large-scale demobilizations, and other approaches (Everly & Mitchell, 1997; Everly et al., 2000; Mitchell & Everly, 1996).

CISD is characterized as a structured technique designed to promote the emotional processing of traumatic events through the ventilation and normalization of reactions, as well as preparation for possible future experiences (Everly & Mitchell, 1997; Mitchell & Everly, 1996). Flexible adaptations of CISD have included applications to individual, family, child, and group therapy (Everly et al., 2000; Miller, 1998, 1999).

The CISD Process

A CISD typically is a peer-led, clinician-guided, group process, although, as noted above, for police officers and military personnel, applications of this approach for individual interventions have proven effective (Miller, 2006c, 2008a, b, 2009a, 2013a, b). The staffing of a debriefing usually consists of at least one licensed mental health professional and one or more *peer debriefers*, that is, fellow police officers, firefighters, paramedics, or other peer personnel who have been trained in the CISD process and who may have been through critical incidents and debriefings in their own careers.

A typical debriefing takes place within 24–72 h after the critical incident and consists of a single group meeting that lasts 2–3 h, although shorter or longer meetings may be dictated by circumstances. Group size may range from a handful to a roomful, usually determined by how many people will have time to fully express themselves in the number of hours allotted for the debriefing. Where large numbers of crisis workers are involved, such as in mass casualty incidents, several debriefings may be held successively over the course of days to accommodate all the personnel involved (Mitchell & Bray, 1990; Mitchell & Everly, 1996).

The standard CISD protocol consists of seven key phases, designed to move from factual and cognitive processing, through emotional engagement, and then back into structured intellectualization and practical recommendations.

1. *Introduction.* The introduction phase of a debriefing is the time in which the team leader—either a mental health professional or peer debriefer, depending on the composition of the group—gradually introduces the CISD process, encourages participation by the group, and sets the ground rules by which the debriefing will operate. Generally, these involve confidentiality, attendance for the full session, non-forced participation in discussions, and the establishment of a non-critical atmosphere.
2. *Fact phase.* During this phase, the group members are asked to briefly describe their job or role during the incident and, from their own perspective, provide some facts regarding what happened. The basic question is: "What did you do?"
3. *Thought phase.* The CISD leader asks the group members to discuss their first and subsequent thoughts during the critical incident: "What went through your mind?"
4. *Reaction phase.* This phase is designed to move the group participants from a predominantly cognitive and intellectual level of processing to a more emotionally expressive and cathartic mode: "What was the worst part of the incident for you?" It is usually at this point that the meeting gets intense, as members take their cues from one another and begin to vent their distress. Clinicians and peer debriefers keep a keen eye out for any adverse reactions among the personnel.
5. *Symptom phase.* This begins the movement back from the predominantly emotional processing level to the cognitive mode. Participants are asked to describe cognitive, physical, emotional, and behavioral signs and symptoms of distress that appeared at the scene or within 24 h of the incident; a few days after the incident; and ongoing, persisting at the time of the debriefing. This allows for the sharing and universalizing of potentially disorienting stress symptoms and reactions in a constructively intellectualized, problem-solving discussion. The question here is: "What have you been experiencing since the incident?"
6. *Education phase.* Continuing the move back toward cognitive processing, information is exchanged about the nature of the stress response and the expected physiological and psychological reactions to critical incidents. The clearest role for the mental health professional in this phase is as a teacher and expert in psychology and the science of traumatic stress effects. This serves to normalize the stress and coping responses and provides a basis for questions and answers.
7. *Re-entry phase.* This is a wrap-up, during which any additional questions or statements are addressed, referral for individual follow-ups are made, and general group bonding is reinforced: "What have you learned?" "Is there anything positive that can come out of this experience that can help you grow personally or professionally?" "How can you help one another in the future?" Indeed, where realistic and appropriate, invoking positivity has been found to have powerful therapeutic effects in many forms of intervention, with diverse populations,

including law enforcement personnel (Galatzer-Levy et al., 2013; Hamling & Jarden, 2017; Miller, 2008b).

This is not to suggest that these phases always follow one another in an unvarying, mechanical sequence. In practice, I have found that once group participants feel comfortable with the debriefing process and start talking, the fact, thought, and reaction phases may start to blend together. Indeed, as Mitchell and Everly (1996) recognize, it would seem artificial and forced to abruptly interrupt someone expressing emotion just because it is not the "right phase." Initially, debriefings should adhere to the stepwise protocol, but as long as the basic rationale and structure of the debriefing are maintained, the therapeutic effect will usually result. In most cases, clinician-team leaders have to assertively step in only when emotional reactions become particularly intense, or where one or more group members begin to blame or criticize others.

Special Modifications and Applications of CISD for Law Enforcement

As noted earlier, for the past quarter century, the standard model of CISD has been used with wide success all over the world, with diverse groups of emergency service, military, and civilian personnel (Dyregrov, 1989; Everly & Mitchell, 1997; Everly et al., 2000; Mitchell & Bray, 1990; Mitchell & Everly, 1996). Police officers, in particular, can be an insular group, often reluctant to talk to outsiders, especially "shrinks." They may be more resistant to showing weakness in front of their peers than other emergency personnel. Officers typically work alone or with a partner, as opposed to firefighters and paramedics, who are trained to have more of a team mentality (Anderson et al., 1995; Blau, 1994; Honig & Roland, 1998; Horn, 1991; Kirschman, 1997; McMains, 1991; Mitchell, 1991; Peak, 2003; Reese, 1987, 1991; Solomon, 1988, 1990, 1995; Toch, 2002; Woody, 2005). This has led to some special adaptations of the CISD approach for law enforcement.

When only one officer has been involved in a critical incident, such as an officer-involved shooting, or as a more focused, individualized follow-up to the general group debriefing, Solomon (1995) recommends that individual debriefings be conducted by a licensed mental health professional. In an individual debriefing, the emotional impact of the incident is assessed and explored as thoughts, feelings, and reactions are discussed. A recommended format for individual debriefing sessions is to go over the incident "frame by frame" with the officer, while they verbalize the moment-to-moment thoughts, perceptions, sensory details, feelings, and actions that occurred during the incident. This can help the officer become aware of, sort out, and understand what happened, get in touch with the perceptions and state of mind experienced during the incident, and understand why certain actions were taken or specific decisions were made. The frame-by-frame approach defuses inappropriate self-blame by helping the officer to differentiate what was under their control from what was not, and what was known at the time from what was impossible to be aware of then, but that may appear painfully clear in hindsight or by subsequent witness testimony and/or video recording (Solomon, 1990, 1995).

For incidents that have had intense or wide-ranging psychological effects, Solomon (1995) recommends what he terms a *critical incident peer support seminar*, in which the involved officers come together for 2 or 3 days in a retreat-like setting to revisit their experience several months following the critical incident. The seminar is facilitated by mental health professionals and peer support officers.

Sewell (1993, 1994) has elaborated a CISD-type adaptation of the CISM model to the particular needs of homicide detectives who investigate multiple murders and other violent crimes. The major objectives of this process are (1) ventilation of intense emotions; (2) exploration of symbolic meanings; (3) group support under catastrophic conditions; (4) initiation of the grief process within a supportive environment; (5) reduction of the "fallacy of uniqueness"; (6) reassurance that intense emotions under catastrophic conditions are normal; (7) preparation for the continuation of the grief and stress process over the ensuing weeks and months; (8) preparing for the possible development of emotional, cognitive, and physical symptoms in the aftermath of a serious crisis; (9) education regarding normal and abnormal stress response syndromes; and (10) encouragement of continued group support and/or professional assistance.

Sewell (1994) regards such interventions as appropriate for two specific groups, at two specific times. First, the stress of the first responders who dealt with the trauma of the original scene must be confronted quickly and decisively. Second, the stress of involved investigators must be handled as needed throughout the course of the crime's investigation and prosecution. In the regular debriefing sessions, whether for the first responders or case investigators, attendance should be mandatory and must be supported by command staff. Where an officer needs additional debriefing or other mental health assistance, this should be administratively encouraged and non-stigmatized.

Because of the often sensitive and secretive nature of their work, in my experience, criminal investigators and other special unit personnel (hostage negotiation, undercover, narcotics interdiction, etc.) may be especially uncomfortable speaking in a group setting for fear of revealing sensitive case material, or even having their identity disclosed to fellow officers or other first responders. In such cases, I typically advise the referring agency that a one-on-one individual debrief with a licensed mental health professional, covered by clinician-patient confidentiality and privilege, may be more appropriate for such personnel—indeed, for any officer whose participation in a group process would be problematic. In such cases, empirically informed flexibility and clinical common sense are usually the best guides (Miller, 2020).

Perhaps the most comprehensive adaptation of the standard CISD process for law enforcement is the one by Bohl (1995), who explicitly compares and contrasts the phases in her program with the phases of the standard model. In Bohl's program, the debriefing takes place as soon after the critical incident as possible. A debriefing may involve a single officer within the first 24 h, later followed by a second, with a group debriefing taking place within 1 week to encourage bonding. This is to address the lower team orientation of most police officers who may not express feelings easily, even—or especially—in a group of their fellow officers (see above).

The Bohl model makes no real distinction between the cognitive and emotional phases of a debriefing. If an officer begins to express emotion during the fact or cognitive phase, there is little point in telling them to stifle it until later. To be fair, as noted earlier, the standard CISD model certainly allows for flexibility and common sense in structuring debriefings, and both formats recognize the importance of responding empathically to the specific needs expressed by the individuals who attend the debriefing, rather than following an arbitrary set of rules.

In the emotion phase itself, what is important in the Bohl model is not the mere act of venting but, rather, the opportunity to validate feelings. Bohl does not ask what the "worst thing" was, because she finds the typical response of cops to be that "everything about it was the worst thing." However, it often comes as a revelation to these law enforcement "tough guys" that their peers have had similar feelings. Still, some emotions may be difficult to validate. For instance, guilt or remorse over actions or inactions may actually be appropriate, as when an officer's momentary hesitation or impulsive action resulted in someone getting hurt or killed. The question then becomes: "Okay, you think you screwed up; now, what are you going to do with that guilt?" That is, "What can be learned from the experience to prevent something like this from happening again?"

The Bohl model inserts an additional debriefing phase, termed the *unfinished business phase*, which has no counterpart in the standard debriefing model. Participants are asked, "What in the present situation reminds you of a past experience? Do you want to talk about that (those) other situation(s)?" This phase grew out of Bohl's observation that the incident that prompted the current debriefing often acts as a catalyst for recalling past events. Participants are reminded of prior critical incidents, probably none of which were followed by a formal debriefing. The questions give participants a chance to talk about incidents that may arouse strong and unresolved feelings. Bohl finds that such multilevel debriefings result in a greater sense of relief and closure than would occur by sticking solely to the present incident.

The education or teaching phase in the Bohl model resembles the standard model in that participants are taught about normal and abnormal stress reactions, how to deal with coworkers and family members, and what to anticipate in the near future. For instance, an officer's child may have heard that their parent shot and killed a suspect and the child may be questioned or teased at school. How to deal with children's responses may, therefore, be an important part of this education phase (Anderson et al., 1995; Kirschman, 1997; Miller, 2007c).

Unlike the standard CISD model, the Bohl model does not ask whether anything positive, hopeful, or growth-promoting has arisen from the incident. Officers who have seen their partners shot or killed, or who have had to deal with horrendous child abuse or other senseless brutality, may find it difficult to see anything hopeful or positive in the experience, no matter how well they have handled this situation. Add to this the potential cumulative demoralization of past encounters with human nature's dark side, and it is understandable that expecting officers to extract some kind of "growth experience" from this kind of tragedy may seem like a sick joke. In my own experience, however, it seems to be the individual personality of the officer that contributes to post-incident hope versus cynicism (Miller, 1998, 2003). And, as noted above, realistic positivity should not be overlooked as a therapeutic force multiplier, as long as it is not forced upon the officers or perceived as trivializing the traumatic experience (Galatzer-Levy et al., 2013; Hamling & Jarden, 2017; Miller, 2006c, 2008b).

A final added phase of the Bohl model is the *round robin*. Each officer is invited to say anything they want. The statement can be addressed to anyone, but others cannot respond directly; this is intended to give participants a feeling of safety. My own concern is that this sometimes provides an opportunity for last-minute gratuitous sniping or doomsaying, which can chip away at the carefully crafted supportive atmosphere built up during the debriefing. In addition, in practice, there does not seem to be anything particularly unique about this round-robin phase to distinguish it from the re-entry phase of the standard model. Finally, adding more and more "phases" to the debriefing process may serve to decrease the forthrightness and spontaneity of its implementation; we do not want this to become a chore. Again, clinical judgment and common sense should guide the process. However, Bohl's (1995) model, as well as those of Sewell (1993, 1994) and Solomon (1988, 1990, 1995), represents important contributions toward tailoring the CISD approach to the specific needs of law enforcement. We need continuing research and more clinically field-tested reports to inform continuing work in this area.

Psychotherapy with Law Enforcement Personnel

In some cases, the psychic cuts go deeper, and the psychological first-aid field dressing of the CISD approach must be supplemented by more intensive and extensive individual psychotherapeutic modalities. This is especially true when a particular traumatic event resonates with prior experiences and unresolved issues from an officer's past (Horowitz, 1992; Rudofossi, 2007, 2011). As with CISD approaches, the particular intervention strategy must be tailored to the job role and personality of crisis intervention specialists we treat.

As noted earlier, police officers have a reputation for shunning mental health services, often repudiating its practitioners as "softies" and "bleeding hearts" who help get guilty criminals off with overelaborate "psychobabble" excuses. Other officers fear being "shrunk," having a view of psychotherapy as akin to brainwashing, a humiliating experience in which they are supposed to lie on a couch and sob about their toilet training. More commonly, the idea of needing "mental help" implies weakness, cowardice, and lack of ability to do the job. In the environment of many departments, some officers realistically fear censure, stigmatization, ridicule, impaired career advancement, and alienation from coworkers if they are perceived as the type who "folds under pressure." Moreover, others in the department who have something to hide may fear a colleague "spilling his guts" to the shrink and blowing the malfeasor's cover. In practice, attempts by personnel to seek mental health intervention of any type should be forthrightly supported by the departmental administration (Anderson et al., 1995; Blau, 1994; Miller, 1995, 2006c; Mitchell & Everly, 1996).

Trust and the Therapeutic Relationship

While essential for any patient, trust is a crucial element in doing effective psychotherapy with police officers, who generally have a strong sense of self-sufficiency and insistence on solving their own problems. Therapists who work with officers may at first need to put up with a lot of probing and testing on the part of their patients: "Why are you doing this?" "What's in it for you?" "Who's going to get this information?" Officers may expose the therapist to mocking cynicism and criticism about the job, baiting the therapist to agree, and thereby hoping to expose the therapist's hidden prejudices about the officer's profession (Silva, 1991).

The development of trust during the establishment of the therapeutic alliance depends on the therapist's skill in interpreting the officer's statements, thoughts, feelings, reactions, and nonverbal behavior. In the best case, the officer begins to feel at ease with the therapist and finds comfort and a sense of predictability from the psychotherapy session. Silva (1991) outlines the following guidelines for the establishment of therapeutic trust:

- *Accurate empathy.* The therapist conveys their understanding of the patient's background and experience (but beware of premature false familiarity and phony "bonding").
- *Genuineness.* The therapist is spontaneous yet tactful, flexible yet creatively structured and adaptive, and tries to communicate as nondefensively as possible.
- *Availability.* The therapist is available, within reason, whenever needed, and avoids making promises and commitments they cannot keep.
- *Respect.* The therapist is tough-minded yet gracious and seeks to preserve the officer's sense of autonomy, control, and self-respect within the therapeutic relationship. Respect is demonstrated by the therapist's overall attitude, language, and behavior, such as indicating regard for rank or job role by initially using formal departmental forms of address, such as "officer," "detective," "lieutenant," and so on, until trust and mutual respect allow the consensual easing of formality. Here it is important to avoid two important traps: (1) overfamiliarity, patronizing, and talking down to the officer or (2) trying to "play cop" or force bogus camaraderie by prematurely or inappropriately assuming the role of a colleague or field commander.
- *Concreteness.* Whether conducting an investigation, making an arrest, or participating in a rescue operation, police officers value action and results. Accordingly, the most effective therapeutic approach will emphasize active, goal-oriented, and problem-solving modalities.

Therapeutic Strategies and Techniques

Aside from administrative referrals for pre-employment screening or fitness-for-duty evaluations (Miller, 2007b, 2015b), most law enforcement and emergency services personnel come under mental health purview in the context of some form of posttraumatic stress reaction or other incidents that abruptly challenge the officer's coping resources. In general, the effectiveness of any intervention will be determined by the timeliness, tone, style, and intent of the intervention. Effective therapy with police officers generally follows the guidelines of brevity and focuses on specific problem areas or conflict issues and practical dysphoric symptom relief, where appropriate (Blau, 1994; Wester & Lyubelsky, 2005).

Blau (1994) recommends that the first meeting between the therapist and a police officer establishes a safe and comfortable working atmosphere by the therapist's articulating: (1) a positive regard for the officer's decision to seek help; (2) a clear description of the therapist's responsibilities and limitations with regard to confidentiality and privilege; and (3) an invitation to the officer to state their concerns in their own way and at their own pace.

A straightforward, goal-directed, problem-solving approach for this patient group includes (1) creating a sanctuary; (2) focusing on critical areas of concern; (3) identifying desired outcomes; (4) reviewing assets; (5) developing a general plan; (6) identifying practical initial implementations; (7) reviewing self-efficacy; and (8) setting appointments for review, reassurance, and further implementation.

Blau (1994) delineates a number of effective individual intervention strategies for police officers:

- *Attentive listening.* This includes good eye contact, an occasional nod, and genuine interest, without inappropriate comments or interruptions.
- *Being there with empathy.* This therapeutic attitude conveys availability, concern, and awareness of the turbulent emotions being experienced by the distressed officer. It is also helpful to provide the officer, in a nonalarming manner, with a reality check as to what he or she may experience in the days and weeks ahead.
- *Reassurance.* This is valuable as long as it is reality-oriented. It should take the form of reassuring the patient that routine matters will be handled, deferred responsibilities will be handled by others, and organizational and command support will be provided. It is always a good idea to ascertain the officer's duty or leave status and to be familiar with departmental rules and regulations.
- *Supportive counseling.* This includes effective listening, restatement of content, clarification of feelings, and reassurance, as well as community referral and networking with liaison agencies, where necessary.
- *Interpretive counseling.* This type of intervention should be used when the officer's emotional reaction is significantly greater than the circumstances of the critical incident or other life crisis seem to warrant. In appropriate circumstances, this therapeutic strategy can stimulate the officer to search for underlying emotional stresses that intensify a traumatic event. In some cases, this may lead to ongoing psychotherapy beyond the initial referral problem.

Not to be neglected is the use of *humor*. While humor has a place in many forms of psychotherapy (Fry & Salameh, 1987), it may be especially useful in working with law enforcement and emergency services personnel (Fullerton et al., 1992; Silva, 1991). In general, if the therapist and patient can laugh together, it may lead to the sharing of more intimate feelings. Humor serves to bring a sense of balance and proportion to a traumatically warped and twisted world. Even sarcastic, gross humor may allow the venting of anger, frustration, resentment, and righteous indignation, foster healthy defensiveness and compartmentalization, and thereby lead to constructive integration and resolution of the traumatic event, or encourage adaptive strategies for dealing with an ongoing crisis (Miller, 2006a, 2008b, 2011, in press). As long as such humor does not degenerate into mean-spirited mockery of victims or colleagues, a mature attitude toward a traumatic event can actually frame the important existential lessons in terms of creative irony. "Show me a man who knows what's funny," Mark Twain said, "and I'll show you a man who knows what's not."

One caveat about humor, however: many traumatized patients may be quite concrete and suspicious at the outset of therapy, so the constructive therapeutic use of humor may have to await the formation of a therapeutic relationship that allows a certain degree of cognitive and emotional latitude. And some things—like the severe abuse of a child or death of a fellow officer—may just not be funny, period. As with all effective therapies, clinicians should respect the individual differences in cognitive style and coping resources of their patients and implement their interventions accordingly.

Summary

Clinicians just starting out in their work with police personnel may be surprised to find that many do not fit the "Officer Hardass" stereotype portrayed in fiction and news media. In fact, psychological intervention with police officers is often quite successful because of two main factors: (1) the initial referral problems, which may relate to the job or to family or other issues, are typically focused and delimited, and thus respond well to structured, cognitive-behavioral and supportive-expressive therapeutic modalities and (2) cops are used to following orders, so they may be even more likely than other patients to show up on time, complete therapeutic homework assignments, and comply with the therapists' recommendations. Working with law enforcement personnel requires skill, intelligence, flexibility, cultural competency, legal literacy, and sometimes a strong stomach, but it can be one of the most interesting and rewarding facets of clinical mental health work.

References

Anderson, W., Swenson, D., & Clay, D. (1995). *Stress management for law enforcement officers*. Prentice Hall.

Belles, D., & Norvell, N. (1990). *Stress management for law enforcement officers*. Professional Resource Exchange.

Benedikt, R. A., & Kolb, L. C. (1986). Preliminary findings on chronic pain and posttraumatic stress disorder. *American Journal of Psychiatry, 143*, 908–910.

Blau, T. H. (1994). *Psychological services for law enforcement*. Wiley.

Bohl, N. (1995). Professionally administered critical incident debriefing for police officers. In M. I. Kunke & E. M. Scrivner (Eds.), *Police psychology into the 21st century* (pp. 169–188). Erlbaum.

Borum, R., & Philpot, C. (1993). Therapy with law enforcement couples: Clinical management of the "high-risk lifestyle". *American Journal of Family Therapy, 21*, 122–135.

Cummings, J. P. (1996, October). Police stress and the suicide link. *The Police Chief, 63*, 85–96.

Curran, S. (2003, January/February). Separating fact from fiction about police stress. *Behavioral Health Management, 23*, 3–4.

Dyregrov, A. (1989). Caring for helpers in disaster situations: Psychological debriefing. *Disaster Management, 2*, 25–30.

Everly, G. S., & Lating, J. M. (2022). *The Johns Hopkins guide to psychological first aid* (2nd ed.). Johns Hopkins University Press.

Everly, G. S., & Mitchell, J. T. (1997). *Critical Incident Stress Management (CISM): A new era and standard of care in crisis intervention*. Chevron.

Everly, G. S., Flannery, R. B., & Mitchell, J. T. (2000). Critical Incident Stress Management: A review of the literature. *Aggression and Violent Behavior, 5*, 23–40.

Fry, W. F., & Salameh, W. A. (Eds.). (1987). *Handbook of humor and psychotherapy*. Professional Resource Exchange.

Fullerton, C. S., McCarroll, J. E., Ursano, R. J., & Wright, K. M. (1992). Psychological responses of rescue workers: Firefighters and trauma. *American Journal of Orthopsychiatry, 62*, 371–378.

Galatzer-Levy, I. R., Brown, A. D., Henn-Hasse, C., Metzler, T. J., Neylan, T. C., & Marmar, C. R. (2013). Positive and negative emotion prospectively predict trajectories of resilience and distress among high exposure police officers. *Emotion, 13*, 545–553.

Hamling, K., & Jarden, A. (2017). Wellbeing and recovery in the emergency services: How do we care for those who care for us? In M. Slade, L. Oades, & A. Jarden (Eds.), *Wellbeing, recovery, and mental health* (pp. 157–168). Cambridge University Press.

Henry, V. E. (2004). *Death work: Police, trauma, and the psychology of survival*. Oxford University Press.

Honig, A. L., & Roland, J. E. (1998, October). Shots fired: Officer involved. *The Police Chief, 65*, 65–70.

Horn, J. M. (1991). Critical incidents for law enforcement officers. In J. T. Reese, J. M. Horn, & C. Dunning (Eds.), *Critical incidents in policing* (Rev ed., pp. 143–148). US Government Printing Office.

Horowitz, M. J. (1992). *Stress response syndromes* (2nd ed.). Jason Aronson.

Kirschman, E. (1997). *I love a cop: What police families need to know*. Guilford Press.

McCafferty, R. L., McCafferty, E., & McCafferty, M. A. (1992). Stress and suicide in police officers: Paradigm of occupational stress. *Southern Medical Journal, 85*, 233.

McFarlane, A. C., Atchison, M., Rafalowicz, E., & Papay, P. (1994). Physical symptoms in post-traumatic stress disorder. *Journal of Psychosomatic Research, 38*, 715–726.

McMains, M. J. (1991). The management and treatment of post-shooting trauma. In J. T. Reese, J. M. Horn, & C. Dunning (Eds.), *Critical incidents in policing* (Rev ed., pp. 191–198). US Government Printing Office.

Miller, L. (1995). Tough guys: Psychotherapeutic strategies with law enforcement and emergency services personnel. *Psychotherapy, 32*, 592–600.

Miller, L. (1998). *Shocks to the system: Psychotherapy of traumatic disability syndromes*. Norton.

Miller, L. (1999). Critical Incident Stress Debriefing: Clinical applications and new directions. *International Journal of Emergency Mental Health, 1*, 253–265.

Miller, L. (2000). Law enforcement traumatic stress: Clinical syndromes and intervention strategies. *Trauma Response, 6*, 15–20.

Miller, L. (2003, May). Police personalities: Understanding and managing the problem officer. *The Police Chief*, 53–60.

Miller, L. (2005a). Police officer suicide: Causes, prevention, and practical intervention strategies. *International Journal of Emergency Mental Health, 7*, 23–36.

Miller, L. (2005b). Hostage negotiation: Psychological principles and practices. *International Journal of Emergency Mental Health, 7*, 277–298.

Miller, L. (2006a). Officer-involved shooting: Reaction patterns, response protocols, and psychological intervention strategies. *International Journal of Emergency Mental Health, 8*, 239–254.

Miller, L. (2006b, October). On the spot: Testifying in court for law enforcement officers. *FBI Law Enforcement Bulletin*, 1–6.

Miller, L. (2006c). *Practical police psychology: Stress management and crisis intervention for law enforcement*. Charles C Thomas.

Miller, L. (2006d). Undercover policing: A psychological and operational guide. *Journal of Police and Criminal Psychology, 21*, 1–24.

Miller, L. (2007a). Line-of-duty death: Psychological treatment of traumatic bereavement in law enforcement. *International Journal of Emergency Mental Health, 9*, 13–23.

Miller, L. (2007b, August). The psychological fitness-for-duty evaluation. *FBI Law Enforcement Bulletin, 76*, 10–16.

Miller, L. (2007c). Police families: Stresses, syndromes, and solutions. *American Journal of Family Therapy, 35*, 21–40.

Miller, L. (2008a). Military psychology and police psychology: Mutual contributions to crisis intervention and stress management. *International Journal of Emergency Mental Health, 10*, 9–26.

Miller, L. (2008b). *METTLE: Mental toughness training for law enforcement*. Looseleaf Law Publications.

Miller, L. (2009a). Criminal investigator stress: Symptoms, syndromes, and practical coping strategies. *International Journal of Emergency Mental Health, 11*, 87–92.

Miller, L. (2009b). You're it! How to psychologically survive an internal investigation, disciplinary proceeding, or legal action in the police, fire, medical, mental health, legal, or emergency services professions. *International Journal of Emergency Mental Health, 11*, 185–190.

Miller, L. (2011). Cops in trouble: Helping officers cope with investigation, prosecution, or litigation. In J. Kitaeff & K. Cather (Eds.), *Handbook of police psychology* (pp. 479–490). Psychology Press.

Miller, L. (2013a). Hostage negotiations. In B. A. Moore & J. E. Barnett (Eds.), *Military psychologists' desk reference* (pp. 86–90). Oxford University Press.

Miller, L. (2013b). Military and law enforcement psychology: Cross-contributions to extreme stress management. In L. Territo & J. D. Sewell (Eds.), *Stress management in law enforcement* (3rd ed., pp. 455–486). Carolina Academic Press.

Miller, L. (2015a). Why cops kill: The psychology of police deadly force encounters. *Aggression and Violent Behavior, 22*, 97–111.

Miller, L. (2015b). Police officers in the legal system. In S. M. F. Clevenger, L. Miller, B. A. Moore, & A. Freeman (Eds.), *Behind the badge: A psychological treatment handbook for law enforcement officers* (pp. 171–183). Routledge.

Miller, L. (2015c). *Posttraumatic Stress Disorder and forensic psychology: Applications to civil and criminal law*. Springer.

Miller, L. (2019). Police deadly force encounters: Psychological reactions and recovery patterns. In L. Territo & J. D. Sewell (Eds.), *Stress management in law enforcement* (4th ed., pp. 115–144). Carolina Academic Press.

Miller, L. (2020). *The psychology of police deadly force encounters: Science, practice, and policy*. Charles C Thomas.
Miller, L. (in press). Force aftermath: Advice for officers and their counselors on coping with the consequences of an adverse/contested use of force action. *AELE Monthly Law Journal*.
Mitchell, J. T. (1983). When disaster strikes: The critical incident stress process. *Journal of the Emergency Medical Services, 8*, 36–39.
Mitchell, J. T. (1988). The history, status, and future of critical incident stress debriefing. *Journal of the Emergency Medical Services, 13*, 47–52.
Mitchell, J. T. (1991). Law enforcement applications for critical incident stress teams. In J. T. Reese, J. M. Horn, & C. Dunning (Eds.), *Critical incidents in policing* (Rev ed., pp. 201–212). US Government Printing Office.
Mitchell, J. T., & Bray, G. P. (1990). *Emergency services stress: Guidelines for preserving the health and careers of emergency services personnel*. Prentice-Hall.
Mitchell, J. T., & Everly, G. S. (1996). *Critical incident stress debriefing: An operations manual for the preservation of traumatic stress among emergency services and disaster workers* (2nd ed.). Chevron.
Peak, K. J. (2003). *Policing in America: Methods, issues, challenges* (4th ed.) Prentice Hall.
Reese, J. T. (1987). Coping with stress: It's your job. In J. T. Reese (Ed.), *Behavioral science in law enforcement* (pp. 75–79). Federal Bureau of Investigation.
Reese, J. T. (1991). Justification for mandating critical incident aftercare. In J. T. Reese, J. M. Horn, & C. Dunning (Eds.), *Critical incidents in policing* (Rev ed., pp. 213–220). US Government Printing Office.
Regehr, C., & Bober, T. (2004). *In the line of fire: Trauma in the emergency services*. Oxford University Press.
Rudofossi, D. (2007). *Working with traumatized police officer-patients: A clinician's guide to complex PTSD syndromes in public safety personnel*. Baywood.
Rudofossi, D. (2011). Police and public safety complex trauma and grief: An eco-ethological existential analysis. In J. Kitaeff (Ed.), *Handbook of police psychology* (pp. 437–468). Routledge.
Russell, H. E., & Beigel, A. (1990). *Understanding human behavior for effective police work* (3rd ed.). Basic Books.
Sewell, J. D. (1993). Traumatic stress in multiple murder investigations. *Journal of Traumatic Stress, 6*, 103–118.
Sewell, J. D. (1994). The stress of homicide investigations. *Death Studies, 18*, 565–582.
Sewell, J. D., Ellison, K. W., & Hurrell, J. J. (1988, October). Stress management in law enforcement: Where do we go from here? *The Police Chief, 55*, 94–98.
Silva, M. N. (1991). The delivery of mental health services to law enforcement officers. In J. T. Reese, J. M. Horn, & C. Dunning (Eds.), *Critical incidents in policing* (pp. 335–341). Federal Bureau of Investigation.
Solomon, R. M. (1988, October). Post-shooting trauma. *The Police Chief*, 40–44.
Solomon, R. M. (1990, February). Administrative guidelines for dealing with officers involved in on-duty shooting situations. *The Police Chief*, 40.
Solomon, R. M. (1995). Critical Incident Stress Management in law enforcement. In G. S. Everly (Ed.), *Innovations in disaster and trauma psychology: Applications in emergency services and disaster response* (pp. 123–157). Chevron.
Solomon, R. M., & Horn, J. M. (1986). Post-shooting traumatic reactions: A pilot study. In J. T. Reese & H. A. Goldstein (Eds.), *Critical incidents in policing* (Rev ed., pp. 383–394). US Government Printing Office.
Toch, H. (2002). *Stress in policing*. American Psychological Association.
Wester, S. R., & Lyubelsky, J. (2005). Supporting the thin blue line: Gender-sensitive therapy with male police officers. *Professional Psychology: Research and Practice, 36*, 51–58.
Woody, R. H. (2005). The police culture: Research implications for psychological services. *Professional Psychology: Research and Practice, 36*, 525–529.
Woody, R. H. (2006). Family interventions with law enforcement officers. *American Journal of Family Therapy, 34*, 95–103.

Mental Health Issues in the Fire Service

Sam J. Buser

> Flipping on my lights and sirens, I accelerate en route to a "Mayday" call for a missing crewman on Engine 26. Making a mental note to advise the Fire Chief on how to notify the family of their missing loved one, I activate the CISM (Critical Incident Stress Management) Team by pager. As a psychologist in the fire service, my "50-minute hour" has been replaced by 24/7 on-call status, emergency dispatch now substitutes for an answering service, and a crisis is not a marital spat, but a line-of-duty death.

Although psychologists have worked in police departments for decades, they have rarely been employed within the fire service. Yet given the high stress nature of firefighting, the exposure of firefighters to traumatic events, and the frequency of suicides among first responders, there is a clear need for mental health services in fire departments. Consequently, firefighter organizations (e.g., the International Association of Firefighters [IAFF], 2023) have called for an increased presence of mental health services.

This chapter concerns the mental health issues and needs of firefighters. It begins with a brief discussion of firefighter culture, noting the ways in which firefighters tend to differ from other first-responder groups. It will review obstacles that may prevent firefighters from seeking mental health care. Additionally, the chapter includes a discussion of some of the more common mental health concerns firefighters experience. While these issues are not necessarily unique to firefighters, they may present differently or with greater frequency among fire service personnel. As a guide to fire departments that want to incorporate mental health services, there is a discussion of the important elements and services that should be included. Finally, the chapter will conclude with tips for mental health providers (MHPs) who seek to provide care to firefighters.

S. J. Buser (✉)
Houston Fire Department (Retired), Houston, TX, USA
e-mail: sam@drsamjbuser.com

M. L. Bourke et al. (eds.), *First Responder Mental Health*,
https://doi.org/10.1007/978-3-031-38149-2_2

Firefighter Culture

Mental health professionals are admonished to be culturally sensitive to their clients. (Pope-Davis, 2003). They are not expected to be experts on all cultures, but they are required to take the client's cultural beliefs and values into account as they provide services. MHPs are encouraged to ask questions of clients about their cultural understanding and to refrain from making assumptions based on stereotyped beliefs.

The concept of culture is often understood as applying to ethnic, racial, or nationality groups, not to occupational roles. One way of defining a culture is that its members set themselves apart, believing they are different from the larger population. There tends to be greater acceptance of others in one's culture/subculture as well as suspicions about those who are not perceived as members.

Although firefighters are part of the broad first responder community, the fire service is a unique subgroup (Avsec, 2013). Firefighters differentiate themselves not only from civilians but also from other first-responder groups. Firefighters are quick to point out that they are not identical to these kindred groups. There is a well-known, sometimes friendly, rivalry between firefighters and law enforcement. Likewise, there are differences and similarities with emergency medical services (EMS) personnel. These groups are not monolithic, and to treat them as such risks being culturally insensitive. When working with firefighters, MHPs are introduced to a culture which is generally quite different from the ones the MHP may have previously encountered.

History

Interestingly, the history of the American Fire Service (Spell, 2021) dates to around 1736 when Benjamin Franklin established the first volunteer fire department in Philadelphia. Eventually, private fire brigades supported by insurance companies were established. These private brigades sometimes competed to provide fire protection to parts of the community. With greater industrialization and societal complexity, it became necessary for the government to provide oversight of fire protection. Municipalities, counties, and other governmental entities took over the funding and direction of fire departments to serve the public's needs. As fire prevention technology has improved, fires have become less common; however, when they occur, they may be more dangerous and deadly because of construction materials such as plastics. Technological advances in firefighting mean that firefighters now wear self-contained breathing apparatus, use infrared cameras to locate fires, and utilize drones to deploy resources. Nevertheless, firefighting remains a dangerous job with about 100 firefighters (NFPA Statistics – Firefighter Deaths, n.d.) dying in the line of duty every year.

Basic Numbers

The National Fire Protection Association (NFPA) estimates there are just over one million firefighters in the USA (Fahy et al., 2022). The same report from the NFPA notes that only about one-third of that number are career firefighters, the rest serve as volunteers. The report also states that there are almost 30,000 different fire departments in the USA but only 18% of those are staffed by career or primarily career firefighters. Yet, again according to this 2022 report from the NFPA, that 18% protect 69% of the US population. The great majority of professional firefighters, then, work in urban areas, while the large majority of American firefighters are volunteers working in rural areas.

Volunteer/Professional

Professional and volunteer firefighters face similar challenges, problems, and dangers. Rural, volunteer departments are usually smaller, and they generally have a much lower volume of responses. However, any given call may be just as difficult or life threatening as in the larger departments. In departments that have some paid staff, those employees often work at other urban departments as well. Rural departments tend to be staffed by volunteers with a small cadre of professional firefighters who serve as officers or chiefs. Not infrequently, those senior managers are retired members from larger, more urban departments. Volunteer firefighters have far less access to both training and support services, including mental health care.

EMS vs Fire

In some locales, fire departments provide only fire-related services, while in others they provide both EMS and fire services (Fahy et al., 2022). In the departments that offer both EMS and fire suppression, most responses are for medical emergencies, not fires. In "combined" departments, there is often tension between EMS and fire suppression providers. Some members of the department may prefer either the EMS or suppression role and may dislike – or even resent – the other role. Within EMS there are other distinctions as well. The term "paramedic" is often used by the media in describing personnel who provide EMS services. In actuality, the providers may be emergency medical technicians (EMTs) offering BLS (basic life support). BLS services are designed for use in traumatic situations such as cardiac arrest, drowning, or choking. They may include techniques such as CPR, the use of an automated external defibrillator (AED), and removing obstructions to the airway. Paramedics are much more highly trained and can provide advanced life support (ALS) enabling them to perform certain invasive procedures (e.g., start an IV, intubation, using a needle to administer medications). Many more firefighters are certified to do BLS with a smaller number qualified to be paramedic ALS providers. In rural areas, a paramedic may be the best trained emergency medical provider available in the area.

Specialty Roles

As with most career fields, there are subspecialities in the fire service. Most firefighters are trained to do suppression duties (i.e., put out fires); however, some are also specialists in dealing with hazardous materials. Dispatch or communication specialists have the role of managing communications for fire response. This role is critical to ensure the right equipment and personnel get to the correct location in the least amount of time. Firefighters working near airports have unique equipment and training to respond to aircraft fires. Wildland fighters, smoke jumpers, and hot shots fight fires in remote wilderness areas. Technical rescue firefighters are the fire service equivalent of police SWAT teams. They utilize special skills, equipment, and training (e.g., ropes, rappelling gear, helicopters) to extricate people who are trapped, perform high-angle rescues (e.g., for window washers), and execute swift water rescues using boats. Each of these special roles comes with its own set of rules, procedures, and potential dangers.

Work Schedules

Most departments utilize a 24-h shift schedule (Waters, 2023), but they vary in how they arrange time off from work. For instance, in some departments firefighters work 24 h on, 48 h off. Others have firefighters work 24 h on, 24 h off, 24 h on again, and then 4 days off. There are many other variations of these schedules. In short, the schedules are very complex and only a member of your crew will share your schedule. The lack of overlap with the lives of other family members wreaks havoc with relationships. As a result of scheduling issues, firefighters frequently miss family gatherings, holidays, and other events involving their children. Their vacation days off must be scheduled in advance, often 1 year ahead of time.

Multiple Jobs

Jobs in the fire service, though dangerous, are not well-paid. According to the US Department of Labor (Occupational Outlook Handbook: U.S. Bureau of Labor Statistics, 2022) the median salary for a firefighter in the USA in 2021 was just under $52,000. It is commonplace for firefighters to work second or even third "side" jobs to support their families. Many side jobs consist of working as a firefighter part-time for another department (e.g., a smaller, suburban department).

Other common side jobs involve providing some level of medical care (e.g., as a paramedic at an emergency room, driving an ambulance, nursing). Construction or mechanical jobs are also popular as many firefighters are skilled in these areas. Departments may require their members to report their side jobs and even to sign contracts clarifying that their primary job will be as a firefighter. For instance, during a natural disaster, firefighters may be required to work as a first responder and may not tend to a side business or report to a part-time job.

Sense of Family

Firefighters often describe their crew as a second family. Firefighters live at the station – sharing meals and cleaning duties, sleeping in communal areas, watching television together, showering, and going to the bathroom. There is little privacy, and the atmosphere is reminiscent of a family home with lots of siblings, or a college fraternity house. Their unique work schedules facilitate them being together even on their days off. Even more than other first-responder groups, firefighters pride themselves on this sense of community. However, as with many families, you may not always get along with some of your "siblings." Conflicts among fellow crew members can escalate quickly, and firefighters often talk about the importance of having a "tight crew."

Paramilitary Structure

Fire departments are arranged along military rather than corporate lines. Superiors are referred to as officers or commanders, and their ranks (lieutenants, captains, chiefs) and assignments (battalions, divisions) have military connotations. Orders are given, the chain of command is followed, uniforms are worn, and decorum is maintained. A station crew operates much like a small unit in the military, and former military members often find comfort and familiarity with this arrangement. Those who have not served in the military may find this system foreign or difficult to adapt to.

Saving a Life

Sculptures that adorn firefighter memorials and the like often feature stylized rescues, typically of a child. To save a life, especially that of a child, is among the greatest experiences a firefighter can have in their career. A save is a cherished moment for firefighters. Conversely, losing a life you thought you could save is among the greatest tragedies for them. Such losses may haunt firefighters – causing them to resign, drink excessively, or develop PTSD. In dealing with the loss of life, firefighters may unfairly blame themselves or perceive they should have done more. Cognitive distortions about the events, pervasive guilt, insomnia, burnout, and depression are common sequelae in these situations. This desire to save someone has far-reaching implications in understanding the personalities of firefighters.

Government Favoring Police over Fire

Politicians and local governments often favor the needs for law enforcement over the needs for fire protection. If crime goes up, it is well-reported in the media. There may be an outcry from the public for more policing and more resources for law enforcement. Fires and natural disasters, though, are low-frequency events, especially in comparison to criminal activity. Furthermore, police and fire departments are expensive components of city and county budgets. The two departments often must compete for scarce tax dollars, and the squeaky wheel of crime tends to get more grease. The need for better equipment or increased numbers of fire personnel is therefore less of a priority for most municipalities. The public tends to appreciate the fire service more during times of natural disaster or in responses to terrorist attacks, but the role of fire departments in reducing insurance costs and preventing fires is harder to quantify and less emotionally appealing. Many people have been affected by crime; fewer have lost their homes or property to fire.

Job Satisfaction

Although their job is dangerous and difficult, most firefighters love their career, and they get a special adrenaline rush when responding to a fire. The combination of danger, teamwork, and overcoming a challenge is typically appealing to firefighters. Many also talk about enjoying station life. The closeness of a tight-knit crew can be very rewarding. If they leave a station because of promotion or transfer, they may mourn that loss and may later seek ways to return to their old assignment.

Self-Reliance

First responders in general, and firefighters in particular, value self-reliance – the ability to take care of problems without the help of others. Firefighters tend to be ingenious problem-solvers, often possessing excellent mechanical and construction abilities. They pride themselves on their improvisation in unique and challenging scenarios. Seeing a counselor is particularly uncomfortable for them because it goes against this notion of self-reliance. Seeking help from an MHP is usually a last resort for them, and the MHP should be mindful of this dilemma.

Mission Priority

As first responders, firefighters may prioritize mission accomplishment over self, family, and even their own safety. It is often the case that to save a life, the first responder must put his or her own life at risk. As others flee the scene, first responders run to the action. Among firefighters this value of mission priority can be quite hazardous. As terrified people scrambled to get out of the World Trade Center following the terrorist attack of 9/11/2001, firefighters were simultaneously climbing the stairs upward to an inferno. FDNY lost 343 firefighters that day, including the Chief of the Department (FireRescue1, 2021).

Natural Disasters

During natural disasters, fire agencies, rather than police, usually provide overall command and control. With their specific training in rescue, handling hazardous materials, and suppression of fires, firefighters are the most involved first responders in emergency responses to natural disasters. Only when the crisis has abated are they able to take care of their own homes and families.

Constant Reminders of Trauma

Firefighters are probably exposed to more traumatic scenes during their careers than most other professions, including even law enforcement. Not all police responses are to traumatic scenes, but most firefighters/EMS responses are to traumatic events: industrial accidents, heart attacks, vehicular injuries, fires, and suicides. Simply driving around their town can remind a firefighter of a traffic fatality they responded to at a particular intersection, the fire at an apartment complex, or the homicide that took place in a home.

Obstacles to Seeking Mental Health Care in the Fire Service

Stigma

If there is a stigma in the public (Corrigan et al., 2014) about seeking mental health services, that stigma is far greater among first responders. A first responder who is mentally unstable will not be trusted to do their job. Indeed, such a first responder is likely to lose their job. Accountants and teachers don't have to pass fitness for duty evaluations! Nor must they pass prescreening evaluations specifically focused on mental health concerns. Both police and fire personnel, however, are always concerned that seeking mental health care could cost them their career. Will they be determined unfit for duty? Naturally, then, they are even more reluctant than most to see a "shrink." To be seen as having "mental problems" in the fire service suggests to your peers that you cannot be counted on in an emergency situation, and this could be potentially life threatening to you and/or your fellow firefighters. The fear of losing the confidence of others, or being prevented from continuing in their career, colors every interaction between a first responder and an MHP.

Confidentiality

Closely related to the issue of stigma are problems surrounding confidentiality. While every MHP is taught to guard client information, the threat of a breach of privacy is especially concerning to first responders. If the MHP is employed by the entity (e.g., the city) that also employs the first responder, there is generally a distrust that the confidential nature of their sessions will be maintained. This fear is especially prominent if the first responder is somehow in trouble (e.g., been charged with DWI). It is essential for MHPs in this role to be very clear with both their firefighter clients and with the command structure regarding how confidentiality will be managed. Clear and formidable barriers must be maintained to prevent any possibility that personal information might be accessible to command staff/officers.

It is a good idea for the MHP to spend more time discussing confidentiality with prospective new first-responder clients than they normally would with other groups of clients. Even then, the MHP should expect the first responder to be skeptical. Any leak of confidential information can be devastating to the long-term viability of mental health services within a department. Furthermore, departments employing MHPs may have to utilize entirely separate computer and recordkeeping systems to prevent any possibility that client information could be hacked or discovered by other employees. Establishing these secure systems requires the support of command staff, IT professionals, and the legal department of the city/municipality. Because of the long legacy of psychology within law enforcement, such protections for confidentiality are often well established among MHPs who work in those departments. However, since fewer fire departments have employed MHPs, these protections may not have been fully considered.

Lack of Mental Health Care in Fire Departments

While law enforcement agencies have incorporated mental health services within their departments for decades (Reese, 1987), and most large police departments employ one or more psychologists or other MHPs, the fire service has been slow to embrace them. Since law enforcement personnel commonly possess firearms and sometimes must use deadly force, it may have appeared more obvious that their mental health should be considered. While firefighters do not typically carry firearms, they, like police, face life-threatening situations and frequently experience trauma. Yet, the need to provide psychological care for them has generally been neglected or minimized.

Many cities and municipalities provide access to employee assistance programs (EAPs) for their firefighters, but these programs are not typically embedded within fire departments in the same way that police psychologists serve within law enforcement agencies. The MHPs employed by EAPs typically are licensed professional counselors who are not specialized in providing care to first responders. Often, the same EAP counselors are tasked with also seeing employees from all the other various city departments (e.g., public works, library, parks). While it is commendable that at least some mental health services are being provided to firefighters, the effectiveness of these services is limited when the MHPs are unfamiliar with the firefighter culture and the needs of this unique population. First responders are notoriously reluctant to share their lives and concerns with outsiders. When the MHP is unfamiliar with the firefighter's experience, good intentions may not be sufficient to overcome the barriers of stigma surrounding mental health treatment and concerns about confidentiality.

Cultural Competence Issues

As indicated, very few MHPs have sufficient familiarity with firefighter culture. Often, they have only vague or stereotyped ideas about the life and work of firefighters. They are unfamiliar with how basic aspects of firefighters' lives such as their work schedules (24-h shifts, rotating days off, prearranged vacation days), communal sleeping and eating, and dealing with death on a frequent basis significantly affect their mental health. For instance, consider how a firefighter with social anxiety might be challenged by working in a setting where there is virtually never any privacy or alone time. Or how fire officers cope with the responsibility of making decisions that can imperil their subordinates. Do they know how firefighters' families are affected by their loved one's frequent exposure to trauma? Or the effect on a crew when they experience a particularly dreadful or gruesome event? If the MHP has little familiarity with firefighter culture, they are apt to not understand or overlook the importance of such cultural variables.

Worse is the MHP who assumes that they understand firefighters because they've treated one in the past or have treated police officers. This is equivalent to an MHP believing that they understand African American culture because they once treated a person of that ethnic group. Some firefighters who seek counseling for the first time may be tempted to try to help the MHP's understanding by describing their job. However, some firefighters have reported that after hearing the details of what they experienced on the job, their MHP "kindly" suggested that they might want to consider a different line of work. Predictably, those firefighters dropped out of treatment.

Common Mental Health Issues Faced by Firefighters

Posttraumatic Stress Disorder (PTSD)

Traumatic exposure is a common experience for firefighters. Yet they typically minimize the significance of repeatedly witnessing violence, suicides, and severe bodily injuries. They commonly remark, "It's part of the job," a comment that implies they have become accustomed to it or have learned to compartmentalize these events. Among themselves, away from the public, they often utilize dark, sarcastic humor to describe their work. To the outsider, the firefighter might seem calloused or uncaring, but the reality is they are trying to cope with being exposed to traumatic scenes. Research on trauma (SAMSHA, 2014) has clearly established that exposure to trauma is bad for one's mental health and that repeated exposure to trauma is worse. Firefighters are no exception to this finding, and they may experience predictable psychological sequelae to traumatic events (Wagner et al., 2010).

Among the factors that can make firefighters more vulnerable to the development of posttraumatic stress disorder (PTSD) is length of service (Soravia et al., 2021). With more service comes more exposure to trauma and consequent risk of developing posttraumatic stress syndrome (PTSS) and PTSD symptoms. It is sometimes debated in the station house whether older, more experienced firefighters are at greater or less risk of developing posttraumatic symptoms than the newer "rookies." "I've seen it before," the veteran firefighter may offer, suggesting they have learned to cope with such events. The research, however, suggests the cumulative effect of multiple exposures to trauma is more problematic for developing PTSD (Jahnke et al., 2016) than the one-time exposure for the novice.

Estimates of the prevalence of PTSD among firefighters have varied widely from 6.5% to 57% (del Ben et al., 2006). A recent review of articles published internationally suggests that the rate of PTSD among firefighters (57%) may be even higher than among combat soldiers (38%) (Obuobi-Donkor et al., 2022). Regardless of the precise statistics, the point is that PTSS and PTSD are occupational hazards for firefighters.

For soldiers, combat is often incredibly terrifying and intense. Typically, though, at some point, their deployment in the combat zone or front lines ends. For firefighters, their deployment ends for this day but resumes on the next shift, a day or so later, for more than 20 years. While firefighters are not the target of an enemy seeking to kill them, fires are no less deadly or dangerous. Fires take no prisoners and show no forgiveness for mistakes. Like the soldier, the firefighter relies upon their protective gear, team, tactics, and equipment to help them survive. As in combat, sometimes those protective systems are not enough.

Alcohol/Substance Abuse

The incidence of illegal drug use among firefighters is low. This is largely because firefighters (as well as other first responders) commonly face random drug screenings as a job requirement. In many departments, failing a drug screening is grounds for automatic suspension. Of course, some firefighters will use drugs and then attempt to avoid getting caught, but in the fire service as a whole, illegal drug use is not a major problem. The trend in the USA to legalize marijuana/cannabis, however, may tempt more firefighters and other first responders to use this class of drugs, particularly because they are often helpful in reducing anxiety symptoms.

Prescription drug overuse, though, can be an issue for firefighters. Sometimes prescription drug problems begin with on-the-job injuries. Given the nature of their work painful burns and orthopedic issues (e.g., broken bones, back problems) are not unusual among firefighters. They may begin the use of pain killers for legitimate reasons but later begin to overuse and even become addicted to them (Jahnke, 2020). Firefighters, not unlike the general population, may also overuse other medications with psychoactive effects (anxiolytics, sleeping medications, stimulants for attention issues) (National Institute of Health: National Institute on Drug Abuse, 2022). These classes of medications all pose a risk for abuse. A MHP in the fire service will almost certainly encounter members who experience problems because of abuse of these prescribed medicines.

The biggest substance abuse issue in the fire service, though, is posed by alcohol (Haddock et al., 2012; IAFF Recoverycenter, n.d.; Jahnke et al., 2014). Levels of alcohol use, abuse, and dependence are considerably higher among firefighters than in the general population. There is a tradition of alcohol use in the fire service both to celebrate events and to commemorate losses. There are historical anecdotes of bars and beer drinking at the station house and the union hall. Social events for firefighters invariably involve alcohol, and since no one other than their fellow crew members share the same schedule, getting together on off days with firefighter buddies will usually include drinking. The shift schedule may promote the use of alcohol on days off, and many firefighters curtail or time their drinking to ensure they will be sober when they return to duty. Some firefighters use alcohol for stress release (Zegel et al., 2019), but they are more likely to minimize this as a reason, and instead describe their alcohol consumption as social drinking. The use of alcohol while on duty is uncommon, but departments vary on how they respond to incidents of alcohol abuse when employees are off duty (e.g., DUIs). In some departments, one DUI results in automatic dismissal, while other departments have more forgiving policies. Haddock et al. (2012) found that 10% of firefighters report they have driven while intoxicated, and less formal surveys have found much higher rates of drinking and driving among firefighters.

Sleep Problems

Sleep problems are almost ubiquitous among firefighters. Their odd work schedules, sleep disruption due to being awakened throughout the night to respond to alarms or emergencies, hours of strenuous physical labor in dangerous conditions, and traumatic exposures all lend themselves to the development of sleep disorders. Research has found that a large percentage of firefighters (37–59%) experience sleep problems (Barger et al., 2015; Carey et al., 2011). Research by Wolkow et al. (2019) found that 49% of firefighters reported they obtained less than 6 h of sleep when working a 24-h shift. Furthermore, in this national sample of 6300 firefighters, 32% reported they got less than 6 h of sleep during the period immediately after a 24-h shift. The researchers found that sleep disorders predicted burnout and emotional exhaustion.

Those who work as an MHP with firefighters will commonly encounter firefighters with sleep problems. These problems may lead to greater use of alcohol and sleep aids to enable the firefighters to fall asleep quickly and to cope with insomnia. The Barger et al. (2015) study also found that firefighter sleep problems were associated with cardiovascular disease risk, depression, anxiety, and motor vehicle accidents.

Relationship and Family Issues

The unusual work schedule of firefighters and the nature of the work itself create common couple and family problems. Being a firefighter means that you miss many of the events (birthdays, Thanksgiving, religious holidays, anniversaries, kids' sports) that are associated with being part of a family. The firefighter's schedule, which often requires them to leave the house before anyone else is awake and return a day or more later, is not conducive to maintaining couple communication or effective parenting. It may seem to the family that the firefighter is more connected with their crew than with their family unit. In addition, the firefighter leaves each day with the family's knowledge that they are going to a dangerous job and that they may not be coming home at the end of the shift. This can be exacerbated by news coverage and social media posts about firefighters in their community engaging in emergency responses to shootings, major fires, floods, explosions, terrorist threats, and the like. Family members quickly become aware of injuries and deaths of firefighters in their department, a knowledge that keeps them on edge about their own loved ones.

When firefighters return home after duty, they frequently feel that they cannot share much with their partner about what has happened to them while they were at work. They seek to protect the family from secondary traumatization, but these protective measures reduce the family's understanding of what they experienced. If the firefighter has experienced something emotionally difficult, the family may be only aware that their partner/parent is acting differently but will not know why. Repeated exposure to severe traumatic scenes negatively affects emotional intimacy and satisfaction in firefighters' relationships (Godfrey et al., 2022). These aspects of firefighter life may fuel couple/marital problems as well as create parenting challenges.

Gender Issues

Firefighting has the highest ratio of men to women of almost any occupation. According to the National Fire Protection Association, nationally, more than 92% of firefighters are male (Fahy et al., 2022). Although this report also notes that there are almost 90,000 women serving as firefighters in the USA, most of these women serve in volunteer departments rather than as career firefighters. The gender imbalance in the fire service exceeds that of other first-responder groups or the military. The challenges this creates for the small percentage of women who join the fire service receive much more (and needed!) attention in a separate chapter in this book. However, men, too, may face considerable gender issues within the fire service. It could be argued that the environment of the fire service is characteristic of the tenets of traditional masculinity as described by Brannon (1985):

- *Antifemininity*: the avoidance of behaviors, interests, and personality traits that are seen as feminine (e.g., emotional vulnerability)
- *Status and achievement:* gaining status through being successful in work, sports, and heterosexual competition
- *Inexpressiveness and independence:* maintaining composure and self-control in all situations, solving problems without help, keeping feelings to themselves, and disdaining any sign of weakness
- *Adventuresomeness and aggressiveness:* a willingness to take physical risks and become violent if necessary

Brooks (2010) has suggested that men who feel pressured to fulfill such traditional masculine roles are at risk of:

- Engaging in risky behavior
- Avoiding health maintenance and prevention
- Fearing being perceived as weak or feminine
- Suppressing tender and vulnerable emotions
- Being less involved in the raising of their children
- Developing unhealthy attitudes toward women

For male firefighters, these gender-related risks may be seen in:

- Putting themselves at greater risk than necessary in doing their jobs
- Engaging in unhealthy habits (e.g., tobacco use, excessive alcohol use)
- Sexism, misogynism, and homophobia in departments or crews

- Anger management problems
- Infidelity and other relationship problems
- A reluctance to seeking help, even when it is clearly needed

Suicide

It is an open secret in the fire service that the suicide rate among firefighters is among the highest of any occupational group (Stanley et al., 2016). The Firefighter Behavioral Health Alliance (2018) estimates that, largely because of stigma, only about 40% of firefighter suicides are reported. They also note that the number of firefighters who die by suicide each year exceeds that of those who die in the line-of-duty (Firefighter Behavioral Health Alliance, n.d.). The suicide rate of firefighters is higher than that of police officers and approximates that of combat veterans (Heyman et al., 2018; Nock et al., 2014). Not long ago, the problem of suicide was largely unaddressed within the fire service, reflecting the general stigma that exists about suicide in the public and the particular reluctance of firefighters to admit that this is a problem for them.

Fortunately, both fire departments and unions now acknowledge that suicide is a major problem. Articles about suicide prevention have been featured in various trade publications (Wilson, 2020), and many departments have developed suicide prevention programs (Finney et al., 2015). Research (e.g., Martin et al., 2017) suggests the suicide problem in the fire service is related to issues of unaddressed depression and traumatic exposure. Moderating variables on this association appear to include the abuse of alcohol (Martin et al., 2017), sleep issues (Healy & Vujanovic, 2021), and emotional regulation (Serrano et al., 2021). The occurrence of a firefighter suicide can be devastating to the morale and effectiveness of a crew or even an entire department.

Line-of-Duty Deaths

The line-of-duty death (LODD) probably has the greatest negative impact of any event on a fire department (Rielage, 2015). As in combat, the death of a comrade shatters any illusion one (or one's family) may have that "this can't happen to me." It is common for firefighters to transfer to another station or to retire after an LODD. Crews, at least for a time, may become unable to perform their mission while the need for their services goes unabated. Emergencies keep happening, but the firefighters may be less able to meet them. Second-guessing decisions made by fireground commanders occurs, both by the commanders themselves and by other members of the department. Official investigations into the circumstances of the LODD, while necessary, prompt defensiveness, feelings of guilt, and – potentially – PTSS/PTSD.

Retirement

First responders often talk about their work not as a career but as a mission or calling. Much of the firefighter's identity tends to revolve around this calling. As previously discussed, firefighters live at the station where they eat, sleep, and work together. They often relate to fellow crew members as family, so it should come as no surprise, then, that retirement may be especially difficult for them. Many retired firefighters maintain relationships with old friends in their departments by dropping in at the station, participating in firefighter retiree organizations, or even going to work for other departments or fire-training organizations.

In addition to potentially losing a sense of identity, firefighter retirees may suffer from conditions related to their service in the department (e.g., posttraumatic stress, job-related injuries, alcohol abuse). In addition, they may be coping with issues common for retirees in other occupations (e.g., depression, loss of purpose, loneliness). But the sad truth is that if mental health services are limited for active-duty firefighters, they are virtually nonexistent for retirees.

Professional firefighters typically start their career in their early 20s and then work for 20–30 years. As a result, they are comparatively young when they retire. Of course, they may retire earlier because of injury or health reasons. The length of time they work often depends on pension benefits in their department. Since professional firefighters retire at a relatively young age, they do not qualify for Medicare. They also may also have health issues related to their service, and they will need continuing, often expensive, medical insurance coverage. In addition, in many states, if they draw a pension, they do not qualify for social security benefits. In places where they are permitted to get social security benefits, firefighter retirees are initially too young to qualify.

Protective Factors Among Firefighters: What Helps?

It is inarguable that firefighters face many difficulties in their job that do not exist in other professions. What helps them cope more effectively? Several protective factors have been identified in the research. *Resilience*, the ability to adapt and cope with adversity, is a trait variable that has been found to reduce the risk of PTSD among firefighters (Lee et al., 2014). A similar concept, *distress tolerance* – the perceived and/or actual ability to endure negative emotional or physical states – also has been found to moderate the effects of occupational stress in this population (Stanley et al., 2018). Sliter et al. (2014) found that coping humor significantly reduced the risk of burnout and PTSD among firefighters. It should be noted that these protective factors all seem to be trait or personality variables that vary among individuals. This suggests there is potential utility in measuring these variables in prospective firefighter candidates in employment prescreening.

Another variable identified as reducing the negative effects of occupational stress among firefighters is perceived social support (Lee, 2019). Firefighters who feel socially supported report less PTSD symptoms and less rumination about negative work events. When firefighters discuss what helps them cope, they often cite a sense of purpose (the meaning they derive from their work) and the cohesion of their unit. Shared danger, close living quarters, and physical exertion all seem to lend themselves to effective coping. In a comprehensive qualitative article by Jacobsson, et al. (2020), researchers identified six themes that promote and maintain firefighter well-being and health:

- Having a strong sense of community (belonging to the "tribe")
- Physical exercise (physical strength and competence to perform the job)
- A balance between emergency work and station work (with sufficient recovery time from dealing with trauma before being asked to respond to another crisis)
- Clarity of roles (what is expected and who is expected to do it). When the crew is responding to an emergency, leadership needs to be clear and decisive, and everyone needs to know their role
- Peer support and tolerance (positive collegial connections with team members)
- The image of firefighters as heroes or helpers (both in the community's perception and the firefighters' self-understanding) creating a positive self-image

Components of an Effective Fire Psychology Program

Counseling

While individual counseling for firefighters is the most obvious mental health service that should be offered, other mental health interventions (e.g., anger management training; smoking cessation; parenting skills classes) may be equally valuable. Although firefighters may present with similar mental health concerns as those expressed by other people (e.g., depression, relationship conflicts, substance use), the issues they experience are always colored by the nature of their work and the culture of the fire service. The firefighter who reports marital problems, for example, is trying to mend their relationship with a partner whom they may go days without seeing. The alcohol abuse problem or depression presented by a firefighter may be fueled by repeated traumatic exposures. The psychological concerns of firefighters cannot be fully understood or addressed outside of the context and culture associated with their career. For that reason, MHPs who treat firefighters need to become well versed in firefighter culture. Generic counseling services offered through an EAP are likely to be ineffective. Furthermore, an effective psychological services program for firefighters needs to also offer counseling services to other members of the fire service community: families and retirees.

Families

The couple and family relationships of firefighters are very affected by their work schedules, the milieu of the fire service, and the hazardous jobs they do. Relationship counseling is frequently requested by firefighters, and the course of that counseling is very much affected by these cultural issues, many of which are impossible to change. Conflicts around parenting, fueled by the frequent absence of the firefighter parent, often occur. While it is probably not feasible for fire departments to offer services such as child therapy, practical guidance on effective parenting can be very helpful in these situations. MHPs who understand the lifestyles of firefighters are much more likely to provide helpful information and interventions. If the services of a child psychologist or psychiatrist are warranted, the MHP also may be able to assist the firefighter by making a referral to the appropriate professional and then providing support to them and their family as they go through the process. This also highlights the importance of the MHP being familiar with other resources in the community and maintaining those connections to facilitate referrals and coordination.

Retirees

Are fire departments obligated to provide mental health care to retirees? From a legal standpoint, they typically would have no such requirement. But is there an ethical responsibility to provide such care to those who put their lives on the line for their community, and who are suffering mentally as a result of that sacrifice? The nation has elected to help military veterans who sustain psychological injuries because of their service. Should our communities do likewise for first responders? The effects of cumulative traumatic exposures do not simply go away with retirement. In fact, some symptoms of PTSS/PTSD may not become apparent until after the person has left the fire service, when the pace slows and previous coping strategies are no longer in place. From a moral standpoint, then, it seems appropriate for MHPs who work within the fire service to consider offering at least some level of services to retired firefighters.

Substance Abuse Abatement

Given that alcohol abuse is common among firefighters, psychological service programs within the fire service need to offer treatment models congruent with their needs (e.g., motivational interviewing Rollnick & Miller, 1995). Often, this will require coordination and familiarity with substance abuse treatment programs (e.g., rehabilitation services, inpatient and outpatient treatment) in the community. Additionally, substance abuse screening, especially for alcohol problems, should be a standard part of assessment of referrals to psychological services. Such screenings should aid members who are willing to seek help for their problems rather than identifying offenders for discipline.

Anger Management

Anger issues can be a disguise for underlying problems with depression, anxiety, and trauma exposure. This is especially true for men (Lynch & Kilmartin, 2013), and, as previously noted, almost all firefighters are male. While firefighters with anger problems can be referred to MHPs outside the department for assistance with anger management, those MHPs are unlikely to be familiar with the lives and work of firefighters. Furthermore, because of their work schedules, firefighters find it difficult to schedule ongoing psychoeducational classes or therapy appointments. The development of anger management classes/programs within the department can alleviate many of the challenges in providing this much needed service to firefighters.

Crisis Intervention

Because firefighters frequently experience traumatic incidents, it is common for departments to provide post-incident crisis intervention services. The goal of these services is to mitigate the deleterious effects of the traumatic events on the firefighters and to return the unit to full mission effectiveness as soon as possible. The department's MHP should be responsible for the development, training, and deployment of these crisis intervention services.

Many departments employ the "Mitchell model" (Everly & Mitchell, 1999) which utilizes a peer-led team (i.e., other firefighters) working under the oversight of an MHP to meet with firefighters after a particularly difficult emergency response (e.g., an LODD, child fatality). All crisis team members must complete standardized training on the model prior to participating in these post-incident interventions. The interventions utilize a group approach attempting to include all emergency response personnel who were present and potentially affected by the event. After the group interventions team members follow up with affected individuals as needed. The International Critical Incident Stress Foundation (ICISF) has continued to develop the "Mitchell model," more accurately referred to as *Critical Incident Stress Management (CISM)* (The International Crisis Incident Stress Foundation, n.d.).

Some studies (Everly & Mitchell, 2000) have questioned the effectiveness of the CISM approach, while others (e.g., Jacobs et al., 2004) have argued that the model has merit for use with emergency services workers. The results of research on the centerpiece of CISM, Critical Incident Stress Debriefing or CISD, have been mixed (Mitchell et al., 2003). Mitchell and colleagues have recommended that future studies on its efficacy need to be better designed to overcome methodological limitations. In Chap. 12 of this handbook, Jeff Mitchell examines the role of CISM and this controversy in greater depth. However, the value of intervening to reduce post-incident stress for firefighters is rarely questioned within the fire service. Departments that do not use the CISM concept usually employ another similar intervention model after major traumatic events.

MHPs within the fire service need to be trained in either the CISM approach or similar methods to participate effectively in ameliorating the negative effects of traumatic incidents. Such events are commonplace for firefighters, and major urban departments will experience multiple severe incidents every year. Personnel who have been involved in these critical incidents are more likely to later experience additional psychological symptoms (Jahnke et al., 2016). By participating in post-incident response teams, the department's MHPs may be able to identify and intervene earlier with firefighters who are the most negatively affected by the incident. While firefighters may talk among themselves about what happened, there is a tendency for them to shut down or to avoid communicating about the incident, especially regarding the emotional content. They may attempt to suppress their feelings about what has happened. They generally will not talk about the events to family members or "civilians," and, as noted earlier, they are unlikely to seek counseling. Unless the department has a preplanned crisis intervention system, many firefighters will attempt to deal with traumatic exposure on their own, often unsuccessfully.

One of the issues faced by the MHP in this role is to determine what incidents require crisis intervention. A large, urban department may respond to emergencies a thousand or more times per day. Every day there will be traumatic events that might warrant a crisis intervention, but resources are limited. Severe injury or death of a firefighter is very debilitating to members of the department and may require an automatic crisis team response. Pediatric emergencies, including injuries, death, or abuse are often the ones that are the most difficult for firefighters, making crisis intervention more necessary in these situations. The MHP must collaborate with the peer members of the team to determine how and when to best respond post-incident.

Consultation

Another valuable role of the MHP within the fire service is to serve as a psychological consultant to officers and command. This might include giving insight to command staff on dealing with major incidents in the department, providing guidance to officers on how to manage members with psychological problems, and translating research findings to practical guidance for chiefs of the department (e.g., What characteristics should be considered in selecting officers for the department? What can we do to reduce the incidence of PTSD among our members?).

Research

To date, there is a paucity of psychological research on the needs and issues of firefighters, so much has yet to be established. The fire service MHP may need to conduct timely and practical research on psychological issues for the department. If the MHP is not well skilled in conducting and analyzing such research, it may be possible for them to collaborate with local universities to plan, execute, and evaluate research on firefighters. Such research should have practical implications for the fire service, rather than serving as exercises in intellectual curiosity. For instance, "What are the most effective stress management techniques for firefighters?" "What is the effect of sleep deprivation on firefighter performance?" "What are the characteristics of an effective paramedic?"

Training

The fire service MHP should serve as the chief trainer for their department on psychological issues. They should plan, develop, and teach on psychologically relevant topics such as suicide prevention, substance use harm reduction, and recognizing mental health issues of peers and subordinates.

Helpful Tips for MHP's Working with Firefighters

- Spend extra time talking about confidentiality, especially if you are working for the same entity (e.g., city) that employs them. Make sure that there are adequate safeguards in place to protect firefighter client records from their employers (e.g., command staff; civilian supervisors).
- If you have previously seen a couple of firefighters in your clinical work, do not assume that you understand their culture.
- Become culturally competent. Seek further training on firefighter culture. Such training can be found from such groups as the IAFF (*iaff.org*), the Center for Firefighter Behavioral Health (*cffbh.org*), and the Fire Psychology Association (*firepsychology.org*). Also seek guidance from senior and respected members of the department so you understand the history and culture of *your* department. In so doing, consult not only with members of the senior command staff but also with officers (e.g., captains and lieutenants) who work in the field at the station. These junior officers are the backbone of the fire service, and they provide critical leadership at the tactical or station level.
- Seek ways to spend time at the fire station and to accompany them on "ride-alongs." Become familiar with their living and working conditions. Where

possible, participate in training exercises with them so that you have some understanding of what it is like to do their job.

- Maintain good relationships with the local union. While union membership is less common today among many occupational groups, firefighters typically belong to a union, especially the International Association of Firefighters (IAFF). This is perhaps because firefighters need an organized body to represent concerns to their employers, usually governmental entities. Governments are often much more responsive to taxpayers and voters than they are to the issues of their employees. Thus, firefighters tend to band together to lobby for such issues as working conditions, pay, and retirement benefits. The union, of course, seeks to protect the interests of their members (i.e., firefighters), and they tend to be suspicious of the role of MHPs. When MHPs develop a negative reputation with local union leaders, it becomes practically impossible to earn the trust of firefighters in the department.
- Training in the treatment of trauma is especially helpful to MHPs working with firefighters. While the source of trauma is different from that experienced by the military or law enforcement, the treatment methods used with those populations are effective with firefighters as well. Empirically supported treatments for trauma like cognitive processing therapy, prolonged exposure, and eye movement desensitization and reprocessing (EMDR) can be utilized with good effect with firefighters.
- Become involved with integrating new firefighters into the department. Develop classes in basic mental health issues faced by firefighters that are incorporated in the orientation and training of new members of the department. New recruits to the fire service have little understanding of the long-term effects of serving as an emergency worker. They are typically focused on being accepted and proving themselves to the more experienced crew members. Offer classes to the family members of new recruits to help them understand what the firefighters experience and to acquaint them with resources to help them if they encounter difficulties.
- Recognize that you have multiple "clients" when you are working with firefighters (or other first responders). For most clinicians, the client is the person in front of you who is seeking help. Whether the client came voluntarily or is coerced into treatment, the client is your primary responsibility. This is true regardless of who is paying for the service: the client themselves, insurance, etc. In contrast, the MHP working with firefighters has multiple levels of responsibility. A firefighter who is suffering from a psychological condition that is impairing their work may imperil the lives of their fellow crew members. The firefighter MHP also has an obligation to those crews. In contrast, as an MHP in most settings, you generally don't have to consider the effects of your client's mental health on co-workers or fellow students. Furthermore, the firefighter/first responder who is psychologically impaired may put the public at risk, as well.
- Sometimes the needs of the individual firefighter client conflict with the needs of their crew or the public. The firefighter MHP must weigh the need to protect others against the individual's rights to privacy and confidentiality. The need to

break confidentiality in these situations might be compared to the duty to warn others of threats (the *Tarasoff* rule) or the requirement to report suspected child abuse.
- From time to time, questions will arise about whether a particular firefighter is psychologically healthy enough to perform their duties (e.g., Have they had a psychotic episode? Do they suffer from a personality disorder that is impairing their ability to get along with others?). The MHP in a fire department must be careful, though, when asked to evaluate the "fitness for duty" of members.
- In some ways, it is logical for the department's MHP to be the one to evaluate the psychological health of members. The fire department MHP will know more about the job demands on firefighters, the work atmosphere of the department/station, and the potential safety risks of firefighters who are struggling psychologically. On the other hand, an MHP who is providing recommendations about fitness for duty to command staff will almost certainly be shunned by firefighters who are interested in obtaining help for their psychological issues. Within the department, the two roles of evaluator and counselor are incompatible. The boundary between these roles must be preserved to have any credibility as a source of help. The MHP, the firefighters, and the department as a whole are all better served when qualified, independent professionals in the community can perform fitness for duty evaluations when the need arises.
- Become familiar with the work of the various subspecialties within the department (e.g., rescue, dispatch, arson). Recognize their needs may be different than those of the rest of the department. In planning training events or interventions, make sure to include them.
- Develop programmatic responses to the mental issues most reported by firefighters (e.g., alcohol overuse, sleep problems) tailoring them to the specific needs of firefighters. Adapt standard interventions for these problems considering the language, working conditions, and culture of firefighters. Use examples based on firefighter experiences, employing firefighter nomenclature.
- Seek connections with local universities to increase staffing and address research needs. Training programs in psychology, counseling, and social work are almost always looking for placement sites for their students. The use of practicum students and interns can multiply the mental health resources available to the department at low cost. Supervision of these students may become a key role for the MHP; thus, the MHP needs to maintain close affiliations with these programs and to hone their skills as a supervisor.

Summary

There is a legitimate need for psychological services within fire departments. This conclusion is based on the extraordinary demands placed on firefighters by the nature of their work. It is a dangerous career where traumatic events are commonly encountered and PTSD is an occupational hazard. Firefighters are at increased risk of developing mental health disorders and substance abuse problems. Their culture is little understood by outsiders, and MHPs are generally unfamiliar with them.

To be effective, the fire service MHP must possess good clinical skills, especially in issues most often presented by firefighters (e.g., posttraumatic stress, alcohol overuse, relationship conflict). The MHP must be culturally fluent in the world of firefighters and proficient in crisis intervention. This requires both an understanding of trauma and group process combined with additional training in how to help first responders who have experienced a critical incident. In addition, the effective fire service MHP must be able to consult with leaders and to utilize research skills to answer questions with practical implications for the department and its members. The fire service MHP will face ethical challenges posed by the need to consider both the needs of individual firefighters and those of their peers and the public at large. The job demands flexibility and innovation, but it offers MHPs the reward of being able to help real heroes.

References

Avsec, R. (2013, December 6). *What is the fire service culture? – Fire & EMS leader pro*. http://www.fireemsleaderpro.org/2013/12/06/what-is-the-fire-service-culture/

Barger, L. K., Rajaratnam, S. M. W., Wang, W., O'Brien, C. S., Sullivan, J., et al. (2015). Common sleep disorders increase risk of motor vehicle crashes and adverse health outcomes in firefighters. *Journal of Clinical Sleep Medicine, 11*(3), 233–240.

Brannon, R. (1985). Dimensions of the male sex role in America. In A. G. Sargent (Ed.), *Beyond sex roles* (pp. 296–316). West.

Brooks, G. R. (2010). *Beyond the crisis of masculinity*. American Psychological Association.

Carey, M. G., Al-Zaiti, S. S., Dean, G. E., Sessanna, L., & Finnell, D. S. (2011). Sleep problems, depression, substance use, social bonding, and quality of life in professional firefighters. *Journal of Occupational and Environmental Medicine, 53*(8), 928–933. https://doi.org/10.1097/JOM.0b013e318225898f

Center for Firefighter Behavioral Health. (n.d.). *Center for firefighter behavioral health home page*. Retrieved from https://cffbh.org/

Corrigan, P. W., Druss, B. G., & Perlick, D. A. (2014). The impact of mental illness stigma on seeking and participating in mental health care. *Psychological Science in the Public Interest, 15*(2), 37–70. https://doi.org/10.1177/1529100614531398

del Ben, K. S., Scotti, J. R., Chen, Y.-C., & Fortson, B. L. (2006). Prevalence of posttraumatic stress disorder symptoms in firefighters. *Work & Stress, 20*(1), 37–48.

Everly, G. S., & Mitchell, J. P. (1999). *Critical incident stress management (CISM): A new era and standard of care in crisis intervention*. http://ci.nii.ac.jp/ncid/BA57034797

Everly, G. S., & Mitchell, J. T. (2000). The debriefing "controversy" and crisis intervention: A review of lexical and substantive issues. *The International Journal of Emergency Mental Health, 2*(4), 211–225. https://pubmed.ncbi.nlm.nih.gov/11217152/

Fahy, R., Evarts, B., & Stein, G. P. (2022). U.S. fire department profile. In NFPA.org. National Fire Protection Association. https://www.nfpa.org/News-and-Research/Data-research-and-tools/Emergency-Responders/US-fire-department-profile

Finney, E. J., Buser, S. J., Schwarz, J., Archibald, L., & Swanson, R. (2015). Suicide prevention in the fire service: The Houston fire department (HFD) model. *Aggression and Violent Behavior, 21*, 1–4. https://doi.org/10.1016/j.avb.2014.12.012

Fire Psychology Association. (n.d.). *Fire psychology association–bridging the gap*. Retrieved July 30, 2022, from https://www.firepsychology.org/

Firefighter Behavioral Health Alliance. (n.d.). https://www.ffbha.org/

FireRescue1. (2021). *How many firefighters died on 9/11?* Retrieved from https://www.firerescue1.com/9-11/articles/how-many-firefighters-died-on-911-SKaClbnYxUtzowuK

Godfrey, D. A., Zegel, M., Babcock, J. C., & Vujanovic, A. A. (2022). Posttraumatic stress disorder and relationship satisfaction among firefighters: The role of emotion regulation difficulties. *Journal of Aggression, Maltreatment & Trauma, 1*, 356. https://doi.org/10.1080/10926771.2022.2043973

Haddock, C. K., Jahnke, S. A., Poston, W. S. C., Jitnarin, N., Kaipust, C. M., Tuley, B., & Hyder, M. L. (2012). Alcohol use among firefighters in the Central United States. *Occupational Medicine (London), 62*, 661–664.

Healy, N. A., & Vujanovic, A. A. (2021). PTSD symptoms and suicide risk among firefighters: The moderating role of sleep disturbance. *Psychological Trauma: Theory, Research, Practice, and Policy, 13*(7), 749–758. https://doi.org/10.1037/tra0001059

Heyman, R. D., Dill, J., & Douglas, R. (2018, April). *The Ruderman white paper on mental health and suicide of first responders*. Ruderman Family Foundation.

IAFF (International Association of Firefighters). (n.d.). *Substance abuse*. Retrieved from https://www.iaffrecoverycenter.com/substance-abuse

International Association of Firefighters. (2023, April 17). *Behavioral health program – IAFF*. https://www.iaff.org/behavioral-health/

International Association of Firefighters Home Page. https://www.iaff.org/

Jacobs, J., Horne-Moyer, H. L., & Jones, R. (2004). The effectiveness of critical incident stress debriefing with primary and secondary trauma victims. *International Journal of Emergency Mental Health, 6*(1), 5–14.

Jacobsson, A., Erlanson, S. B., Brulin, C., & Sjolander, A. E. (2020, October, 1–12). *Promoting and hindering health and well-being in firefighter discourse*. Sage Open. https://doi.org/10.1177/2158244020979170

Jahnke, S. A. (2020, December 18). *Opioid addiction: The epidemic's impact on firefighters*. FireRescue1. Retrieved May 12, 2023, from https://www.firerescue1.com/opioids/articles/opioid-addiction-the-epidemics-impact-on-firefighters-ETPqgmqu1e6AsL1l/

Jahnke, S. A., Poston, W. S., & Haddock, C. K. (2014). Perceptions of alcohol use among US firefighters. *Journal of Substance Abuse: Alcohol, 2*(2), 1012.

Jahnke, S. A., Poston, W. S., Haddock, C. K., & Murphy, B. (2016). Firefighting and mental health: Experiences of repeated exposure to trauma. *Work, 53*(4), 737–744. https://doi.org/10.3233/WOR-162255

Lee, J. H. (2019). Perceived social support functions as a resilience in buffering the impact of trauma exposure on PTSD symptoms via intrusive rumination and entrapment in firefighters. *PLOS One, 14*(8), e0220454. https://doi.org/10.1371/journal.pone.0220454

Lee, J.-S., Ahn, Y.-S., Jeong, K.-S., Chae, J.-H., & Choi, K.-S. (2014). Resilience buffers the impact of traumatic events on the development of PTSD symptoms in firefighters. *Journal of Affective Disorders, 162*, 128–133.

Lynch, J. R., & Kilmartin, C. (2013). *The pain behind the mask: Overcoming masculine depression* (2nd ed.). Routledge.

Martin, C. E., Tran, J. K., & Buser, S. J. (2017). Correlates of suicidality in firefighter/EMS personnel. *Journal of Affective Disorders, 208*, 177–183.

Mitchell, A. M., Sakraida, T. J., & Karmeg, K. (2003). Critical incident stress debriefing: Implications for best practice. *Disaster Management & Response, 1*(2), 46–51.

National Institute of Health: National Institute on Drug Abuse. (2022, May 28). *Misuse of prescription drugs research report: What is the scope of prescription drug misuse in the United States?* https://Nida.Nih.Gov/, https://nida.nih.gov/publications/research-reports/misuse-prescription-drugs/what-scope-prescription-drug-misuse

NFPA statistics - Firefighter deaths. (n.d.). https://www.nfpa.org/News-and-Research/Data-research-and-tools/Emergency-Responders/Firefighter-fatalities-in-the-United-States/Firefighter-deaths

Nock, M. K., Stein, M. B., Heeringa, S. G., Ursano, R. J., Colpe, L. J., Fullerton, C. S., Hwang, I., Naifeh, J. A., Sampson, N. A., Schoenbaum, M., Zaslavsky, A. M., Kessler, R. C., & Army STARRS Collaborators. (2014). Prevalence and correlates of suicidal behavior among soldiers: Results from the Army study to assess risk and resilience in servicemembers (Army STARRS). *JAMA Psychiatry, 71*(5), 514–522.

Obuokj-Donkor, G., Oluwasina, F., Nkire, N., & Agyapong, V. I. O. (2022). A scoping review on the prevalence and determinants of post-traumatic stress disorder among military personnel and firefighters: Implications for public policy and practice. *International Journal of Environmental Research and Public Health, 19*(3), 1565. https://doi.org/10.3390/ijerph19031565

Occupational Outlook Handbook: U.S. Bureau of Labor Statistics. (2022, November 3). https://www.bls.gov/ooh/protective-service/firefighters.htm

Pope-Davis, D. B. (2003). *Handbook of multicultural competencies in counseling and psychology*. http://ci.nii.ac.jp/ncid/BA65128477

Reese, J. T. (1987). *A history of police psychological services*. U.S. Department of Justice, Federal Bureau of Investigation.

Rielage, R. (2015, November 3). *How to handle a firefighter LODD*. Firerescue1.Com. https://www.firerescue1.com/exclusives-1/articles/how-to-handle-a-firefighter-lodd-oIZdLjVsJOov01NQ/

Rollnick, S. & Miller, W. R. (1995). What is motivational interviewing. *Behavioural and Cognitive Psychotherapy, 23*(4), 325–334.

SAMSHA. (2014). TIP 57: Trauma-informed care in behavioral health services. *samhsa.gov*, SMA14-4816. https://textbooks.whatcom.edu/cdpresources/chapter/tip-57-trauma-informed-care-in-behavioral-health-services-2/

Serrano, D. M., Rufino, K. A., Tran, J. K., & Vujanovic, A. A. (2021). The association of sleep disturbance and suicide risk among firefighters: Exploring emotion regulation dimensions. *Archives of Suicide Research*, 1–13. https://doi.org/10.1080/13811118.2021.1982093

Sliter, M., Kale, A., & Yuan, Z. (2014). Is humor the best medicine? The buffering effect of coping humor on traumatic stressors in firefighters. *Journal of Organizational Behavior, 35*(2), 257–272. https://doi.org/10.1002/job.1868

Soravia, L. M., Schwab, S., Walther, S., & Müller, T. (2021). Rescuers at risk: Posttraumatic stress symptoms among police officers, fire fighters, ambulance personnel, and emergency and psychiatric nurses. *Frontiers in Psychiatry, 11*. https://doi.org/10.3389/fpsyt.2020.602064

Spell, J. (2021). *A brief history of the fire service: From ancient equipment to modern technology*. FireRescue1.

Stanley, I. H., Horn, M. A., & Joiner, T. E. (2016). Suicide mortality among firefighters: Results from a large, urban fire department. *American Journal of Industrial Medicine, 59*(11), 942–947. https://doi.org/10.1002/ajim.22587

Stanley, I. H., Boffa, J. W., Smith, L. J., Tran, J. K., Schmidt, N. B., Joiner, T. E., & Vujanovic, A. A. (2018). Occupational stress and suicidality among firefighters: Examining the buffering role of distress tolerance. *Psychiatry Research, 266*, 90–96.

The International Crisis Incident Stress Foundation. (n.d.). The International Critical Incident Stress Foundation. Retrieved July 30, 2022, from https://icisf.org

Wagner, S. L., McFee, J. A., & Martin, C. A. (2010). Mental health implications of fire service membership. *Traumatology, 16*(2), 26–32. https://doi.org/10.1177/1534765610362803

Waters, R. (2023). Firefighter shift schedules: A comprehensive guide. *Firefighter connection*. https://firefighterconnection.com/understanding-a-firefighter-workschedule/#:~:text=24%2F48%20Schedule%3A%20Widely%20used,of%2010%20days%20per%20month

Wilson, H. (2020, December 11). *It could never happen here: Preventing suicides in the volunteer fire department*. Fireengineering.Com. https://www.fireengineering.com/health-safety/it-could-never-happen-here-preventing-suicides-in-the-volunteer-fire-department/#gref

Wolkow, A. P., Barger, L. K., O'Brien, C. S., Sullivan, J. P., Qadri, S., Lockley, S. W., Czeisler, C. A., & Rajaratnam, S. M. W. (2019). Associations between sleep disturbances, mental health outcomes and burnout in firefighters, and the mediating role of sleep during overnight work: A cross-sectional stud. *Journal of Sleep Research, 28*(6). https://doi.org/10.1111/jsr.12869

Zegel, M., Tran, J. K., & Vujanovic, A. A. (2019). Posttraumatic stress, alcohol use, and alcohol use motives among firefighters: The role of distress tolerance. *Psychiatry Research, 282*, 112633. https://doi.org/10.1016/j.psychres.2019.112633

Psychological Health of Correctional Workers

Krystal Lowe, Marc Patry, Philip R. Magaletta, and Eleni Travers

Working within the correctional setting is both physically and psychologically demanding, with employees facing stressful and often precarious work circumstances (Johnston et al., 2022). Correctional work ranges from mundane and repetitive to unpredictable and arduous (Ricciardelli et al., 2021a, b), with all correctional workers (CW) in general experiencing repeated exposure to traumatic incidents. These incidents may occur directly, as the target of violence, or indirectly, through witnessing or hearing assaults, murders, and suicides (Carelton et al., 2018; Konda et al., 2012; Ricciardelli et al., 2021a, b). In the 24 h a day, 7 days a week environment, CW provide both custody of and care to offenders. They are not only *first* responders – they are *the only* responders.

Scholars specifically studying corrections officers (CO) find that compared to other law enforcement colleagues such as police, CO are just as likely, if not more so, to experience potentially traumatic events (Carelton et al., 2018). Moreover, those working in correctional systems are exposed to occupational hazards unique to the correctional environment, such as increased exposure to potentially infectious contaminants through the weaponization of bodily fluids and the ongoing risk of physical violence, including high rates of workplace homicide (Bick, 2007; Konda et al., 2012). To illustrate, CO in the United States account for the highest number of work-related injuries compared to all other government employees (Konda et al., 2013). Correspondingly, violent acts accounted for the majority of occupational injuries for CO between the years 1999 and 2008 (Konda et al., 2012).

K. Lowe (✉) · M. Patry
Saint Mary's University, Halifax, NS, Canada
e-mail: Krystal.Lowe@smu.ca

P. R. Magaletta
ICF, Columbia, MD, USA

E. Travers
Federal Bureau of Prisons, Ayer, MA, USA

M. L. Bourke et al. (eds.), *First Responder Mental Health*,
https://doi.org/10.1007/978-3-031-38149-2_3

According to the Bureau of Labor Statistics (2017), approximately 431,000 individuals are employed by correctional institutions in the United States. However, a vast amount of the existing literature has focused on CO, ignoring the ecological framework in which all CW function. Prior estimates for the correctional workforce indicate that nearly two-thirds of employees are CO (BJS, 2008), leaving a third of the workforce unexamined. In addition, empirical research on the psychological health of CW more globally is lacking, and what does exist is limited by an almost exclusive reliance upon self-report survey data. This gap introduces a problem within the literature: despite the notion that trauma exposure experienced by all CW are mediated by the same environmental factors, it prevents us from generalizing findings.

Although this presents challenges for understanding the psychological health needs of CW, one can at least delineate the CW category. Correctional workers include staff in various roles throughout a correctional institution, such as correctional officers; service providers such as psychologists and medical staff; managerial and governance staff (wardens, superintendents); parole/probation officers; and administrative or executive staff and leaders (Carelton et al., 2018). While there are differences between occupational roles within the institution, all workers serve within the same setting and are thus exposed to potentially traumatic circumstances (Fusco et al., 2021). Arguably, the majority of these workers, while perhaps performing different roles, are influenced by the same organizational and environmental factors that make correctional work stressful and dangerous. Nevertheless, CW collectively remain unnoticed as a subgroup of public safety and first-responder personnel requiring assistance with specific psychological health needs. Although the field of psychology has recognized the unique treatment needs of first responders such as police officers, it has failed to do the same for those working among correctional organizations (Ferdik & Smith, 2017).

The oversight of such treatment needs in this particular subgroup is problematic as CW have a significant and often overlooked role within society. Issues surrounding the psychological health and workplace stress of CW have a detrimental impact on society, thwarting efforts at developing therapeutic or working relationships with justice-involved people (Fusco et al., 2021; Lambert & Hogan, 2018). Correctional workers are assigned with the inherently stressful undertaking of maintaining social order amidst a population of individuals confined against their will (Finn, 2000); they are required to quickly respond to critical incidences on foot and without a weapon, often relying on their ability to listen, make prompt decisions, and take decisive action. Likewise, they are confronted with workplace demands and threats of ongoing violence that contribute to the excessive stress rooted in correctional work. These levels of workplace adversity, which are arguably unique to corrections, contribute to physical and psychological illnesses and burnout and may lead to an inability of workers to properly carry out their duties (Finn, 2000; Jaegers et al., 2019).

All CW face numerous challenges within the confines of their workplace. These may be delineated into clinical disorders, psychological distress (e.g., suicide risk and secondary traumatic stress), and occupational stress. This chapter will take an intentionally broad approach to correctional employees and utilize the term "CW," moving beyond the narrow focus on CO. In instances where references solely related to CO are utilized, this distinction will be noted to emphasize the notion that CW do not serve their communities in a vacuum. Instead, they are a part of a much larger, interdependent system that exists out of sight from the rest of society. These first-and-only responders provide custody to and care for offenders as a public service, thus protecting society and keeping communities safe. Accordingly, it is vital that the psychological health and treatment needs of this under examined group of first responders are recognized. This recognition begins with elucidating the clinical disorders, psychological distress, and occupational stress reported in research studies; proposes approaches to prevention, treatment seeking and intervention; and concludes with recommendations for future research.

Clinical Disorders

Research on clinical disorders among CW is limited, with the majority of existing literature relying heavily on self-selected samples and suffering from self-report bias. Despite this, the existing studies provide us with valuable insights into the psychological health of CW. Additionally, we are confident that individuals in these occupations experience psychological health challenges similar to, if not go beyond, those experienced by other first responders such as paramedics, police officers, and firefighters.

Contemporary research examining the prevalence of psychological health challenges in diverse samples of correctional workers has found high frequencies of symptoms associated with clinical disorders (Carelton et al., 2018; Ricciardelli et al., 2021a, b). A recent systematic review identified six studies that, albeit limited, point toward a high prevalence of posttraumatic stress disorder (PTSD), major depressive disorder (MDD), and generalized anxiety disorder (GAD) in international samples of CO (Regehr et al., 2021). For instance, in Canada, it is estimated that 29.1% of CO struggle with symptoms related to PTSD, which is on par with prevalence estimates for the Royal Canadian Mounted Police (30%; Carelton et al., 2018). In France, 240 randomly selected correctional workers responded to a battery of questionnaires evaluating PTSD, burnout, and inmate-to-staff assaults. According to Boudoukha et al. (2013), 15% of the sample experienced symptoms characteristic of GAD. Moreover, participants reported frequent experiences of traumatic events and high scores on measures of PTSD. Additionally, in China, Liu et al. (2013) discovered high levels of depression among front-line CO (n = 943; 59.7%) and other prison staff (n = 475; 56.2%).

In another Canadian study, Ricciardelli et al. (2021a, b) explored the relationship between psychological health disorders and uncertainty intolerance – a negatively reinforcing factor related to the development of emotional and behavioral problems – among specific occupational roles within corrections. The sample (n = 842) consisted of a broad range of employees, including those working in wellness and training roles (social workers, psychologists, nurses, program coordinators), governance (superintendents, managers), community (parole and probation officers), administration (records officers, assistants), and CO. Similarly to the current chapters' conceptualization of CW, Ricciardelli et al. (2021a, b) argue that while the roles of correctional employees vary, they are entrenched within the same system and thus influenced by similar ecological factors. For instance, despite the highly structured environment of corrections, all workers are subject to uncertainty and varying levels of control over the environment in which they work.

In Ricciardelli et al.'s (2021a, b) study, participants were assessed for PTSD, GAD, MDD, panic disorder, and alcohol-use disorder. Results indicated that uncertainty intolerance did not moderate the association between occupational roles and psychological health disorders. However, results did reveal high prevalence rates of clinical symptoms among the combined CW group. The results from this study suggest that heightened risk of mental illness is not limited to CO and includes workers serving in institutional governance positions and parole/probation officers. For instance, more than half (55.8%) of the sample screened positive for at least one of the five disorders measured. Additionally, prevalence estimates varied depending on the occupational role, with those serving in institutional governance roles experiencing significantly higher rates of PTSD and alcohol-use disorder. Given that there were more mid-to-later career individuals in this subgroup, the authors report: "These findings shed light on the cumulative trauma that correctional workers face throughout their career…" (p. 14).

Despite current advances in the literature surrounding CW psychological health and well-being, all of the abovementioned studies suffer from common methodological flaws grounded in issues of external validity. For instance, while the majority of studies reported by Regehr et al. (2021) utilized empirically validated measures such as the PTSD Checklist for DSM-5 (PCL-5), no studies included randomized control trials or structured clinical interviews and are therefore limited by self-report data. Similarly, Ricciardelli et al.'s (2021a, b) study suffers from issues of generalizability given its reliance on a self-selected sample and self-report data. As such, the sample itself may be more reflective of the roles of CO due to the unequal participation of each occupational group.

Psychological Distress

Suicide Risk

The risk of death by suicide is a relevant area of concern for CW. Between 1998 and 2008, 38% of work-related fatalities for CO in the United States were the result of suicide (Konda et al., 2013). In New Jersey, from 2003 to 2007, 55 law enforcement officers died by suicide, 30% of whom were CO (New Jersey Police Suicide Task Force, 2009). Moreover, in a larger sample of Canadian correctional staff ($n = 974$),

Carleton et al. (2021) explored prevalence estimates of suicidality (thoughts, planning, and attempts), discovering that 26.6% of the sample had experienced a history of suicidal thoughts, 11.9% had planned an attempt, and 5.2% had attempted suicide.

Research on rates of suicidality among CW is sparse; however, many of the risk factors that apply to police officers also apply to those working in the correctional environment (Frost et al., 2020). Among these are direct and indirect incidences of trauma exposure, organizational stress, and substance use (Chae & Boyle, 2013). In a mixed-methods study of suicidality, Frost et al. (2020) evaluated the antecedents of suicides in 20 case studies of American CW. The researchers then conducted interviews with a random sample of 440 CW, 45 of whom were new recruits, to examine rates of suicidality among those currently working in the institutions. A thematic analysis of the first study suggested that unique organizational and individual factors combined to elevate the risk for suicide and that risk levels increased following exposure to trauma within the institution.

Interviews with those still working within corrections revealed that one-quarter of the sample displayed clinically relevant levels of anxiety and PTSD, with 4% of the sample flagged as high risk for suicide. Correctional workers who had personally known a colleague who died by suicide were increasingly more likely to experience psychological distress. New recruits did not display similar levels of psychological distress and were not considered at risk for suicide. These findings suggest that the organizational environment plays a significant role in the development of suicidality.

Secondary Traumatic Stress

Recent empirical evidence suggests a strong association between repeated exposure to violence and the ramifications on a person's psychological health (Lerman et al., 2022). Given that CW are tasked with the public service of keeping communities safe by housing criminal offenders, much of their role consists of mitigating violence. Moreover, they have a responsibility to ensure the safety of both offenders and themselves. Thus, the level of exposure to violence within corrections precedes that of others working in the realm of public safety. For context, in a sample of CW in California ($n = 4300$), 67% of workers reported that they had witnessed someone killed or seriously injured, 60.5% observed or handled dead bodies, and nearly 18% had been seriously injured themselves (Lerman et al., 2022). With that said, the reality of correctional work does not simply consist of exposure to primary trauma but rather a combination of direct and indirect trauma (Cassidy & Bruce, 2019).

Indeed, CW are indirectly exposed to traumatic events throughout the organization. This type of exposure is referred to as secondary traumatic stress (STS, and it is a known risk factor for the development of DSM-5 diagnoses such as PTSD (Sprang et al., 2021). Secondary traumatic stress can profoundly influence the psychological health and well-being of individuals working in helping professions

(Kim et al., 2021) and, furthermore, impact the quality of care offenders receive, as well as the occupational environment as a whole (Kessler et al., 2008). Furthermore, recent research has outlined an increased risk of developing STS symptoms among service providers who work with violence and trauma (Kim et al., 2021). By nature of the environment, CW are exposed to these factors at unprecedented rates compared to the general population.

The potential for secondary traumatic exposure among CW ranges from listening to the victimization and transgressions of offenders to the traumatic experiences of their colleagues (Rhineberger-Dunn et al., 2016). Researchers have also proposed that compassion fatigue, a phenomenon associated with physical, emotional, and spiritual depletion, may occur as a consequence of STS (Kim et al., 2021). Symptoms of STS include hypervigilance, avoidant behaviors, difficulty concentrating, and fluctuations in mood and are often the outcome of witnessing or working closely with individuals who are suffering. For instance, Rhineberger-Dunn et al. (2016) found that STS was present among parole/probation officers and was associated with increased time spent with offenders. Furthermore, Lewis et al. (2013) investigated traumatic stress due to indirect exposure to violence, injury, and death in a sample of 309 American probation officers. Participants were asked how many secondary traumatic events they had experienced throughout their career, and responses indicated that 48% of the sample had experienced four or more incidences of STS.

Additionally, many of the incidences of STS reported by participants included offender suicides, offender recidivism involving homicide or sexual offences against children, injury or death of a colleague, and delivering death notices. Lastly, in a sample of CO ($n = 356$) and institutional wellness employees ($n = 68$), Fusco et al. (2021) found that all officers reported multiple exposures to traumatic events in the workplace. Some of these included witnessing or learning about the suicide of a coworker and witnessing life-threatening incidents or severe workplace injuries.

Given the working environment's unpredictable and sometimes hazardous conditions, some scholars have argued that correctional organizations may generate transactional and collective STS (Handran, 2015; Horman & Vivian, 2005; Sprang et al., 2021). That is to say, the conditions and policies of the organization, including its response to employee STS, can serve to inflict more harm on workers (transactional), and workers' STS may serve to influence the social and emotional dynamics of their cohorts (collective). Johnston et al. (2022) elaborated on institutional responses to psychological health concerns and argued that organizational barriers might lead to increased symptom severity and undiagnosed mental illnesses. The authors surveyed 870 CW and found that most of the sample felt as though reliable access to psychological health services in the institution was lacking, and those that did exist took a reactive rather than proactive approach. These findings suggest that the organization itself can play an integral role in addressing worker STS.

Occupational Stress

Occupational stress, while having received wide attention within and across disciplines, is pervasive among CW and is a function of aggregate factors related to job demands including, but not limited to, mandatory overtime and understaffing, safety hazards (threats and actions of violence), and interpersonal factors (conflict with coworkers and manipulation by inmates) (Finn, 2000). Lambert and Hogan (2018) provide a summary of the occupational stress construct and underscore the influence of work-family conflict, role conflict, and role overload. Work-family conflict functions in two directions, that is, issues at work influence the dynamics of the home and vice versa. For instance, mandatory overtime is a common area of strain for CW and inevitably affects the workers' home life. Moreover, behavioral role expectations at work are incongruent with those expected in one's domestic life. Role overload also encompasses the multiple occupational demands faced by workers and the often-limited resources they have to perform their duties.

As can be expected, there are numerous consequences of job-related stress for this population, including low levels of motivation at work, decreased support of offenders, and increased risk for occupational burnout (Elliot et al., 2015). According to Maslach and Jackson (1981), occupational burnout is a consequence of (a) emotional exhaustion, (b) depersonalization, and (c) a reduced sense of personal accomplishment. Furthermore, psychological ramifications of burnout include symptoms characteristic of depression and PTSD (Lambert et al., 2015). There is a well-documented link between occupational burnout and STS (Cieslak et al., 2014). The causal relationship between burnout and STS remains unclear, but it is nonetheless relevant to CW who experience work related stress and burnout at higher levels than the general population (Lambert & Hogan, 2018).

Prevention, Treatment Seeking, and Intervention

The burden to seek treatment falls on the employee if and when they experience psychological distress as a result of STS, which can be exceptionally challenging given a culture that places a premium on psychological imperviousness. Nevertheless, exposure to traumatic events, in combination with stigma surrounding psychological health issues, may further influence treatment-seeking behavior among CW (Ricciardelli et al., 2021a, b). At times, the culture of correctional work may discourage help-seeking behaviors by virtue of the hypermasculine culture that minimizes trauma as something they have "signed up for" (Wills et al., 2021). Moreover, CW may forgo reaching out for help in fear of how it will impact their employment, for instance, being perceived as incompetent or unfit (Wills et al., 2021). To illustrate, Ricciardelli et al. (2021a, b) surveyed 1017 prison staff in Canada and found that, out of all occupational roles, CO were less likely to seek treatment out of fear that it would impact their employment. Additionally, male staff were most likely to exhibit psychological health stigma and less likely to seek help if they experienced psychological distress.

The unique working environment of CW requires specifically tailored and targeted services for worker psychological health and well-being. Unfortunately, previous research has brought into question the effectiveness of interventions for these purposes, with meta-analytic data suggesting that current interventions do not improve the psychological health or stress levels of CW (Evers et al., 2020). With that said, recent advances in the general STS literature offer promising directions for the development of effective prevention and intervention approaches. Experts have also recommended that similar approaches to detecting and preventing PTSD can be utilized in the context of STS and that these approaches should be cognizant of the particular needs of the target group (Sprang et al., 2018).

By adapting evidence-based prevention and treatment programs traditionally directed toward screening for a treating PTSD, organizations and service providers can circumvent the stigma associated with psychological health and treatment seeking (Sprang et al., 2018). For instance, Sprang et al. (2018) have proposed a two-pronged approach to addressing and preventing STS that may prove to be of value for CW. This approach borrows from a framework introduced by the Institute of Medicine (IOM, 1994), which suggests that prevention efforts must be considered in a broader context. The frameworks' underlying assumption is that a universal approach to prevention begins with an understanding that all individuals within a given population may experience equivalent risk factors. Recently, Sprang et al. (2018) have suggested a framework that involves combining a universal prevention and selective treatment approach to combating STS.

Universal Approach

Applied to the correctional setting (see Table 1), the universal approach is grounded in primary prevention and recognizes the importance of having everyone at the organizational level understand that correctional work is a high-risk profession. This approach requires buy-in at the institutional level and would target staff in all occupations to reduce risk factors and increase protective factors (Sprang et al., 2018). As a strategy, the universal approach has the advantage of being proactive in directing prevention toward the entire group of employees prior to the onset of individual risk. Universal prevention strategies focus on environmental and population-based interventions, including the development of education, programs, and policies (Institute of Medicine, 1994). The universal approach to evidence-based prevention should be a top priority when considering the issues of psychological health among CW. As mentioned previously, some data suggest that baseline levels of psychological distress for entry-level employees are much lower than that of senior workers (Frost et al., 2020). This finding, while in need of replication, suggests that the ecology of correctional work has the capacity to influence the psychological health of

Table 1 Prevention, treatment seeking, and intervention

Levels of prevention and treatment	Definition	Examples[a]
Universal	Prevention effort to reach the entire CW population	Annual training events to review the benefits and costs to psychological health of correctional setting work for CW; review of when to get help; review of how to get help "Lunch room" flyers; brown bag lunches Introduction to techniques/academy type session
Selective	Prevention and treatment efforts to reach a subgroup of CW at potentially greater risk of developing problems with psychological health	Pre-brief; post-brief for those assigned to isolated posts (tower duty) Pre-brief; post brief for those assigned to units with violent populations (restricted housing units) Additional identification of resources, services, peer-support for groups of individuals as risk for relapse – including correctional workers in recovery from alcohol and substance use disorders; those who experienced trauma in a previous role; those who may have served as an active-duty service member; those nearing retirement
Indicated	Prevention and treatment efforts to reach CW who experienced psychologically distressing incidents; or who are involved in disciplinary actions; who were involved in critical incident response	Recommendations for psychological first-aid (PFA); employee assistance program (EAP) services after witnessing suicide of staff to inmates; homicide of staff or inmate; other acts of violence and/or natural disasters

[a]Note: Examples are provided as broad and general guidelines for systems, human resource professionals, and service providers including chaplains and psychologists. They may be used to guide strategy and policy in the creation and maintenance of a psychologically heathy correctional workforce

workers. Moreover, it is a strong indicator of a need for more universal and proactive approaches to intervention and treatment.

Selective Approach

Moving from prevention to intervention, selective approaches focus on entire subgroups of individuals with a potentially higher risk of clinical disorder, such as those who have endured STS or have responded to critical incidences. With this strategy, individual personal risk is not assessed; instead, this approach is based on their membership to a specific group that has been recognized as high risk (Institute of Medicine, 1994). In the correctional context, this could include CW serving in environments with violent populations, such as restricted housing. Strategies for intervention at this level may include pre- and post-briefing for individuals working in higher risk environments, peer support for individuals at risk of relapse, and identifying additional resources for CW who have experienced trauma in previous roles. Borrowing from Sprang et al. (2018), this approach would also include motivational interviewing and cognitive therapy directed at particular STS symptoms experienced by service providers.

Indicated Approach

The third and final approach, indicated, is designed to prevent the onset of disorders among those with problematic behaviors or who are already experiencing psychological distress (Institute of Medicine, 1994). Programs at this level address individual risk factors, and approaches should be utilized and applied in contexts where correctional workers have experienced direct or indirect trauma, provide indications of early clinical disorder, or are involved in disciplinary action. An example of this approach would include employee assistance programs for CW prior to witnessing staff or inmate suicides, homicides, or natural disasters.

While the selective and indicated approaches provide important secondary prevention and intervention, the Institute of Medicine (2012) has recognized that emphasizing population-level and nonclinical strategies is necessary for better health outcomes. Correspondingly, Sprang et al. (2018) emphasized the value of a universal approach for several reasons, including its potential to influence organizational culture and ultimately decrease the risk of symptoms related to STS. Ultimately, the underlying goal of prevention and intervention strategies is to reduce the onset and severity of symptoms related to clinical disorder while improving individuals' psychological health.

Conclusion

The majority of research to date has focused on more salient categories of first responders, such as paramedics and police officers, often overlooking the population of individuals within corrections who are tasked with patrolling the border between public safety and health. However, CW are not immune to the psychological risks inherently involved in public safety work. In fact, they are exposed to occupational and psychological hazards at an unprecedented rate. They are frequently the target of violence while also bearing witness to both direct and indirect trauma. Despite the risks of violence and psychological distress, CW must maintain their ability to respond effectively to critical incidences, mitigate violence, and offer support to those who are involved with the criminal justice system.

While occupational roles within corrections may be qualitatively different, the overall correctional environment creates a leveled playing field, regardless of title, that results in equal impact for all staff. In this chapter, we have suggested that the ecology of correctional work, in large part, creates the stimulus for clinically relevant phenomena and disorders. We have also argued that these stimuli are not unique to CO and that they apply to the broader context of CW, and this points the way forward for future research in this arena.

As has been illustrated thus far, and for a variety of compelling reasons, there is a great need for research to more extensively evaluate the diverse service needs of CW. Taking a socioecological perspective to correctional work, scholars will be better positioned to develop a more comprehensive understanding of how to support the psychological health of those engaged in correctional work. More recently, researchers in Canada have attempted to capture the interconnected and interdependent nature of correctional work and its influence on first responders in various roles beyond CO (Carelton et al., 2018, 2021; Ricciardelli et al., 2021a, b). These efforts mark the start of a growing body of research that may have powerful implications for the overall psychological health and well-being of all correctional works. In addition, it may point the way for more nuanced CW sub-typing beyond occupational roles such as those who are transitioning into law enforcement/correctional work from active-duty service in the military, or individuals who are in recovery from alcohol and substance abuse.

Future research will also benefit from higher degrees of rigor than has been commonly observed. For instance, studies must explicitly use gold standard, clinical interviews (semi-structured, qualitative interviews across groups) when examining clinical disorders, be stringent in operationalizing nonclinical disorders such as STS and compassion fatigue, and employ random assignment of CW (i.e., those who participate in survey research via emails may be more motivated to participate due to personal views). Finally, it is imperative to examine psychological distress and service needs across the developmental career spectrum for CW. This calls for a necessary focus on the unique and distinctive stressors along the trajectory of early-mid-, and late-career, as well as retired CW.

References

Bick, J. A. (2007). Infection control in jails and prisons. *Clinical Infectious Diseases, 45*(8), 1047–1055. https://doi.org/10.1086/521910

Boudoukha, A. H., Altintas, E., Rusinek, S., Fantini-Hauwel, C., & Hautekeete, M. (2013). Inmates-to-staff assaults, PTSD, and burnout: Profiles of risk and vulnerability. *Journal of Interpersonal Violence, 28*(11), 2332–2350. https://doi.org/10.1177/0886260512475314

Bureau of Justice Statistics [BJS]. (2008). *Census of State and Federal Correctional Facilities, 2005* (Appendix table 12. All employees and correctional officers in correctional facilities). http://bjs.ojp.usdoj.gov/content/pub/pdf/csfcf05.Pdf

Bureau of Labor Statistics. (2017). *Occupational employment and wages, May 2016: 33-3012 Correctional officers and jailers.* Retrieved from https://www.bls.gov/oes/current/oes333012.htm

Carelton, R. N., Afifi, T. O., Turner, S., Taillieu, T., Duranceau, S., LeBouthillier, D. M., Sareen, J., Ricciardelli, R., MacPhee, R. S., Groll, R., Hozempa, K., Brunet, A., Weekes, J. R., Griffiths, C. T., Abrams, K. J., Jones, N. A., Beshai, S., Cramm, H. A., Dobson, K. S., Hatcher, S., Keane, T. M., Stewart, S. H., & Asmundson, G. J. G. (2018). Mental disorder symptoms among public safety personnel in Canada. *The Canadian Journal of Psychiatry, 63*(1), 56–64. https://doi.org/10.1177/0706743717723825

Carelton, R. N., Ricciardelii, R., Taillieu, T., Stelnicki, A. M., Groll, D., & Afifi, T. O. (2021). Provincial correctional workers: Suicidal ideation, plans, and attempts. *Canadian Psychological Association., 63*, 366. https://doi.org/10.1037/cap0000292

Cassidy, T., & Bruce, S. (2019). Dealing with Death in Custody: Psychosocial Consequences for Correctional Staff. *Journal of Correctional Health Care, 25*(4), 304–312. https://doi.org/10.1177/1078345819879752

Chae, M. H., & Boyle, D. J. (2013). Police suicide: Prevalence, risk, and protective factors. *Policing: An International Journal of Police Strategies & Management, 36*(1), 91–118. https://doi.org/10.1108/13639511311302498

Cieslak, R., Shoji, K., Douglas, A., Melville, E., Luszczynska, A., & Benight, C. C. (2014). A meta-analysis of the relationship between job burnout and secondary traumatic stress among workers with indirect exposure to trauma. *Psychological Services, 11*(1), 75–86. https://doi.org/10.1037/a0033798

Elliot, D., Kuehl, K., El Ghaziri, M., & Chemiack, M. (2015). Stress and correction: addressing the safety and well being of correctional officers. *Corrections Today, 77*, 40–44.

Evers, T. J., Ogloff, J. R. P., Trounson, J. S., & Pfeifer, J. E. (2020). Well-being interventions for correctional officers in a prison setting: A review and meta-analysis. *Criminal Justice and Behaviour, 47*(1), 3–21. https://doi.org/10.1177/0093854819869975

Ferdik, F. V., & Smith, H. P. (2017). *Correctional officer safety and wellness literature synthesis.* National Institute of Justice.

Finn, P. (2000). *Addressing correctional officer stress: Programs and strategies.* National Institute of Justice. Retrieved from https://www.ojp.gov/pdffiles1/nij/183474.pdf

Frost, N. A., Monteiro, C. E., Stowell, J. I., Trapassi, J., & St. Louis, S. (2020). *The impact of correctional officer suicide on the institutional environment and on the well-being of correctional employees.* National Institute of Justice. Retrieved from https://nij.ojp.gov/library/publications/impact-correction-officer-suicide-institutional-environment-and-wellbeing

Fusco, N., Ricciardelli, R., Jamshidi, L., Carelton, R. N., Barnim, N., Hilton, Z., & Groll, D. (2021). When our work hits home: Trauma and mental disorders in correctional officers and other correctional workers. *Frontiers in Psychiatry, 11*(2), 1–10. https://doi.org/10.3389/fpsyt.2020.493391

Handran, J. (2015). Trauma-informed systems of care: The role of organizational culture in the development of burnout, secondary traumatic stress, and compassion satisfaction. *Journal of Social Welfare and Human Rights, 3*(2), 1–22. https://doi.org/10.15640/10.15640/jswhr.v3n2a1

Horman, S., & Vivian, P. (2005). Toward an understanding of traumatized organizations and how to intervene in them. *Traumatology, 11*(3), 159–169. https://doi.org/10.1177/153476560501100302

Institute of Medicine. (1994). *Reducing risk for mental disorders: Frontiers for prevention intervention research.* National Academy Press.

Institute of Medicine. (2012). *An integrated framework for assessing the value of community-based prevention.* The National Academies Press.

Jaegers, L. A., Matthieu, M. M., Werth, P., Ahmad, S. O., Barnidge, E., & Vaughn, M. G. (2019). Stressed out: Predictors of depression among jail officers and deputies. *The Prison Journal, 100*(2), 240–261. https://doi.org/10.1177/0032885519894658

Johnston, M. S., Ricciardelli, R., & McKendy, L. (2022). Improving the mental health of correctional workers: Perspectives from the field. *Criminal Justice and Behavior*, 1–20. https://doi.org/10.1177/00938548221081468

Kessler, R., White, L. A., Birnbaum, H., Qiu, Y., Kidolezi, Y., Mallet, D., & Swindle, R. (2008). Comparative and interactive effects of depression relative to other health problems on work performance in the workforce of a larger employer. *Journal of Occupational and Environmental Medicine, 50*, 809–816. https://doi.org/10.1097/jom.0b013e318169ccba

Kim, J., Chesworth, B., Franchino-Olsen, H., & Macy, R. J. (2021). A scoping review of vicarious trauma interventions for service providers working with people who have experienced traumatic events. *Trauma, Violence, & Abuse*, 1–24. https://doi.org/10.1177/1524838021991310

Konda, S., Reichard, A., & Tiesman, H. (2012). Occupational injuries among U.S. correctional officers, 1999-2008. Journal of Safety Research, 43(3), Lambert, E. G., & Hogan, N. L. (2018). Correctional staff: The issue of job stress. In M. Ternes, P. R. Magaletta, & M. W. Patry (Eds.), *The practice of correctional psychology* (pp. 259–281). Springer Nature Switzerland AG). https://doi.org/10.1007/978-3-030-00452-1_12

Konda, S., Tiesman, H., Reichard, A., & Hartley, D. (2013). U.S. corrections officers killed or injured on the job. *Corrections Today, 75*(5), 122–123.

Lambert, E. G., & Hogan, N. L. (2018). Correctional staff: The issue of job stress. In M. Ternes, P. Magaletta, & M. Patry (Eds.), *The practice of correctional psychology*. Springer. https://doi.org/10.1007/978-3-030-00452-1_2

Lambert, E. G., Hogan, N. L., Griffin, M. L., & Kelley, T. (2015). The correctional burnout literature. *Criminal Justice Studies, 28*(4), 397–443. https://doi.org/10.1080/1478601X.2015.1065830

Lerman, A., Harney, J., & Sadin, M. (2022). Prisons and mental health: Violence, organizational support, and the effects of correctional work. *Criminal Justice and Behavior, 49*(2), 181–199. https://doi.org/10.1177/00938548211037718

Lewis, K. R., Lewis, L. S., & Garby, T. M. (2013). Surviving the trenches: The personal impact of the job on probation officers. *American Journal of Criminal Justice, 38*, 67–84. https://doi.org/10.1007/s12103-012-9165-3

Liu, L., Hu, S., Wang, L., Sui, G., & Ma, L. (2013). Positive resources for combating depressive symptoms among Chinese male correctional officers: Perceived organizational support and psychological capital. *BMX Psychiatry, 13*(1), 89. https://doi.org/10.1186/1471-244XX-13-89

Maslach, C., & Jackson, S. (1981). The measurement of experienced burnout. *Journal of Organizational Behavior, 2*(2), 99–113. https://doi.org/10.1002/job.4030020205

New Jersey Police Suicide Task Force. (2009). *New Jersey police suicide task force report*. New Jersey Police Suicide Task Force. Retrieved from https://www.nj.gov/oag/library/NJPoliceSuicideTaskForceReport-January-30-2009-Final(r2.3.09).pdf

Regehr, C., Carey, S., Wagner, S., Alden, L. E., Buys, N., Corneil, W., Fyfe, T., Fraess-Phillips, A., Krutop, E., Matthews, L., Randall, C., White, M., & White, N. (2021). Prevalence of PTSD, depression and anxiety disorders in correctional officers: A systematic review. *Corrections, 6*(3), 229–241. https://doi.org/10.1080/23774657.2019.1641765

Rhineberger-Dunn, G., Mack, K. Y., & Baker, K. M. (2016). Secondary trauma among community corrections staff: An exploratory study. *Journal of Offender Rehabilitation, 55*(5), 293–307. https://doi.org/10.1080/10509674.2016.1181132

Ricciardelli, R., Mitchell, M., Taillieu, T., Angehrn, A., Afifi, T., & Carelton, R. (2021a). Pervasive uncertainty under threat: Mental health disorders and experiences of uncertainty for correctional workers. *Criminal Justice and Behavior*, 1–19. https://doi.org/10.1177/00938548211050112

Ricciardelli, R., Haynes, S. H., Burdette, A., Keena, L., McCreary, D. R., Carelton, R. N., Lambert, E. G., & Groll, D. (2021b). Mental health, stigma, gender, and seeking treatment: Interpretations and experiences of prison employees. *Applied Psychology in Criminal Justice, 16*(1), 108–127.

Sprang, G., Ford, J., Kerig, P., & Bride, B. (2018). Defining secondary traumatic stress and developing targeted assessments and interventions: Lessons learned from research and leading experts. *Traumatology, 25*(2), 72–81. https://doi.org/10.1037/trm0000180

Sprang, G., Lei, F., & Bush, H. (2021). Can organizational efforts lead to less secondary traumatic stress? A longitudinal investigation of change. *American Journal of Orthopsychiatry, 91*(4), 443–453. https://doi.org/10.1037/ort0000546

Wills, C., Bates, K., Frost, N., & Monteiro, C. E. (2021). Barriers to help-seeking among correction officers: Examining the influence and institutional culture and structure. *Criminal Justice Studies, 34*(4), 423–440. https://doi.org/10.1080/1478601X.2021.1997276

Crime Scene Investigators

Brittany A. Plombon, Teresa Bryant, and Caroline M. Haskamp

Crime scene investigators (CSIs) are an integral part of law enforcement and research suggests that law enforcement work is among the most stressful occupations in the world, impacting officers by a variety of physiological and psychological symptoms and problems (Kelty & Gordon, 2015; Marshall, 2006; McCraty & Atkinson, 2012; Sollie et al., 2017; Vivona, 2013). Across the world, tragedies happen every day that threaten people, property, and society. Therefore, one is reliant on first responders to restore safety and security within the community. The crime scene is one of the most crucial aspects of an investigation conducted by law enforcement. The personnel who are responsible for examining, evaluating, documenting, collecting, and processing evidence at crime scenes for forensic analysis are known as CSIs (International Crime Scene Investigators Association, n.d.). A CSI is defined as an individual whose job is to process crime scenes (Dutelle, 2020). However, the term also refers to any personnel who may refer to themselves as an "evidence technician," "criminalistics officer," "crime scene technician," "scenes of crimes officer," "crime scene examiner," and "forensic investigator" (International Crime, n.d.). This varying terminology represents the diverse work within law enforcement agencies and CSIs internationally. Crime scene processing is the act of processing the crime scene in the field, which includes examining, photographing, sketching, and using field techniques to identify, evaluate, document, process, and collect physical, testimonial, and fingerprint evidence.

Previous research suggests that first responders, such as police officers, firefighters, and emergency medical personnel, often experience stress. However, there is a modicum of literature on the unique stressors surrounding CSIs' mental health.

B. A. Plombon (✉) · C. M. Haskamp
College of Psychology, Nova Southeastern University, Fort Lauderdale, FL, USA
e-mail: bp789@mynsu.nova.edu; ch1894@mynsu.nova.edu

T. Bryant
Forensic Psychology, Walden University, Minneapolis, MN, USA

M. L. Bourke et al. (eds.), *First Responder Mental Health*,
https://doi.org/10.1007/978-3-031-38149-2_4

Flannery (2015) proposed several reasons why first responders, in general, have received less attention: (a) media are not focused on the needs of first responders; (b) first responders are action-oriented and self-contained; complaining is unacceptable behavior, and seeking mental health counseling is typically not considered; (c) the reality of the work leaves limited time for processing one critical incident before a second call for assistance at the next is received; (d) distress is often self-medicated through substance abuse, the basic trauma remaining unaddressed; and (e) fewer resources are allocated toward addressing their treatment needs. Recently, there has been an increase in research on CSIs due to a global initiative from countries (e.g., Australia, Israel, Korea, Norway, Netherlands, Slovenia, the United Kingdom, the United States) to further recognize, assess, and identify coping strategies because of the effects of stress and trauma on CSIs.

First responders rarely experience a single traumatic event (whether directly or indirectly) but rather a series of incidents that have accumulated over the course of their career (Marshall, 2006). CSIs do not typically experience the speed and intensity of emergency work as other first responders. Yet, they experience work-related incidents that involve the same types of violence, trauma, and personal tragedy (Roth & Vivona, 2010). CSIs are the closest to the crime scene and must occupy the scene longer than responding police officers (Leone & Keel, 2016). CSIs also encounter death at higher rates than most people, including exposure to bloody scenes, decomposing bodies, mangled corpses, and autopsies (Henry, 2004; Pavšič Mrevlje, 2016; Roth & Vivona, 2010). According to Kelty and Gordon (2015), CSIs encounter violent scenes of death with the requirement to examine, smell, and touch bodies, body parts, and fluids. Research further indicates first responders operating under intense stress are at an increased risk of producing errors, accidents, and overreactions that can compromise their performance, endanger public safety, and pose substantial liability costs to the organization (McCraty & Atkinson, 2012). Stress and trauma may manifest itself differently and vary in forms of maladaptive behaviors or symptoms, which have the potential to become dangerous if unaddressed.

Types of Crime Scene Investigators

As of 2019, 30.5% of the nation's full-time law enforcement employees were civilians (US Department of Justice, 2020). CSIs comprise a very small percentage of the overall population of law enforcement personnel in the United States (Roth & Vivona, 2010). The organizational placement and recognition of CSIs varies within police agencies. Whereas some CSIs are academy trained and certified sworn law enforcement officers, in other agencies, CSIs may be non-sworn, civilian trained personnel (Leone & Keel, 2016). The term sworn law enforcement officer refers to personnel who have completed a police academy course of instruction, are certified to enforce laws, have arrest powers, and are licensed to carry a firearm (Anderson et al., 2002; Sewell, 1994). CSIs are usually civilian employees who respond to death investigations and collect evidence. Boyd et al. (2003) found significant differences between sworn and non-sworn personnel in their levels of stress, specifically in the areas of job satisfaction and morale. Non-sworn personnel are not trained police officers; therefore, they do not have the same training and support in place to deal with law enforcement-related stressors (Adderley et al., 2012). Research on CSIs may be sparse due to the consideration of CSIs as civilians and not as first responders.

Duties and Procedures for Search Operations

CSIs need to always be available to respond to incidents as their workload is dependent on requests from law enforcement agencies who determine whether or not CSIs are needed at the scene. A forensic team leader designates specific CSIs and briefs them upon arrival to the crime scene. The amount of information known prior to arrival is varied. However, information concerning the location (public or private), scene (indoor or outdoor), safety (e.g., drugs, violence, other substances), and tactical information are important (van den Eeden et al., 2017). Like other first-responder groups, CSIs often work in shifts (day, night, on call). Depending on an agency's schedule, CSIs have considerable exposure to critical incidents and attend scenes of accidental or natural deaths, fatal traffic crashes, suicides, murders, thefts, burglaries, assaults, arsons, shootings, drug factories, armed robberies, sexual assaults, and explosions (Fowler, 2006; Roth & Vivona, 2010).

CSIs have a profound duty and responsibility to ascertain truth and to bring to justice those who commit criminal offenses (Roth & Vivona, 2010). Julian et al. (2012) provided guidelines on how to process a crime scene effectively: (a) maintain the integrity of the crime scene and a consistent chain of evidence and (b) ensure the integrity of any physical and/or scientific evidence that is gathered. Before a piece of evidence is collected, it must be documented in the CSI's notes, measured and sketched, and logged in each of the crime scene logs (crime scene photography, evidence log, etc.) before recovery is attempted (Blozis, 2010). After completion of the investigation, administrative work includes writing an official report, processing forensic samples, carrying out further tests, and adding the results of these tests to the forensic files (Sollie et al., 2017). CSIs spend a significant amount of time on administrative duties while spending only 20% of their time at the crime scene (Sollie et al., 2017).

Review of the Literature

Stress

Workplace stress has been associated with law enforcement departments after exposure to stressful or traumatic events. CSIs encounter a variety of stressors, most of which are unique to their profession. These can affect a CSI's mental health and leave them at an increased risk for experiencing elevated levels of stress. Kelty and Gordon (2015) defined stress as, "a response that occurs when an individual perceives a situation as having a personal impact, and where the demands of that situation exceed the individual's coping resource repertoire" (p. 273). Law enforcement has not always required or offered mental health services to personnel who are exposed to stressful or traumatic events, and often the most neglected personnel are CSIs (Leone & Keel, 2016). Identified sources of stress include occupational, organizational, and personal stressors with an accumulation of increased working demands. The cumulation of these identified stressors may undermine the CSI's physical, mental, and emotional health over their careers while jeopardizing their work performance and personal life (Marshall, 2006; Yoo et al., 2013). Increased levels of stress deplete the physical and psychological resources needed when exposed to traumatic events; therefore, individuals become more vulnerable to stressors when they are fatigued (Yoo et al., 2013). The levels of stress-related symptoms reported by CSIs are significantly greater than one would expect to find in the general population (Van Patten & Burke, 2001). Stress often manifests itself through a variety of symptoms, which are found to have an increased effect on workplace-related accidents, absenteeism, substance abuse, and early retirement in CSIs (Kelty & Gordon, 2015).

Occupational Stress

CSIs are a unique profession embedded within law enforcement agencies. Therefore, they experience different stressors related to their job that entails unpredictable circumstances. Occupational stress is both constant and interactive for CSIs, where individual factors can serve to exacerbate the effect of workplace stress (Leone & Keel, 2016). Research has identified a sizable number of occupational stressors specific to CSIs including extended and irregular work hours, diverse locations, poor weather conditions, exposure to human suffering, decision-making, dirty and physically demanding circumstances at the crime scene (Sollie et al., 2017) and dealing with emotionally distressed crime victims, working alone, and vandalization of their vehicles (Adderley et al., 2012). CSIs encounter a variety of difficult and challenging circumstances. The working conditions of a crime scene can be extremely unpleasant, with physical disgust and stench of decomposing corpses, contact with bodily fluids, dismembered body parts, attending autopsies, digging through garbage dumpsters, and removing bodies burned beyond recognition from fire scenes (Sollie et al., 2017). CSIs are required to be readily available when working on-call shifts. Sollie et al. (2017) noted sleep deprivation, poor quality of sleep, fatigue, irritability, and impaired concentration impact CSIs' stress levels and have a negative effect on their work quality. CSIs who are on-call reported higher levels of stress than those who engaged in routine work (Clark et al., 2015). Crime scenes are often associated with tragedy and death, which may inflict emotional connectedness: empathizing with and imagining what the families of the bereaved are experiencing (Kelty & Gordon, 2015; Vivona, 2014).

Organizational Stress

CSIs report several organizational stressors which have profound effects on their stress levels. Specifically, they identify long work hours, heavy workload, job insecurity, conflicts with coworkers, exposure to highly charged and/or emotional incidents, discrimination and workplace bullying, staff shortages resulting in additional shifts, and canceling rostered days off as organizational stressors (Kelty & Gordon, 2015; Leone & Keel, 2016). These were often intensified in situations of large, popularized crimes due to administrative pressures to solve them, inequities in the workplace, and conflicts over due process (Clark et al., 2015). Shift work and staff shortages have been identified by researchers as the greatest causes of stress due to budget cuts and salary issues (Leone & Keel, 2016) that impact staff morale, the ability to effectively manage unexpected increases in the number of crime scenes, and changes in work procedures (Kelty & Gordon, 2015).

The unpredictability of the day-to-day aspects of the job can be particularly stressful when CSIs are called out to new crime scenes and the administrative work associated with the previous scene is not yet completed (Sollie et al., 2017). Administrative duties and colleagues continue to play a factor in CSI's stress levels. Some CSIs have referred to colleagues as a source of more stress than the actual work at the crime scene due to their inability to reflect critically on their actions, their drawing of erroneous conclusions, their mishandling of crime scene procedures and evidence, their overlooking of safety regulations, and their inability to be open to feedback (Sollie et al., 2017). An ongoing challenge for CSIs is the lack of recognition, availability of resources, and outlets for stress relief. Clark et al. (2015) found that only 36% of CSIs reported that their department appreciated their work; in addition, 37% felt that they could talk to their fellow officers about any troubles they might be having; and 30% felt they could talk to a supervisor about problems with their work. Disregard from administrative officials has impacted CSIs' mental health and stress levels as shown by their lack of support and limited availability of services.

Sewell (1993) identified several pressures unique to law enforcement, including the administrative challenge to rapidly solve crimes while continuing to carry out daily routine tasks. Clark et al. (2015) found 52% of 51 CSIs reported unmanageable amounts of work, and 50% felt that making even one mistake in processing the crime scene may result in losing the case. The constant pressure of perfection is reflected in CSIs' concern that colleagues may not have sufficient skills to carry out a high standard of quality work. CSIs experience intense pressure to produce physical evidence that will assist in the identification and conviction of offenders (Roth & Vivona, 2010). Julian et al. (2012) recognized that CSIs undergo high levels of pressure when processing a crime scene and handling evidence due to possible errors resulting in wrongful criminal indictments, as well as additional pressures from multiple agencies to provide supportive evidence. Crime scenes often involve different law enforcement agencies at a scene which may serve as additional sources of stress due to conflicting interests during the investigation (Sollie et al., 2017).

Personal Stress

The personal life of a CSI is frequently disrupted due to the strenuous demands from their job. The nature of the job can often lead to both work-related and personal stress, with work stress often eclipsing personal stress (Clark et al., 2015). In particular, the disruption of on-call shifts can affect a CSI's relationship with partners, children, relatives, and friends (Sollie et al., 2017). Shift work was identified as one of the primary sources of stress for CSIs that diminished their ability to make plans or keep appointments (Kelty & Gordon, 2015). Indeed, 56% of CSIs felt their work decreased the amount of time spent with family members, 42% indicated their work disrupted the quality of family life, and 38% reported they were unable to discuss what they did with their loved ones (Clark et al., 2015).

Issues at the Crime Scene

A crime scene presents an unknown and unpredictable set of circumstances. CSIs are often confronted with human vulnerability and the consequences of human suffering, concerning the circumstances of death (Sollie et al., 2017). When CSIs encounter a deceased person, there are four possibilities of the cause of death: (a) a natural death, (b) an accident, (c) a suicide, or (d) a crime (Sollie et al., 2017). Sollie et al. (2017) distinguished five main triggers of stress for CSIs when confronting human suffering at a crime scene: (a) the type of victim, (b) the way in which the crime was committed, (c) identifying with the victim, (d) the circumstances of the death, and (e) contact with bereaved relatives. Leone and Keel (2016) contend that the most stressful experience for a CSI is investigating the death of an officer followed by mass fatalities, while the least stressful circumstances consisted of weather-related conditions and intimate partner violence. Similarly, Kelty and Gordon (2015) found CSIs identified the presence of a victim's relatives or friends at the crime scene as one of the most significant sources of stress in their work. Vivona (2014) noted that each CSI mentioned child victimization as the most troubling crime scene to work. CSIs may become bewildered and angered by the forms of violence endured by victims, especially those who were considered defenseless or innocent (Sollie et al., 2017). This type of exposure can elicit feelings of confusion, helplessness, and unfairness. It is not uncommon for a CSI to identify with the victim of a crime scene, such as someone in their community (e.g., a family member, friend, acquaintance, or neighbor). CSIs may be exposed to the emotional pain and suffering of the victim's bereaved family members or friends, inflicting different emotional reactions (Sollie et al., 2017). Leone and Keel (2016) indicated that repeated exposures to stressful events tended to diminish the subjective stress associated with the crime scene and thus create desensitization.

Acute Stress Disorder

The *Diagnostic and Statistical Manual of Mental Disorders*, 5th edition Text Revision (DSM-5-TR; American Psychiatric Association [APA], 2022), defines acute stress disorder as:

> Exposure to actual or threatened death, serious injury, or sexual violation in one (or more) of the following ways: (1) directly experiencing the traumatic event(s); (2) witnessing, in person, the event(s) as it occurred to others; (3) learning that the event(s) occurred to a close family member or close friend, in cases of actual or threatened death of a family member or friend; (4) experiencing repeated or extreme exposure to aversive details of the traumatic event(s) (e.g., first responders collecting human remains; police offices repeatedly exposed to details of child abuse). (p. 271)

Other characteristics of acute stress disorder include intrusion symptoms, negative mood, dissociative symptoms, avoidance symptoms, and arousal symptoms (APA, 2022). The duration of symptoms of acute stress disorder ranges from 3 days to 1 month following the traumatic event(s). Stressors occur soon after the traumatic event has occurred. Acute stress disorder commonly manifests in catastrophic or extremely negative thoughts about the individual's role in the traumatic event, their response to the traumatic experiences, or the likelihood of future harm (APA, 2022).

Extant research has closely identified acute stress disorder and posttraumatic stress as similar conditions. Posttraumatic stress is caused by extreme stress from experiencing traumatic accidents and fatalities, which is a considerable threat to one's mental health (Yoo et al., 2013). Posttraumatic stress can be a common and adaptive response to experiencing a traumatic event that eventually subsides. The prevalence of acute stress disorder varies according to the nature and context of the event, and research has found higher rates occurring in cases involving interpersonal trauma (APA, 2022). The experience of acute stress is inherent in police work when there is an inability to effectively cope with stressful events which can result in adverse psychological and physiological symptoms, chronic stress, burnout, and attrition (Anshel, 2000).

Clark et al. (2015) found 63% of CSIs reported experiencing a moderate or high level of posttraumatic stress symptoms following a crime scene investigation. Further, they observed that 43% of CSIs experienced fatigue because of their job, 27% felt tense and "uptight" at work, and 78% reported at least one physical symptom (e.g., headache, loss of appetite, upset stomach, fatigue, shortness of breath). Research also reveals that most CSIs experience acute stress and symptoms of posttraumatic stress following a crime scene with increased levels of associated violence and morbidity. Most notably, the symptoms of stress were significantly greater for those involved with crime scenes reminding them of loved ones compared to incidents of aggravated robbery, felony assault, and arson (Clark et al., 2015). Yoo et al. (2013) found that CSIs who experienced three to four homicides a week had the highest levels of posttraumatic stress; CSIs who experienced one to two homicides a week appeared to accept the traumatic event(s) rationally; and CSIs who experienced five or more homicides a week seemed to be desensitized to the stress due to frequent exposure. Posttraumatic stress scores were positively correlated with personality type, fatigue from work, and death related anxiety and negatively correlated with career length and emotional intelligence (Yoo et al., 2013).

Posttraumatic Stress Disorder

The *Diagnostic and Statistical Manual of Mental Disorders, 5th edition Text Revision* (APA, 2022), defines posttraumatic stress disorder (PTSD) as:

> Exposure to actual or threatened death, serious injury, or sexual violence, in one (or more) of the following ways: (1) directly experiencing the traumatic event(s); (2) witnessing, in person, the event(s) as it occurred to others; (3) learning that the traumatic event(s) occurred to a close family member or close friend; (4) experiencing repeated or extreme exposure to aversive details of the traumatic event(s) (e.g., first responders collecting human remains; police offices repeatedly exposed to details of child abuse). (p. 271)

Additional symptoms of PTSD may include recurrent and distressing memories, dreams, and dissociative symptoms, persistent avoidance of stimuli, negative cognitions and mood, and marked changes in arousal and reactivity (APA, 2022). The duration of symptoms must exceed 1 month from the traumatic event(s). PTSD may manifest itself as an acute, chronic, or delayed response to the traumatic event (Van Patten & Burke, 2001). PTSD often involves substantial functional impairment and is frequently comorbid with other mental health conditions such as depression, generalized anxiety disorder, and substance use.

The *DSM-5-TR* criteria for PTSD include first responders who are involved in criminal investigations and the collection of human remains. The impact of these traumatic risk factors and repeated exposures may evolve into PTSD or other mental health-related conditions, causing severe emotional distress and feelings of sadness, anger, depression, and devastation (Yoo et al., 2013). There are substantial variations in individual responses to traumatic events. Carlson and Dalenberg (2000) proposed factors that influence an individual's response to trauma to include biological variables, developmental level, severity of the stressor, social context, and prior exposure to trauma. Evans et al. (2013) found that incidents causing the most distress for police officers were those that had personal relevance, which heightened their perceptions of their self-and/or their loved ones. In another study, CSIs reported that their most traumatic crime scene included a case that was at least 1 year old (67%) and included the death of an adult (60%) and/or death of a minor (45%) (Pavšič Mrevlje, 2018). Mitchell and Hogg (1997) found that CSIs only reported being affected when they allowed themselves to become too emotionally involved with the crime scene.

Collective research suggests the investigation of crime scenes may evoke varying levels of traumatic stress in CSIs. Pavšič Mrevlje (2018) estimated an average workload in Slovenia of 97 cases a year. It is important to consider the different criminal laws, crime rates, populations, regions, and types of crime scenes investigated in various countries before generalizing internationally. PTSD symptoms were found in 17% of CSIs with an additional 12% of CSIs indicating elevated PTSD symptomology (Pavšič Mrevlje, 2018). A similar study conducted by Sollie et al. (2017) found 13% of CSIs had been diagnosed with PTSD symptomology due to crime scene investigations. In the United States, the projected lifetime risk for PTSD using the *DSM-V* criteria by age 75 is 8.7% (APA, 2013). Another study has shown that 5.9 to 22% of first responders who respond to crime scenes may develop PTSD, evoking stress and trauma that impacts their mental health (Flannery, 2015). The aforementioned research conducted on CSIs is consistent with the suggested statistics concerning other first responder groups (i.e., police officers, firefighters, detention deputies, and dispatchers) who are diagnosed with PTSD. However, these studies only suggest that CSIs are characterized by PTSD symptomology and do not necessarily meet the full PTSD criteria. Posttraumatic symptomology may appear suddenly, intensely, and persistently yet will not necessarily meet PTSD criteria (Marshall, 2006). Pavšič Mrevlje (2018) argued that most CSIs do not meet the criteria for PTSD according to the *DSM-V*, and consequently, their problems may go unattended until further, more serious complications develop.

PTSD can give rise to the significant problems associated with vicarious trauma and secondary traumatic stress (STS). First responders often encounter traumatic incidents; therefore, it is not surprising that those who assist with the investigations may become traumatized themselves. The term *secondary traumatic stress* (STS) refers to the emotional consequences of working with traumatized individuals. It was described by Figley (2002) as "a state of tension and preoccupation with traumatized patients by re-experiencing the traumatic events, avoidance/numbing of reminders and persistent arousal associated with the patient" (p. 1435). Bourke and Craun (2014) found that the most common symptoms of STS were (a) thinking about work when not intending to; (b) becoming easily irritated; (c) feeling emotionally numb; and (d) experiencing sleep difficulties. Research on first responders and CSIs support findings that STS impacts psychological functioning and is clearly present in these professions. Perez et al. (2010) found that 18% of police officers experienced moderate levels of STS, and another 18% had high levels of STS. In a study of CSIs, Hyman (2004) found low to medium levels of STS with intrusion being significantly associated with psychological distress and avoidance. Finally, Craun et al. (2014) observed police officers' STS to be stable over time, with little variation between the average scores. Coping tactics that involve social support appeared to be helpful in impacting the immediate effects of STS, while long-term support from supervisors and refraining from denial were identified as having the biggest impact.

Physiological Factors

CSIs are exposed to a variety of stressful and traumatic events which impact their physiological functioning. They are exposed to additional and sometimes greater physical stressors than other first-responder groups which results from exposure to toxins and other residues associated with the crime scene (Jackson et al., 2004). The deleterious physical and psychological effects of stress have been connected through the general adaptation syndrome (Selye, 1936), which consists of the body's stress response stage of alarm, resistance, and exhaustion. In the alarm stage, the onset of stress is immediate and fast-acting. During the resistance stage, the body attempts to resist or adjust to prolonged stress. Over the course of the exhaustion stage, the body's physical resources are depleted, and organ function begins to weaken due to the prolonged effects of the psychological stressors. Not only is the body depleting its resources, other internal systems, such as the immune system, may become weakened, leading to infections or other diseases (Leone & Keel, 2016). Other common effects include heart attacks and strokes due to increased blood pressure which is often accompanied by prolonged stress (Selye, 1936).

Police officers have a reputation for being hardy and capable of coping with challenges. Therefore, it may lead them to neglect signals of work strain, which may result in subjective health complaints (Fyhn et al., 2016). Anderson et al. (2002) conducted a longitudinal study of law enforcement which showed officers had significantly elevated levels of cortisol, body mass, depressive symptoms, cardiovascular disease, and early mortality related to long-term exposure to severe stressful incidents. Research on police officers also reveals that the most frequently reported problems are high blood pressure, divorce, high cholesterol, migraines, chronic back problems, chronic or severe gastrointestinal disturbances, chronic sleep difficulties, increased anxiety, and depression (Bradway, 2009). Investigations of CSIs has shown that those who are repeatedly exposed to traumatic events at a crime scene failed to modify their behaviors in accordance with their changing contextual demands, where they reacted in similar ways to aversive conditions with both high and low intensities, producing a higher resting heart rate suggesting stress reactivity during routine crime scenes (Adderley et al., 2012; Levy-Gigi et al., 2016).

Burnout

Burnout is a chronic form of psychological strain and emotional exhaustion that is increasingly common in professionals who have increased levels of interactions with the public (Maslach & Jackson, 1981). Further, burnout is associated with various self-reported indices of personal distress, including physical exhaustion, insomnia, increased use of alcohol and drugs, and marital and family problems (Maslach & Jackson, 1981). Emotional exhaustion is the core component of burnout and is characteristic of a depletion of energy and empathy that results from an accumulation of stress and inundation of personal and work-related demands (Maslach & Jackson, 1981). Depersonalization, another component of burnout, refers to feelings of detachment, having a decreased interest in one's work, and engaging in negative or cynical attitudes towards the work or others (Maslach & Jackson, 1981).

Due to the nature of CSIs' work, it is reasonable to expect that the cumulative impact of crime scene exposure may lead to harmful psychological effects, such as burnout and fatigue (Hyman, 2004; Kelty & Gordon, 2015; Pavšič Mrevlje, 2016). And, because of the repetitive exposures and disturbances of a crime scene, burnout may pose a safety concern for the CSI. Kelty and Gordon's (2015) found that results of burnout included (a) psychological reactions (anger, anxiety, frustration, job dissatisfaction); (b) physical reactions (dizziness, headache, heart pounding, stomach distress, illnesses); and (c) behavioral reactions (accidents, smoking, substance use, turnover, or absenteeism, lengthened sick leave). Risk factors for burnout may be a result of individual factors (e.g., demographics, education, age, personality), occupational characteristics (e.g., high levels of cynicism, low levels exhaustion), or organizational characteristics (e.g., hierarchies, operating rules) (Maslach et al., 2001).

In some CSI studies, reported attrition rates were 50% over a 3-year period (e.g., Kelty & Gordon, 2015). Fatigue is common in CSIs due to unpredictable callouts and shift work. Yoo et al. (2013) reported that CSIs rated fatigue levels as a 6.6 out of 10, which is considered severe. Sollie et al. (2017) noted that the stress of the job or circumstances in their personal life became too much for a group of CSIs to cope, which lead to 6 of the 30 participants quitting their profession. Alternately, Fyhn et al. (2016) found no significant differences regarding burnout and sickness absence scores. However, CSIs reported significantly higher scores on subjective health complaints, with musculoskeletal pain receiving the highest scores. Occupational stress and job burnout in CSIs also result in high organizational and individual costs from a financial and physiological perspective (Kelty & Gordon, 2015).

Job Satisfaction

Crime scene work environments tend to be undesirable, and CSIs often see the worst of society in terms of violence and its outcomes. Due to the daunting and often gruesome tasks, one may expect CSIs to experience less job satisfaction. Nonetheless, the totality of their work is associated with higher levels of job satisfaction. All CSIs voluntarily apply for the position; however, it can be a difficult decision due to the significant mental and physical strain associated with this work (Sollie et al., 2017). It is impractical, if not impossible, to eliminate the stressful circumstances in crime scene investigations; consequently, stress is an inherent part of the job. Prior research on law enforcement job satisfaction suggests taking a multidimensional approach examining officer demographics, job tasks, and organizational characteristics (Johnson, 2012). Findings on police officers have highlighted their preference for working where they can use their own discretion to best handle difficult situations. However, stress and role conflict were deemed significant contributors to low job satisfaction (Johnson, 2012); and ill-fated relationships, employee disengagement, and administrative estrangement effected turnover (Brunetto et al., 2012). Sollie et al. (2017) supported the findings that working as a CSI is fulfilling. They reported that CSIs evaluated their investigative work experience as an 8.3 out of 10 (10 = feeling fulfilled) and denied motivational problems doing their assigned work-related tasks. Overall, more than 70% of CSIs indicated they would take the same job without hesitation if they had to restart their careers and that they were generally satisfied with their profession (Clark et al., 2015).

Recruitment/Skills

When recruiting personnel for crime scene work, it is imperative to select the right person due to the required repeated exposures to violence and gruesome details (Kelty & Gordon, 2015). Certain characteristics are desirable when working on crime scenes, for example, an individual who can develop positive coping mechanisms, which serve as protection from psychological stress and trauma. Recruitment guidelines have recommended a multistep process including psychometric assessments, written and oral examinations, and medical evaluations (Kelty, 2012). A set of skills that appear to be requisite to effective performance in critical situations for law enforcement in general, and CSIs in particular, appear to be commitment, confidence, arousal control, attention control, imagery, self-talk, and cognitive restructuring (Miller, 2006). Kelty and Gordon (2015) presented seven key attributes that characterize a high-performing CSI: (a) cognitive abilities, i.e., the ability to think on their feet, respond quickly to changing situations, problem-solve; (b) knowledge base, i.e., educational degree, awareness of criminal justice process, legal aspects of evidence collection; (c) life experience, i.e., background as a police officer or other emergency personnel, and maturity; (d) work orientation, i.e., self-motivated learner, good time management, persistence, dedication; (e) resilience and a positive approach to life, i.e., work/life balance, active, support system, self-awareness; (f) communication skills, i.e., active listener; verbal, interpersonal, writing skills; and (g) professional demeanor, i.e., positivity, respectful; leadership qualities.

Kelty (2012) demonstrated the shortcomings of employing poor-performing CSIs who were inept with poor skills or who were less diligent in their roles, thus directly impacting the morale and occupational stress levels of their colleagues. In order to ensure competent processing of crime scenes, departments would benefit from having highly qualified and trained CSIs because (a) attrition rates would decrease through hiring CSIs who are more resilient to stress and (b) employment of CSIs with increased scientific knowledge and the ability to collect higher quality evidence reduces the risk of negatively impacting a case.

Coping and Defense Mechanisms

CSIs are exposed to a wide range of stressful stimuli that affect each person differently. To diminish exposure to potentially stressful and traumatic events, there are three different types of coping: (a) problem-focused, i.e., ability to gather information, problem-solve, and make decisions; (b) emotion-focused, i.e., the ability to regulate emotion through support, distancing, or avoidance; and (c) meaning-focused, i.e., values and beliefs enabling effective strategies (Kelty & Gordon, 2015). Competent CSIs have been characterized by mental hardiness or toughness to perform their duties as a criminal investigator, in which they are able to block out or compartmentalize unpleasant thoughts, emotions, or visualizations (Miller, 2009). A CSI's ability to cope with stress is dependent on their (a) appraisal of the stressful work-related situation; (b) implemented coping strategy; and (c) availability of resources (Sollie et al., 2017). CSIs utilizing less efficacious coping mechanisms (e.g., low social support, lack of exercise, use of alcohol and/or tobacco) were found to have higher levels of secondary traumatic stress over time (Craun et al., 2014).

CSIs with repeated exposure to traumatic events have performed work-related tasks under pressure better than unexposed individuals. However, CSIs who are repeatedly exposed to traumatic events as a part of their job-related tasks fail to modify their behavior in accordance with changing contextual demands (Levy-Gigi et al., 2016). This impaired performance may account for their tendency to be highly alert and use extra caution not only in emergency situations but also in safe environments when such a response is no longer adequate (Levy-Gigi et al., 2016). These findings suggest that repeated traumatic exposure can lead to both positive and negative consequences in a CSI's ability to understand and perform work-related assignments. Few CSIs reported using negative coping strategies, such as excessive drinking (less than 30%) and verbally (8%) or physically (2%) lashing out at others (Clark et al., 2015). A few studies indicate that despite frequent exposure to potentially distressing circumstances at crime scenes, most CSIs accomplish their investigative work without problems (Hyman, 2004; Kelty & Gordon, 2015; Pavšič Mrevlje, 2016).

Mental Resilience

Sollie et al. (2017) defined *mental resilience* as "the outcome of a coping process in which internal and external resources enable a criminal investigator to continue to function during stressful situations and to recover from such situations in sustainable manner, while retaining their motivation to carry out investigative work" (p. 1584). Mental resiliency is an important part of a CSI's work due to the repeated exposure to violence, allowing them to control their emotions in overwhelming circumstances. CSIs cannot predict when or where a criminal investigation is going to occur; however, they can control how they react to the situation. Overall, CSIs have been shown to perform well given the stressful nature of their occupation regarding emotional consistency and stress resilience. In particular, they report greater levels of self-efficacy than police recruits and the general population (Kelty & Gordon, 2015). Mental resiliency allows CSIs to develop a persistent toughness needed to respond and adapt to adverse situations. Mental resiliency in CSIs does not mean that they will demonstrate the same level of resiliency across situations (Sollie et al., 2017). CSIs with diminished mental resiliency appear to be due to (a) self-neglect (e.g., lack of self-reflection, not defending one's own interest, inability to reveal vulnerabilities); (b) poor teamwork (e.g., conflict, disagreement, lack autonomy); (c) organizational shortcomings (e.g., lack of training, resources, or professional support); and (d) life events, which can have a negative impact on their mental health and family (Sollie et al., 2017).

Emotional Distancing

CSIs are frequently exposed to disturbing crime scenes and given the task of collecting, processing, and analyzing evidence. Emotional distancing may be used as a technique to manage thoughts at a crime scene and decrease psychological stress or discomfort. CSIs indicated it is crucial that they prevent themselves from being affected by disturbing or distressing scenes they witness (Sollie et al., 2017). Kelty and Gordon (2015) found that CSIs were more likely than college students to compartmentalize their thoughts from interfering with their work, easily initiate work on tasks, and were more likely to effectively maintain focus on a task until complete. This appears to suggest that CSIs who have exposure to distancing techniques are less distracted and more flexible in their cognitive demeanor. When at a crime scene, CSIs must practice self-control to manage their thoughts in order to focus on their assignments by remaining calm and buffering negative impacts (Sollie et al., 2017). However, this coping strategy is not always sufficient to suppress emotions as CSIs are not always able to maintain an emotional distance from the crime scene.

Visualization

As a form of mental preparation, CSIs have employed visualization as a coping strategy. A sense of uncertainty is pervasive in CSIs prior to arriving at the crime scene; thus, any information received prior to their arrival about the scene is crucial. This information may include what has been found at the scene, the type of victim involved, any actions that have been implemented to enable the CSI to prepare themselves for what they are about to witness, and any stressful tasks they will need to perform. For visualization to be implemented as a coping strategy, CSIs need accurate information prior to arrival, and they must be able to utilize their prior experience at crime scenes. The last component may make visualization a difficult coping mechanism for inexperienced CSIs because they are unable to mentally prepare themselves.

Social Support

Social support is defined as "an exchange of resources between at least two individuals perceived by the provider or the recipient to be intended to enhance the well-being of the recipient" (Shumaker & Brownell, 1984, p. 14). Social support includes friends, family, colleagues, or other people who one can depend on in times of need through sharing emotions. CSIs are not immune to emotional distress, and most have expressed a need to talk to colleagues about their experience and its impact after working a crime scene. Rapport with colleagues is imperative due to the importance of sharing experiences and emotions with those who have worked at the same scene. A supportive relationship among colleagues promotes safe, open, and direct communication without concerns about confidentiality. According to Craun et al. (2014), social support from colleagues was related to lower levels of secondary traumatic stress. Social support factors have been found to be beneficial to CSIs across their professional careers, especially when exposed to particularly traumatic crime scenes (Craun et al., 2014). CSIs also acknowledged the importance of participation in activities and outside interests that were meaningful to them to help manage stress (Kelty & Gordon, 2015). Social support is recognized as an important coping strategy; however, CSIs with a limited social life or support are at risk for job burnout due to the stressful nature of the crime scenes they must process.

Stigma

Law enforcement has long been considered a high-risk profession for mental health concerns, and CSIs are no different based on their repeated trauma exposure. While police departments have dedicated increased time and funding toward the development and implementation of mental health training programs, CSIs' mental health has largely been neglected. First, there is a stigma associated with seeking mental health assistance, and CSIs must find the courage to reveal their own vulnerabilities or weaknesses when asking for help (Sollie et al., 2017). Second, it is not uncommon for CSIs to receive derogatory comments and ridicule from colleagues for seeking assistance (Sollie et al., 2017). Third, CSIs may perceive asking for help as a personal failure because they do not fit the ideal image of a "strong" law enforcement professional (Sollie et al., 2017). CSIs have reported reasons for not seeking support from their supervisors stating the following: (a) talking with a colleague is enough; (b) experiencing significant emotional distance from supervisors; and (c) feeling mistrust caused by previous conflicts or fear of possible negative career consequences (Sollie et al., 2017).

Avoidance

CSIs may experience difficult and distressing work with which they must learn to cope. However, there may come a time when they no longer want to be exposed to certain feelings, thoughts, or tragedies. Therefore, CSIs may avoid certain stimuli as an attempt to escape difficult work situations, both cognitively and physically (Anshel, 2000). The avoidant strategies dominate the other coping styles for CSIs, which is understandable since their profession includes criminal investigations entailing forensic evidence in which they need to perform to the best of their ability without distractions (Pavšič Mrevlje, 2016). Avoidance prevents anxiety from becoming debilitating and allows the CSIs to perform their tasks efficiently (Pavšič Mrevlje, 2016).

According to the cognitive processing model, intrusions are part of the adjustment process to traumatic events, and avoidance is the defense against the intrusions of the traumatic experience (Hyman, 2004). Intrusions are unexpected, recurring memories of experienced trauma. This model further contends that intrusions and avoidance are linked to psychological distress, which has been found to be significantly related to work exposures in CSIs (Hyman, 2004). CSIs may begin to think about themselves or their work environment differently, and these cognitions may lead to negative emotions and diminished work performance.

Considering the work of CSIs, avoidance may be perceived as a positive coping mechanism; however, due to repeated exposures to traumatic events, it is likely to be harmful over time. Avoidance strategies have proven least effective when dealing with traumatic experiences and are related to more physical health problems (Pavšič Mrevlje, 2018).

Humor

Martin (2007) defined *humor* as an "emotional response of mirth in a social context that is elicited by a perception of playful incongruity and is expressed through smiling and laughter" (p. 177). CSIs are exposed to many complexities of death, trauma, and tragedy and experience them in a more intimate manner than most other law enforcement professionals (Vivona, 2013). Investigating death and other heinous crimes is a serious matter, and the average person would be appalled to hear laughter coming from those working a crime scene, noting behaviors in the CSI culture may not be acceptable to onlookers (Roth & Vivona, 2010). Klein (1998) made three observations relevant to humor and CSIs: (a) death itself is not funny, but things that revolve around it may be humorous; (b) those who work with tragedy understand the need for humor; and (c) no matter how serious a situation might be, humor can help get them through the experience. Several studies have identified humor as a beneficial outlet for CSIs in coping with work-related stress (Hyman, 2004; Kelty & Gordon, 2015; Pavšič Mrevlje, 2016; Roth & Vivona, 2010; Vivona, 2013, 2014).

Humor can also provide CSIs with a mental break in times they need to be resilient from emotional distress (Roth & Vivona, 2010). This may allow for CSIs to cognitively shift or restructure their mindset. Indeed, CSIs who engage in humor were found to be more resilient and mentally stable (Vivona, 2014).

Types of Humor Law enforcement officers describe using various types of humor: (a) affiliative jokes, funny stories, and spontaneous banter that may be used to build social cohesion; (b) self-enhancing a humorous outlook on life, amusement by incongruities one faces, and humorous perspective under stress; (c) aggressive humor used to criticize others with sarcasm and ridicule; and (d) self-defeating humor amusing others by saying funny things at their own expense (Martin, 2007). Each type of humor style can be distinguished as beneficial or detrimental, depending on how the jokes are used, the situation, the tasks CSI must perform, and the working conditions (Martin, 2007).

Gallows humor is one of the most misunderstood styles due to its ambiguity and emotionally threatening response (Vivona, 2014). It originates from making fun of people who are in dangerous situations in a satirical way. Conversely, Thorson and Powell (1993) indicate that gallows humor may be described as a joke involving people who are exposed to death. CSIs are exposed to violent and heinous crime scenes, and their emotions and tension may build, making simple work-related tasks difficult to perform, thus using humor to compensate. CSIs report only using gallows humor in "extreme situations" (Vivona, 2014). CSIs who use gallows humor do not necessarily mean to make light of the victim or show disrespect, although their statements are intentional (Vivona, 2014). When humor becomes gallows and less jovial, caution is warranted due to the unknown circumstances or situation eliciting the humor (Craun & Bourke, 2014). Finally, Roth and Vivona (2010) suggested CSIs who use aggressive or self-defeating humor may be having difficulty coping with distressing circumstances of the crime scene or long-term repeated exposure to tragedy.

Function of Humor Humor can be distinguished in a variety of contexts (e.g., jokes, pranks, humorous situations, banter), with CSIs employing jokes as a means of relaxation and tension reduction to focus on their job (Vivona, 2014). CSIs also have relayed that humor is a source of stress relief and is used as a barometer of emotional burdens between colleagues at the crime scene (Vivona, 2014). Humor is recognized as an important coping mechanism for CSIs who are exposed to violence and tragedy. CSIs signified that humor in the workplace distinguished a sense of normalcy when their senses have been overloaded at a crime scene (Roth & Vivona, 2010). CSIs' culture is like other law enforcement agencies where a team approach is ideal. However, CSIs are often isolated from colleagues and other first responders. For them, humor serves to (a) solidify team membership and socialize new members; (b) relieve stress and tension; and (c) act as an overt display of the joking culture of this group (Vivona, 2013).

Humor in the Workplace Humor is stabilized across multiple settings for CSIs (e.g., during crime scenes, paperwork, and debriefings). Culture is largely enmeshed within a CSI's workplace, in which humor plays a distinct role. The emotional and physical work employed by CSIs is challenging especially with showing whether one's humor will assimilate with the work culture (Vivona, 2014). Humor is employed by CSIs who share a common understanding of stress and trauma, which can contribute to their sense of professional identify (Roth & Vivona, 2010). Even with humor and joking behaviors characterizing the CSI's culture, some colleagues may find it inappropriate or callous.

Humor within the CSI's work environment has been encouraged as it has a positive effect on group cohesion and reduces stress (Craun & Bourke, 2014). It is important to note that humor and joking are not indications of a CSI's lack of seriousness perpetrated toward their tasks. CSI supervisors need to understand the underpinnings of humor and how it can be a helpful coping mechanism for handling stress and trauma (Roth & Vivona, 2010).

Summary and Conclusions

There are several limitations to the current body of literature on stress and trauma in CSIs. Despite the burgeoning body of research in this field, estimates of stress and trauma in CSIs may be underestimated, possibly because of first-responder culture, perceptions of potential occupational repercussions, limited self-reflection, and social desirability. Consequently, it may be difficult to recruit participants for research due to skepticism or fear that information will not remain confidential. The stigma attached to emotional and psychological vulnerability remains a barrier across first-responder groups. There are also shortcomings in strategies employed to assess stress and mental health problems in first responders. Specifically, there is a lack of instrumentation designed, normed, and validated on first-responder samples. Based on the review of the literature to date, there are currently no measures developed specifically for the evaluation of stress and trauma in CSIs.

Further, there is often no distinction between subgroups of CSIs. For instance, within CSIs, differences between sworn and non-sworn CSIs may contribute to disparities in stress and trauma. In addition, research on CSIs reflects a wide range of activities occurring in the lab, field, and office (e.g., crime scene investigator, latent print examiner, DNA analyst, blood stain analyst, ballistics/firearms/toolmarks, computer forensics, forensic toxicology, forensic odontology, digital forensics, medical examiner investigator, anthropology). The differences in occupational responsibilities, exposure to traumatic events, organizational stressors, and supervisor support, among other factors, could potentially contribute to differences in stress and trauma symptomatology.

CSIs are a frequently neglected group of first responders who experience unique stressors and traumatic events that impact their mental health. They are routinely exposed to, and spend the longest time interacting with, the scene of the crime. When stressors were integrated into domains, occupational and organizational stressors were identifiable along with the psychological deficits imposed by long-term stress and repeated exposure to traumatic incidents. CSIs appear to employ coping mechanisms including social support and humor and utilize resources available that contribute to their mental resiliency. Although CSIs experience varying levels of stress, research shows that CSIs have higher levels of resiliency than the general population. It is important to note the limited research that has been conducted specific to the mental health and wellness of CSIs.

Appendix

Recommendations for CSIs (Sollie et al., 2017).

Six recommendations are offered for law enforcement agencies, managers, and personnel to invest in CSIs to help promote resiliency and long-term sustainability while reducing the risk of health problems:

1. Let CSIs choose to do this work of their own volition, because self-assessment and self-selection are key factors in the experience of stress among CSIs. Therefore, refine the recruitment process of CSIs by organizing information meetings, professional assessments, and short-term internships.
2. Facilitate autonomy during distressing cases, so that CSIs can manage their own workload and apply coping strategies of their own choosing.
3. Encourage and facilitate peer support by investing in psychoeducation (i.e., information about stressors, coping, resources, and stress reactions) and dialog techniques with regard to discussing sensitive topics. It is also advisable to invest in the resources from investigators' personal lives, for example, providing psychoeducation to their partners.
4. Continue to invest in adequate forensic resources and training; this is what gives CSIs the confidence to know that they are able to make the right decisions at the crime scene and can find personal meaning in their stressful work.
5. Facilitate professional support; set up regular meetings with an independent psychologist who is familiar with the work context. This offers CSIs an opportunity for reflection and taking precautionary measures where necessary.
6. Periodic monitoring of mental resilience.

References

Adderley, R., Smith, L. L., Bond, J. W., & Smith, M. (2012). Physiological measurement of crime scene investigator stress. *International Journal of Police Science & Management, 14*(2), 166.

American Psychiatric Association. (2013). *Diagnostic and statistical manual of mental disorders* (5th ed.). American Psychiatric Association.

American Psychiatric Association. (2022). *Diagnostic and statistical manual of mental disorders* (5th ed., Text Rev ed.). American Psychiatric Association.

Anderson, G. S., Litzenberger, R., & Plecas, D. (2002). Physical evidence of police officer stress. *Policing: An International Journal of Police Strategies & Management, 25*(2), 399.

Anshel, M. H. (2000). A conceptual model and implications for coping with stressful events in police work. *Criminal Justice and Behavior, 27*(3), 375–400.

Blozis, J. (2010). Forensic DNA evidence at a crime scene: An investigator's commentary. *Forensic Science Review, 22*(2), 121–130.

Bourke, M. L., & Craun, S. W. (2014). Secondary traumatic stress among internet crimes against children task force personnel: Impact, risk factors, and coping strategies. *Sexual Abuse: A Journal of Research and Treatment, 26*(6), 586–609.

Boyd, C. M., Dollard, M. F., Dormann, C., Winefield, A. H., & Winefield, H. R. (2003). Unique aspects of stress in human service work. *Australian Psychologist, 38*(2), 84–91.

Bradway, J. H. (2009). Gender stress: Differences in critical life events among law enforcement officers. *International Journal of Criminal Justice Sciences, 4*(1), 1–12.

Brunetto, Y., Teo, S. T. T., Shacklock, K., & Farr-Wharton, R. (2012). Emotional intelligence, job satisfaction, well-being and engagement: Explaining organizational commitment and turnover intentions in policing. *Human Resource Management Journal, 22*(4), 428–441.

Carlson, E. B., & Dalenberg, C. J. (2000). A conceptual framework for the impact of traumatic experiences. *Trauma, Violence, & Abuse, 1*(1), 4–28.

Clark, R., Distelrath, C., Vaquera, G., Winterich, D., & DeZolt, E. (2015). Critical-incident trauma and crime scene investigation: A review of police organizational challenges and interventions. *Journal of Forensic Identification, 65*(6), 929–951.

Craun, S. W., & Bourke, M. L. (2014). The use of humor to cope with secondary traumatic stress. *Journal of Child Sexual Abuse, 23*(7), 840–852.

Craun, S. W., Bourke, M. L., Bierie, D. M., & Williams, K. S. (2014). A longitudinal examination of secondary traumatic stress among law enforcement. *Victims & Offenders, 9*(3), 299–316.

Dutelle, A. W. (2020). *An introduction to crime scene investigation*. Jones & Bartlett Learning.

Evans, R., Pistrang, N., & Billings, J. (2013). Police officers' experiences of supportive and unsupportive social interactions following traumatic incidents. *European Journal of Psychotraumatology, 4*, 9.

Figley, C. R. (2002). Compassion fatigue: Psychotherapists' chronic lack of self-care. *Journal of Clinical Psychology, 58*(11), 1433–1441.

Flannery, R. B., Jr. (2015). Treating psychological trauma in first responders: A multi-modal paradigm. *Psychiatric Quarterly, 86*(2), 261–267.

Fowler, S. (2006). A crime scene investigator in the police force. *Biological Sciences Review, 18*(3), 38–41.

Fyhn, T., Fjell, K. K., & Johnsen, B. H. (2016). Resilience factors among police investigators: Hardiness-commitment a unique contributor. *Journal of Police and Criminal Psychology, 31*(4), 261–269.

Henry, V. E. (2004). *Death work: Police, trauma, and the psychology of survival*. Oxford University Press.

Hyman, O. (2004). Perceived social support and secondary traumatic stress symptoms in emergency responders. *Journal of Traumatic Stress, 17*(2), 149–156.

International Crime Scene Investigators Association. (n.d.). *What is ICSIA?* Retrieved from https://www.icsia.org/what-is-icsia/

Jackson, B. A., Baker, J. C., Ridgely, M. S., Bartis, J. T., & Linn, H. I. (2004). *Protecting emergency responders, volume 3: Safety management in disaster and terrorism response*. RAND Corporation.

Johnson, R. R. (2012). Police officer job satisfaction: A multidimensional analysis. *Police Quarterly, 15*(2), 157–176.

Julian, R., Kelty, S., & Robertson, J. (2012). Get it right the first time: Critical issues at the crime scene. *Current Issues Criminal Justice, 24*(1), 25–37.

Kelty, S. F. (2012). Professionalism in crime scene examination: Recruitment strategies using the seven key attributes of top crime scene examiners. *Forensic Science Policy and Management, 2*, 198–204.

Kelty, S. F., & Gordon, H. (2015). No burnout at this coal-face: Managing occupational stress in forensic personnel and the implications for forensic and criminal justice agencies. *Psychiatry, Psychology and Law, 22*(2), 273–290.

Klein, A. (1998). *The courage to laugh: Humor, hope and healing in the face of death and dying*. Penguin Putnam.

Leone, M. C., & Keel, R. (2016). Occupational stress and the crime scene investigator. *Journal of Law and Criminal Justice, 4*(1), 63–74.

Levy-Gigi, E., Richter-Levin, G., Okon-Singer, H., Kéri, S., & Bonanno, G. A. (2016). The hidden price and possible benefit of repeated traumatic exposure. *Stress, 19*(1), 1–7.

Marshall, E. K. (2006). Cumulative career traumatic stress (CCTS): A pilot study of traumatic stress in law enforcement. *Journal of Police and Criminal Psychology, 21*(1), 62–71.

Martin, R. A. (2007). *The psychology of humor: An integrative approach*. Elsevier.

Maslach, C., & Jackson, S. E. (1981). The measurement of experienced burnout. *Journal of Organizational Behavior, 2*(2), 99–113.

Maslach, C., Schaufeli, W. B., & Leiter, M. P. (2001). Job burnout. *Annual Review of Psychology, 52*, 397–422.

McCraty, R., & Atkinson, M. (2012). Resilience training program reduces physiological and psychological stress in police officers. *Global Advances in Health and Medicine, 1*(5), 44–66.

Miller, L. (2006). *Practical police psychology: Stress management and crisis intervention for law enforcement*. Charles C Thomas Publisher.

Miller, L. (2009). Criminal investigator stress: Symptoms, syndromes, and practical coping strategies. *International Journal of Emergency Mental Health, 11*(2), 87–92.

Mitchell, M., & Hogg, I. (1997). The emotional impact of collecting crime evidence: The work of the scenes of crime officers. *Issues in Criminological & Legal Psychology, 29*, 35–40.

Pavšič Mrevlje, T. (2016). Coping with work-related traumatic situations among crime scene technicians. *Stress and Health, 32*(4), 374–382.

Pavšič Mrevlje, T. (2018). Police trauma and Rorschach indicators: An exploratory study. *Rorschachiana, 39*(1), 1–19.

Perez, L. M., Jones, J., Englert, D. R., & Sachau, D. (2010). Secondary traumatic stress and burnout among law enforcement investigators exposed to disturbing media images. *Journal of Police and Criminal Psychology, 25*(2), 113–124.

Roth, G. L., & Vivona, B. (2010). Mirth and murder: Crime scene investigation as a work context for examining humor applications. *Human Resource Development Review, 9*(4), 314.

Selye, H. (1936). A syndrome produced by diverse nocuous agents. *Nature, 138*, 32.

Sewell, J. D. (1993). Traumatic stress of multiple murder investigations. *Journal of Traumatic Stress, 6*(1), 103–118.

Sewell, J. D. (1994). The stress of homicide investigations. *Death Studies, 18*(6), 565.

Shumaker, S. A., & Brownell, A. (1984). Toward a theory of social support: Closing conceptual gaps. *Journal of Social Issues, 40*(4), 11–36.

Sollie, H., Kop, N., & Euwema, M. C. (2017). Mental resilience of crime scene investigators: How police officers perceive and cope with the impact of demanding work situations. *Criminal Justice and Behavior, 44*(12), 1580–1603.

Thorson, J. A., & Powell, F. C. (1993). Sense of humor and dimensions of personality. *Journal of Clinical Psychology, 49*(6), 799–809.

U. S. Department of Justice. (2020). *Uniform crime report, crime in the United States, 2019*. https://ucr.fbi.gov/crime-in-the-u.s/2019/crime-in-the-u.s.-2019/tables/table-75/table-75-overview.pdf

van den Eeden, C. A. J., de Poot, C. J., & van Koppen, P. J. (2017). From emergency call to crime scene: Information transference in the criminal investigation. *Forensic Science Policy & Management, 8*(3–4), 79–89.

Van Patten, I. T., & Burke, T. W. (2001). Critical incident stress and the child homicide investigator. *Homicide Studies: An Interdisciplinary & International Journal, 5*(2), 131–152.

Vivona, B. D. (2013). Investigating humor within a context of death and tragedy: The narratives of contrasting realities. *The Qualitative Report, 18*(50), 1–22.

Vivona, B. D. (2014). Humor functions within crime scene investigations: Group dynamics, stress, and the negotiation of emotions. *Police Quarterly, 17*(2), 127–149.

Yoo, Y., Cho, O., Cha, K., & Boo, Y. (2013). Factors influencing post-traumatic stress in Korean forensic science investigators. *Asian Nursing Research, 7*(3), 136–141.

Emergency Communications Operators

Angela T. Beamer, Tara D. Thomas, Sheri L. White, and Vincent B. Van Hasselt

> I remember I was dispatching and a K9 unit responded to a domestic violence call. When officers attempted to break up the fight, the dog was stabbed in the face. The dog was transported with lights and sirens to a nearby city where the animal hospital was. It was the middle of the night and we were calling to get the veterinarian to respond as quickly as possible. I was coordinating officers to blockade roads because when a K9 gets injured, it is treated the same as when an officer is down. I had only been on the job for four months.

The True First Responders

Emergency communications operators (ECOs) are considered the true first responders in critical incident response (Blankenship, 1990). However, due to ECOs not being physically present at the scene of the critical incident, other first responder groups often do not acknowledge the levels of stress and trauma that ECOs experience. Historically, individuals tasked with answering 911 calls were often police officers who were injured and on light duty, or secretaries. As the number of 911 calls increased, it was evident there was a need for specialized training in emergency response (e.g., providing instructions on how to perform CPR), and the current system of ECOs trained as professionals emerged (Sheehan, 1995). ECOs deal with difficult situations including communication difficulties, uncertainty, and insufficient resources; but knowledge, skills, and experience help to manage these situations (Forslund et al., 2004). According to the Bureau of Labor Statistics, U.S. Department of Labor (2021), there are approximately 99,500 ECOs employed in the United States. ECOs can also be referred to as dispatchers (police, fire,

A. T. Beamer (✉) · V. B. Van Hasselt
College of Psychology, Nova Southeastern University, Davie, FL, USA

T. D. Thomas · S. L. White
Regional Communications Division, Broward Sheriff's Office, Fort Lauderdale, FL, USA

M. L. Bourke et al. (eds.), *First Responder Mental Health*,
https://doi.org/10.1007/978-3-031-38149-2_5

medical), 911 operators, and telecommunicators. ECOs are typically in civilian positions and are expected to receive incoming calls, correctly route these calls to coordinate an appropriate response, help the caller remain calm, and occasionally provide emergency lifesaving instructions over the phone (Klimley et al., 2018). Examples of these types of calls include drownings, fires, shootings, sick or injured individuals, motor vehicle accidents, and suicides (Trachik et al., 2015). ECOs must be able to remain calm and have an accurate and timely response. These decisions are made while dealing with individuals who are emotionally distressed, while multitasking other responsibilities, and, typically, without consulting with coworkers or supervisors due to time constraints (Davis, 2005; Franklin & Hunt, 1993; Steinkopf et al., 2018). Some ECOs also dispatch over police and fire radio channels to convey real-time information about units, locations, and details of the evolving event. Shifts and roles may vary depending on the department and the day (e.g., 12 hours divided between 911 operator and police/fire channel dispatching). The ECO may not know their schedule until the moment they walk in for roll call, especially if they are working in a relief position (i.e., providing breaks to other ECOs). In recent years, due to the increase in school shootings, some communications centers have also been tasked with monitoring panic buttons in schools. These buttons were implemented to create a real-time silent method for communicating various types of emergencies that require police, fire, and/or rescue response without dialing 911. ECOs are a critical aspect of emergency response, and without their assistance, police, fire, and rescue units would not have the vital information they need to be able to respond on-scene.

Occupational Hazards

ECOs experience stressors related to job tasks as well as stressors from within the organization itself. These can include shift work, low pay, lack of organizational support, lack of control, perceived lower rank than other first responders, decreased support from supervisors, and inadequate training (Blankenship, 1990; Burke 1995; McCarty & Skogan, 2013; Payne, 1993; Quinn & Shepard, 1974; Sewell & Crew, 1984; Wahlgren et al., 2020). In addition to stress, factors unique to this occupation, including back-to-back calls, lack of resolution, helplessness due to handling the situation over the phone, and creating a graphic mental picture of the scene, all contribute to psychological and physiological effects.

Stress: Psychological and Physiological Effects

ECOs regularly experience stress as part of their occupation. Stress is both a physical and psychological reaction that occurs when an individual believes that the situational demands are so high, it compromises their ability to respond to the threat

(Lazarus, 2000; Lazarus & Folkman, 1984). ECOs may have shifts that range from dull and boring to highly stressful with few breaks. Their work schedules often rotate, and they may be asked to work overtime with very little notice. Dealing with calls that involve traumatic events, pain, and death can also lead to PTSD due to regular exposure to these types of events at work (Shakespeare-Finch et al., 2015). Steinkopf et al. (2018) found that ECOs experience psychological distress, occupational stress, and subthreshold PTSD at similar or higher rates than police officers. PTSD is positively correlated with work-related stress and difficulty expressing feelings in ECOs (Wojciechowska et al., 2021). Trauma responses can be subjective, due to individual personality differences, prior trauma exposure, and the social context the trauma occurs (Carleton et al., 2019; Ricciardelli et al., 2020):

> Sometimes the incident that causes trauma is not even your call. I remember I pulled a recording for an investigator and in the tape you could hear a woman who called 911 from a locked bedroom. She was saying, 'He's coming in. He's going to rape me.' You could hear him break the door, then her screaming, and the bed squeaking. The next thing you could hear were the police officers coming in and then a tussle. The operator was able to stay on the line and coordinate a police response. This man was suffering from PTSD, and while he was on leave from the military, he raped his own wife. It was the worst call I ever heard, and I still remember it even 32 years later.

There is limited research on suicidal ideation and attempts in ECOs. One study of Canadian ECOs found there was a lifetime suicide ideation rate of 28% (Carleton et al., 2018b). Stress will manifest differently depending on the individual, and healthy coping strategies are not always adopted. Lack of exercise, consuming excessive amounts of alcohol, and binge eating over the course of their career can have extremely detrimental effects on an ECO's physical health (Smith et al., 2019). Chronic stress can contribute to mental health problems, such as depression, anxiety, PTSD, substance abuse, sleep problems, and hyperarousal, as well as physical health problems (e.g., high blood pressure, weight fluctuation, a weakened immune system, chronic pain) (Carleton et al., 2018a; Dallman et al., 2003; Glaser & Kiecolt-Glaser, 2005; Hall et al., 2004; Kindermann et al., 2020; Marin et al., 2011; McEwen, 1998; Pendleton et al., 1989; Perez et al., 2021; Vrijkotte et al., 2000). Over time, this can lead to burnout, increased employee absenteeism, and subsequent turnover (Kirmeyer & Dougherty, 1988; Maslach, 2003; McAleavy et al., 2021; McCarty & Skogan, 2013). Sometimes these rates of burnout can even exceed that of police officers (Roberg et al., 1988). ECOs were found to have elevated cortisol levels at all times of the day that were correlated with the subjective perception of emotional stress (Weibel et al., 2003). Significantly higher heart rates and irregular heartbeat variability were also present in ECOs (Oldenburg et al., 2014). These high rates of stress, combined with low job satisfaction, affect overall quality of life.

Call-Taking

ECOs may feel out of control due to the fact that they are de-escalating these events over the phone (Ksionzky & Mehrabian, 1986). Pierce and Lilly (2012) reported that one third of calls that ECOs receive cause peritraumatic stress. This is a type of intense fear and helplessness that can lead to posttraumatic stress disorder (PTSD) (Brunet et al., 2001). Trauma can accumulate over years of service and thousands of calls. The "good" calls do not outweigh the "bad" calls, but what is critically important, is how the individual recovers from those "bad" calls. During a critical incident (e.g., an airport shooting) a worker may be hiding for hours, and the operator must make a choice to stay on the line, or ensure the civilian is in a safe location, direct them to call back if the situation deteriorates, and answer other emergency calls. This system of triaging calls can be very stressful and may lead to feelings of guilt and helplessness (Adams et al., 2015; de Nooij, 2013). One of the most stressful types of calls for an ECO is hearing an officer screaming for help when they are injured. This type of call causes unique distress because officers are thought of as heroes who are invincible:

> A dispatcher was listening to a conversation between a helicopter pilot and a police officer who was riding with him. The helicopter pilot was dipping the plane to have fun and scare the officer, when a wire was accidentally pulled. Suddenly, the dispatcher could not hear their voices, and thinking there may be an issue with her headset, she unplugged it. Screams from the officer that the helicopter was going down echoed throughout the communications center. All of the dispatchers in the room heard the screams from the men that the helicopter was crashing into the ocean and they knew they were dying. The officer's wife was an ECO at the communications center.

Working as an ECO taking calls is highly stressful and fast-paced (Franklin & Hunt, 1993). Kirmeyer (1988) found interruption of work tasks and handling simultaneous demands contributed significantly to stress in ECOs. Although some calls are aggravating or emotionally distressing, the ECO does not always have the luxury of taking a break because they have to answer the next incoming call. Police officers and firefighters may stay on the same scene for hours or remain on a call while parked to write their report. However, ECOs must remain in the same room and answer back-to-back calls while dealing with trauma and the resulting emotions (Smith et al., 2019).

Additionally, ECOs may not have a resolution because they are not usually informed of the outcome of the call. ECOs hear a mother screaming as she discovers her toddler in the pool, assist the mother through the steps of administering CPR, and then hear the phone disconnect as the police arrive. The ECO is not updated on whether the child started breathing again or if they will live. Traumatic events without closure continue to play in the minds of ECOs, even if it is a call they heard about but did not handle directly. One way ECOs attempt to get a resolution is by reading the notes of the call, calling the on-scene sergeant, or, if it was a larger incident, watching the news report later in the day. During the Marjory Stoneman Douglas shooting in Parkland, Florida, dispatchers heard the radio traffic about kids being injured and killed but did not find out for hours how many casualties there were. ECOs were fielding calls from frantic parents trying to get in touch with their children with little to no information.

Due to not being physically present on-scene, the ECO envisions what the trauma may look like, and this image may be more graphic than the actual event. These mental pictures can also have a traumatic effect because the individual does not have an ability to experience, and, therefore, process the scene firsthand. These images, in combination with the audio the ECO experienced, can result in flashbacks and nightmares, even though the images were manufactured by the individual's own mind.

Law Enforcement Culture

Law enforcement agencies have unique cultural aspects such as hyper-masculinity, within-group mentality, social pressure to conform, and lack of help-seeking behavior. First responders are seen as heroes who assist others, and they often do not acknowledge when they require help themselves. The stigma of seeking mental health treatment is stronger in this population because any perceived sign of weakness or injury may be an indication that they are unable to perform their job (Haugen et al., 2017). Drew and Martin (2021) found that even if a police officer is willing to seek help, and finds it helpful, the stigma is not reduced, thereby making the interventions less effective. Law enforcement agencies are considered paramilitary organizations, and some models applied to military populations have theorized that stigma can take several forms. Ben-Zeev et al. (2012) theorized there is *public stigma* (individuals' awareness of stereotypes from the public about people who seek mental health treatment), *self-stigma* (the individual applying these stereotypes to themselves, resulting in loss of power and value), and *label avoidance* (individuals denying symptoms and treatment to avoid the stigma of receiving a diagnosis). This culture permeates not only law enforcement officers but also the civilians who work at the agency (McCall et al., 2021). The trauma and stress ECOs experience get exacerbated due to lack of help-seeking behavior. These social norms and pressure to conform from the group create a toxic culture of self-reliance that leads to psychological and physical consequences (Crowe et al., 2017).

Tesser et al. (1983) found conformity was positively associated with self-doubt and negatively associated with attention. When applying this to ECOs mental health symptoms, the ECO may be more likely to doubt their intuition that the symptoms warrant help, and, therefore, pay less attention to them. Individuals create norms, in part, due to a need to be accepted (Argyle, 1957). First responders often complete individual tasks, but function as part of a larger team. Being accepted by the group is central to the social roles that play a part in their identities. Research indicates that social theories can explain differences in how individuals respond to stress (Carr & Umberson, 2013). Biddle (1979) theorized that the social roles we adopt for everyday activities, such as through our occupation, are accompanied by unstated expectations and norms that may lead to role overload or role conflict. Females in law enforcement agencies are at particular risk for role conflict when they are aligned with their gender identity while working in a masculine environment. This can lead to additional stress, placing females at greater risk for poor mental health outcomes when they adopt the same lack of help-seeking behaviors as their male counterparts. This is especially relevant for dispatchers since, historically, a majority of ECOs are female.

Resilience

ECOs are under enormous pressure to perform their jobs well, despite the occupational and organizational stressors they face. Their stress levels are largely maintained by cultural norms that reinforce a pressure to keep moving forward even when they need to engage in self-care. Additional research is needed to develop strategies to increase ECO resilience. *Resilience* refers to an individual's ability to maintain relatively stable, healthy levels of psychological and physical functioning when faced with adverse events (Bonanno, 2004; Connor & Davidson, 2003), and has been found to have a central role in coping with stressors and trauma (Almedom, 2005; Bartone, 2006; Bonanno, 2004; Bonanno et al., 2006; Collins, 2007; Honig & Sultan, 2004; Lightsey, 2006; Miller et al., 2017). Resilience can be learned and has been found to protect individuals against job burnout and related conditions in other job professions (Bartone, 2006). Factors, such as optimism, social support, and hope, have been identified as significant contributors to psychological well-being (Reivich & Seligman, 2011), as well as individual resilience (Masten, 2001; Reivich & Seligman, 2011). Several prevention and intervention programs have had success in providing coping strategies and decreasing stress in law enforcement personnel (Anshel et al., 2013; Boothroyd et al., 2019; Edgelow, et al., 2022; Fay et al., 2006; Henderson et al., 2018; Scully, 2011; Steinkopf et al., 2016; Van Hasselt et al., 2019, 2020).

There has been a generational shift in career longevity with an increase in individuals changing jobs multiple times over their lifetime. Job turnover is high, and geographical relocation for one's occupation is increasing. Individuals are motivated more often by internal satisfaction (i.e., does this job bring me happiness) versus external rewards (i.e., pension, benefits). Job satisfaction and altruism are motivating factors for ECOs to stay in the profession. Perceived job satisfaction, or lack thereof, contributes to ECO stress and occupational burnout (Burke, 1995). Factors that increase job satisfaction in ECOs include decreased work-related stress, feeling content with salary and benefits, equality in the workplace, and feelings of acceptance (Alderden & Skogan, 2014). Focusing on the "good" calls, such as delivering a baby, instructing someone in CPR, and hearing someone gasp for air after nearly drowning, are reminders of why the individual may have entered this profession. It is critically important to assist ECOs in discovering the reason they started working in the field and why they have remained.

Social Support

First responders often work as part of a team and specific social-cultural norms are prevalent, such as within-group mentality and lack of help-seeking behavior from outside mental health professionals. Interventions that bolster social support have been shown to directly impact the mental health of first responders (Prati & Pietrantoni, 2010, Regehr et al., 2013). Social support is characterized as, "An exchange of resources between at least two individuals perceived by the provider or the recipient to be intended to enhance the wellbeing of the recipient" (Shumaker & Brownell, 1984, p. 13). Zimet et al. (1988) revealed the level of social support is directly related to the reported severity of psychological and physical symptoms. It has been posited that social support may serve a buffering function through direct effects on self-perceptions and other cognitive activities, or changes in problem-solving behaviors (Horton & Wallander, 2001). High levels of social support are associated with a sense of control and predictability in life, self-esteem, lower levels of stress, and higher resilience. Additionally, it has been demonstrated that encouragement of social support through training has positive effects on social networks and prosocial behavior, which has been linked to improved job performance and overall well-being (Southwick & Charney, 2012). Social support has been theorized to account for well-being (i.e., social causation theory), and well-being has also been theorized to determine social support (i.e., social selection theory) (Dohrenwend, 2000; Johnson et al., 1999). In a study by Crowe et al. (2017), first responders recognized that positive coping and resilience were related to social support. Social connectedness and support have been found to be protective factors against stress, anxiety, depression, PTSD, and suicide (Hilbrink, 2022; Kshtriya et al., 2020). Specifically, in a study on ECOs, social support coping explained 10% of the variance in intrusion symptoms of PTSD (Jenkins, 1997). Support from friends and family, peer support, employee assistance programs (EAP) programs, and Critical Incident Stress Management (CISM) are all recommended forms of social support for ECOs (Bourgeois et al., 2021; Fay et al., 2006; Golding et al., 2017).

Friends and Family

Research has demonstrated that friends and family can provide valuable types of social support (e.g., emotional, instrumental, appraisal, and informational) (Tjin et al., 2022). Although some first responders are hesitant to share aspects of their job with their family members to protect them from secondary trauma or because it is cumbersome to explain the details, family members are the most easily accessible group that most first responders share general stressors with on a daily basis (O'Toole et al., 2022). Research indicates 74% of ECOs would first access a spouse, followed by 67% accessing ECO leaders, and between 43 and 60% accessing a mental health professional (Carleton et al., 2020). Family members are often the first to notice changes in loved ones, and the longer the ECO is on the job, the more stress, mood changes, and social withdrawal occurs (peaking around 10 years on the job) (Camaro et al., 2020). It is imperative for ECOs to maintain friendships outside of their chosen field so they can relate to others who have varied interests, and conversational topics are not always centered around work. However, it is equally as important to have friends that are peers because other ECOs will truly empathize and understand the various aspects of the job. Some forms of "dark humor" that ECOs engage in with each other can be therapeutic in relieving stress (Tracy & Tracy, 1998). Maintaining a balanced social group and a life outside of their career will allow the individual to have a career that supports their lifestyle versus viewing their career as their sole purpose in life.

Peer Support

Another valuable resource for ECOs is peer support, which has been found to be effective in reducing stigma and promoting treatment-seeking when there is a foundational level of trust (Horan et al., 2021). It is important to have trained individuals who are on-site and readily available to assist with crisis intervention. Peer support is especially important because it helps individuals discuss the event in the context the trauma occurred (i.e., using 10 codes and signals). Some peers may have a tendency to say, "What is the big deal? Just take the next call." This is why training for specialized peer support teams is invaluable. Staffing agencies with administrators who have worked as operators and/or dispatchers in the past allows them to relate to others' experiences on a personal level. Supervisors can assist peer support teams by facilitating leave for an employee who needs to take time off:

> After a "bad" call, the dispatcher talks to the supervisor and the supervisor asks what the dispatcher needs. Sometimes they want to talk and other times they want to go home. A lot of the time they say, "I'm good", but then they realize an hour later after taking other calls that they are not feeling ok. Each situation has to be handled individually because some people are immediately emotional and others will never have a reaction to the call. If the dispatcher is consistently having a negative response to calls and cannot handle the stress of the job, command can refer them to the EAP program. We also have a quiet room with recliners where dispatchers can sit and process their emotions and/or talk to a peer support member or EAP employee who responds to the communications site. Some agencies are implementing mental health days that can also be used if a peer support team member identifies an employee who is struggling. The peer support member can advocate for the dispatcher to have time off. The EAP stigma has lessened over time and ECOs in this generation want to know what the agency is offering for their wellbeing.

Critical Incident Stress Management

Critical Incident Stress Management (CISM) is a model that provides defusings (i.e., an immediate group process for crisis intervention provided within a few hours of a critical incident) and debriefings (i.e., a group process to discuss the critical incident typically within 72 hours) to mitigate suicidal ideation and PTSD symptoms (Everly & Mitchell, 1999). During large events, such as the Marjory Stoneman Douglas shooting, many resources such as EAP, chaplains, and peer support teams were responding directly to the scene. However, due to ECOs being located off-site, the defusing did not happen immediately. Supervisors are trained to debrief after a large call such as a shooting or a pursuit, and peer support can be requested to respond to communications immediately, while trained CISM facilitators may arrive later. Debriefings may separate supervisors and operators/dispatchers so employees feel like they can speak openly about what happened. Supervisors may be multitasking during a large event, and it is critical to ensure supervisors also attend a debriefing, especially when dealing with the death of an employee. It should be cautioned that even if shift change is about to occur, employees should not be released to go home until someone has checked in with them to provide a defusing. Encouraging attendance at debriefings where facilitators use psychoeducation to inform participants of possible reactions to traumatic events is useful. It would be impractical to have police and firefighters working the road assemble in a location with dispatchers who are off-site, even if they have handled the same event. However, after defusings are provided immediately to each group, gathering all first responder groups together to discuss the event on another date would help ECOs feel included and integrated with other first responders. Allowing for additional staffing to "cover the road" while these debriefings occur would also allow for this participation.

Mental Health Clinicians

Research indicates even those who have strong support systems, and a belief they possess the ability to handle their stress, still experience effects from stress (Bundy, 2020). Some ECOs find relief in expressing their emotions or talking to a mental health clinician. In order to gain an understanding and appreciation of what first responders face on a daily basis, clinicians have the opportunity to attend ride-longs and clinician awareness programs where they learn what specific stressors firefighters and police officers encounter in the field. However, many clinicians do not have this same opportunity to experience a day in the life of a dispatcher at communications centers. Clinicians who want to work with this population should arrange to spend time alongside ECOs to gain a better understanding of the job requirements. Future wellness programs could provide an on-site clinician who is dedicated to the employees at the communications center. ECOs would have the opportunity to become familiar with this clinician and build trust, so the clinician could be an immediate resource in times of crisis. For those ECOs who still find it difficult to speak to a mental health clinician, some communications centers are also incorporating the use of therapy dogs who work alongside these clinicians to decrease stress (Dvoskina & Cole, 2020).

Summary

Although communications centers can be hectic, there is also downtime where dispatchers joke with one another, share meals, and function like a second family. They are protective and loyal due to their shared comradery. Although they may not always get along, when crisis occurs, everyone comes together and performs their job seamlessly. Many ECOs express a sense of pride in their occupation but feel overwhelmed by the workload and undervalued by other first responders (Coxon et al., 2016). Future studies should investigate the role of social support (i.e., peers, friends, family) across a variety of mental disorders in ECOs to prevent and treat stress and job-burnout in this highly important, but historically underserved group of first responders. This research will also benefit emergency response organizations by providing them with empirical data concerning factors that could assist with these issues. Heuristic coping strategies, organizational reform, and educational measures can be proactively and successfully implemented to teach stress management and promote resilience to allow for a lower incidence of stress-related physical, behavioral, and emotional problems, as well as job-related burnout in ECOs. It is equally as important to support efforts to correctly classify ECOs as *first responders*, because in certain states their job descriptions are still affiliated with administrative professionals, along with their retirement benefits. Emergency Communications Operators are the lifeline for civilians, police officers, firefighters, and paramedics:

> We do not have the option to stay at home in an emergency and this is why during the COVID pandemic we were mandated first responders. What if we were not there to answer the call of someone breaking into your house or the baby not breathing? When one of our own dispatchers died of COVID she was recognized as a first responder because she was mandated to work. We are the true first responder. Everything starts with communications.

References

Adams, K., Shakespere-Finch, J., & Armstrong, D. (2015). An interpretative phenomenological analysis of stress and well-being in emergency medical dispatchers. *Journal of Loss and Trauma, 20*(5), 430–448.

Alderden, M., & Skogan, W. G. (2014). The place of civilians in policing. *Policing: An International Journal of Police Strategies & Management, 37*(2), 259–284.

Almedom, A. (2005). Resilience, hardiness, sense of coherence, and posttraumatic growth: All paths leading to 'light at the end of the tunnel'? *Journal of Loss and Trauma, 10*, 253–265. https://doi.org/10.1080/15325020590928216

Anshel, M. H., Umscheid, D., & Brinthaupt, T. M. (2013). Effect of a combined coping skills and wellness program on perceived stress and physical energy among police emergency dispatchers: An exploratory study. *Journal of Police and Criminal Psychology, 28*(1), 1–14.

Argyle, M. (1957). Social pressure in public and private situations. *The Journal of Abnormal and Social Psychology, 54*(2), 172–175. https://doi.org/10.1037/h0040490

Bartone, P. T. (2006). Resilience under military operational stress: Can leaders influence hardiness? *Military Psychology, 18*, 131–148.

Ben-Zeev, D., Corrigan, P. W., Britt, T. W., & Langford, L. (2012). Stigma of mental illness and service use in the military. *Journal of Mental Health, 21*(3), 264–273. https://doi.org/10.3109/09638237.2011.621468

Biddle, B. J. (1979). *Role theory: Expectations, identities, and behaviors*. Academic.

Blankenship, B. (1990, November). Dispatching units: Improvements for the 'first line'. *FBI Law Enforcement Bulletin, 59*, 12–13.

Bonanno, G. A. (2004). Loss, trauma, and human resilience: Have we underestimated the human capacity to thrive after extremely aversive events? *American Psychologist, 59*(1), 20.

Bonanno, G. A., Galea, S., Bucciarelli, A., & Vlahov, D. (2006). Psychological resilience after disaster: New York City in the aftermath of the September 11th terrorist attack. *Psychological Science, 17*(3), 181–186.

Boothroyd, R. A., Green, S., & Dougherty, A. (2019). Evaluation of operation restore: A brief intervention for first responders exposed to traumatic events. *Traumatology, 25*(3), 162–171.

Bourgeois, P. J., Hotz, E., Perrott, S., & Bigelow, T. (2021). Stress and wellbeing in emergency dispatchers. *Annals of Emergency Dispatch and Response, 9*(3), 12–18.

Brunet, A., Weiss, D. S., Metzler, T. J., Best, S. R., Neylan, T. C., Rogers, C., Fagan, J., & Marmar, C. R. (2001). The Peritraumatic Distress Inventory: A proposed measure of PTSD criterion A2. *American Journal of Psychiatry, 158*(9), 1480–1485.

Bundy, W. L. (2020). Emergency medical dispatchers: PTSD and preventing it. *Crisis, Stress, and Human Resilience: An International Journal, 1*(4), 192–214.

Bureau of Labor Statistics, U.S. Department of Labor. (2021). *Occupational outlook handbook, public safety communicators*. Retrieved 10 Mar 2023, from https://www.bls.gov/ooh/office-and-administrative-support/police-fire-and-ambulance-dispatchers.htm

Burke, T. W. (1995). Dispatcher stress. *FBI Law Enforcement Bulletin, 64*, 1.

Camaro, A., Belmonte, E., Demar, D. J., & Timm, A. (2020). The impact of 911 telecommunications on family and social interaction. *Annals of Emergency Dispatch & Response, 8*(3), 4–10.

Carleton, R. N., Afifi, T. O., Taillieu, T., Turner, S., El-Gabalawy, R., & Sareen, J. (2018a). Anxiety-related psychopathology and chronic pain comorbidity among public safety personnel. *Journal of Anxiety Disorders, 55*, 48–55.

Carleton, R. N., Afifi, T. O., Turner, S., Taillieu, T., Lebouthillier, D. M., Duranceau, S., Sareen, J., Ricciardelli, R., MacPhee, R. S., Groll, D., Hozempa, K., Brunet, A., Weekes, J. R., Griffiths, C. T., Abrams, K. J., Jones, N. A., Beshai, S., Cramm, H. A., Dobson, K. S., et al. (2018b). Suicidal ideation, plans, and attempts among public safety personnel in Canada. *Canadian Psychology, 59*(3), 220–231.

Carleton, R. N., Afifi, T. O., Taillieu, T., Turner, S., Krakauer, R., Anderson, G. S., MacPhee, R. S., Ricciardelli, R., Cramm, H. A., Groll, D., & McCreary, D. R. (2019). Exposures to potentially traumatic events among public safety personnel in Canada. *Canadian Journal of Behavioural Science, 51*(1), 37–52.

Carleton, R. N., Afifi, T. O., Turner, S., Taillieu, T., Vaughan, A. D., Anderson, G. S., Ricciardelli, R., MacPhee, R. S., Cramm, H. A., Czarnuch, S., Hozempa, K., & Camp, R. D. (2020). Mental health training, attitudes toward support, and screening positive for mental disorders. *Cognitive Behaviour Therapy, 49*(1), 55–73.

Carr, D., & Umberson, D. (2013). The social psychology of stress, health, and coping. In J. DeLamater & A. Ward (Eds.), *Handbook of social psychology* (pp. 465–487). Springer Science + Business Media. https://doi.org/10.1007/978-94-007-6772-0_16

Collins, S. (2007). Social workers, resilience, positive emotions and optimism. *Practice: Social Work in Action, 19*, 255–269.

Connor, K. M., & Davidson, J. R. T. (2003). Development of a new resilience scale: The Connor-Davidson Resilience Scale (CD-RISC). *Depression and Anxiety, 18*, 76–82.

Coxon, A., Cropley, M., Schofield, P., Start, K., Horsfield, C., & Quinn, T. (2016). 'You're never making just one decision': Exploring the lived experiences of ambulance emergency operations centre personnel. *Emergency Medicine Journal, 33*(9), 645–651.

Crowe, A., Glass, J. S., Lancaster, M. F., Raines, J. M., & Waggy, M. R. (2017, January-March). A content analysis of psychological resilience among first responders and the general population. *SAGE Open*, 1–9. https://doi.org/10.1177/2158244017698530

Dallman, M. F., Pecoraro, N., Akana, S. F., la Fleur, S. E., Gomez, F., Houshyar, H., Bell, M. E., Bhatnagar, S., Laugero, K. D., & Manalo, S. (2003). Chronic stress and obesity: A new view of 'comfort food'. *Proceedings of the National Academy of Sciences, 100*(20), 11696–11701.

Davis, J. B. (2005). Finding calm after the call. *ABA Journal, 91*(3), 75.

de Nooij, J. (2013). Emergency dispatch: Quo Vadis? (Where are you going?). *Annals of Emergency Dispatch and Response, 1*(1), 9–10.

Dohrenwend, B. (2000). The role of adversity and stress in psychopathology: Some evidence and its implications for theory and research. *Journal of Health and Social Behavior, 41*, 1–19.

Drew, J. M., & Martin, S. (2021). A national study of police mental health in the USA: Stigma, mental health, and help-seeking behaviors. *Journal of Police and Criminal Psychology, 36*, 295–306. https://doi.org/10.1007/s11896-020-09424-9

Dvoskina, M., & Cole, G. (2020). Introduction of facility therapy dogs to 911 communication centers: A proposal. *Traumatology, 26*(1), 147–151.

Edgelow, M., Scholefield, E., McPherson, M., Mehta, S., & Ortlieb, A. (2022). A review of workplace mental health interventions and their implementation in public safety organizations. *International Archives of Occupational and Environmental Health, 95*, 645–664.

Everly, G. S., Jr., & Mitchell, J. T. (1999). *Critical Incident Stress Management (CISM): A new era and standard of care in crisis intervention*. Chevron Publishing Corporation.

Fay, J., Kamena, M. D., Benner, A., & Buscho, A. (2006). A residential milieu treatment approach for first-responder trauma. *Traumatology, 12*(3), 255–262.

Forslund, K., Kihlgren, A., & Kihlgren, M. (2004). Operators' experiences of emergency calls. *Journal of Telemedicine and Telecare, 10*, 290–297.

Franklin, A. L., & Hunt, E. (1993). An emergency situation simulator for examining time-pressured decision making. *Behavior Research Methods, Instruments, and Computers, 25*(2), 143–147.

Glaser, R., & Kiecolt-Glaser, J. K. (2005). Stress-induced immune dysfunction: Implications for health. *Nature Reviews Immunology, 5*(3), 243.

Golding, S. E., Horsfield, C., Davies, A., Egan, B., Jones, M., Raleigh, M., Schofield, P., Squires, A., Start, K., Quinn, T., & Cropley, M. (2017). Exploring the psychological health of emergency dispatch centre operatives: A systematic review and narrative synthesis. *PeerJ, 5*(10), 1–29.

Hall, M., Vasko, R., Buysse, D., Ombao, H., Chen, Q., Cashmere, J. D., Kupfer, D., & Thayer, J. F. (2004). Acute stress affects heart rate variability during sleep. *Psychosomatic Medicine, 66*(1), 56–62.

Haugen, P. T., McCrillis, A. M., Smid, G. E., & Nijdam, M. J. (2017). Mental health stigma and barriers to mental health care for first responders: A systematic review and meta-analysis. *Journal of Psychiatric Research, 94*, 218–229. https://doi.org/10.1016/j.jpsychires.2017.08.001

Henderson, S., Burns, A., Van Hasselt, V. B., & LeDuc, T. J. (2018, September). FIRST response: The firefighter intervention and response support team. *Fire Engineering, 171*, 8–10.

Hilbrink, D. (2022). The role of social connectedness in protecting first responder mental health and wellbeing. *The Australian Journal of Emergency Management, 37*(4), 65–68.

Honig, A. L., & Sultan, S. E. (2004). Reactions and resilience under fire: What an officer can expect. *The Police Chief, 71*(12), 54–60.

Horan, K. A., Marks, M., Ruiz, J., Bowers, C., & Cunningham, A. (2021). Here for my peer: The future of first responder mental health. *International Journal of Environmental Research and Public Health, 18*, 11097. https://doi.org/10.3390/ijerph182111097

Horton, T. V., & Wallander, J. L. (2001). Hope and social support as resilience factors against psychological distress of mothers who care for children with chronic physical conditions. *Rehabilitation Psychology, 46*(4), 382–399.

Jenkins, S. R. (1997). Coping and social support among emergency dispatchers: Hurricane Andrew. *Journal of Social Behavior and Personality, 12*(1), 201–216.

Johnson, J. G., Cohen, P., Dohrenwend, B., Link, B., & Brook, J. (1999). A longitudinal investigation of social causation and social selection processes involved in the association between socioeconomic status and psychiatric disorders. *Journal of Abnormal Psychology, 108*, 490–499.

Kindermann, D., Sanzenbacher, M., Nagy, E., Greinacher, A., Cranz, A., Nikendei, A., Friederich, H.-C., & Nikendei, C. (2020). Prevalence and risk factors of secondary traumatic stress in emergency call-takers and dispatchers – A cross sectional study. *European Journal of Psychotraumatology, 11*(1), 1799478.

Kirmeyer, S. L. (1988). Coping with competing demands: Interruption and the type a pattern. *Journal of Applied Psychology, 73*(4), 621–629.

Kirmeyer, S. L., & Dougherty, T. W. (1988). Work load, tension, and coping: Moderating effects of supervisor support. *Personnel Psychology, 41*(1), 125–139.

Klimley, K. E., Van Hasselt, V. B., & Stripling, A. M. (2018). Posttraumatic stress disorder in police, firefighters, and emergency dispatchers. *Aggression and Violent Behavior, A Review Journal, 43*, 33–44.

Kshtriya, S., Kobezak, H. M., Popok, P., Lawrence, J., & Lowe, S. R. (2020). Social support as a mediator of occupational stressors and mental health outcomes in first responders. *Journal of Community Psychology, 48*, 2252–2263. https://doi.org/10.1002/jcop.22403

Ksionzky, S., & Mehrabian, A. (1986). Temperament characteristics of successful police dispatchers: Work settings requiring continuous rapid judgments and responses to complex information. *Journal of Police Science & Administration, 14*(1), 45–48.

Lazarus, R. S. (2000). Toward better research on stress and coping. *American Psychologist, 55*, 665–673.

Lazarus, R. S., & Folkman, S. (1984). *Stress, appraisal, and coping*. Springer Publishing Company.

Lightsey, O. R., Jr. (2006). Resilience, meaning, and well-being. *The Counseling Psychologist, 34*(1), 96–107.

Marin, M. F., Lord, C., Andrews, J., Juster, R. P., Sindi, S., Arsenault-Lapierre, G., Fiocco, A. J., & Lupien, S. J. (2011). Chronic stress, cognitive functioning and mental health. *Neurobiology of Learning and Memory, 96*(4), 583–595.

Maslach, C. (2003). *Burnout: The cost of caring*. Prentice-Hall.

Masten, A. S. (2001). Ordinary magic: Resilience processes in development. *American Psychologist, 56*(3), 227–238. https://doi.org/10.1037//0003-066X.56.3.227

McAleavy, T., Choi, B., & Arlikatti, S. (2021). Faceless heroes: A content analysis of determinants for the recruitment, career development and retention of emergency medical dispatchers in the United States of America. *International Journal of Disaster Risk Reduction, 61*(2), 102335.

McCall, H. C., Beahm, J. D., Foumier, A. K., Burnett, J. L., Carleton, R. N., & Hadjistavropoulos, H. D. (2021). Stakeholder perspectives on internet-delivered cognitive behavioural therapy for public safety personnel: A qualitative analysis. *Canadian Journal of Behavioural Science, 53*(3), 232–242.

McCarty, W. P., & Skogan, W. G. (2013). Job-related burnout among civilian and sworn police personnel. *Police Quarterly, 16*(1), 66–84.

McEwen, B. S. (1998). Stress, adaptation, and disease: Allostasis and allostatic load. *Annals of the New York Academy of Sciences, 840*(1), 33–44.

Miller, A., Unruh, L., Zhang, N., Liu, X., & Wharton, T. (2017). Professional quality of life of Florida emergency dispatchers. *International Journal of Emergency Services, 6*(1), 29–39.

O'Toole, M., Mulhall, C., & Eppich, W. (2022). Breaking down barriers to help-seeking: Preparing first responders' families for psychological first aid. *European Journal of Psychotraumatology, 13*(1), 2065430. https://doi.org/10.1080/20008198.2022.2065430

Oldenburg, M., Wilken, D., Wegner, R., Poschadel, B., & Baur, X. (2014). Job-related stress and work ability of dispatchers in a metropolitan fire department. *Journal of Occupational Medicine and Toxicology, 9*, 31.

Payne, D. M. (1993). Role disequilibrium among police dispatchers. *Police Studies: International Review of Police Development, 16*, 99.

Pendleton, M., Stotland, E., Spiers, P., & Kirsch, E. (1989). Stress and strain among police, firefighters, and government workers: A comparative analysis. *Criminal Justice and Behavior, 16*(2), 196–210.

Perez, R. A., Jetelina, K. K., & Reingle Gonzalez, J. M. (2021). The chronic health effects of work-related stressors experienced by police communications workers. *Safety and Health at Work, 12*, 365–369.

Pierce, H., & Lilly, M. M. (2012). Duty-related trauma exposure in 911 tele-communicators: Considering the risk for posttraumatic stress. *Journal of Traumatic Stress, 25*(2), 211–215.

Prati, G., & Pietrantoni, L. (2010). The relation of perceived and received social support to mental health among first responders: A meta-analytic review. *Journal of Community Psychology, 38*(3), 403–417.

Quinn, R. P., & Shepard, L. G. (1974). *The 1972–1973 quality of employment survey: Continuing chronicles of an unfinished enterprise* (pp. 90–97). Institute for Social Research, University of Michigan.

Regehr, C., LeBlanc, V. R., Barath, I., Balch, J., & Birze, A. (2013). Predictors of physiological stress and psychological distress in police communicators. *Police Practice and Research, 14*(6), 451–463.

Reivich, K. J., & Seligman, E. P. (2011). Master resilience training in the U.S. Army. *American Psychologist, 66*(1), 25–34.

Ricciardelli, R., Czarnuch, S., Afifi, T. O., Taillieu, T., & Carleton, R. N. (2020). Public safety personnel's interpretations of potentially traumatic events. *Occupational Medicine, 70*, 155–161.

Roberg, R. R., Hayhurst, D. L., & Allen, H. E. (1988). Job burnout in law enforcement dispatchers: A comparative analysis. *Journal of Criminal Justice, 16*(5), 385–393.

Scully, P. J. (2011). Taking care of staff: A comprehensive model of support for paramedics and emergency medical dispatchers. *Traumatology, 17*(4), 35–42.

Sewell, J. D., & Crew, L. (1984). The forgotten victim: Stress and the police dispatcher. *FBI Law Enforcement Bulletin, 53*(3), 7–12.

Shakespeare-Finch, J., Rees, A., & Armstrong, D. (2015). Social support, self-efficacy, trauma and well-being in emergency medical dispatchers. *Social Indicators Research, 123*(2), 549–565.

Sheehan, K. M. (1995). Reflections on dispatching: Improving dispatcher training. *FBI Law Enforcement Bulletin, 64*(6), 17–21.

Shumaker, S. A., & Brownell, A. (1984). Toward a theory of social support: Closing conceptual gaps. *Journal of Social Issues, 40*(4), 11–36.

Smith, E. C., Holmes, L., & Burkle, F. M., Jr. (2019). Exploring the physical and mental health challenges associated with emergency service call-taking and dispatching: A review of the literature. *Prehospital and Disaster Medicine, 34*(6), 619–624.

Southwick, S., & Charney, D. S. (2012). The science of resilience: Implications for the prevention and treatment of depression. *Science, 338*(5), 79–82.

Steinkopf, B., Klinoff, V., Van Hasselt, V. B., Leduc, T., & Couwels, J. (2016). Behavioral health training for fire rescue personnel. *Fire Engineering, 169*(12), 59–67.

Steinkopf, B., Reddin, R. A., Black, R. A., Van Hasselt, V. B., & Couwels, J. (2018). Assessment of stress and resiliency in emergency dispatchers. *Journal of Police and Criminal Psychology, 33*(4), 398–411.

Tesser, A., Campbell, J., & Mickler, S. (1983). The role of social pressure, attention to the stimulus, and self-doubt in conformity. *European Journal of Social Psychology, 13*, 217–233.

Tjin, A., Traynor, A., Doyle, B., Mulhall, C., Eppich, W., & O'Toole, M. (2022). Turning to 'trusted others': A narrative review of providing social support to first responders. *International Journal of Environmental Research and Public Health, 19*, 16492. https://doi.org/10.3390/ijerph192416492

Trachik, B., Marks, M., Bowers, C., Scott, G., Olola, C., & Gardett, I. (2015). Is dispatching to a traffic accident as stressful as being in one? Acute stress disorder, secondary traumatic stress, and occupational burnout in 911 emergency dispatchers. *Annals of Emergency Dispatch and Response, 3*(1), 27–38.

Tracy, S. J., & Tracy, K. (1998). Emotion labor at 911: A case study and theoretical critique. *Journal of Applied Communication Research, 26*(4), 390–411.

Van Hasselt, V. B., Klimley, K. E., Rodriguez, S., Themis-Fernandez, M., Henderson, S. N., & Schneider, B. A. (2019). Peers as Law Enforcement Support (PALS): An early prevention program. *Aggression and Violent Behavior, A Review Journal, 48*, 1–5.

Van Hasselt, V. B., Klimley, K. E., & Geller, S. (2020, September). Behavioral health training for police officers: A prevention program. *FBI Law Enforcement Bulletin, 89*, 1–8.

Vrijkotte, T. G., Van Doornen, L. J., & De Geus, E. J. (2000). Effects of work stress on ambulatory blood pressure, heart rate, and heart rate variability. *Hypertension, 35*(4), 880–886.

Wahlgren, K., Fraizer, A., Taigman, M., Gay, M., Williscroft, R., Faudere, D., Jones, A., & Olola, C. (2020). Factors contributing to stress levels of emergency dispatchers. *Annals of Emergency Dispatch and Response, 8*(3), 11–16.

Weibel, L. W., Gabrion, I., Aussedat, M., & Kreutz, G. (2003). Work-related stress in an emergency medical dispatch center. *Annals of Emergency Medicine, 41*(4), 500–506.

Wojciechowska, M., Jasielska, A., Ziarko, M., & Sienski, M. (2021). Mediating role of stress at work in the relationship of alexithymia and PTSD among emergency call operators. *International Journal of Environmental Research and Public Health, 18*, 12830.

Zimet, G. D., Dahlem, N. W., Zimet, S. G., & Gordon, K. F. (1988). The multidimensional scale of perceived social support. *Journal of Personality Assessment, 52*(1), 30–41.

Part II
Assessment and Prevention

Psychological Evaluations in Public Safety Settings

Brian Mangan

The objective of this chapter is to provide evaluators and agency personnel a general overview of the purpose, process, and legal considerations of pre-employment psychological evaluations and psychological fitness for duty evaluations in public safety settings. Qualified evaluators will gain a broad understanding of these specialized evaluations and how to better serve their public safety agencies. However, this overview will not include in-depth information regarding various standardized objective test instruments, interpretation of profiles, and research to support the use of evidence-based instruments. Qualified evaluators should seek continuing education and reliable source materials to gain a strong understanding in the use of standardized testing. Additionally, evaluators should be familiar with federal and state laws when conducting these evaluations. In general terms, a pre-employment psychological evaluation assesses whether a candidate is suitable for the specific job applied for, including but not limited to police officer, correctional officer, firefighter, or communications operator. A psychological fitness for duty evaluation (FFDE) looks for the presence or absence of a psychological condition or impairment that would prevent an incumbent employee from performing job duties in a safe and effective manner.

The legal framework in conducting these evaluations is established by laws such as the Americans with Disabilities Act of 1990 (ADA), ADA Amendments Act of 2008 (ADAA), the Health Insurance Portability and Accountability Act (HIPAA, 1996; Privacy Rule, 2000; Final Omnibus Rule, 2013), Genetic Information Nondiscrimination Act of 2008 (GINA), Uniformed Services Employment and Reemployment Rights Act of 1994 (USERRA), and Family Medical Leave Act of 1993 (FMLA). Additionally, evaluators must rely on primary legal statutes and

B. Mangan, PsyD, ABPP (✉)
Board Certified in Police & Public Safety Psychology, Law Enforcement Psychological & Counseling Associates, Inc, Medley, FL, USA
e-mail: bmangan@lepca.com

M. L. Bourke et al. (eds.), *First Responder Mental Health*,
https://doi.org/10.1007/978-3-031-38149-2_6

administrative codes within the state they practice. Although some states do not mandate psychological pre-employment evaluations for law enforcement officers, it is now the standard of practice nationwide for agencies to conduct these psychological evaluations, including FFDEs. Further, several well-respected law enforcement organizations, such as the International Association of Chiefs of Police (IACP), Department of Justice (DOJ), and Commission on Accreditation for Law Enforcement Agencies (CALEA), strongly support these services.

Evaluators should make ongoing efforts to maintain and develop areas of competence based on education, training, and professional experience and seek appropriate consultation, supervision, and/or specialized knowledge to address pertinent issues outside areas of competence that may arise during psychological evaluations (EPPCC 2.01, 2.03). Seeking membership or certification in national police and public safety psychology organizations can provide the ongoing education, support, and networking necessary to develop and maintain competence within this specialized field. These organizations include, but are not limited to, the International Association of Chiefs of Police-Police Psychological Services Section (IACP-PPSS), American Board of Police and Public Safety Psychology (ABPPSP), American Psychological Association Division 18 Psychologists in Public Service-Police and Public Safety Section (APA Div. 18), and Society for Police and Criminal Psychology (SPCP). Additionally, evaluators will benefit from regular attendance at local, state, and national professional conferences. Through these conferences, organizational listservs, and professional networking, evaluators will optimize their ability to remain cognizant of new research and updates with guidelines, practice standards, and legal considerations when providing evaluation services to public safety agencies.

Evaluators should understand that guidelines and/or principles are aspirational in nature and recommend professional behavior, endeavors, or conduct for evaluators, while standards are mandatory and may be accompanied by an enforcement mechanism. The guidelines identified in this section and discussed in this chapter are intended to reflect the commonly accepted practices of the evaluators experienced in police and public safety psychological evaluations and the agencies they serve. Evaluators will benefit from maintaining awareness of updated and pertinent information from National Institute of Justice publications, California Commission on Peace Officer Standards and Training, and US Equal Employment Opportunity Commission (EEOC) published opinions, as well as the following guidelines and standards:

- APA Professional Practice Guidelines for Occupationally Mandated Psychological Evaluations (2018)
- APA Multicultural Guidelines: An Ecological Approach to Context, Identity, and Intersectionality (2017)
- Ethical Principles of Psychologists and Code of Conduct (EPPCC)
- IACP Pre-employment Psychological Evaluation Guidelines (2020)
- IACP Psychological Fitness-for-Duty Evaluation Guidelines (2018b)

- California Commission on Peace Officer Standards and Training (2014, Revised 2022)

The psychological evaluation of police and public safety candidates and incumbent personnel is a specialized assessment that has unique dimensions, which overlaps other psychological specialties of clinical, forensic, industrial, and organizational psychology. As an evaluator conducting screenings, a primary goal is to address the basic referral questions from the public safety agencies by utilizing valid, reliable, ethical, and legally defensible protocols and procedures. Virtually all states, local governmental boards, prominent law enforcement organizations, and several local and national court rulings have clearly created an expected standard for the appropriate utilization of psychological services by public safety agencies, especially in the hiring process with psychological pre-employment evaluations and in justified FFDEs of incumbent public safety personnel. The absence of these types of psychological services can seriously expose agencies to legal culpability and large payouts to plaintiffs for both negligent hiring and retention lawsuits.

Pre-employment Psychological Evaluations

The purpose of the pre-employment psychological evaluation is to deselect candidates who do not meet minimum standards and is aimed at determining if a candidate is at a low risk for engaging in ineffective or counterproductive job behavior. These evaluations are not intended as a prediction that the candidate will exhibit high levels of performance. Very important legal rulings such as McKenna v. Fargo (1978) and Bonsignore v. City of New York (1982) established the purpose and need for psychological evaluations for public safety employees. The rulings in these cases determined that pre-employment psychological screening is appropriate and in fact, if not done, could lead to a finding of negligent hiring. Bonsignore v. City of New York (1982) is the landmark case in establishing the need for evaluations to ensure that police officers are psychologically fit to perform their designated job duties, with failure to do so leading to the potential for civil liability. In support, the following two cases involved agencies that did not conduct pre-employment psychological evaluations. Individual officers for those agencies were involved in false arrests, with alleged physical and/or emotional harm. In Hild v. Bruner (1980), the court's opinion was that the department's failure to conduct a psychological evaluation of its police officers constituted gross negligence. In addition, Woods v. Town of Danville (2010) involved a department that hired a candidate with known background and anger issues. However, the agency did not conduct pre-employment psychological evaluations as a standard practice. Additional cases that reinforced or expanded upon the Bonsignore decision include Nilsson v. City of Mesa (2007) and Lewis v. Goodie (1992).

Evaluators and agency personnel should be aware of specific federal laws that significantly impact the provision of pre-employment screening services. The ADA is a far-reaching law that is multifaceted and aims to prevent hiring and workplace discrimination against persons with a covered disability under the law. In 2008, the ADAAA expanded the definition of who is covered by the law as disabled and clarified what is medical versus nonmedical. As a result, the law includes specific legal requirements for hiring of employees, which includes sequencing requirements for the collection and use of nonmedical vs. medical information during the selection process. Consider a ninth Circuit Court case, Leonel v. American Airlines (2005) as the closest authoritative legal ruling that succinctly and logically provides direction on how the ADA expects agencies to bifurcate their collection and use of nonmedical and medical information during the hiring process. In summation, the ruling states that all nonmedical information must be collected, evaluated, and used before a bona fide Conditional Offer of Employment (COE) can be provided to the job applicant. This is consistent with how the EEOC (2020) defines a bona fide job offer in the document *Enforcement Guidance on Disability-Related Inquiries and Medical Examinations of Employees under the ADA* (2000), which states a job offer as "real" if the employer has "evaluated all relevant non-medical information which it reasonably could have obtained and analyzed prior to giving the offer." The EEOC has commented that the only exceptions to this rule are when certain components cannot be collected or completed in a timely manner, for instance, contacting references or when collecting nonmedical information, such as military records. However, consistent with the ADA, the assessment of normal-range personality traits, behaviors, and characteristics is an integral part of the evaluation process; therefore, these traits may be included in the pre-employment psychological evaluation conducted post-COE (Corey & Zelig, 2020).

Information considered to be medical under the ADA must be collected, evaluated, and used only in a final post-COE phase of the hiring process. During the post-COE medical phase, collecting and using new nonmedical information, or revisiting information supposedly reviewed during the pre-offer phase, would likely be a violation of ADA and possibly expose the agency and/or evaluator to potential legal challenges. Although the outcome of Leonel v. American Airlines (2005) is precise in defining ADA's intent with the selections and hiring process, many public safety agencies are not aware of, or overlook, this case entirely. The law does seem to provide some latitude around bifurcation if the agency can demonstrate that bifurcation will unduly extend the hiring process or place an increased financial burden on the agency. Nonetheless, the legal burden is still on the agency to prove these assertions, which likely would require an in-depth and objective analysis of these issues. Disregarding the ADA and the EEOC's guidance could result in potential litigation and possible liability. Therefore, it is always wise for evaluators to educate agencies and seek a formal opinion from an agency's legal counsel.

The Civil Rights Act of 1964 and 1991 prohibits discrimination based on race, color, religion, etc. Additionally, the Uniform Guidelines on Employee Selection Procedures (1978a, b) describe the federal government's position on how tests should be used in making employment decisions which are consistent with federal equal employment opportunity (EEO) laws. As a result, evaluators should be aware of the potential for adverse impact regarding procedures utilized and final determinations provided. To monitor this, it would be prudent to maintain an evaluation database including demographic data for each candidate tested. At regular intervals, the evaluator can extract data for the specified timeframe and conduct an analysis, typically using the 4/5ths rule, which states that if the selection rate for a certain group is less than 80% of that of the group with the highest selection rate, there is adverse impact on that group.

Additional federal law that impacts pre-employment evaluations include HIPAA (1996) and GINA (2008). The purpose of HIPAA (1996) was to establish standards for the protection, use, and disclosure of protected healthcare information (PHI). The law strengthens an individual's right to privacy and obligates healthcare providers to clearly explain any limits of confidentiality and how PHI is to be used or shared. This necessitates the use of appropriate consent and release of information forms consistent with HIPAA standards and requirements, acknowledging that information obtained in the evaluations will be shared with the referring agency for the determination of suitability for employment or returning to work. Thus, the referring agency is the client of record, the applicant/candidate (pre-employment) or employee (FFDE) is the subject of record, and the psychologist is examiner of record.

GINA (2008) "prohibit[s] discrimination on the basis of genetic information with respect to health insurance and employment." GINA defines "genetic information" to include an individual's family medical history, the results of an individual's or family member's genetic tests, the fact that an individual or an individual's family member sought or received genetic services, genetic information of a fetus carried by an individual or an individual's family member, and genetic information of an embryo lawfully held by an individual or family member receiving assistive reproductive services. Because of this act, evaluators and agencies must refrain from asking questions about family medical history and genetic information, such as the manifestation of a disease or disorder in family members. Therefore, personal history questionnaires, interview questions, and test items must be carefully reviewed to remove applicable items, such as direct questions regarding a family history of mental health, suicide, or alcohol/substance use concerns. Additionally, GINA admonishments should be included on all consent forms during the evaluation process, including any request of treatment information forms provided during employment evaluations. In cases where the candidate or treatment provider inadvertently discloses information without solicitation, the information is considered protected under GINA, is not recorded or disclosed in documentation to agency, and is not considered when making employment decisions (Corey & Zelig, 2020).

Guidelines and Standards

With the legal framework in place, it is important to engage in practice with consideration for the universal guidelines and standards developed and recognized by the professionals in the field of public safety evaluation. The IACP PPSS

Pre-employment Psychological Evaluation Guidelines (2020) are clear, concise, and effective. Relying on these guidelines to correspond with agencies, educate on the scope and limitations of services, and develop communication in reports is a safe and appropriate practice. These guidelines define a pre-employment psychological evaluation as a "specialized examination to determine whether a public safety candidate meets the requirements for psychological suitability mandated by jurisdictional statutes and regulations, as well as any other psychologically relevant criteria established by the hiring agency." More directly, the purpose of the evaluation is to determine the potential presence of a psychological impairment that may negatively affect and/or interfere with the candidate's ability to perform the defined job responsibilities and effectively manage the demands of the position. Furthermore, agencies should utilize qualified evaluators trained and experienced specifically in conducting pre-employment psychological evaluations for public safety positions and who are committed to continued education and training within this specialized area of practice.

A pre-employment psychological evaluation typically occurs post COE, unless the process is bifurcated with the nonmedical portion taking place prior to COE and medical portion taking place post-COE. The evaluation process includes the administration of standardized objective test instruments, including a standard personal history questionnaire, and a clinical interview with a licensed, qualified evaluator after standardized objective test results, questionnaires, and any additional supportive documents are completed and reviewed. The standardized objective testing should include instruments with documented reliability, validity, and evidence supporting use, assessing both normal and abnormal traits, and should be supported in the use for public safety pre-employment screening through established scientific research and professional knowledge. If an agency bifurcates the screening procedures, the standardized objective test instruments measuring normal traits and questionnaires addressing nonmedical information may be administered prior to COE, while test instruments measuring abnormal traits and questionnaires addressing medical information must be administered post-COE. The sequencing of pre-employment testing was also clarified in Barnes v. Cochran (1996), which ruled that a psychologist cannot administer standardized tests measuring medical/abnormal traits or review medical records until after a COE is provided to the job applicant.

The purpose of the interview during the evaluation process is to gather and review with candidate all information related to personal background history, including legal, traffic, work, credit, school, military, substance use, mental health, etc. The use of a standard personal history questionnaire or similar instrument and a semi-structured interview should be utilized during this process. During this information gathering and review, the candidate may reveal additional information, such as previous mental health treatment or service-connected disability. In order to conduct a comprehensive and thorough evaluation, the evaluator should request and carefully review this information and request additional information or clarification if necessary. This will require use of proper consent to release treatment information forms and/or use of the Department of Veterans Affairs Form 10-5345 Request for and Authorization to Release Health Information. With these evaluations, the candidate has a primary goal of presenting as suitable for hire and it is not uncommon for them to withhold or minimize noteworthy background information, including past mental health treatment or concerns. A failure to review treatment records or condition ratings could result in missing crucial information regarding a candidate's mental health history, as well as indicate a concern for integrity with providing honest background information, which could lead to an imprecise determination and negligent hiring.

The evaluator should have a clear understanding of job-related traits when integrating data gathered during the evaluation. The California Commission on Peace Officer Standards and Training (POST) Job Task Analysis provides a set of job-related traits widely accepted by qualified police and public safety evaluators. The ten dimensions in the final set of the POST Peace Officer Psychological Screening Dimensions (2014) include (1) social competence, (2) teamwork, (3) adaptability/flexibility, (4) conscientiousness/dependability, (5) impulse control/attention to safety, (6) integrity/ethics, (7) emotional regulation/stress tolerance, (8) decision-making/judgment, (9) assertiveness/persuasiveness, (10) avoiding substance abuse and other risk-taking behaviors.

For additional guidance, the California POST Peace Officer Screening Manual (2014) provides definitions, positive behaviors, counterproductive behaviors, and levels of effectiveness during critical incidents. The evaluator can use this information to communicate potential deficits and concerns to the hiring agency through integrating evidence-based results, behavioral anchors from background information, and other data sources gathered during the evaluation process.

Interview Process

The evaluation interview provides a source for observations regarding a candidate's interpersonal style, presentation, and approach to testing. Moreover, the interview and review of background information allow the evaluator to identify potential behavioral patterns of concern that may interfere with a candidate's ability to safely and effectively perform the duties of the position applied for. The semi-structured interview may include job-relevant open-ended questions to determine a candidate's insight, accountability, emotional intelligence, multicultural awareness, and any evidence of bias. Through additional inquiry and exploration during the interview, an evaluator may be able to gain insight into the candidate's locus of control, emotional intelligence, ability to accept constructive criticism/feedback, and the potential for any inconsistencies or evasiveness with background information. The evaluator can then use the interview data to integrate with standardized objective test results to mitigate or substantiate concerns.

As an evaluator, the standardized objective test results provide tremendous guidance in the interview, particularly regarding areas for review or additional questioning. Specific item responses and patterns of responding are very useful in consideration of a candidate's evaluation profiles; however, the specific item content should never be disclosed to the candidate to protect test integrity (EPPCC, 9.11). Instead, the evaluator should review theme content with the candidate, being mindful not to reveal specific items or influence a particular response during the interview or future psychological pre-employment evaluations. Additionally, reviewing theme content or response patterns provides the evaluator an opportunity to reconcile inconsistent profiles or critical item content that appears divergent from other data sources, including interview and background information. Item response concerns that are reconciled by determining the candidate exhibited multiple reading errors, carelessness with the test process, or poor reading comprehension will be valuable information when determining suitability for the applied for position. Nevertheless, when considering responses to standardized testing, the evaluator must also take into consideration a candidate's language proficiency, academic ability, and reading comprehension with the support from other data gathered from personal history and background review.

Integration of Data Sources

The evaluator's main role is to integrate multiple sources of information gathered during the evaluation process. The California POST Peace Officer Screening Manual (2014) recommends a useful model of six sequential steps for a systematic data review, which reduces the influence of subjectivity and evaluator bias. These six sequential steps are comprehensive and very useful to provide evaluators with a solid framework when determining a final risk rating or recommendation. To improve decision-making, the following steps and related data sources should be considered according to relevance and reliability (Corey & Zelig, 2020; Heilbrun et al., 2009). A review of standardized objective test results should begin with investigating test profiles for evidence of response inconsistency, infrequency, over-reporting, and/or under-reporting, which determines the reliability of profiles. Assuming profiles are reliable, the evaluator can then identify and interpret relevant findings using standard community norms and public safety norms, depending on the instruments used and the position in consideration. Relevant personal history information from all sources, including personal history questionnaire, agency background investigations, and/or polygraph, should be reviewed to determine if information is convergent with, divergent from, or complementary of relevant test findings. In essence, the evaluator seeks to identify behavioral anchors demonstrated by the candidate to corroborate with standardized objective test results.

Additionally, the evaluator reviews relevant clinical observations gathered during the evaluation and interview process to determine how they are convergent with, divergent from, and/or complementary of relevant test findings and personal history information. Based on this integration, the evaluator must determine whether the weight of the aggregate data and information supports or refutes the final determination regarding a candidate's suitability. Finally, the evaluator seeks to obtain feedback from the hiring agency to determine the status of hired candidates through initial phases of employment, including academy, field training, and probation and adjust the prediction strategy as necessary, otherwise known as a feedback loop.

Final Reports

The pre-employment psychological evaluation reports should clearly communicate the suitability of the candidate for the position based upon an integration of all psychological material including standardized objective test data, information gathered during the interview, and any ancillary information provided by agency. The evaluator should actively collaborate with the referring agency and background investigator to gather all available information related to the employment evaluation to provide comprehensive and integrated results. Conclusions concerning a candidate's qualifications should be based on consistencies and patterns across data sources rather than from a single source. All agency personnel directly involved in the hiring process should be given access to the evaluator's final report and, importantly, should be trained in understanding the purpose, content, and limitations of the report. The agency should be directed to incorporate the psychological evaluation findings with all other selection materials, which varies by state, including oral board results, background investigations, and polygraph or controlled voice stress analysis results. Failure to provide such training could lead to misunderstanding of evaluation findings and ultimate misuse of the report.

Reports to the agency should contain a risk rating and/or recommendation for employment based upon the results of the screening. The evaluator's risk rating system should be clearly defined and explained to the agency, which reduces the risk for misunderstanding and potential error in hiring decisions. Further, each report should include the justification for risk rating or hiring recommendation and any potential limitations or reservations regarding reliability of the results. This could be due to the candidate taking a defensive approach to standardized objective testing, guarded/evasive approach to interview, ongoing and open investigations, or limited/incomplete background information received from the referring agency. In these cases, it is important for the evaluator to document and communicate the limitations of the report, including the potential that background investigations or other selection procedures reveal important and noteworthy information not disclosed during the pre-employment psychological evaluation process. The evaluator should state in the report that it is imperative for the referring agency to provide any inconsistent or withheld information discovered during investigations, as it could impact the overall final rating after integration with gathered data. Further, in some cases, the evaluator may find it necessary to provide an "indeterminant" final rating when important information is not accessible or available for review, or investigations involving the candidate are still pending. Ultimately, the direct written communication with the agency regarding limitations may lead to subsequent investigation and clarification for a more comprehensive final determination.

Importantly, the evaluator should also communicate with agencies and include statements in the evaluation report that the findings should be valid for no longer than 1 year from completion of the evaluation, unless another time period is established by policy or regulation, and results should not be used for public safety positions or agencies not explicitly considered by the psychologist at the time of evaluation (IACP Guidelines, 2020). Further, the reports should not be used to question a candidate's ability to perform a job they may hold in good standing with the same agency or another employer, and reports should not be used for subsequent disciplinary matters. Evaluators should educate agency personnel on how to store and manage reports, as well as how to respond to potential requests for information related to the evaluation. Providing sensitive information contained in the report or a copy of the report to a candidate raises clear concerns about test information security, potential for misuse of the report, and the possibility that report access may provide sensitive information to covertly assist a candidate on future evaluations. It is imperative for the evaluator and agency to work together to protect the integrity of the evaluation process (EPPCC 9.04, 9.10), which includes requests by the candidate for feedback or an explanation of the test results.

The agency should be clear that with these employment evaluations, the agency is the client of record, the candidate is subject of record, and the psychologist (or other qualified licensed professional) is examiner of record. HIPAA and ADA generally support an individual's right to have access to their health records and reports, especially when the evaluation or report involves PHI. However, employment-related evaluations are unique and are not intended for treatment or continuity of care, and the candidate is not the client of record. In terms of court rulings involving job candidates and rights to these type reports, the rulings vary and are not conclusive. For instance, Cremer v. City of Macomb Board of Fire and Police Commissioners (1996) ruled that a rejected firefighter candidate was entitled to learn the results of his pre-employment psychological evaluation, and Siegfried v. City of Easton (1992) ruled that these pre-employment evaluations are not confidential and must be provided during discovery. On the other hand, Mason v. Stock (1994) and Delaurentos and Miami-Dade County v. Peguero (2010) ruled that pre-employment psychological reports were not discoverable in their respective cases. Ultimately, through the use of proper consent forms, candidates are not entitled to these records provided they knowingly signed a waiver of their access rights as provided under state and federal law (California POST Peace Officer Psychological Screening Manual, 2014).

Psychological Fitness for Duty Evaluation

The IACP-PPSS Psychological Fitness for Duty Evaluation Guidelines define an FFDE as "a formal, specialized examination of an incumbent employee that results from: (1) objective evidence that the employee may be unable to safely or effectively perform a defined job, and (2) a reasonable basis for believing that the cause may be attributable to a psychological condition or impairment." Further, the guidelines help define for evaluators and agency personnel what is considered "objective evidence," which includes documented incidents, events, and observations, as opposed to conjecture and unconfirmed information or reports. Due to the nature of the evaluation, an FFDE is considered a medical examination under ADA, and all final documents should be stored in a secure medical file separate from public record personnel files.

The following specific cases have affirmed an agency's legal authority to order FFDEs of incumbent officers when appropriate justification has been documented. In the landmark case Watson v. City of Miami Beach (1999), the court ruled in support of an agency's right to conduct FFDEs under a wide range of circumstances. This case determined, based on the fact that agencies place armed police officers in situations where they can do harm if acting in an irrational manner, the agency can order an FFDE due to reasonable concerns, including behavior perceived as oppositional, hostile, paranoid, etc. Additional important court rulings that support and elaborate on an agency's right to mandate FFDEs when an officer exhibits potential serious emotional difficulties are Conte v. Horcher (1977), Brownfield v. City of Yakima (2010), and McKnight v. Monroe Co. (2002).

In discussion of ADA and the impact on FFDEs, the ADA permits agencies to order FFDEs, but the agency must demonstrate through objective observations and facts that the employee's job performance is impaired, and reasonably believes that an underlying psychological condition or medical condition is the cause. The FFDE must also be shown to be job relevant and of business necessity. Again, the cases of Watson v. Miami Beach (1999) and Broomfield v. City of Yakima (2010) support the ordering of an FFDE as a preventive tool to intervene in certain job situations, especially for employees in safety sensitive, armed, and/or dangerous public safety positions in which potential impairment could lead to serious and dire consequences. The ADA also specifies that protections are not afforded to employees who are unable to perform essential job functions, even with requested accommodations (Valdes v. City of Doral, 2013). The term "qualified individual" means an individual who, with or without reasonable accommodation, can perform the essential functions of the employment position that such individual holds or desires (42 U.S.C § 12111).

Conte v. Horcher (1977) stated FFDEs should not be disciplinary in nature and agencies have a responsibility to order FFDEs when warranted, with failure to order an evaluation under those circumstances leading to potential liability if a future negative incident should occur. As a result of ADA guidelines and these court cases, a provider may consider declining agency requests for FFDEs when objective documentation is lacking, other less restrictive measures could be taken, or the FFDE is going to be punitive or misused. Further, an evaluator and agency would be wise to document the reasons why an FFDE was not justified or ordered.

Issues at times arise with FFDEs in consideration of the Family and Medical Leave Act of 1993 (FMLA) and the Uniformed Services Employment and Reemployment Rights Act of 1994 (USERRA). FMLA permits eligible employees of covered employers to take unpaid, job-protected leave for specified family and medical and/or psychological reasons. The employee is required to provide documentation of the issue qualifying for FMLA, so the employer can provide the employee with notice concerning their eligibility, as well as information regarding the employee's rights and responsibilities. In the case of public safety personnel who take leave under FMLA, once the mental health or medical professional determines the public safety employee has addressed the issues requiring leave, the individual is entitled to be returned to their position or an equivalent position. Relatedly, USERRA is a federal law protecting military service members and veterans from employment discrimination on the basis of their service and allows them to regain their civilian jobs following a period of uniformed service.

In Albert v. Runyon (1998), the court held that an employer cannot require an FFDE of any employee who has been certified by a treating healthcare provider to return to work, unless post-leave behavior justifies it. However, while FMLA protects the individual from being required to participate in an FFDE with an independent professional prior to returning to work, a more recent court ruling determined that agencies have the option to require an individual to undergo an FFDE before being returned to full-duty status, provided they are first reinstated, which may be accomplished in a light-duty position (White v. County of Los Angeles, 2014). Additionally, an agency can lawfully refer an individual for an independent FFDE if the individual exhibited concerning behavior prior to taking FMLA that would have resulted in a referral for an FFDE if the leave was not taken (Carrillo v. National Council of Churches of Christ in the U.S., 1997; White v. County of Los Angeles, 2014). Similarly, under USERRA, if an agency has objective concerns regarding the potential that a returning service member may have psychological concerns that would interfere with their ability to safely and effectively perform the duties of their public safety civilian position, they must be first reinstated to their former position prior to ordering an evaluation.

As discussed, HIPAA and the ADA both emphasize an individual's right to privacy and an obligation on the part of the examining doctor to limit inquiries, comments, and recommendations to the referral question at hand. GINA (2008) also applies to FFDEs and provides direction on how psychologists and agencies should revise questionnaires and interviews based on the prohibition of "intentional acquisition and use of genetic information in making employment decisions regarding applicants and employees." Therefore, GINA admonishments should be included on all consent forms during the evaluation process, including any request of treatment information forms provided to the employee being evaluated. These laws place limits on what kind and how much information is provided to the employer from an assessment such as an FFDE. Legal cases such as Pettus v. Cole (1996) and McGreal v. Ostrov (2004) both support this position and require that an evaluator avoid revealing sensitive personal or intimate information in reports to employers that is not relevant to the referral question. As a result, public safety evaluation reports should be limited to addressing the job-relevant referral question(s), and an attempt is made to be precise with narrative comments. Undoubtedly, in cases where there is a negative recommendation, the examiner should judge and use commonsense in providing enough supportive information, data, and examination results to adequately support conclusions.

Procedures

FFDEs are complex and exhaustive evaluations that have many implications for the subject of the evaluation, the employer, fellow coworkers, and the public. It is important for the agency to choose a qualified evaluator experienced with these type evaluations and who possesses strong knowledge of work in public safety positions. The evaluator should request the specific job description for the employee being evaluated to ensure a comprehensive understanding of areas to evaluate during an FFDE. Due to the varying potential employment and safety-related outcomes of the FFDE, the evaluator should pay “maximum attention to the relevant legal, ethical, and practice standards and guidelines. Such standards include, but are not limited to, the American Psychological Association's (APA's) Ethical Principles of Psychologists and Code of Conduct. Guidelines include the APA Professional Practice Guidelines for Occupationally Mandated Psychological Evaluations. Examiners also consider and are guided by statutory and case law applicable to the employer's jurisdiction” (IACP Psychological Fitness for Duty Guidelines, 2018b).

Evaluators should be familiar with the standard process of conducting an FFDE and advise agencies forthrightly on the proper process during a pre-conference meeting. FFDEs are psychological investigations and invasive by nature, and agencies may benefit from clarification of less restrictive measures utilized in a progressive manner that may mitigate noted concerns. Conversely, agencies may present as misguided with their understanding of the purpose of an FFDE, believing that the FFDE is a vehicle to termination. Depending on the circumstances leading to concerns, if the agency appears determined that they have enough evidence to move toward an outcome of termination with the employee, the evaluator should exercise extreme caution and reconsider involvement. The evaluator should always consult with the agency and encourage dialogue with legal counsel, both the agency's and their own, if necessary, to determine the appropriate level of intervention and to provide a clear understanding of the purpose of an FFDE.

Due to unfortunate misperceptions and misinformation that may exist within agencies, public safety employees sometimes view FFDEs as a threat to their career and professional image, which may lead to additional and unnecessary stress or concern. Understandably, a determination of unfit for duty may negatively impact an employee's job status, depending on the severity of the condition(s) or circumstance(s) interfering with the ability to perform job duties in a safe and effective manner. However, as Kudrick and Schlosser (2021) discuss, this perspective can perpetuate the negative stigma of psychological services and interventions, which may influence an employee's defensive posture during the evaluation process, viewing the evaluator as an adversary. Moreover, helping agency personnel better understand the purpose and scope of an FFDE when other interventions are ineffective can prove very valuable for all involved. A competently performed FFDE can have a profound impact on the direction of the employee's mental health, career, personal life, and the overall wellness of the agency.

Initiating the process for an FFDE involves a designated official of the agency documenting incidents, behavior, activities, etc., which provide objective evidence and raise legitimate concerns about an employee's psychological state of mind to perform the full duties of the job description in a safe, effective, and competent manner. Along with this initial document, the agency should provide ancillary information if available, including job performance evaluations, letters of counseling, written reprimands, internal affairs investigations, witness statements, commendations, previous remediation efforts, citizen complaints, disciplinary actions, past involvement with shooting incidents, reports of any triggering events, prior psychological evaluations, and any other potentially relevant background information related to the employee's psychological fitness for duty (Section 7.4 IACP Guidelines, 2018b). This information should be provided to the qualified evaluator in advance to review and determine whether the referral meets the necessary threshold for an FFDE or if any additional information is needed.

Prior to moving forward with FFDEs, evaluators should be aware of any potential for conflict of interest or multiple relationships that could reasonably be expected to impair their objectivity, competence, or effectiveness in performing their functions as psychologists (EPPCC 3.05, 3.06). This could include previous involvement in treatment interventions with the employee or professional/personal relationship that could reasonably impair objectivity. In addition, pending investigations may limit the evaluator's ability to conduct a thorough and comprehensive evaluation and may limit the employee's ability to provide vital information that would directly impact the final fitness determination. Furthermore, the failure of an agency to provide all information related to the question of an employee's fitness for duty could directly interfere with the accuracy of the report outcome and could further jeopardize the safety and well-being of employee, agency, fellow coworkers, and general community, which could result in liability for the involved agency (Colon v. City of Newark, 2006). The agency and evaluator should discuss and agree on the purpose and nature of the evaluation, the referral question(s) to be addressed, report format, intended use of the report, and the possible inclusion of a "back to work" plan, if applicable and requested by the agency.

When the threshold for FFDE is met, an appropriate administrative order (AO) from the agency should be presented to the employee requiring they undergo the FFDE. In general, the AO should briefly describe the reason for the evaluation and the limits of confidentiality and that a written report of findings concerning the employee's psychological ability to perform specific job duties will be provided to the agency. The AO should also require the employee to cooperate with the evaluator's requests while undergoing the evaluation, including completion of proper consent forms, personal history questionnaire, standardized objective testing, and clinical interview. Assuming the employee complies, the AO should be signed by the employee verifying receipt of the AO. If the employee refuses to sign the AO or insists that the evaluation is not warranted or illegal, then those issues should be dealt with based on agency policy and/or input from the agency's legal counsel. Importantly, the employee should provide all credentials to agency personnel (e.g., badge, agency identification card, access cards), and depending on the public safety position, the agency should secure all firearm(s) from the employee, or at a minimum, agency firearms. Lastly, the employee should be relieved of full-duty status and placed on paid administrative leave pending the FFDE outcome.

The FFDE process will include administration of standardized objective test instruments, mental status assessment, and clinical interview, which will allow for a thorough review of the employee's self-reported personal history and ancillary background information provided by the agency. The evaluator will then integrate all available data to make a final determination regarding the employee's ability to perform the assigned job duties in a safe and effective manner. The final determination and any limitations therein should be clearly defined by the evaluator and reviewed with the referring agency. As stated previously, information provided in the report to the agency should not include sensitive, personal, or intimate information that is not relevant to the referral question (McGreal v. Ostrov, 2004; Pettus v. Cole, 1996).

Generally, the final determination of an FFDE will be "fit for full-duty" or "unfit for full-duty," but at times, some evaluators may include other qualifiers, such as "temporarily unfit," "permanently unfit," or "fit with restrictions." The evaluator should be clear and concise with the rating system utilized and make sure the agency is educated of this system during preconference discussion. Depending on the outcome and supportive information, the agency should clarify with the evaluator any request for a "back to work" plan. Based on the aggregate information gathered during the evaluation process, and if requested by the agency, the evaluator may provide suggested procedures and steps an agency may consider to potentially remediate psychological concerns and impairments to restore an employee to full duty. Although this plan may include psychological intervention such as mental health counseling or evaluation for medication management by qualified professionals, the precise treatment plan, frequency, schedule, and goals for treatment should be determined by the treating professionals and not the evaluator conducting the FFDE (EPPCC, 3.05). Preferably, the treatment providers selected should be familiar with public safety employment, specific job duties, and safety requirements and may benefit from access to the FFDE report through proper consent to fully understand the issues experienced by the employee that warranted the FFDE referral and contributed to evaluation results.

FFDE Versus Critical Incident Stress Debrief

As mentioned throughout this chapter, the qualified evaluator will often provide education and direction for agency personnel who are not as familiar with the standards of practice, guidelines, and legal/ethical implications of these psychological evaluations. A critical incident stress debriefing (CISD) is a specialized counseling/

educational session utilized with public safety personnel who have experienced an unusual, abnormal, or potentially traumatic job-related event. Typically, officers are most often referred for this service after discharging their firearm in the performance of their duties. However, as emotional health and wellness have become more supported and accepted in the public safety community, so does an agency's awareness that critical incidents and events can vary greatly and affect personnel in many different ways. Therefore, any incident viewed as impactful by a supervisor or an affected public safety employee may warrant referral for CISD. For instance, an officer responding to the scene of a murdered child, traffic homicide, or fellow officer who was seriously injured or killed can have serious emotional repercussions for officers, firefighters, crime scene investigators, victim advocates, dispatchers, etc. Responding to critical incidents is part of the routine job description of many public safety employees and should not ordinarily trigger serious concerns about an employee's emotional fitness or ability to safely and effectively perform duties. In many medium- to large-sized agencies, the CISD program with a qualified licensed practitioner specializing in public safety psychology is often an integrated part of comprehensive psychological services.

Importantly, according to International Association of Chiefs of Police (IACP) Officer-Involved Shooting Guidelines (2018a), critical incident stress debriefings as post-incident interventions are "separate and distinct from any fitness-for-duty assessments or administrative or investigative procedures." Additionally, "In general, mental health professionals refrain from rendering fitness-for-duty opinions when they are not conducting an FFDE, such as when providing debriefings in the context of an officer-involved shooting or similar services in other situations when return to duty is at issue." A CISD is conducted for the benefit of the public safety employee and is never to be confused with a formal FFDE. The client of record for the CISD is the employee, while in an FFDE referral, the agency is the client of record, and a formal evaluation is conducted that includes extensive standardized testing, review of ancillary background materials, and a comprehensive written report of findings is provided to the agency. It is important for psychology professionals and qualified evaluators to understand the clear differences with these interventions and educate agency personnel to limit confusion and mismanagement of critical situations.

References

42 U.S.C § 12111(8).

American Psychological Association. (2017). *Ethical principles of psychologists and code of conduct*. APA. (2002, amended effective June 1, 2010, and January 1, 2017).

American Psychological Association. (2018). Professional practice guidelines for occupationally mandated psychological evaluations. *American Psychologist, 73*(2), 186. https://www.apa.org/pubs/journals/features/amp-amp0000170.pdf

Americans with Disabilities Act Amendments Act of 2008. Pub. L. No. 110-325, 122 Stat. 3553 (2008).

Americans with Disabilities Act of 1990. Pub. L. No. 101-336, §2, 104 Stat. 328 (1991).
Civil Rights Act of 1964. Pub.L. 88-352, 78 §241 (1964).
Civil Rights Act of 1991 § 109, 42 U.S.C. Stat. 2000e et seq (1991).
Corey, D. M., & Zelig, M. (2020). Evaluations of police suitability and fitness for duty. In T. Heilbrun & A. M. Goldstein (Eds.), *Best practices in forensic mental health assessment*. Oxford University Press.
EEOC. (1978a). *Uniform guidelines of employee selection procedures*. 43 FR (August 25, 1978); 29 CFR Part 1607, Section 4.
EEOC. (1978b). *Uniform guidelines on employee selection procedure*. 43 FR (August 25, 1978); 28 CFR 50.14.
EEOC. (2020). *Enforcement guidance: Pre-employment disability-related questions and medical examinations*. ADA, Rehabilitation Act, 29 CFR Part 1630, 29 CFR Part 1614 (2000).
Family and Medical Leave Act of 1993. 29 U.S.C. § 2601–2654 (1993).
Genetic Information Nondiscrimination Act of 2008. Pub. L. No. 110-223, 122 Stat. 881, 42 U.S.C. 2000 (2008).
Health Insurance Portability and Accountability Act of 1996. Pub. L. No. 160, General Administrative Requirements.
Health Insurance Portability and Accountability Act (HIPAA) Privacy Rule. (2000). Title 45, Subtitle A, Subchapter C, Part 160, Part 164, Subparts A-E, Privacy of Individually Indentifiable Health Information.
Health Insurance Portability and Accountability Act (HIPAA) Final Omnibus Rule. (2013). Vol. 78, FR 5566.
Heilbrun, K., Grisso, T., & Goldstein, A. M. (2009). *Foundations of forensic mental health assessment*. Oxford University Press.
IACP Police and Psychological Services Section. (2018a). *Officer-involved shooting guidelines*. https://www.theiacp.org/sites/default/files/2019-05/Officer%20Involved%20Shooting%20Guidelines%202018.pdf
IACP Police and Psychological Services Section. (2018b). *Psychological fitness-for-duty evaluation guidelines*. https://www.theiacp.org/sites/default/files/2019-05/Fitness%20for%20Duty%20Evaluation%20Guidelines%202018.pdf
IACP Police and Psychological Services Section. (2020). *Pre-employment psychological evaluation guidelines*. https://www.theiacp.org/resources/document/pre-employment-psychological-evaluation-guidelines
Kudrick, A., & Schlosser, L. (2021, May). Psychological fitness-for-duty evaluations. *Police Chief, 88*(5), 54–57.
Spilberg, S. W., & Corey, D. M. (2014, Revised 2017, 2018, 2019, 2020, 2022). *Peace officer psychological screening manual*. California Commission on Peace Officer Standards and Training (POST) Standards, Evaluation, and Research Bureau.
Uniformed Services Employment and Reemployment Rights Act of 1994. 38 U.S.C. § 4301–4333.

Legal Citations

Albert v. Runyon, 6 F. Supp. 2d 57 (D. Mass. 1998).
Barnes v. Cochran, 944 F. Supp. 897 (S.D. Fla. 1996).
Bonsignore v. City of New York, 521 F. Supp. 394 (S.D.N.Y. 1982).
Brownfield v. City of Yakima, 612 F.3d 1140, 1144 (9th Cir. 2010).
Carrillo v. National Council of Churches of Christ in the U.S., 976 F. Supp. 254, 256 (S.D.N.Y, 66 1997).
Colon v. City of Newark, #A-3260-03T23260-03T2, 2006 WL 1194230 (N.J.A.D. 2006).
Conte v. Horcher, 50 Ill. App. 3d 151 (1977).

Cremer v. City of Macomb Board of Fire and Police Commissioners, 281 Ill. App.3d 497, 499, 666 N.E.2d 1209, 1210 (1996).
Delaurentos & Miami-Dade County v. Peguero, 47 So. 3d 879 (Fla. Dist. Ct. App. 2010).
Hild v. Bruner, 496 F. Supp. 93 (D.N.J. 1980).
Leonel v. American Airlines, 400 F.3d 702 (9th Cir. 2005).
Lewis v. Goodie, 798 F. Supp. 382 – Dist. Court, WD Louisiana 1992.
Mason v. Stock, 869 F. Supp. 828 (D. Kan. 1994).
McGreal v. Ostrov, 368 F.3d 657 (7th Cir. 2004).
McKenna v. Fargo, 451 F. Supp. 1355 (D.N.J. 1978).
McKnight v. Monroe County, 2002 – McKnight v. Monroe Cty. Sheriff's Dep't, IP 00-1880-C-B/F, 2002 U.S. Dist. LEXIS 18148 (S.D. Ind. Sep. 23, 2002).
Nilsson v. City of Mesa, 503 F. 3d 947 – Court of Appeals (9th Circuit 2007).
Pettus v. Cole, 49 Cal.App.4th 402, 57 Cal. Rptr. 2d 46 (Cal. Ct. App. 1996).
Siegfried v. City of Easton, 146 F.R.D. 98 (E.D. Pa. 1992).
Valdes v. City of Doral, 2013 – Valdes v. City of Doral, 662 F. App'x 803 (11th Cir. 2016).
Watson v. City of Miami Beach, 1999 – Watson v. City of Miami Beach, 177 F.3d 932 (11th Cir. 1999).
White v. County of Los Angeles, 2014 – White v. Cty. of L.A., 225 Cal. App. 4th 690, 170 Cal. Rptr. 3d 472 (2014).
Woods v. Town of Danville, WV, 712 F. Supp. 2d 502 – Dist. Court, SD West Virginia 2010.

Behavioral Health Training and Peer Support Programs

Hannah Pressley, Jessica R. Blalock, and Vincent B. Van Hasselt

For first responders (police officers, firefighters, emergency medical personnel, crime scene investigators, and emergency communication operators), the stresses of the job can become overwhelming and result in a higher risk for physical and mental health problems. Indeed, a burgeoning body of research has demonstrated that these populations are characterized by a variety of physical and mental health risks (Mona et al., 2019). These health concerns are reinforced over the course of their careers as they experience repeated exposure to traumatic events, shift work, disrupted sleep, and command/administrative inequities, to name but a few of the challenges inherent in their work (McCoy & Aamodt, 2010). Additionally, first responders are typically provided little to no recovery time after involvement in a particularly difficult call or event, compounding the issues that often lead to higher rates of mental health problems, in particular (see Klimley et al., 2018; Van Hasselt et al., 2020). To help first responders better identify and prevent the negative sequelae of their critical incident exposure, Behavioral Health and Peer Support Training programs have garnered increased attention, as reflected by their growing utilization in law enforcement and fire rescue agencies. The present chapter describes efforts in this area that have been conducted over the past several years and provides illustrations of their purpose, components, and utility. While still in the nascent stage, these programs exhibit considerable heuristic value as part of broad-spectrum mental health endeavors with first-responder populations.

H. Pressley (✉) · J. R. Blalock · V. B. Van Hasselt
College of Psychology, Nova Southeastern University, Davie, FL, USA
e-mail: hp462@mynsu.nova.edu

M. L. Bourke et al. (eds.), *First Responder Mental Health*,
https://doi.org/10.1007/978-3-031-38149-2_7

Behavioral Health Training

Behavioral Health Training (BHT) for first responders is a preventive strategy focused on: (1) increasing awareness of the signs and symptoms of stress- and mental health-related problems, (2) providing psychoeducation related to risk and protective factors for potential difficulties, and (3) discussing early identification efforts and intervention resources available for first responders experiencing any mental health difficulty. The training can serve as a model for first responder agencies to utilize when collaborating with internal and community resources to provide education and awareness for first responder personnel (Van Hasselt et al., 2020).

Ideally, BHTs should begin at the academy level and continue to be included in mandatory departmental training. This will ensure that all first responder personnel receive the training and are made aware of the available resources. The more exposure a first responder has to behavioral health resources, the more likely that individual will seek help before their distress has life-threatening impacts. Additionally, annual refresher training may help reduce the stigma of stress and mental health-related issues and increase peer awareness and support (Van Hasselt et al., 2020).

BHT materials need to be presented in a manner that fits within the first responder culture. This can be achieved in the description and content of the course, presentation style, and selection of training instructors (Van Hasselt et al., 2020). Since the use of humor has been an effective way to reduce stress in first responders (Sollie et al., 2017; Vivona, 2014), Behavioral Health Training should include media (e.g., videos and pictures) that will maintain an upbeat and relaxed learning environment. The use of a lighthearted approach can be helpful when trying to keep first responders engaged with the material.

BHTs can also assist qualified mental health professionals who want to help first responders interact with a population that traditionally has proven difficult to infiltrate (Van Hasselt et al., 2020). As facilitators of the training, the mental health professionals can begin to build rapport, understand the unique first responder culture, and gradually work to dismantle the stigma surrounding mental health care. Given that first responders are at a high risk of developing mental health issues over the course of their career, it is imperative that Behavioral Health Training focus on the most common concerns. The following section will briefly discuss recommended Behavioral Health Training modules regarding common mental health concerns first responders experience.

Behavioral Health Training Modules

As previously mentioned, first responders experience a higher risk of developing serious mental health concerns compared to other professions due to field-specific stressors. These field-specific stressors tend to exacerbate personal stressors-increasing divorce rates, burnout, poor sleep quality, and lack of positive coping mechanisms within first responders (McCoy & Aamodt, 2010). The Council of State Governments Justice Center (CSGJS, 2019) indicated the importance of collaboration between first responders and mental health. Though this research concerns responding to mental health calls, it also highlights the importance of education across these diagnoses and intervention options (CSGJS, 2019). Not only do first responders experience mental health calls frequently, they also experience a high prevalence of mental health concerns among themselves. In turn, the lack of awareness and available resources exacerbate mental health concerns. Mumford et al. (2015) identified the most prominent mental health concerns of first responders as posttraumatic stress symptoms, substance abuse, depression, suicide, and sleep disturbances.

More recently, a two-hour BHT program was developed in collaboration between a local police agency and a University psychology department. The training targets specific information utilizing prior law enforcement research and personal experience of mental health and police professionals. Each section focuses on significant issues that police officers often face – stress, depression, substance use, sleep disturbances, anxiety, Posttraumatic Stress Disorder (PTSD), and suicide. Outside resources for additional help are also presented (Van Hasselt et al., 2020). Additionally, to help decrease the stigma of mental health concerns within the first responder culture, facilitators briefly discuss common myths or misconceptions about mental health diagnoses. While initially developed for law enforcement, this BHT model has been adapted to serve other first responder personnel, including fire and rescue, corrections, emergency communication operators (Beamer, in press), and crime scene investigators (Plombon et al., 2020). For this chapter, each module will be discussed with all first responder populations in mind.

Curriculum

Stress

Prevalence BHT first focuses on stress because of its correlation with other areas of concern. Over the past decade, job-related illnesses caused 22% of law enforcement officer deaths (National Law Enforcement Officers Memorial Fund, 2023). Among firefighters, over 50% of deaths are due to extreme exhaustion and stress (Stanley et al., 2017). For these reasons, BHT discusses the fight-or-flight response, physiological effects of stress, and its correlation to negative health outcomes.

Presentation in First Responders Occupational stressors specific to first responders may include departmental oversight, insufficient equipment, and rotating work schedules. Personal stressors, such as family problems and financial difficulties, are likely weighing on first responders concurrently. Numerous studies have reported the association between high perceived stress and emotional distress, including anxiety and depression (Besharat et al., 2020), and PTSD (Wang et al., 2019). Prior research has also differentiated between acute and chronic stress and how physical (e.g., sedentary hours, running) and psychosocial (e.g., coping skills, isolation) aspects of policing impact the body (Anderson et al., 2002). When considering all first responders, these findings indicate the effects of acute stress persist after the end of the shift (Anderson et al., 2002), and chronic stress can result in burnout and lead to cynicism and detachment (Maslach & Leiter, 2016; Schaible & Six, 2015). Additionally, the public pressure to protect their community because of political and societal expectations can further exacerbate stress (Purba & Demou, 2019).

Depression

Prevalence A recent study examined rates of general mental health concerns among first responders after experiencing a global pandemic (Huang et al., 2022). Researchers found 31% of the first responders in the analysis reported experiencing depressive symptoms. Of the 31% who reported depressive symptoms, 16% endorsed severe depression. Overall, these researchers concluded the prevalence of depression, anxiety, and stress has increased in the past several years due to unique workplace stressors (i.e., lack of personal protective equipment and increase in calls). Brooks et al. (2016) examined the available literature on factors impacting psychological distress in first responders when providing disaster relief. With the increase in calls observed over the past several years, first responders are spending more time on scene, thereby increasing their risk of developing depressive-like symptoms. They further discussed the importance of proactive steps to increase first responder resiliency, support, and training opportunities (Brooks et al., 2016). Emergency medical personnel reported the highest rate of depression, with paramedics at 37% and emergency medical services at 28%. Additionally, 22% of law enforcement in the study reported depressive symptoms (Huang et al., 2022).

Presentation in First Responders Depression in first responders presents in a different manner than social withdrawal and depressed mood. Rather, first responders often report feelings of fatigue, loss of enthusiasm or drive, and feelings of guilt or hopelessness (Marston-Salem, 2019). Behavioral Health Training should emphasize how first responders present in a different manner than the stereotypical representation of depression. Common stereotypes regarding depression in first responders should also be covered in this section. Specifically, facilitators should work toward debunking the stigma regarding mental health issues as a weakness but rather a medical condition (Steinkopf et al., 2016). First responders should be cautioned of the potential increased irritability and sexual impulsivity or sexual acting out (Steinkopf et al., 2016). By providing psychoeducation on the differences in depressive symptoms for first responders versus the general public, it should help to reduce the stigma and increase help-seeking behaviors.

Substance Use

Prevalence Present research suggests one in four law enforcement officers endorse hazardous drinking patterns (Syed et al., 2020). Further, firefighters and emergency medical services personnel that participated in a Substance Abuse and Mental Health Services Administration (SAMHSA, 2018) survey endorsed patterns of problematic drinking. Of the firefighters who participated in the study, 88.9% endorsed alcohol use within the past month. With alcohol as a culturally accepted form of coping, this likely factors into current prevalence rates. BHT should define the differences between substance use, overuse, and abuse, and bring awareness to its prevalence within the field. Further, it is imperative to teach when drinking patterns become problematic and how to identify those patterns within themselves and fellow first responders. Syed et al. (2020) reported maladaptive coping, occupational stress, and poor social support as global risk factors for first responders developing mental health concerns. Yet, first responders often believe alcohol use and dependence are utilized to help cope with the underlying mental health concerns (Al-Humaid et al., 2007; SAMHSA, 2018). Therefore, to help alleviate alcohol overuse and dependence, underlying mental health concerns must be addressed throughout the provision of adequate care.

Presentation in First Responders It is common knowledge that within the first responder culture, social support and after-hour gatherings typically include alcohol. Accordingly, alcohol use has become a widely accepted and relied upon form of coping. Specifically, first responders reported utilizing alcohol as a primary method of coping with on-the-job stressors, prior to alcohol overuse and abuse (Al-Humaid et al., 2007; SAMHSA, 2018). This further highlights the prevalence and acceptance of substance use and indicates first responders exhibit problematic drinking patterns. Consequently, BHT should utilize this section as an opportunity to discuss the myths associated with substance abuse in first responders. These myths include alcohol improves sleep quality and quantity, and alcoholism is only present in those with physical signs (i.e., 'beer belly'; Steinkopf et al., 2016). BHT should also differentiate between problematic drinking and social drinking.

Sleep Disturbances

Prevalence First responders across the nation face the repercussions of shiftwork. These stressors are unique in that first responders are required to engage in unknown situations daily, and many have rotating shifts or required "midnights." The nature of this career requires physical and mental wear and tear and requires hyperarousal, as they must be ready to react at a moment's notice. On the other hand, first responders working rotating shifts are unable to train their body to sleep or relax at appropriate times (Cleveland Clinic, 2021). The Cleveland Clinic (2021) recognizes shift work as a form of sleep disorder, as the impact of the hyperarousal significantly impacts the body's central nervous system.

Presentation in First Responders After experiencing prolonged sleep disturbances, first responders may experience mood-related problems, increased work-related errors, and poor physical health (Cleveland Clinic, 2021). Further, since they do not achieve normal sleep cycles, they are unable to train their body to sleep or relax at appropriate times (Cleveland Clinic, 2021). This prevents their bodies from resetting during REM sleep, in turn increasing the likelihood of mood changes, increased irritability, and overall fatigue. Further, short- and long-term sleep loss or deprivation can lead to higher risks of hypertension, depression, poor cardiovascular health, and diabetes (Medic et al., 2017).

Anxiety

Prevalence A recent meta-analysis (Huang et al., 2022) reported the overall prevalence of anxiety among first responders was estimated to be 32%. Interestingly, the prevalence of anxiety varied among different first responder groups, with 38% for paramedics, 28% for emergency medical personnel, and 19% for police. Within the US general population, prevalence rates of generalized anxiety disorder ranges between 1.6% and 5% (Spitzer et al., 2006), with the latest estimates of 2.9% (American Psychiatric Association, 2022).

Presentation in First Responders Aspects of being a first responder are inherently anxiety-provoking. For example, low perceived safety and dealing with serious injuries or deceased bodies have been linked to increased anxiety (Brooks et al., 2016). In a small sample of emergency medical service providers, increases in PTSD, depression, and anxiety symptoms were predicted by poor sleep and lower social support (Feldman et al., 2021). Additionally, physical pain and discomfort has been proven to be significantly correlated with somatic, cognitive, and general anxiety (Bergen-Cico et al., 2015). While a substantial portion of first responders experience anxiety, the specific environment they work in may normalize it, and not allow for the first responder to recognize it cognitively, regardless of how their body responds. Simply put, it may be easier for first responders to both accept and acknowledge physical pain or discomfort as opposed to identifying the experience of anxiety related symptoms.

Posttraumatic Stress Disorder

Prevalence Due to the magnitude of critical incidents first responders experience, they are predisposed to the development of posttraumatic stress symptoms, with 5.9–22% developing trauma symptoms or PTSD (Flannery, 2015). A recent review examining the rates of PTSD and posttraumatic symptoms in first responders found approximately 10% of first responders in the US have symptoms consistent with a stress disorder (Klimley et al., 2018). While they may not meet the full criteria, these symptoms met partial or subthreshold criteria for a diagnosis of PTSD (Klimley et al., 2018). Further, studies have shown that experiencing multiple events was greater than any single event in predicting PTSD, and first responders are subjected to more critical incidents now than ever before (Breslau et al., 1999; Klimley et al., 2018). With both the occupational risk and the increase in witnessing a larger magnitude of critical incidents, first responders are at a significantly higher risk of developing symptoms consistent with PTSD than civilians (Lewis-Schroeder et al., 2018). The accumulation of traumatic events further predisposes first responders to develop severe pathological reactions (Jørgenson & Elklit, 2022), including long-term physical and mental health outcomes such as high cholesterol, hypertension, diabetes, gastrointestinal disorders, and sleep apnea (Mumford et al., 2021).

Presentation in First Responders Common misconceptions among first responders regarding stress and trauma exposure are that stress motivates them to complete the job and to normalize trauma exposure as an expectation of the job (Steinkopf et al., 2016). However, it is important to note that symptoms may present differently in first responders than in the general public. For example, The Institute of Health (2022) indicated first responders engage in higher rates of emotional numbing and avoidance. Avoidance symptoms could be seen through absences at work, increased alcohol use, and irritability. Emotional numbing leads to insensitivity toward workplace requirements and irritability or anger toward their work crew/unit. These symptoms often act as a protective factor for first responders yet lead to interpersonal difficulties, alcohol abuse, and workplace stress (McCoy & Aamodt, 2010). BHT should focus on providing psychoeducation on how stress-related disorders may look within first responders and encourage departmental or agency awareness. This awareness will help to identify those who are struggling with these symptoms to receive appropriate services.

Suicide

Prevalence While suicide rates of first responders are often under-reported, in 2017, more first responders died by suicide than in the line of duty (U.S. Fire Administration, 2021). Further, the U.S. Fire Administration (2021) reported EMS personnel are 1.39 times more likely to die by suicide than individuals in the general public. Blue H.E.L.P. (2022), a not-for-profit organization, compiled annual data to bring awareness to the prevalence of suicide among first responders. The organization outlines suicide rates by state, type of first responder, age, and gender. In 2021, there were 182 reported deaths by suicide by first responders across the U.S. (Blue H.E.L.P., 2022). Of the 182 deaths by suicide, 138 were law enforcement officers, 22 were correctional officers, 18 were fire, and 4 were EMS (Blue H.E.L.P., 2022).

These rates of suicide highlight the need for more BHT and mental health awareness in this population. More specifically, these findings emphasize the importance of recognizing warning signs and symptoms on the peer-to-peer level in agencies (Steinkopf et al., 2016). Further, BHT should focus on identifying these warning signs and encouraging first responders to have open conversations about suicide, potentially increasing awareness and access to resources for suicide prevention.

Presentation in First Responders Research suggests law enforcement officers are at the highest risk among first responders for death by suicide (Blue H.E.L.P., 2022). This is likely due to various factors, such as stigma, access to firearms, and lack of positive coping mechanisms. Regarding stigma, many first responders avoid discussing suicide as they believe there is nothing to be done, or they may put the idea in the individual's mind (Steinkopf et al., 2016). While it warrants mention that first responders show signs of suicidal ideation similar to that of the general public, the means of death is fatal as they have easier access to firearms (EMS World, 2022). Specifically, social isolation and mood changes (i.e., improved mood, enthusiasm) are common warning signs for suicidal ideation (Steinkopf et al., 2016). Further, BHT should caution first responders to be mindful of anniversaries that are particularly difficult for individuals that they had a close connection to, as these tend to be particularly tough times for first responders.

Additional Training Modules

Treatment/Intervention Options

Despite first responders presenting at higher risk for developing mental health concerns, research indicates this population has difficulty utilizing mental health professionals as a form of intervention (Jones et al., 2020). Therefore, this section of BHT should briefly discuss the various treatment options available for mental health concerns. Further, research highlighted challenges in both reaching first responders and establishing policies to delineate when to provide mental health resources (Kleim & Westphal, 2011). When providing Behavioral Health Training, it is imperative to first discuss the prevalence of mental health concerns and the tendency to self-rely, then provide additional intervention options. Providing general information decreases the reluctance and ambiguity surrounding treatment options. Typically, first responders believe medication to be the only method of intervention. In response, BHT should provide explicit information regarding the current treatment options as it may help to debunk this myth. Further, BHT facilitators should briefly discuss the importance of the mind-body connection. As it is common to visit a doctor for a physical health need, it is also equally important to speak to someone regarding mental health needs.

Available Resources

Finally, Behavioral Health Training should provide open access to nationwide resources, such as hotlines and websites (Steinkopf et al., 2016). Any information regarding agency-specific resources (i.e., employee assistance programs and insurance-approved clinicians) should be included to provide individualized assistance (Steinkopf et al., 2016). Information regarding peer support programs within the agency should also be promoted within this section of training to encourage first responders to utilize peer interaction as a supportive mechanism during mental health needs. This is beneficial and an essential part of BHT as it is more difficult to find mental health treatment when going through a crisis, as knowledge of resources serves as a facilitator to help-seeking (Jones et al., 2020). This section of BHT should cover who to contact when mental health concerns arise, how to contact them, and limits of confidentiality, if any. This will give first responders a sense of agency and remove ambiguity from the process/expectations of seeking mental health treatment or resources when needed, in turn reducing the stigma associated (Jones et al., 2020).

Discussion

By implementing BHT at an academy level, first responders will have access to mental health training and resources available within their agency. Although first responders are generally apprehensive about engaging in mental health care, providing psychoeducation, debunking common misconceptions, and promoting awareness may be beneficial in helping them identify changes on a peer-to-peer level.

Effectiveness

At present, there is no standard practice for BHT across the United States; however, implementation has been effective. Steinkopf et al. (2016) conducted a program evaluation of the BHT completed with Firefighters in Broward County, Florida. The researchers examined the modules covered and conducted a pre- and postevaluation. They found overall, the firefighters accurately identified the information learned and found it to be helpful. Given that providing first responders with digestible psychoeducation is one of the aims of BHT, it appears this model was effective in reaching its goal (Steinkopf et al., 2016; Van Hasselt et al., 2020). To help provide more qualitative data regarding the effectiveness of BHT, it is essential to implement a pre- and posttest evaluation within the agency. This will allow facilitators to receive feedback based on the material covered, make improvements, and provide more individualized mental health care.

Additionally, BHT assists in destigmatizing mental health concerns. By providing accurate information to first responders regarding mental health concerns, BHT helps debunk the myths reinforcing the stigma. These misconceptions and the first responder culture play significant roles in perpetuating their mental health concerns. For example, Stanton (2022) reported that nearly half of the first responders they interviewed believed there would be repercussions at work for getting mental health care. While this is a possibility, it is not the normal response from agencies. Therefore, BHT is beneficial in that it provides an opportunity to create awareness of the potential barriers to help-seeking behaviors.

Finally, to understand what barriers exist that are preventing first responders from receiving care, the cultural stigma among first responders and the utilization of mental health professionals needs must be assessed within each agency. Jones et al. (2020) reported three patterns that impact first responders from seeking mental health care: knowledge of resources, barriers (i.e., culture, potential confidentiality breach, prior negative experience, and family burden), and facilitators to help-seeking. By providing a detailed understanding of the departmental or agency resources, BHT can attempt to reduce barriers to seeking services and increase first responder knowledge of who they can contact to receive help. Additionally, BHT facilitators should address the cultural challenges that occur within the population regarding mental health. Promoting mental health resources at an academy level is the first step to remedying the stigma and self-reliance that often occurs (Jones et al., 2020; Soomro & Yanos, 2019).

Limitations

While the primary limitation remains the lack of empirical data on BHT and its efficacy, there are two mechanisms that can help offset this need. First, agencies must have buy-in to protect their employees' mental health needs (Rutkow et al., 2011). To achieve such buy-in, it is imperative to have culturally competent BHT facilitators to increase the participation and engagement of the agency and the individuals. Through utilizing culturally competent clinicians, BHT helps to break down some of the barriers seen in accessing mental health care. Training facilitators must understand the impact of the stigma, how these diagnoses present and are viewed by first responders, and provide resources that are beneficial and easily accessible. This will, in turn, increase mental health services that are utilized by first responders, establish trust between providers and first responders, and increase awareness of the available resources.

Peer Support Programs

Society regularly relies on first responders to perform their duties effectively and make sound judgments in response to highly stressful, life-threatening situations. Due to a combination of trauma exposure (e.g., repeated call-outs to traumatic scenes, domestic disputes, disorderly conduct, civil disorder), occupational stress (e.g., shift work, rotating schedules, personnel shortages), and a persistent stigmatized culture, there is a heightened risk for the development of various mental and physical health disorders compared to the general population. Specifically, first responders are at an increased risk for alcohol abuse (Ballenger et al., 2011; Ménard & Arter, 2013), post-traumatic stress disorder (Klimley et al., 2018), depression (Hartley et al., 2013), cardiovascular disease (Hartley et al., 2013), marital discord and domestic violence (Kirschman et al., 2015), and suicide (Chae & Boyle, 2013; Violanti et al., 2013). Thus, the need for effective psychological and behavioral health intervention is imperative to the overall well-being of first responders. In the following sections, we examine the current and relevant literature regarding implementation methods and attitudes toward peer support programs within the first responder community.

Overview

Peer support programs (PSP), a broad term used to describe services delivered by people with lived experience, are now regarded as a hallmark of recovery-oriented care (Davidson et al., 2012), which is currently viewed as an essential additional resource for rehabilitative and ongoing continued care. Within the existing literature, anticipated mechanisms of peer services include: "increased participant social bonds and activity, an emphasis on recovery-oriented attitudes such as hope and empowerment, and promotion of awareness, trust, and engagement in mental health care" (Kumar et al., 2019, p. 416).

Many peer support programs rely on the established and frequent interaction among peers within the first responder agencies. Working long shifts together qualifies them to take notice of any behavioral or psychological changes in their peers. The established rapport and close nature of the work may allow for the peer to feel more comfortable discussing any difficulties they have been experiencing; and, a conversation coming from a concerned colleague may be better received than an immediate referral to outside services. Similarly, there is an underlying commonality that may serve to unify a response coming from someone who understands the culture and may have lived through similar experiences. Without serving as a therapist or providing any professional assistance, a peer may assist an individual in recognizing a problem that has impacted some aspect of their ability to perform their job duties, and serve as the first step toward determining the best avenue for appropriate assistance.

Guidelines

The increase in awareness and implementation of peer support programs has grown at a quicker rate than most agencies' abilities to develop guidelines. As a result, research into specific peer support programs yields relatively insufficient information, and program descriptions are often either advertised within the agency or occasionally as a supplemental resource on the agency website. For that reason, little consensus exists regarding the most basic concepts and procedures for peer support programs (Creamer et al., 2012). In response, researchers developed evidence-informed peer support guidelines for use in high-risk organizations designed to increase consistency around goals and procedures and provide a foundation for a systematic approach to evaluating the program (Creamer et al., 2012). They found peer supporters should (a) provide an empathic, listening ear; (b) provide low-level psychological intervention; (c) identify peers who may be at risk to themselves or others; and (d) facilitate pathways to professional help. They noted the use of spontaneous or informal peer support during the day was considered an important aspect of peer support programs. It was agreed that peer supporters should not limit their activities to high-risk incidents but rather should be part of routine employee health and welfare. The consensus to become a peer supporter was that the individual should be a member of the target population, with considerable experience in the field of work, and should be respected by their peers. It was agreed that potential peer supporters undergo a formal application and selection process.

In 2016, The International Association of Chiefs of Police (ICAP) provided peer support guidelines that included sections detailing the purpose, definitions, administration, selection/deselection, consultation services from mental health professionals, confidentiality, role conflict, and training. The guidelines were intended to provide all public safety employees in an agency the opportunity to receive emotional and tangible support through times of personal or professional crisis and to help anticipate and address potential difficulties. The guidelines were also intended to provide information and recommendations on forming and maintaining a peer support structure for sworn and civilian personnel in law enforcement agencies (ICAP, 2020).

In 2020, Police Executive Research Forum provided a document detailing occupational risk and outlined what every police agency should do to prevent suicide among personnel (Martin, 2020). Within this lengthy document, peer support is highlighted as a recommended action to prevent suicide. It recommends that agencies should provide a range of programs, including employee assistance programs and peer support, to assist personnel who may need help. Further, they should train employees on how to access those services and identify and support fellow personnel showing signs of stress, depression, or behavioral crisis. The goal of peer support is highlighted as a confidential service that is intended to help the officers accept professional help from a qualified clinician. Essentially, peer support provides the first responders the transition to do just that.

PSPs have garnered increased interest and support in the first responder community (Cnapich et al., 2022). Within organizations that have created peer support programs to enhance the mental health and well-being of first responders, training topics often include the long-term psychological effects of repeated exposure to traumatic events and job stress, the benefits of peer support training and what constitutes a successful peer support team, and the key objectives of the program (Cnapich et al., 2022). To date, most of the research related to peer support focuses on qualitative feedback and the perceived impact of the program. While it is crucial to know whether the peers find the interaction beneficial, more research is warranted to determine whether peer involvement is mitigating any long-term potential consequences associated with FR work.

Advantages

In recent years, the implementation of peer support training as a strategy for identifying and intervening in psychological and behavioral issues has become widely accepted among the first responder community (Henderson et al., 2018). PSPs are based on the notion that those who have experienced and overcome the negative impacts of traumatic and stressful events are uniquely qualified to help others dealing with similar experiences. This is believed to be done through increased awareness and vigilance, empathic responding, and personal validation (Repper & Carter, 2011).

Several advantages of peer support programs include training in the identification of risk factors for behavioral health problems, reducing stigma as the "first line of defense" by assuring seeking help is not a sign of weakness, facilitating easier approachability for peers initially relaying any problems, and providing outside resources for additional care. These advantages are likely to contribute to the overall goals of peer support programs, which include but are not limited to (a) providing an informal resource for peers in their personal or professional lives, (b) fostering social, physical, and emotional health of fellow FR, (c) recognize and evaluate conflicts, utilize active listening skills, and offer support, (d) demonstrate and promote communication, encouragement, trust, and confidentiality in those receiving peer services, and (e) identify and serve as a liaison between peers who need help, and the appropriate resources (see Van Hasselt et al., 2019).

Disadvantages

While the majority of the literature discusses the potential benefits of PSP, there is limited information regarding potential disadvantages. From a peer supporter perspective, there may be an increased potential for the development of burnout, as they are continuing to be exposed to regular trauma during their own work hours but subsequently are consoling and attending to peer trauma. Within the profession, in conjunction with other life stressors, FR suffer from a high degree of compassion fatigue (Figley, 1999) and burnout (Alexander, 1999). Burnout can result from emotionally-draining interactions with other people, which likely includes peer interactions. Interventions to combat secondary trauma and burnout, or limit the effects of vicarious and secondary trauma may limit the potential of indirect trauma interactions within work environments (Palm et al., 2004).

Disenfranchised grief or complex bereavement may also arise from the ongoing interactions with peers who may be experiencing differing levels of grief that may resemble a similar instance for the peer supporter. For this reason, consensus shows that a mental health professional should occupy the role of clinical director and should be involved in training and supervision of the peer support programs (Creamer et al., 2012). Having a professional resource to encourage self-care and provide a supervisory role may help to reduce the capacity, at least to some degree, of experiencing the effects of vicarious or secondary trauma. The inclusion of information regarding the risk factors and awareness of the potential dangers of peer support programs should be discussed prior to the initiation of a program.

Utilization

In organizations with peer support programs, approximately half of the participants, and half of those who had not participated, stated they would be likely to very likely to seek peer support in the future. Over half of the participants reported the peer support programs directly or indirectly helped them to perform their job better and/or improve their home life (Digliani, 2018). Some evidence indicates that peer support programs have a higher utilization rate than employee assistance programs (EAPs) and mental health professionals (Goss, 2013). The rationale for these programs is that consulting with a peer may reduce the resistance and stigma associated with seeking help. More specifically, the rationale for the provision of peer support programs often includes the goals of meeting the moral and legal duty of care for their employees, in addition to addressing several barriers to standard care (i.e., stigma, lack of trust, poor access to resources) (Creamer et al., 2012). While research concerning the efficacy of peer support programs is lacking, there has been evidence that shows enhancing and protecting social support can increase an individual's ability to deal with a potentially traumatic event (Norris & Stevens, 2007). Thus, within high-risk populations, such as first responders, peer support programs represent an attempt to operationalize social support.

Personnel Attitudes and Perceptions

Many peer support programs have been implemented in first responder agencies to the satisfaction of their personnel (Andersen et al., 2015; Digliani, 2018). Beneficial interactions include perceived degree of satisfaction regarding program interaction;

reported direct or indirect help to improve their job duties and/or home life; reduced feelings of stigma regarding seeking services; increased utilization of resources provided by peer support; acknowledgment of future participation and fellow peer referral. These attitudes were often measured utilizing self-report instruments and questionnaires based on either hypothetical programs or regarding the recent implementation of a PSP. It should be noted that there is no clear or consistent outcome measurement that provides data to address whether these programs are in fact beneficial to the population they serve. Further, there appears to be no assessment measure that adequately assesses the efficacy of PSP. One study, however, conducted by Heffren and Hausdorf (2016), utilized the Distress Disclosure Index (DDI) and concluded that police officers found it easier to talk to other officers within a supportive environment. In conjunction with the FR culture and inhouse mentality, the attitudes reflect a preference for communicating among themselves rather than to an outside referral or resource.

Digliani (2018) conducted a survey to inquire whether peer support programs work. Of the 631 employees that completed the survey, 48% reported having participated in peer support. Of that group, over half of the participants reported it directly or indirectly helped them to perform their job better and/or improve their home life. Nearly nine out of 10 reported peer support interactions to be helpful to very helpful. Nearly eight out of 10 reported they would seek peer support again, if necessary. Nearly nine out of 10 reported they would recommend peer support to a coworker known to be dealing with stressful circumstances. Finally, nearly six out of 10 participants who did not indicate participating in peer support stated they would be likely to very likely to seek peer support in the future if necessary.

Millard (2020) conducted a qualitative small-sample study focused on the utilization and impact of peer support programs. A sample of nine police peer support team members perceived peer support as being more than just a conversation. It was considered an "indispensable tool for helping police officers learn about themselves, mental health, and the importance of seeking help early" (p. 7). This study provided emergent themes and subthemes of peer support effectiveness that included: mental health literacy, stigma reduction, police culture, internal policy, and provincial standards. Participants strongly agreed that organizations need to implement internal policies regarding peer support, which include the need to develop an adequacy standard for peer support and mental health training.

Current Program Methods

The term peer support includes programs that provide various service types with different organizational structures. However, there appears to be an overall consensus regarding several general elements of peer support programs. The main goals of peer support are: "(a) to provide an empathic, listening ear; (b) to provide low-level psychological intervention; (c) to identify peers who may be at risk to themselves or others; and (d) to facilitate pathways to professional help" (Creamer et al., 2012,

p. 137). It is evident that the goals of peer support relate to psychological well-being more broadly and do not relate solely to recovery from a highly stressful situation or traumatic incident.

From a selection standpoint, a formal application or referral procedure is highly recommended. More specifically, a member of the target population with experience within the field is essential to ensure the credibility of the peer supporter (Creamer et al., 2012). Once selection of the appropriate individuals has been made, required training ensues with an emphasis on behavioral and psychological constructs. Learning modules often include in-depth educational lectures on behavioral and psychological constructs such as stress, active listening skills, depression, substance use, anxiety and posttraumatic stress disorder, and suicide (Van Hasselt et al., 2019). Further, the introduction of role-play scenarios following the educational component of training has proven to be a useful tool in assessing the competencies of basic skills (such as active listening). To our knowledge, there do not appear to be any other peer support programs that formally use role-play scenarios in the initial and ongoing training. Following training, the focus remains on varying degrees of continued education, supervision, and consultation policies.

When determining a peer support team, the following six objectives should be established: (a) serve as a resource for **peers** during times of crisis; (b) foster **peer** emotional health; (c) recognize and evaluate conflicts, use active listening skills, and offer **support;** (d) demonstrate and provide encouragement and trust; (e) identify problem signs and symptoms that may indicate the need for help; and (f) provide options and referrals for outside mental health resources when needed (Van Hasselt et al., 2019). Training modules should focus on active listening skills, stress, depression, substance use, anxiety and PTSD, suicide, and resilience. Additionally, role-play scenarios may be included at the end of each module to incorporate and practice newly acquired information and skills (Van Hasselt et al., 2019).

Law Enforcement

Based on the increased risk of suicide among law enforcement, peer support programs among this first responder population have been more widely researched. A 2015 survey of Finnish police officers sought to answer the following questions: (a) What do police officers know about stress, trauma, and health? (b) Are police officers interested in attaining more knowledge (and in what ways) about stress, trauma, and health? and (c) Are police officers open to seeking help for trauma and/or stress-related issues, and if so, where do they prefer to seek help? They found officers were open to learning more about both traditional (e.g., peer support) and alternative therapeutic techniques (e.g., relaxation). And, many reported a willingness to enroll in such programs if offered by the organization. Further, with regard to the ways in which participants wanted to learn about posttrauma interventions, most stated they preferred basic training (39.4%), followed by debriefing practices (33.4%), formal peer support (33.3%), and handbooks (31.5%) (Andersen et al., 2015).

Van Hasselt et al. (2019) developed the Peers as Law Enforcement Support (PALS) program in collaboration with a local police agency and a University psychology department. PALS is voluntary peer support training whose goals are to provide police officers the opportunity to assist each other in times of professional or personal crisis, and to help each other keep mentally healthy. The purpose of this program is to reduce the stigma of seeking help in the context of police culture, which views mental health service providers with suspicion. The program emphasizes that peer team members be sensitive to issues of trust, confidentiality, and anonymity for peers seeking assistance. The goals of PALS training of peer support personnel are to: (a) provide a resource for peers during times of crisis in their personal or professional lives; (b) foster social, physical, and emotional health of fellow police officers; (c) learn to recognize and evaluate conflicts, utilize active listening skills, and offer support; (d) demonstrate and provide communication, encouragement, trust, and confidentiality in officers receiving peer services; (e) identify and serve as a liaison between peers who need help, and provide the appropriate resources.

Training modules cover the topics of stress, active listening skills, depression, substance use, anxiety and posttraumatic stress disorder, suicide, tactical wellness, relationships/work-life balance, and scenario-based training. In a pilot study, a preliminary evaluation of participants' perceptions of the quality of course content and instructor effectiveness was carried out. Results indicated that the activities were practical and aided in the learning of material/skills and provided information that could be used on the job. Further, the participants viewed the trainers as well-prepared, engaging, knowledgeable, and encouraging of discussion throughout the program.

Fire Rescue

Gulliver et al. (2019) examined access, attitudes, and preferences regarding behavioral health programs among individuals in the fire service. Results indicate that the most commonly endorsed barriers to behavioral health programs were clinician unfamiliarity with the work culture (53%), fear of breach in confidentiality (51%), and stigma (43%) (Gulliver et al., 2019). Despite the availability of behavioral health or other psychological support services from most departments, the majority of the firefighters in this study indicated a preference for seeking out a spouse or family member, or a private professional service. However, over the course of their career in the fire service, firefighters became less likely to seek assistance from their immediate social support (i.e., spouse/family member, coworker, and officer). Instead, they were more likely to seek help from a private, professional service or a department-related EAP service (Gulliver et al., 2019). This finding reiterates the need for clinicians to consider individual preferences, and potential generational or otherwise age-related influences, in the determination of help-seeking behaviors.

Emergency Dispatchers

Findings from a National Wellness Survey indicated ECOs were as likely to seek support from a mental health professional as they were from a peer. Supportive interaction with vocational peers may be particularly helpful for dispatchers because of the potential increase in rapport due to shared historical experiences, capability to normalize, reduced stigma, and implicit understanding of the unique occupational situations (Forster & Haiz, 2015). However, gaps still exist in the current empirical literature regarding treatment comparisons and outcome measurements for peer support programs. Ideally, peer support should be a supplementary resource in conjunction with adequate mental health programs to ensure the proficiency of services (Van Hasselt et al., 2019). Understanding the tendency to seek out peers at the same rate as mental health professionals can be instrumental in determining whether a combination of the two can be established as a potential efficacious treatment option that emergency communication operators will be more receptive to.

Differences Among First Responder Groups

While job duties and exposure to trauma differ among the various first responder groups (i.e., police, fire and rescue, emergency medical services, and emergency dispatch), it may be worth evaluating whether specific first responder jobs have an impact on the peer support interaction. There is certainly variability across agencies on several factors, such as funding, geographic location, and department size; thus, implications from one agency may not be generalizable to another. It could be argued that having someone who understands the first responder community could be beneficial. However, whether their lived work experience is exactly like that of the peer may alter the interaction. Similar backgrounds may serve to facilitate easier discussion and understanding related to the experience. However, they may also serve to increase the likelihood of comparing traumas and result in vicarious or compounding trauma. Further, specifics related to the peer's difficulty may be unique and not benefit from being equated with a similar experience of a colleague. A "rookie" firefighter may also dismiss their reaction to an event as being less significant than that of a seasoned firefighter, which may further decrease their motivation to seek help.

Summary

Peer support following traumatic incidents may be of direct benefit to the affected individuals and also contribute to a culture of caring, further benefiting the well-being of all agency personnel (Feuer, 2021). PSPs are designed to provide emotional, social, or practical support, and referrals to professional services when needed (IACP, 2020).

PSPs have the potential to influence a paradigm shift within professions traditionally prone to minimal disclosure. Supportive interaction with vocational peers may be particularly helpful for law enforcement officers because of the potential increase in rapport due to shared historical experiences, capability to normalize, reduced stigma, and implicit understanding of unique occupational situations. However, gaps still exist in the current empirical literature regarding treatment comparisons and outcome measurements for peer support programs. Efforts to ensure PSP efficacy should include pre- and posttest role-play assessments and knowledge acquisition measures to compare and adequately measure the progress of the program during its development. Training and ongoing evaluation should continue on a regular basis to remain current regarding the relevant research and to maintain assurance that the PSP is beneficial to its organization and the members it serves. Peer support should be a supplementary resource in conjunction with adequate mental health programs to ensure proficiency of services. In addition, further research should consider the potential risk of vicarious, co-occurring, or compounding psychological interactions between peer supporters as it pertains to the efficacy of peer support programs serving the first responder population.

References

Alexander, C. (1999). Police psychological burnout and trauma. In J. M. Violanti & D. Paton (Eds.), *Police trauma: Psychological aftermath of civilian combat* (pp. 54–64). Charles C. Thomas.

Al-Humaid, H., El-Guebaly, N., & Lussier, D. (2007). Substance use and the police: An international workplace experience. *Addictive Disorders and Their Treatment, 6*(3), 107–115. https://doi.org/10.1097/01.adt.0000210728.38509.3d

American Psychiatric Association. (2022). *Diagnostic and statistical manual of mental disorders: DSM-5-TR*. American Psychiatric Association.

Andersen, J. P., Papazoglou, K., Koskelainen, M., & Nyman, M. (2015). Knowledge and training regarding the link between trauma and health. *SAGE Open, 5*(2). https://doi.org/10.1177/2158244015580380

Anderson, G. S., Litzenberger, R., & Plecas, D. (2002). Physical evidence of police officer stress. *Policing: An International Journal of Police Strategies & Management, 25*(2), 399–420. https://doi.org/10.1108/13639510210429437

Ballenger, J. F., Best, S. R., Metzler, T. J., Wasserman, D. A., Mohr, D. C., Liberman, A., Delucchi, K., Weiss, D. S., Fagan, J. A., Waldrop, A. E., & Marmar, C. R. (2011). Patterns and predictors of alcohol use in male and female urban police officers. *The American Journal on Addictions, 20*(1), 21–29. https://doi.org/10.1111/j.1521-0391.2010.00092.x

Beamer, A. (in press). Emergency communication operators. In M. L. Bourke, V. B. Van Hasselt, & S. Buser (Eds.), *First responder mental health: A clinician's guide*. Springer.

Bergen-Cico, D., Lane, S., Thompson, M., Wozny, S., Zajdel, M., Barduhn, M., & Noce, J. (2015). The impact of post-traumatic stress on first responders: Analysis of cortisol, anxiety, depression, sleep impairment and pain. *International Paramedic Practice, 5*(3), 78–87. https://doi.org/10.12968/ippr.2015.5.3.78

Besharat, M.-A., Khadem, H., Zarei, V., & Momtaz, A. (2020). Mediating role of perceived stress in the relationship between facing existential issues and symptoms of depression and anxiety. *Iranian Journal of Psychiatry*. https://doi.org/10.18502/ijps.v15i1.2442

Blue H.E.L.P. (2022). *The numbers* [Infograph]. https://bluehelp.org/the-numbers/

Breslau, N., Chilcoat, H. D., Kessler, R. C., & Davis, G. C. (1999). Previous exposure totrauma and PTSD effects of subsequent trauma: Results from the Detroit Area Survey of Trauma. *American Journal of Psychiatry, 156*(6), 902–907. https://doi.org/10.1176/ajp.156.6.902

Brooks, S. K., Dunn, R., Amlot, R., Greenberg, N., & Rubin, G. J. (2016). Social and occupational factors associated with psychological distress and disorder among disaster responders: A systematic review. *BMC Psychology, 4*, 18. https://doi.org/10.1186/s40359-016-0120-9

Chae, M. H., & Boyle, D. J. (2013). Police suicide: Prevalence, risk, and protective factors. *Policing: An International Journal of Police Strategies & Management, 36*(1), 91–118. https://doi.org/10.1108/13639511311302498

Cleveland Clinic. (2021, February 25). Shift work sleep disorder. *Cleveland Clinic*. https://my.clevelandclinic.org/health/diseases/12146-shift-work-sleep-disorder#:~:text=What%20are%20the%20symptoms%20of,shift%20worker%20suffers%20from%20SWSD

Cnapich, E., Rodriguez, S., Schuhmann, B., Couwels, J., Van Hasselt, V., & Blalock, J. (2022). First responder peer support programs. *FBI Law Enforcement Bulletin*, 1–9.

Council of State Governments Justice Center. (2019, April). *Police- mental health collaborations: A framework for implementing effective law enforcement responses for people who have mental health needs.* https://csgjusticecenter.org/wp-content/uploads/2020/02/Police-Mental-HealthCollaborations-Framework.pdf

Creamer, M. C., Varker, T., Bisson, J., Darte, K., Greenberg, N., Lau, W., Moreton, G., O'Donnell, M., Richardson, D., Ruzek, J., Watson, P., & Forbes, D. (2012). Guidelines for peer support in high-risk organizations: An international consensus study using the Delphi method. *Journal of Traumatic Stress, 25*(2), 13–141. https://doi.org/10.1002/jts.21685

Davidson, L., Amy, C. B., Guy, K., & Er, R. A. (2012). Peer support among persons with severe mental illnesses: A review of evidence and experience. *World Psychiatry, 11*(2), 123–128. https://doi.org/10.1016/j.wpsyc.2012.05.009

Digliani, J. (2018, March 15). *Police peer support: Does it work?* Law Enforcement Today. http://www.lawenforcementtoday.com/police-peer-support-work/

EMS World. (2022, June 22). *Study: First responders more likely to die by suicide than in line of duty*. https://www.hmpgloballearningnetwork.com/site/emsworld/news/study-first-responders-more-likely-die-suicide-line-duty

Feldman, T. R., Carlson, C. L., Rice, L. K., Kruse, M. I., Beevers, C. G., Telch, M. J., & Josephs, R. A. (2021) Factors predicting the development of psychopathology among first responders: A prospective longitudinal study. *Psychological Trauma: Theory Research Practice and Policy, 13*(1) 75–83. https://doi.org/10.1037/tra0000957

Feuer, B. S. (2021). First responder peer support: An evidence-informed approach. *Journal of Police and Criminal Psychology, 36*(3), 365. https://doi.org/10.1007/s11896-020-09420-z

Figley, C. R. (1999). Police compassion fatigue (PCF): Theory, research, assessment, treatment, and prevention. In J. M. Violanti & D. Paton (Eds.), *Police trauma: Psychological aftermath of civilian combat* (pp. 37–53). Charles C. Thomas.

Flannery, R. B. (2015). Treating psychological trauma in first responders: A multi-modal paradigm. *Psychiatric Quarterly, 86*(2), 261–267. https://doi.org/10.1007/s11126-014-9329-z

Forster, E., & Haiz, A. (2015). Paediatric death and dying: Exploring coping strategies of health professionals and perceptions of support provision. *International Journal of Palliative Nursing, 21*(6), 294–301. https://doi.org/10.12968/ijpn.2015.21.6.294

Goss, C. L. (2013). *Utilizing the brotherhood of law enforcement personnel: The need for a statewide peer officer support model.* Doctoral dissertation, State University of New York Empire State College.

Gulliver, S. B., Pennington, M. L., Torres, V. A., Steffen, L. E., Mardikar, A., Leto, F., Ostiguy, W., Zimering, R., & Kimbrel, N. A. (2019). Behavioral health programs in fire service: Surveying access and preferences. *Psychological Services, 16*(2), 340–345.

Hartley, T. A., Gu, J., Baughman, P. J., Violanti, J. M., Andrew, M. E., Fekedulegn, D., & Burchfiel, C. M. (2013). *Comparisons of cardiovascular health in police officers, U.S. general population and U.S. employed population.* PsycEXTRA Dataset. https://doi.org/10.1037/e577572014-379.

Heffren, C. D., & Hausdorf, P. A. (2016). Post-traumatic effects in policing: Perceptions, stigmas and help seeking behaviours. *Police Practice and Research, 17*(5), 420–433. https://doi.org/10.1080/15614263.2014.958488

Henderson, S., Burns, A., Van Hasselt, V. B., & LeDuc, T. J. (2018). FIRST response: The firefighter intervention and response support team. *Fire Engineering, 171*, 8–10.

Huang, G., Chu, H., Chen, R., Liu, D., Banda, K. J., O'Brien, A. P., Jen, H.-J., Chiang, K.-J., Chiou, J.-F., & Chou, K.-R. (2022). Prevalence of depression, anxiety, and stress among first responders for medical emergencies during COVID-19 pandemic: A meta-analysis. *Journal of Global Health, 12*. https://doi.org/10.7189/jogh.12.05028

Institute of Health. (2022). *PTSD in first responders*. https://institutesofhealth.org/ptsd-in-firstresponders/#:~:text=First%20responders%20with%20PTSD%20sometimes,alcohol%20use%20or%20substance%20abuse

International Association of Chiefs of Police. (2020). *An occupational risk – Police executive research forum*. https://www.policeforum.org/assets/PreventOfficerSuicide.pdf

Jones, S., Agud, K., & McSweeney, J. (2020). Barriers and facilitators to seeking mental healthcare among first responders: "Removing the darkness". *Journal of the American Psychiatric Nurses Association, 26*(1), 43–54. https://doi.org/10.1177/1078390319871997

Jørgensen, L. K., & Elklit, A. (2022). Trauma and critical incident exposure in law enforcement. In *Police psychology* (pp. 87–111). Academic.

Kirschman, E., Kamena, M., & Fay, J. (2015). *Counseling cops: What clinicians need to know*. Guilford Publications.

Kleim, B., & Westphal, M. (2011). Mental health in first responders: A review and recommendation for prevention and intervention strategies. *Traumatology, 17*(4), 17–24. https://doi.org/10.1177/1534765611429079

Klimley, K. E., Van Hasselt, V. B., & Stripling, A. M. (2018). Posttraumatic stress disorder inpolice, firefighters, and emergency dispatchers. *Aggression and Violent Behavior, 43*, 33–44. https://doi.org/10.1016/j.avb.2018.08.005

Kumar, A., Azevedo, K. J., Factor, A., Hailu, E., Ramirez, J., Lindley, S. E., & Jain, S. (2019). Peer support in an outpatient program for veterans with posttraumatic stress disorder: Translating participant experiences into a recovery model. *Psychological Services, 16*(3), 415–424. https://doi.org/10.1037/ser0000269

Lewis-Schroeder, N. F., Kieran, K., Murphy, B. L., Wolff, J. D., Robinson, M. A., & Kaufman, M. L. (2018). Conceptualization, assessment, and treatment of traumatic stress in first responders: A review of critical issues. *Harvard Review of Psychiatry, 26*(4), 216–227. https://doi.org/10.1097/HRP.0000000000000176

Marston-Salem, N. (2019, August 21). Signs of depression in your first responder loved one. *Fountain Hills Recovery*. https://fountainhillsrecovery.com/blog/first-responder-depression/

Martin, S. (2020). *Peer support as a powerful tool in law enforcement suicide prevention*. https://www.theiacp.org/sites/default/files/2020-10/244736_IACP_NOSI_PeerSupport_p5.pdf

Maslach, C., & Leiter, M. P. (2016). Burnout. In *Stress: Concepts, cognition, emotion, and behavior* (pp. 351–357). Academic. https://doi.org/10.1016/b978-0-12-800951-2.00044-3

McCoy, S. P., & Aamodt, M. G. (2010). A comparison of law enforcement divorce rates with those of other occupations. *Journal of Criminal Psychology, 25*, 1–16. https://doi.org/10.1007/s11896-009-9057-8

Medic, G., Wille, M., & Hemels, M. E. H. (2017). Short- and long-term health consequences of sleep disruption. *National Science of Sleep, 9*, 151–161. https://doi.org/10.2147/NSS.S134864

Ménard, K. S., & Arter, M. L. (2013). Police officer alcohol use and trauma symptoms: Associations with critical incidents, coping, and social stressors. *International Journal of Stress Management, 20*(1), 37–56. https://doi.org/10.1037/a0031434

Millard, B. (2020). Utilization and impact of peer-support programs on police officers' mental health. *Frontiers in Psychology, 11*. https://doi.org/10.3389/fpsyg.2020.01686

Mona, G. G., Chimbari, M. J., & Hongoro, C. (2019). A systematic review on occupational hazards, injuries and diseases among police officers worldwide: Policy implications for the South African Police Service. *Journal of Occupational Medicine and Toxicology, 14*(1), 1–15. https://doi.org/10.1186/s12995-018-0221-x

Mumford, E. A., Taylor, B. G., & Kubu, B. (2015). Law enforcement officer safety and wellness. *Police Quarterly, 18*(2), 111. https://doi.org/10.1177/1098611114559037

Mumford, E. A., Liu, W., Taylor, B. G., & Ramey, S. (2021). Profiles of US law enforcement officers' diagnosed health conditions: Results from a probability- based sample of officers. *Journal of Occupational & Environment Medicine, 63*(5), 422–431. https://doi.org/10.1097/JOM.0000000000002162

National Law Enforcement Officers Memorial Fund. (2023, March 24). *Causes of law enforcement deaths*. Retrieved April 1, 2023, from https://nleomf.org/memorial/facts-figures/officer-fatality-data/causes-of-law-enforcement-deaths/

Norris, F. H., & Stevens, S. P. (2007). Community resilience and the principles of mass trauma intervention. *Psychiatry: Interpersonal & Biological Processes, 70*(4), 320–328. https://doi.org/10.1521/psyc.2007.70.4.320

Palm, K. M., Polusny, M. A., & Follette, V. M. (2004). Vicarious traumatization: Potential hazards and interventions for disaster and trauma workers. *Prehospital and Disaster Medicine, 19*(1), 73–78.

Plombon, B.A., Bryant, T., & Van Hasselt, V.B. (2020, January–March). Behavioral health training for crime scene investigators. *Florida Division of the International Association for Identification News* (pp. 30–35).

Purba, A., & Demou, E. (2019). The relationship between organisational stressors and mental wellbeing within police officers: A systematic review. *BMC Public Health, 19*(1). https://doi.org/10.1186/s12889-019-7609-0

Repper, J., & Carter, T. (2011). A review of the literature on peer support in mental health services. *Journal of Mental Health, 20*(4), 392–411.

Rutkow, L., Gable, L., & Links, J. M. (2011). Protecting the mental health of first responders: Legal and ethical considerations. *Journal of Law, Medicine, & Ethics, 39*(21), 56–59. https://doi.org/10.1111/j.1748-720X.2011.00567.x

Schaible, L. M., & Six, M. (2015). Emotional strategies of police and their varying consequences for burnout. *Police Quarterly, 19*(1), 3–31. https://doi.org/10.1177/1098611115604448

Sollie, H., Kop, N., & Euwema, M. C. (2017). Mental resilience of crime scene investigators: How police officers perceive and cope with the impact of demanding work situations. *Criminal Justice and Behavior, 44*(12), 1580–1603. https://doi.org/10.1177/009385481776959

Soomro, S., & Yanos, P. T. (2019). Predictors of mental health stigma among police officers: The role of trauma and PTSD. *Journal of Police and Criminal Psychology, 34*(2), 175–183. https://doi.org/10.1007/s11896-018-9285-x

Spitzer, R. L., Kroenke, K., Williams, J. B., & Löwe, B. (2006). A brief measure for assessing Generalized Anxiety Disorder: the GAD-7. *Archives of Internal Medicine, 166*(10), 1092–1097. https://doi.org/10.1001/archinte.166.10.1092

Stanley, I. H., Boffa, J. W., Hom, M. A., Kimbrel, N. A., & Joiner, T. E. (2017). Differences in psychiatric symptoms and barriers to mental health care between volunteer and career firefighters. *Psychiatry Research, 247*, 236–242. https://doi.org/10.1016/j.psychres.2016.11.037

Stanton, C. (2022, June 10). *Police, firefighters die by suicide more often than in line of duty. Why rates remain high.* USA Today. https://www.usatoday.com/story/news/nation/2022/06/10/high-suicide-rate-police-firefighters-mental-health/7470846001/

Steinkopf, B. L., Klinoff, V. A., Van Hasselt, V. B., Leduc, T. J., & Couwels, J. (2016). Behavioral health training for fire rescue personnel. *Fire Engineering, 169*, 59–67.

Substance Abuse and Mental Health Services Administration. (2018, May). *First responders: Behavioral health concerns, emergency response and trauma.* Disaster Technical Assistance Center Supplemental Research Bulletin, SAMHSA. https://www.samhsa.gov/sites/default/files/dtac/supplementalresearchbulletin-firstresponders-may2018.pdf

Syed, S., Ashwick, R., Schlosser, M., Jones, R., Rowe, S., & Billings, J. (2020). Global prevalence and risk factors for mental health problems in police personnel: A systematic review and meta-analysis. *Occupational Environmental Medicine, 77*, 737–747. https://doi.org/10.1136/oemed-2020-106498

U.S. Fire Administration. (2021, September 23). *Suicide prevention and awareness resources.* https://www.usfa.fema.gov/blog/ig-092321.html

Van Hasselt, V. B., Klimley, K. E., Rodriguez, S., Themis-Fernandez, M., Henderson, S. N., & Schneider, B. A. (2019). Peers as law enforcement support (PALS): An early prevention program. *Aggression and Violent Behavior, 48*, 1–5. https://doi.org/10.1016/j.avb.2019.05.004

Van Hasselt, V. B., Klimley Margres, K. E, Geller, S., & Rodriguez, S. (2020, September 10). Behavioral health training for police officers: A prevention program. *FBI Law Enforcement Bulletin, 89*, 1–8.

Violanti, J. M., Robinson, C. F., & Shen, R. (2013). Law enforcement suicide: A national analysis. *International Journal of Emergency Mental Health and Human Resilience, 15*(4), 289–298.

Vivona, B. D. (2014). Humor functions within crime scene investigations: Group dynamics, stress, and the negotiation of emotions. *Police Quarterly, 17*(2), 127–149. https://doi.org/10.1177/1098611114531418

Wang, Q., Xu, W., Ren, L., Wang, W., & Wang, Y. (2019). The relationship between hope and post-traumatic stress disorder in Chinese Shidu parents: The mediating role of Perceived stress. *Journal of Affective Disorders, 251*, 23–30. https://doi.org/10.1016/j.jad.2019.03.049

Psychological Safeguarding and First Responder Wellness

Michael L. Bourke

It goes without saying that first responders are exposed to traumatic circumstances at a much greater frequency than the average person; indeed, they are literally called to situations where they are expected to become directly involved in matters involving violence, loss, and depravity. As the name implies, first responders are not mere witnesses; they cannot cross their arms, shield their eyes, or walk away for a bit when things become difficult. They serve on the "thin lines" of our society – the blue line of the police, the red of the fire services, the white of EMTs and paramedics, the gold of emergency communication personnel, and the silver of the men and women who work in correctional institutions. First responders are the people in charge – the ones who handle the problems. They are our community's helpers, protectors, enforcers, and guardians.

First responders see human behavior at its worst, and the consequences of being regularly exposed to violence, suffering, and morally abhorrent behavior can be significant. For instance, many who work in law enforcement are familiar with the statistic that more officers die by their own hand than are killed in the line of duty. What is lesser known is the problem is worsening and that this observation is also true for firefighters and other first responders. The percentage of firefighters and EMS personnel who have contemplated suicide, for example, is ten times the rate of American adults (Abbott, et al., 2015). And the effects of large-scale stressors (e.g., pandemics, social justice protests, attitudes toward police) on public safety personnel are still unfolding.

Recently the Fairfax County Police Department in Northern Virginia, the Behavioral Analysis Unit of the United States Marshals Service, and Nova Southeastern University came together to determine how to assess these – and many other – issues facing first responders. We distributed anonymous online self-report surveys to 165 fire and EMS departments, police agencies, emergency

M. L. Bourke (✉)
Michael Bourke, Ph.D., PLLC, Springfield, VA, USA

M. L. Bourke et al. (eds.), *First Responder Mental Health*,
https://doi.org/10.1007/978-3-031-38149-2_8

communication operators (i.e., dispatchers), and correction officers across the United States. More than 8,700 respondents completed the measure. The survey, named the National Wellness Survey (NWS) for Public Safety Personnel, incorporated a demographic questionnaire and a number of empirically validated assessment measures that assess psychological symptoms, suicidality, PTSD and secondary traumatic stress, job burnout, social desirability, and substance use. Our[1] goal was to shed light on these and other important questions relating to the mental well-being of first responders.

Suicidal Ideation

Results, while not entirely unexpected, were nonetheless sobering. 7.8% of first responders indicated they were contemplating suicide (by comparison, the rate of suicidal thoughts in the general population is thought to be around 3%). This is particularly remarkable since the population of first responders is presumably healthier than the general population when they start their careers; most undergo psychological screening and then participate in a rigorous selection process. Those who endorsed suicidal thoughts were more likely to suffer from reactions to traumatic experiences; the more reactions they experienced, the more likely they were to report suicidal thoughts. These findings are consistent with extant research in repeated exposure to trauma (FEMA, 2018; Jahnke et al., 2016; Levy-Gigi et al., 2014). First responders who reported three out of five types of traumatic reactions were twice as likely to have suicidal thoughts, and those who experienced all five types of trauma were four times as likely to be actively considering taking their lives.

Depression

With regard to depressive symptoms, almost 1 in 4 respondents said they suffered depression as a consequence of their work. Depression tended to affect experienced personnel more than colleagues with less than 5 years on the job. Although seasoned first responders were much more likely to indicate they wanted help, they felt pessimistic or hopeless that things would improve. Not surprisingly, they were far more likely than their younger counterparts to think about retiring or leaving the profession.

It is noteworthy that most research in this area has been conducted with police officers and firefighters. Although studies have found that approximately one-quarter of emergency dispatchers (Lilly & Pierce, 2013) and one-third of correctional officers (Burhanullah et al., 2022) report depressive symptoms, research on these

[1] This author was a codeveloper of the NWS.

populations' suicide risk and mental health has lagged. A search on Google Scholar with the terms "depression" and "police officers" resulted in 18,400 citations, and replacing "police officers" with "firefighters" resulted in 12,600 citations; in contrast, searches using "depression" and "correctional officers" or "dispatchers" resulted in only 3190 and 1420 citations, respectively.

First-Responder Wellness

As awareness of the psychological issues faced by first responders has grown, an increasing number of departments have begun to develop plans to address these concerns. Resources vary from one agency to the next; one department might employ in-house psychologists, whereas another might rely on contract clinicians. Still others could use a model that consists solely of peer support, or they might avail themselves of the services of a police chaplain. These models are discussed elsewhere in this book, and it likely goes without saying that what works for one department may not be the best choice for another. It is also worth noting that hybrid models allow the greatest degree of flexibility and options for first responders. In any case, what clearly does *not* work is to offer no services – to bury our heads in the sand and pretend it "doesn't apply to this agency," or to adopt the mindset that if a first responder "can't cut it," they are better off finding another line of work.

What Stops First Responders from Seeking Help

Even when services are available, barriers exist that make it difficult for first responders to seek help. The National Wellness Survey assessed what stopped the first responders from getting assistance when they knew they needed it; the more common impediments follow.

"Treatment will be used against me." Many survey respondents expressed fears that seeking help from a mental health professional could hurt their career, future employment, or their ability to secure/maintain a security clearance. This concern is not entirely misplaced, despite the assertions of many online resources that indicate the problem is no longer an issue. Certainly some progress with regard to security clearances has been made; for example, as the result of a 2017 update to federal form SF-86, federal applicants and employees currently are not required to report certain forms of counseling (e.g., marital therapy) as mental health treatment. While that was a step in the right direction, by no means did the change remedy the issue. Further, state and local agencies may still require treatment – in any form – to be disclosed. As observed in a report to Congress by the US Department of Justice's Community Oriented Policing:

> Their fears [that seeking help will lead to sanctions or loss of professional opportunities] may not be without merit; some departments have policies requiring mental health treatment be reported, especially if it involves medication. Even when that is not the case, the small and communal nature of many departments, along with regressive attitudes about emotional health, can render stigmatization a real threat. (Spence, et al., 2019, p. 26)

Clinicians should recognize that the issue of whether mental health treatment can be "used against" the first responder will remain a valid concern no matter what policies are put in place. As a federal agent once explained to this author:

> When I apply to be on SWAT, the form will ask if I've ever received any kind of mental health treatment or counseling. I know I do not have to disclose why I sought therapy, and I know my therapist must keep my diagnosis confidential. But confidentiality doesn't matter. As soon as I check the box I will immediately be seen as potentially less stable than all the agents I'm competing against for this spot who did *not* check that box. So while I'm legally protected from being forced to disclose why I sought help, it's irrelevant. I'm done.

"Shrinks are for the weak." Given the hyper-masculine climate in many first-responder settings, the stigma persists that needing help can be a sign of weakness (Spence et al., 2019). This stigma can be reduced, however, and even reversed. To illustrate, about a decade ago an Internet Crimes Against Children (ICAC) taskforce commander in the Midwest became interested in wellness after he noticed the detrimental effects the work was having on his team. He researched safeguarding practices and then made changes to increase resilience and facilitate healthy coping. For instance, he strongly encouraged his employees to seek therapy as a precautionary measure – not to "fix" them but to help them "offload" the horrors they had encountered each week. Several years later, one of the team members disclosed to this author that *everyone* on the team was receiving therapy. He said:

> It used to be if someone was in therapy they'd be an outlier. Now if a new investigator joins the taskforce and mentions they are 'fine' and 'don't need therapy,' we all look at him or her and say, 'You get oil changes for your car, right? You get tune-ups? You don't wait until the car is breaks down, right? This is the same. You don't want to wait until things get bad. And why on earth would you want to take this [stuff] home with you on the weekend?'

In 2 years, they managed to completely reverse the stigma's polarity, so that therapy is now seen as what strong people do, rather than as something weak people need.

"I'm self-sufficient. I got this." The third impediment to seeking assistance was the belief by some first responders that they can handle almost anything all by themselves. On the NWS, three in ten first responders indicated they felt a need to "tough it out" or mitigate stressors on their own. This is more often witnessed in law enforcement circles rather than fire services or EMS, where nearly everything is done in teams and each firefighter/EMT/paramedic typically relies on others to accomplish important tasks. The toxic self-sufficiency in police departments, however, can also influence relationships with spouses and partners. Many officers claim they do not talk about work at home because their significant other would not understand; others say they try to "leave work at work" by refusing to discuss what they experienced that day, or they indicate they are "protecting" their family from the hazards of their job. The reality is this is a pervasive myth – first responders can absolutely discuss their day, including difficult experiences, without going into explicit detail. And they should. Such communication would likely lead to closer relationships with their partners as well as provide the first responder with a pathway to obtain support when needed.

The mindset that "no one outside the job can possibly understand what I do" can also interfere with help-seeking from professionals: "I respect psychologists, and I'm sure they help normal people. But there's no way they could possibly understand what we see and do every day. Do they actually think they can understand our world simply because they've read a lot of books?" Some clinicians have reinforced this belief by attempting to apply "traditional" stress management techniques (e.g., progressive muscle relaxation, diaphragmatic breathing) when a first responder has experienced a crisis. Techniques that may be useful to, say, help students reduce test anxiety will typically annoy and frustrate first responders. As one police officer told this author, "The first time she told me I just needed to take a time out after a call to imagine myself in a 'safe place,' I was gone."

I am not suggesting clinicians must have lived experience in areas where they provide psychotherapeutic services. With first responders, however, it is essential to have at least a decent understanding of the work they do and to have an appreciation for their subculture. I am reminded of two very similar stories I have heard from online (ICAC) investigators who said they went to see clinicians who did not specialize in work with first responders. They said they spent the first 10 min of the session explaining what they did each day and then the next 40 min "putting the therapist back together" because they became upset at the horrific abuse material the investigator was describing.

Too often clinicians believe they are qualified to work with first responders simply because they have a license. By pretending their degrees have made them experts in working with all psychological conditions, they alienate the population, and word gets out very quickly. Put simply, if you cannot listen to stories involving the horrors of war, do not work with veterans. If you cannot hear stories of egregious violence and mindless exploitation and sadistic acts against children, do not work with child abuse detectives or online investigators. If you do not want to hear stories involving serious injury and death, do not work with *any* first responder. Know the boundaries of your professional expertise, as well as your ability to establish and work within a suitable protective frame.

It is critical for clinicians who work with first responders to convey competence and expertise without coming across as condescending. Do not pretend you understand what it is like to be their particular kind of first responder, or use their jargon, if you have never done the job. First responders can be slow to trust, but they are better than most clients with "sizing you up," and they are quick to recognize poseurs. If you are approachable and humble, and they view you as helpful and genuine, they will come to you.

"Things are only confidential until they aren't." An additional impediment pertains to concerns about confidentiality. This issue is discussed in other chapters in this book, but the suspicions of first responders can increase if they perceive that their agency and the clinician are connected in such a way that the clinician's allegiance is uncertain. Do they believe the "doc" is loyal to first responders, or to the chief officer who supervises them or manages their contract? How could the clinician be truly independent from those who are in positions to increase their salary, renew their contract, or give them other "perks"? Whose side will the therapist take if senior leadership sees a first responder as a problem and wants a bit of information about "how they are adjusting" or "whether they are a good fit"? Is it safe to discuss certain "hot button" stressors (e.g., sexual harassment, racial discrimination) without the clinician feeling ethically compelled to run to senior officers, or to Human Resources?

Of course, the key to addressing these concerns is with the truth. Any ambiguity needs to be clarified (and ideally memorialized in writing) so that everyone is on the same page. The boundaries must be clearly defined (e.g., "These are the circumstances that justify or require me to break confidentiality"). Certain roles must be established by the clinician and communicated to departmental staff, such as whether the clinician will serve on promotional or team selection boards, since these can cause ethical dilemmas. As one officer stated:

> Let's say I told the doc I was having suicidal thoughts two years ago, but no longer. And then this year I apply for the Bomb Squad. Even if I'm no longer having those thoughts, how can she *not* take my past disclosures into consideration? If it's between me and some other officer who has never mentioned to her that they had those thoughts, are you telling me she would pick me? No way. Better to say nothing.

Posttraumatic Stress Disorder

First responders work in environments characterized by traditional workplace stressors (e.g., high workload, internal administrative and bureaucratic battles) as well as occupation-specific stressors such as exposure to death and violence (Collins & Gibbs, 2003; Cubrich et al., 2022). Direct physical threats include assaults, car accidents, acts of violence, and exposure to toxins and pathogens (Donnelly et al., 2015). This makes public safety professionals particularly vulnerable to various forms of job strain including burnout and PTSD (Bakker & Hueven, 2006; Gershon et al., 2009). In a study by Lilly and Pierce (2013), 17% of emergency communications operators had symptoms of PTSD; in more recent research, Burhanullah et al. (2022) found a startling 45% of correctional officers were experiencing PTSD symptoms.

While it is unnecessary to list all the criteria for PTSD found in the DSM-5-TR (American Psychiatric Association [APA], 2022), it is worth summarizing that the first two criteria refer to exposure to "actual or threatened death, serious injury or sexual violence" that is directly experienced, and the third is learning a traumatic event has happened to a close family member or friend. These criteria are consistent with the way PTSD was conceptualized prior to the publication of this latest iteration of the DSM-5. In this author's view, however, the fourth criterion is problematic:

> Experiencing repeated or extreme exposure to aversive details of the traumatic event(s) (e.g., first responders collecting human remains; police officers repeatedly exposed to details of child abuse). **Note:** Criterion A4 does not apply to exposure through electronic media, television, movies, or pictures, unless this exposure is work related. (APA, 2022, p. 271)

The examples provided are confusing. The first is consistent with the theoretical basis for the construct – one can see how collecting human remains could be a repeated traumatic experience. Importantly, however, these acts would be experienced firsthand, in real time – the trauma would evolve as the first responder repeatedly viewed, touched, handled, smelled, etc. the remains. In contrast, the second example is less conceptually consistent. Police investigators who are exposed to "details of child abuse" typically view child sexual exploitation material[2] (CSEM), or read about or view the abuse after the fact. Thus, they are *secondarily* witnessing the traumatic event. While one could argue they are "nearly there" in the sense they are viewing a vivid memorialization of actual traumatic acts, it is also important to distinguish that the trauma is not happening in real time, and they are witnessing behaviors vicariously through an artificial (electronic) medium. The trauma is *vicarious*.

This is not hairsplitting and by no means is this writer minimizing the traumatic nature of viewing CSAM. On the contrary, the insidious nature of secondary traumatization makes it particularly harmful, and I am a fierce advocate for protecting those who view potentially traumatic material.[3] My issue is only what I view as an awkward attempt to force the square pegs of secondary traumatic stress (STS) and vicarious traumatization (VT) into the existing round hole of PTSD. The extant research and this author's clinical experience support the view that VT and PTSD are distinct constructs. In fact, Charles Figley, the researcher who first coined the term *vicarious trauma*, indicated that while VT is related to PTSD, there are unique characteristics that differentiate the two. He noted, "VT is a syndrome with symptoms nearly identical to PTSD except that exposure to a traumatizing event experienced by one person becomes a traumatizing event for a second person" (Figley, 1999, p. 4).

The note in the fourth DSM-5 criterion is also perplexing. The authors indicate the criterion applies to exposure via electronic media only if it is "work related." Does the brain somehow refuse to be traumatized when it is away from the office? This writer was working in a federal prison during the attacks on 9/11; in the days following, inmates began getting into altercations with staff and each other with increasing frequency. Initially, this phenomenon was attributed to the shock and stress that was universally experienced across the nation. When the altercations increased, it was blamed on the inmates' inadequate problem-solving techniques

---

[2] In the field of child exploitation, the term "child pornography" is considered outdated, minimizing, and not victim-centric. The preferred terms are "child sexual abuse material" or "child sexual exploitation material."

[3] In addition to CSEM, I would include material relating to the atrocities of war, terrorism, and images from manmade or natural disasters.

and poor stress management skills. In addition, staff recognized that many inmates were having difficulty as they attempted to check on the welfare of relatives in the New York City and Washington, DC, areas. Eventually, however, it became apparent the inmates were experiencing significant STS as a consequence of repeatedly watching the news footage (inmates watch a lot of television, and little else was airing on the limited channels offered). They were becoming "pickled" in the horrific scenes that were looped over and over. The decision was made to turn off the televisions, and although some prisoners viewed the removal of the televisions as an undeserved "punishment," almost immediately tensions abated and the violence dramatically dropped off. This exposure was not "work related," and the inclusion of the caveat seems unnecessary.

From a wellness or safeguarding standpoint, the distinction of whether the trauma is experienced firsthand or secondarily is critical. It is inarguably important to recognize that a person viewing potentially traumatic image and video files, or reading accounts involving pain, death, and exploitation, may be exposed to sights and sounds of significant violence and depravity. But the fact the exposure is vicarious provides an opening for the clinician to use tools to help the first responder combat what historically has been dismissed with a shrug of the shoulders – the inevitable consequence of working in that space. With the right interventions, STS's otherwise inevitable march toward VT can be stopped in its tracks.

Secondary Traumatic Stress

As indicated, something does not have to be experienced firsthand to result in symptoms similar to those found in posttraumatic stress disorder (PTSD). Various terms are used in the extant literature to describe these secondhand effects – *vicarious stress*, *vicarious trauma*, *vicarious stress reactions*, *compassion fatigue*, *secondary trauma*, *secondary traumatic stress*, and others. Unfortunately, these terms are often used interchangeably, which complicates research efforts and prevents conceptual clarity.

It is strongly suggested that any clinician who works with first responders avoid treating primary traumas and secondary traumas as if they are synonymous. For instance, following a critical incident, some departments use a version of *critical incident stress debriefing* (CISD; Mitchell, 1983).[4] Although the efficacy of debriefing is controversial, and some departments may not strictly adhere to the seven steps that comprise the "Mitchell model" (Mitchell & Everly, 1996), CISD and critical incident stress management (CISM), a more holistic approach than CISD, are nevertheless the starting point for first-responder agencies, schools, and other organizations (Everly & Mitchell, 1997).

[4] See also Mitchell and Everly's chapter in this book.

Clinicians who work in the ICAC space may be tempted to use the CISM/CISD model to safeguard investigators and analysts, but in most cases, they will find themselves quickly running into difficulties. Unlike those who experience direct traumas, ICAC investigators may have difficulty identifying the critical incident. Is each image or video file of child sexual exploitation material a critical incident? Is it only the worst file encountered that day or that week? Or perhaps every period when potentially traumatic material is viewed collectively should be considered a critical incident, no matter how many files are viewed? Depending on the answers to those questions, the clinician then must decide how often to debrief the investigators – every day? Each week? Once per quarter? These questions are difficult to answer. Certainly, some cases can stand out as particularly upsetting, and there may be specific sights and sounds from the potentially traumatic material that an investigator or analyst cannot get out of their head (Feuer [2021] refers to these as "imprints of horror" [p. 366]). But while these images and video files are inarguably upsetting, they typically are insufficient, by themselves, to cause PTSD.

The detectives and agents who investigate crimes against children usually describe their symptoms arising from a completely different process – they say they emerge from the "gradual accumulation of evil" – a layering of STS. I often describe the difference between PTSD and VT by using a metaphor of burns. If someone touches their hand to a hot stove and immediately gets burned, this would be analogous to an acute psychological stressor. And there may thereafter be a scar in the shape of the object they touched – the equivalent of the psychological scarring of PTSD. But one's skin can also get burned from being exposed to the sun's radiation. Becoming sunburned is not acute, it is gradual; like VT, it results from a gradual accumulation of invisible but potentially harmful factors.

I possess an ongoing worry that clinicians will inadvertently cause harm if they treat secondary stressors using research and treatment models designed for primary stressors. After more than two decades working in the child exploitation space, we are still learning how to increase resilience – the "sunscreen" that serves to protect first responders from the toxic effects of what they are exposed to. And we have yet to create best practices for how to best cope with potentially traumatic material that manages to worm through our psychological defenses. For instance, I am clear that the practice of sitting around a circle and "processing" what each person witnessed that week is not cathartic, and I would argue it is not particularly therapeutic. At best, it is only a temporarily release. And even if it was cathartic – if it allowed investigators and analysts to "release" the STS in some way where it did not boomerang back – then at the end of the session each participant would find they had given up one layer, only to gain another from each of the other members of the group. Such group "debriefings" only result in additional exposure to more harmful radiation – adding more layers of upsetting things to each person's plate before they go home for the weekend.

The STS I am referring to in this chapter – the primary target of safeguarding and resiliency efforts – is the equivalent of the ancient Chinese practice of *lingchi*, or death by a thousand cuts. In the ICAC world, the cuts are each image, video file, chat log, or story that form building blocks of STS – sedimentary layers that gradually accrete. These emotional wounds result from exposure to a seemingly endless stream of horrific stories, chats, images, video footage, and sounds depicting the abuse of children.

For other first responders, the blocks are similarly comprised of pain that is witnessed and absorbed. In the fire services and EMS, the emotional sequelae include the after effects from repeated calls to respond to car accidents, traffic fatalities, and medical events involving severely injured children. It includes the anger that results when the drunk driver is driven away unscathed but leaves critically injured or deceased persons behind, as well as the sadness when the system has insufficient resources to protect a child or an elderly person. It includes the sense of helplessness when the first responder hears the teenager they saved from an overdose last week was just found deceased. Every first responder can name the calls that tend to get underneath their armor, the cases they cannot let rest, and the people they will never forget.

Vicarious Trauma

Whether offline or online, the layering continues until it causes a transformation in one's worldview, spirituality, and relationships (Pearlman & Saakvitne, 1995). Once the STS has set down roots – once it has begun to transform an individual's sense of self and/or their worldview – it signals the move to a more profound construct. It is at this point the sufferer is experiencing vicarious trauma. Baird and Kracen (2006) define vicarious trauma as "harmful changes that occur in professionals' views of themselves, others, and the world as a result of repeated exposure to graphic and/or traumatic material" (p. 182).

For firefighters, becoming trapped in an engulfed structure, backdraft situations, and other emotional punches (e.g., locating a child's body under the bed) can be critical incidents. The effects of systemic racism in the department, or the effects from working car crashes caused by impaired drivers, could be examples of secondary stress. With secondary stress, the effects are cumulative and they accumulate gradually. While none are necessarily crises in the same way as becoming trapped after a partial building collapse, the layers endure and may be long-lasting.

Emergency communication operators/dispatchers are a unique group of first responders who experience regular doses of both primary and secondary stress. For instance, there are times when they may secondarily follow a major incident as they listen to radio traffic. They often worry and experience stress when one of "their" firefighters or officers has not checked in to say they are okay. Similarly, during a vehicle pursuit, they are obviously not careening down the road, and they may not even be the individual with primary duties for communicating with the officers engaged in the pursuit, but they are, in every other sense of the word, "there." Yet moments later they may be on the phone with someone in an emergent crisis – they may find themselves advising a woman how to prepare to deliver a child herself if the ambulance can't get there in time. Or asking a suspected hostage of a domestic violence incident "yes or no" questions to ascertain what it happening without putting the caller in danger. Or they may hear the gunshot after speaking with a suicidal caller. The latter examples not only occur in real time, but they involve firsthand involvement. Although the nature and timing of the next crisis is unknown, they must immediately adapt, calm the caller, gather information, give directives, and then communicate relevant information to responding units. Their risk for experiencing secondary traumatic stress is compounded by the lack of closure they often receive; once the other first responders arrive at the door, they hang up.

Safeguarding

The term safeguarding may be familiar to readers outside the United States as referring to the protection of children from harm. This writer, however, was introduced to the word in reference to adults, specifically, ensuring the well-being of law enforcement officers who are in positions in which they are likely to experience intense and unique pressures (e.g., undercover officers) and/or investigators who are exposed to potentially traumatic material (e.g., child sexual abuse images). In fact the unit developed by the FBI to protect their ICAC agents is named the Undercover Safeguard Unit (Krause, 2009), and the National Center for Missing and Exploited Children set up a similar initiative they call the Safeguard Program (Holmes & Bowers, 2015).

Although there are well-established methods for increasing resilience and reducing general workplace stress, the application of these principles to specific missions and tasks is by no means standardized and perhaps with good reason. This writer has assisted federal government agencies, private companies, and nongovernmental organizations in developing effective safeguard programs, and no two have been the same. The demands of the job, the costs involved in implementing certain recommendations, and the resources of each group (to name only a few variables) can significantly differ and affect what the programs become. Thus, it is beyond the scope of this chapter to offer everything that should be taken into consideration, but the following are suggested areas of focus for any clinician who intends set up and/or maintain a safeguard program for first responders.

Online Investigation

Because online investigators, computer forensic analysts, and prosecutors have much more control over when and how they view the evidence, they can use tools to help ensure their well-being that first responders on a call, or handling an emergent crisis, cannot implement. For instance, they can stop a video clip when they need to take a break or implement a safeguard tool to "reset" before they come back to continue their review. They can choose which file or series of images to review at a given time and decide when to switch to another task. They can also adjust the media – change the colors to black and white, alter the size, turn off the sound, and even view the images sideways or upside-down. They can scan images in rapid succession or, in the case of victim identification, more carefully scrutinize the tiniest details within a particular image. These simple techniques remind their brain that they are not looking through a window; this is not happening in real time.

Peer Support

Extant research, as well as anecdotal reports from first responders of all types, has shown that relationships with peers and the support of command staff are among the most important factors related to resiliency. Clinicians should seek to strengthen these support systems, especially if command staff do not understand the work performed by the first responders (it is common in the ICAC space, e.g., for the investigator's chain of command to be unfamiliar with their work; if they spent their career in other areas of policing, they may only superficially appreciate the difficulties inherent in this particular mission).

Environmental Factors

Clinicians should view safeguarding as holistically as possible and thus consider the work environment. While everyone wants the window office, it is particularly important for those who work with the darkest areas of humanity to be provided with windows to the outdoors. Clinicians should advocate for ICAC taskforces, child abuse squads, and vice crimes units to bring them out of the basement (whether literally or figuratively) to avoid the insinuation their work is "dirty." For staff who are at particular risk for STS, the need for balance and periodic rest may require them to have greater flexibility with their work schedules. Clinicians may find themselves working with the police union to adjust certain policies and procedures, or securing funding for specialized software designed to reduce the level of traumatic material investigators must review. Such advocacy likely was not taught in graduate school, but it is appropriate in the context of the role of safeguarding professional.

Check-Ins with the Safeguard Clinician

When command staff first attempt to implement a safeguard program, one of the questions frequently posed is, "How often should personnel be required to check in with the psychologist?" In my opinion, the best way to address this issue is by offering various avenues through which the first responder can communicate with the safeguard clinician.

First, employees should be formally checked, at a minimum, no less than four times per year. Note that no research has been conducted on the efficacy of mental health checks – at any interval – for first responders (Spence et al., 2019), but proactive mental health checks have become a growing practice. These checks do not have to be 1-hour therapy sessions (and they should not be; safeguarding is not a substitute for psychotherapy). Rather, these are "well-being checks" to see how staff are doing.

Second, safeguard clinicians should maintain an open-door policy whereby staff can stop by for informal sessions ("Do you have any tricks for getting rid of nightmares?") or to update the safeguard clinician on something that was brought up in the previous session ("Remember when I told you I was stressed out about my mom's medical test? Well, everything came back negative. I'm so relieved!"). These "drive-by" sessions help diffuse stress between formal sessions and can help enhance the relationship.

Third, in addition to established meetings, safeguard clinicians should also see staff at random intervals. There are two reasons for such unscheduled sessions. First, public safety professionals tend to be nosy, and sometimes they will pick up on the fact that one of their colleagues has gone to see the "shrink" more often than usual. If consistent intervals are avoided, then no one bothers to keep track of how often their colleagues are seen, and no one knows if the extra sessions were requested or if they were random. The second reason is that the "random" sessions can be prompted by something relayed to the safeguard clinician by someone in the first responder's support system. For instance, a coworker or supervisor may notice the person has seemed depressed, lately, or that they suffered a loss. This could prompt the safeguarding clinician to invite the person in for an unscheduled wellness check.

These meetings should be positive, supportive conversations, not sessions staff dread attending because they are afraid they will be considered "unfit" to continue working in the field. Confidentiality should apply as it would in a therapy session to ensure personnel feel comfortable discussing what they are truly experiencing. If sufficient rapport and trust are not present, staff will simply begin lying. I once spoke with a federal agent who was forced to participate in a safeguard program we both believed was dysfunctional. She told me:

> We don't tell the safeguard psychologists the truth about what we're going through, because they'll put something in our file or tell us we can't do the work, anymore. And you can't completely lie and say everything's awesome, because that makes them suspicious. So you have to give them a little morsel – like tell them you've had some nightmares, or you're having trouble sleeping, or you've been irritable with your spouse or something. Then they give you some tips on sleep hygiene or progressive muscle relaxation or whatever, and they're happy they were able to help. And you don't get pulled off the job. But it's kind of a game because we don't really trust them.

Safeguarding is not going to work if sufficient trust is not in place or if the clinician is in a "dual role" where they are also evaluating whether the investigator should continue to do the work (essentially an informal fitness for duty evaluation).

Independence

Obviously, no one benefits if the intended beneficiaries do not trust those who are expected to look after them, or if they see the process as a game to manipulate. Part of the issue in the situation described above is the safeguard psychologists worked for supervisory special agents who were not mental health professionals and knew nothing about safeguarding or the ethical standards the psychologists endeavored to maintain. Some were viewed as agency "stair-climbers" who were more invested in their careers than in ensuring employee well-being. Whether that opinion was warranted or not is irrelevant – there was too much at risk.

Generally speaking, the more safeguard professionals are separated from the department or agency, the better. Ideally, the safeguard staff should be contracted mental health professionals with no other ties or allegiances to the agency; their only job should be ensuring the wellness of the first responders. The safeguard clinician should not serve on promotional boards, help decide whom should be selected for elite teams, engage in fitness for duty evaluations, or work with internal affairs. The moment the safeguard professional is seen as someone who will run to management, or who is on any "side" other than that of the first responder in front of them, is the moment when first responders will collectively shut down and will stop telling the truth during sessions.

Feedback

This does not mean safeguard professionals cannot provide feedback to management. Of course they can, and they should. But they must do so without violating the confidence of their clients. Aggregate data can be offered, if the pool is large enough. General suggestions can be offered without indicating if staff have complained about the issue (to avoid global retaliation). Of course, if the safeguard professional works with different departments, (e.g., fire services, police officers, dispatchers, and jail staff), it can be easier to describe general trends without pointing a finger at any particular group. If the safeguard professional works for more than one first-responder department, it may also be possible to mention issues that every chief officer should keep in mind, even if it has only reached critical levels in one or two agencies.

Assessment

It is inappropriate, and possibly unethical, to regularly administer certain psychological assessment measures to employees to measure "how they are doing." For instance, one large agency administered the MMPI-2 to investigators every 6 months as part of their safeguard program. The MMPI-2 was not designed for this purpose, and the repeated administration of a measure of personality to "monitor" well-being is concerning. Guideline 6 of the American Psychological Association's Ethical Guidelines for Psychological Assessment and Evaluation (2020) states:

> Psychologists who conduct psychological testing, assessment, and evaluation endeavor to select (a) assessment tools that demonstrate sufficient validity evidence for their uses, sufficient score reliability, and sound psychometric properties and (b) measures that are fair and appropriate for the evaluation purpose, population, setting, and context at hand. (p. 16)

I recommend only the use of instruments that closely align with constructs of concern, such as the Secondary Traumatic Stress Scale (STSS; Bride et al., 2004), the Maslach Burnout Inventory (MBI; Maslach et al., 1997), and the Professional Quality of Life Scale (ProQOL; Stamm, 2010), among others.

The Catch-22

Clinicians who work in public safety settings sometimes find a surprising Catch-22, that, is, many first responders do not want to leave jobs that they suspect (or know) are hurting them. As one ICAC investigator noted:

> My work has caused tremendous stress on my family and relationships. It creates distrust, emotional distance, anger, fatigue, depression and overall cynicism. I have lost the majority of my hope and trust in people. Even a good deed plants a seed of doubt into my mind as to what the motive is behind it… I often feel like I have worked so hard to save the children of the "world" that I neglected my own children by working on holidays, weekends, and late hours … My work has taken away time from the two children who matter the most to me because I was out trying to save the ones I don't even know … and yet, it is my passion and I love my job. I can't imagine doing anything else.

This quote captures the commitment and passion that can hold first responders hostage. The rewards can outweigh the sacrifices. The sense of meaning the work offers can trump any simmering and creeping cynicism. And the belief that one is acting in the interest of justice, or helping those who are suffering and saving lives – the knowledge that one is doing the right thing for the right reasons – is what keeps the first responders on the job. Safeguarding therefore is not merely enhancing morale, or teaching stress management skills. It is a holistic approach to ensuring that first responders balance their sacrifices with ways to recharge. The alternative is that the work will emotionally drain them until there is nothing left.

Clinical Competence

A clinician may have an advanced degree in mental health and possess certain impressive credentials, but this does not mean he or she is competent to work as a safeguard clinician/wellness professional. Some professionals think they can simply read up on the literature and then walk in and do the job. This is far from accurate, and this approach will likely backfire. You have to understand the culture and speak with humility, leaving your ego at the door. You must always admit when you do not know something and when you make a mistake. You must be genuine.

If you are currently working with first responders, or intend to, and have not worked in the setting, yourself, then take time to learn the job. Not from a book, but by getting out there. Go on ride-alongs – on every shift, and in every part of the city (this applies to police and sheriff's departments as well as fire departments). Sit with a surveillance team on a freezing, rainy day. Go out with a warrant team at 3:00 AM. Participate in the citizen's police academy. Observe a confined space exercise or swift water rescue. Help out. Chip in. If you want first responders to trust you, meet them in their world. Word that you are "okay" will get out much faster if you stay after a meeting and help stack chairs than if you tell people you know what white spaces mean on a Rorschach.

Conclusion

It is clear from the results of the NWS that first responders are quietly suffering. As one of my colleagues, a police psychologist and co-developer of the NWS, noted, "On the worst day of their lives, they are the first to respond and the last to seek help." (C. Mills, personal communication, August 24, 2022). Safeguard clinicians must turn this around. The good news is, for most agencies that have implemented focused safeguard programs, the anecdotal reports are positive. Even the more cynical first responders who believe it is a waste of time often acknowledge they know others on their team who benefited from the program. And they admit they appreciate "at least the bosses care enough to try."

The job of taking care of first responders is multifaceted and complex. Clinicians who enter this area of practice should expect to wear a number of hats: advocate, counselor, educator, and liaison, to name only a few. They should keep in mind that in some ways safeguarding is a departure from the traditional clinical role. The model is more preventive than reactive – clinicians help them "armor up" before they go into battle so that, hopefully, there is less caring for psychological wounds later on down the road.

References

Abbott, C., Barber, E., Burke, B., Harvey, J., Newland, C., Rose, M., & Young, A. (2015). *What's killing our medics?* Ambulance Service Manager Program. Retrieved from www.revivingresponders.com/originalpaper

American Psychiatric Association. (2022). *Diagnostic and statistical manual of mental disorders* (5th, Text Rev ed.). American Psychiatric Association. https://doi.org/10.1176/appi.books.9780890425787

Baird, K., & Kracen, A. C. (2006). Vicarious traumatization and secondary traumatic stress: A research synthesis. *Counselling Psychology Quarterly, 19*(2), 181–188.

Bakker, A. B., & Heuven, E. (2006). Emotional dissonance, burnout, and in-role performance among nurses and police officers. *International Journal of Stress Management, 13*(4), 423.

Bride, B. E., Robinson, M. R., Yegidis, B., & Figley, C. R. (2004). Development and validation of the secondary traumatic stress scale. *Research on Social Work Practice, 14*, 27–35.

Burhanullah, M. H., Rollings-Mazza, P., Galecki, J., Van Wert, M., Weber, T., & Malik, M. (2022). Mental health of staff at correctional facilities in the United States during the COVID-19 pandemic. *Frontiers in Psychiatry, 12*. https://doi.org/10.3389/fpsyt.2021.767385

Collins, P. A., & Gibbs, A. C. (2003). Stress in police officers: A study of the origins, prevalence, and severity of stress-related symptoms within a county police force. *Occupational Medicine, 53*(2), 56–64.

Cubrich, M., Sodhi, K., Petruzzelli, A., & Doverspike, D. (2022). Who rescues the rescuers? Multilevel challenges facing first responder organizations. In D. Svyantek (Ed.), *Crisis and chaos and organizations: The coronavirus and lessons for organizational theory* (pp. 65–96). Information Age Publishing.

Donnelly, E. A., Siebert, D., & Siebert, C. (2015). Development of the emergency medical services role identity scale (EMS-RIS). *Social Work in Health Care, 54*(3), 212–233.

Everly, G. S., & Mitchell, J. T. (1997). *Critical incident stress management (CISM): A new era and standard of Care in Crisis Intervention*. Chevron.

FEMA. (2018). *The effect of repeated exposure trauma on firefighters*. Retrieved from www.usfa.fema.gov/blog/ci-011718.html

Feuer, B. S. (2021). First responder peer support: An evidence-informed approach. *Journal of Police and Criminal Psychology, 36*, 365–377. https://doi.org/10.1007/s11896-020-09420-z

Figley, C. R. (1999). Compassion fatigue: Toward a new understanding of the costs of caring. In B. H. Stamm (Ed.), *Secondary traumatic stress: Self-care issues for clinicians, researchers, and educators* (pp. 3–28). Sidran.

Gershon, R. R., Barocas, B., Canton, A. N., Li, X., & Vlahov, D. (2009). Mental, physical, and behavioral outcomes associated with perceived work stress in police officers. *Criminal Justice and Behavior, 36*(3), 275–289.

Holmes, L. J., & Bowers, D. T. (2015). *The National center for missing and exploited children: The safeguard program*. Office of Justice Programs. Retrieved from https://ovc.ojp.gov/sites/g/files/xyckuh226/files/media/document/imp_ncmec_safeguard_program-508.pdf

Jahnke, S. A., Poston, W. S. C., Haddock, C. K., & Murphy, B. (2016). Firefighting and mental health: Experiences of repeated exposure to trauma. *Work, 53*(4), 737–744. https://doi.org/10.3233/wor-162255

Krause, M. (2009). History and evolution of the FBI's undercover safeguard program. *Consulting Psychology Journal: Research and Practice, 61*(1), 5–13. https://doi.org/10.1037/a0015280

Levi-Gigi, E., Richter-Levin, G., & Szabolcs, K. (2014). The hidden price of repeated traumatic exposure: Different cognitive deficits in different first responders. *Frontiers in Behavioral Neuroscience, 8*, 281. https://doi.org/10.3389/fnbeh.2014.00281

Lilly, M. M., & Pierce, H. (2013) PTSD and depressive symptoms in 911 telecommunicators: The role of peritraumatic distress and world assumptions in predicting risk. *Psychological Trauma: Theory Research Practice and Policy, 5*(2), 135–141. https://doi.org/10.1037/a0026850

Maslach, C., Jackson, S. E., & Leiter, M. P. (1997). Maslach burnout inventory: Third edition. In C. P. Zalaquett & R. J. Wood (Eds.), *Evaluating stress: A book of resources* (pp. 191–218). Scarecrow Education.

Mitchell, J. T. (1983). When disaster strikes…The critical incident stress debriefing. *Journal of Emergency Medical Services, 13*(11), 49–52.

Mitchell, J. T., & Everly, G. S. (1996). Critical incident stress debriefing: An operations manual for the prevention of traumatic stress among emergency services and disaster workers. Ellicott City, MD: Chevron.

Pearlman, L. A., & Saakvitne, K. W. (1995). *Trauma and the therapist: Countertransference and vicarious traumatization in psychotherapy with incest survivors*. W. W. Norton & Co.

Spence, D. L., Fox, M., Moore, G. C., Estill, S., & Comrie, N. E. A. (2019). *Law enforcement and mental health and wellness act: A report to congress*. U.S. Department of Justice.

Stamm, B. H. (2010). *The concise ProQOL manual* (2nd ed.). ProQOL.org.

Wellness, Resilience, and Mindfulness

Antoine Lebeaut, Maya Zegel, Elizabeth Anderson Fletcher, and Anka A. Vujanovic

First responders are exposed to high rates of potentially traumatic and stressful emergency events (Jahnke et al., 2016; Jones et al., 2018) and work in a demanding profession that includes long shift work, wearing and manipulating heavy work-related equipment, and engaging in physically intensive tasks. As a result, first responders are disproportionally susceptible to occupational injuries and fatalities, work-related burnout, and various psychological symptoms and disorders compared to other working professions (Jones, 2017; Reichard & Jackson, 2010). Compared to the general population, first responders experience greater job-related pain (Carleton et al., 2018; Nazari et al., 2020) and increased rates of posttraumatic stress disorder (PTSD) symptoms, depression, suicidal ideation and behaviors, and problematic alcohol use (Jones et al., 2018; Stanley et al., 2016). Considering these factors and the nature of first responder occupations, a proactive and preventative approach to addressing the mental health and well-being of first responders has garnered significant interest and support among emergency service organizations.

Defining Wellness, Resilience, and Mindfulness

Strategies for mitigating mental and physical health risks and supporting the well-being of first responders include the development of programs focused on building resilience, mindfulness, and wellness. While these factors tend to overlap in the

A. Lebeaut (✉) · M. Zegel · A. A. Vujanovic
Department of Psychology, University of Houston, Houston, TX, USA
e-mail: amlebeaut@uh.edu

E. A. Fletcher
Department of Decision and Information Sciences, University of Houston, Houston, TX, USA

M. L. Bourke et al. (eds.), *First Responder Mental Health*,
https://doi.org/10.1007/978-3-031-38149-2_9

literature and share related features, there are varied approaches across emergency service organizations and departments to bolster them. Therefore, defining resilience, mindfulness, and wellness within the context of first responder work may provide a better understanding of these strategies.

Resilience

Resilience is a dynamic process broadly defined as the ability to effectively manage and adapt to mentally and/or physically aversive situations (Luthar & Cicchetti, 2000). Resilience in the aftermath of potentially traumatic life events is comprised of key competencies, including the ability to invoke resilience-focused beliefs (e.g., hope and realistic optimism) and efficiently navigate and use coping techniques (e.g., diaphragmatic breathing) and resources (e.g., peer support networks; Crane et al., 2021). Extant literature focused on civilians (Joyce et al., 2018), first responders (Denkova et al., 2020; Mahaffey et al., 2021), and military service members and/or veterans (Kahn et al., 2016) underscores both the malleability of resilience and the benefit of explicitly targeting mechanisms to bolster resilience. Building resilience is important because it enables first responders to "bounce back" from challenging situations (e.g., marital conflicts, personnel shortages, long shifts) and potentially traumatic events (e.g., natural disasters, fires, motor vehicle accidents). First responders who build their resilience are better able to adapt to change, cope with stress, and recover from adversity. Moreover, with greater resilience, first responders may be better able to manage their emotions, maintain healthy relationships, and have a more positive outlook on life and their occupation.

Mindfulness

A promising target for resilience training programs (RTPs) among first responders is mindfulness, defined as purposeful awareness of the present moment and non-judgmental acceptance of adverse emotional states (Baer et al., 2006). Programs focused on improving mindfulness have been developed and tested among various populations, including first responders, and have demonstrated strong utility and outcomes (Joyce et al., 2018, 2019). Theoretically, increasing mindfulness, via RTPs or mind-body interventions (e.g., yoga-based interventions; Floyd et al., 2022), can help first responders better regulate negative affective states and experiential avoidance, particularly after traumatic emergency calls (e.g., Reffi et al., 2019). For instance, improving mindfulness may elicit adaptive cognitions and affective responses (i.e., acceptance and improved emotion regulation), enhance strategies to cope with negative emotional states and experiences, and increase cognitive flexibility (e.g., Bravo et al., 2018). Improved mindfulness may also promote greater nonjudgmental awareness of thoughts, emotions, and physical sensations, which can help first responders identify and address negative thought patterns and/or behaviors that may hinder resilience. Accordingly, mindfulness may serve to buffer the consequences of occupational stressors typically faced by first responders, and RTPs that incorporate mindfulness-based strategies can effectively promote mental health, well-being, reduce absenteeism, increase job satisfaction, and build resilience.

Wellness

Along with RTPs, national first-responder organizations as well as local and regional emergency service departments have sought to improve quality of life and well-being via wellness initiatives. These initiatives aim to address first responders' wellness, described as the state of an individual's physical, mental, and emotional readiness for duty (IAFF, 2018). As such, wellness programs aim to strengthen these states through periodic assessments and routine exercises that examine, maintain, and improve physical, mental, and emotional capabilities. For instance, for US fire departments, the National Fire Protection Agency (NFPA) has established guidelines (i.e., NFPA 1582 Standard on Comprehensive Occupational Medical Program for Fire Departments; NFPA 1583 Standard on Health-Related Fitness Programs for Fire Department Members) for wellness programs meant to ensure firefighters are capable and ready for the physical and mental rigor of the job (NFPA, 2022). However, many fire departments, particularly small and/or rural departments, do not adopt these standards, which may amplify the risks associated with emergency service work. Additionally, the number of wellness programs for other types of first responders is limited. Departments are increasingly making wellness curricula available, including access to peer support programs, yoga and exercise programs, mental health counseling on-site, and in-service training on wellness and behavioral health. Despite these strides, wellness initiatives are still in early stages of development and uptake, and implementation across departments nationally is highly variable.

The goal of this chapter is threefold. First, we will provide an overview of the resilience, mindfulness, and wellness literature among first responders, generally, and among each emergency service profession, specifically, including (1) law enforcement officers (LEOs), (2) firefighters, (3) emergency medical service (EMS) personnel (e.g., emergency medical technicians [EMTs] and paramedics), and (4) public safety/emergency dispatchers. Second, we will review relevant programs that aim to examine, maintain, and/or improve resilience, mindfulness, and/or wellness in first responders, along with their implementation in practice across various public safety settings. Finally, we will outline an approach to large-scale as well as client-focused implementation, discuss notable limitations, and provide suggestions for future directions to better inform prevention and treatment approaches.

Resilience, Mindfulness, and Wellness in First Responders: A Brief Literature Review

Initiatives to improve mental health and well-being via resilience and wellness programs have primarily been developed and tested among specific professions within emergency service work (i.e., firefighters *or* LEOs); however, some research utilizes mixed samples of first-responder professions (e.g., samples that include firefighters and LEOs; e.g., Kaplan et al., 2017; Wild et al., 2020). Therefore, the relevant literature is organized and reviewed below by first-responder type with some exceptions.

Law Enforcement Officers

LEOs are routinely exposed to a high level of potentially life-threatening and dangerous events and, as such, are at elevated risk for developing work-related stress and burnout, problems with substance use, suicidal thoughts and intentions, and symptoms of depression, anxiety, and PTSD (Syed et al., 2020). LEOs are also at increased risk to develop cardiovascular complications (e.g., cardiac arrest), diabetes, obesity, and other adverse medical conditions (Hartley et al., 2011). Taken together, the mental and physical health consequences faced by LEOs due to the nature of their work can negatively impact on- and off-duty performance and quality of life. Thus, there has been increased attention and support in the USA to develop and implement resilience and wellness programs for LEOs.

Treatments and Interventions

Effective RTPs for LEOs have utilized components of mindfulness and stress management techniques in light of robust associations between (1) resilience and mindfulness and (2) mindfulness and mental and physical health outcomes among LEOs (Kaplan et al., 2018, 2020; Williams et al., 2010). Accordingly, these studies offer a framework for mental health professionals who are considering implementing a resilience-focused and/or mindfulness-based program for first responders, whether in a single department or across multiple departments. For instance, in a pilot study of 43 Pacific Northwestern US LEOs, Christopher et al. (2016) tested the feasibility and efficacy of a mindfulness-based resilience training (MBRT) intervention (no control/comparison group was included) to reduce mental and physical health risks (i.e., fatigue, organizational stress, burnout, sleep disturbance, and mindfulness). MBRT was delivered across eight weekly 2-hour group sessions and included psychoeducation (e.g., information on strategies to manage stressors in police work) and opportunities to learn about and practice mindfulness-based exercises (e.g., body scans, meditation, breathing exercises, mindful movement). Results indicated that LEOs who received MBRT reported significant improvements in mindfulness, resilience, perceived stress, burnout, and overall mental and physical health; these findings were replicated in additional work (Grupe et al., 2021). Given the promise of these interventions and the potential durability of outcomes, opportunities to support and reinforce routine engagement with mindfulness and stress reduction exercises via check-ins and follow-up refresher sessions may serve to bolster these gains.

Wellness Programs and Initiatives

Similar to RTPs, wellness programs and initiatives for LEOs aim to support physical health through regular assessments and trainings that aim to examine, maintain, and improve physical, mental, and emotional capabilities. In 2018, the US government established the Law Enforcement Mental Health and Wellness Act of 2017 (LEMHWA), which recognized the crucial need to promote mental health and well-being among LEOs and improve the delivery of mental health and wellness services for federal, state, and local LEOs (Congress, 2018). As part of this act, the Department of Justice (DOJ) is required to submit periodic reports to Congress that identify extant mental health services delivered in the US Departments of Defense and Veterans Affairs that could be adopted by law enforcement agencies and highlight recommendations. In 2021, 65 state, tribal, and local law enforcement agencies were awarded funding (totaling $7 million in grants) under the LEMHWA to develop, implement, and embed peer support mental health and wellness pilot programs among their agencies (DOJ, 2021).

Successful wellness programs for law enforcement tend to (1) develop formal policies geared toward promoting wellness and mental health, (2) include supportive department leaders who are educated on best practices for mental health care and wellness, (3) recruit mental health professionals who are trained specifically to work with LEOs and understand law enforcement culture, and (4) implement prevention-focused programs that are mandatory and require routine mental health evaluations (Taylor, 2022). Various departments in the USA have successfully established wellness programs, which has helped to reduce stigma associated with seeking mental health care and improve service utilization (e.g., Lapum, 2020; Rachele et al., 2014). However, the availability of these programs and their uptake among LEOs remain low across law enforcement agencies. Approximately 11% of agencies did not offer wellness programs, and for those that did, there were inconsistencies in the development and implementation of these programs (Thoen et al., 2020).

Interestingly, approximately 25% of the 144 US LEOs interviewed were not aware of their own agency's wellness programming options (Thoen et al., 2020). Thus, there is a clear need for not only the implementation of wellness programs but also for a greater focus on advertising and encouraging participation in existing programs available to first responders. Strategies to improve participation may include emailing department listservs, circulating paper flyers with QR codes and posting them in private spaces, and/or asking personnel (e.g., station captains and department chiefs) to endorse and encourage participation. Additional strategies may include developing online content and anonymous participation to facilitate ease of access.

Firefighters

Research on firefighters has demonstrated the link between mindfulness and other facets of mental health and wellness. A study of 114 Australian firefighters found that mindfulness was negatively associated with depression and anxiety symptoms and positively associated with psychological well-being after controlling for age and years of service (Counson et al., 2019). Studies of firefighters in the USA and worldwide have established negative (i.e., inverse) associations between mindfulness and various mental health symptoms, including anxiety, depression, PTSD, suicidal ideation and risk, and alcohol use (Huang et al., 2019; Lebeaut et al., 2021; Setti & Argentero, 2014; Smith et al., 2011). Given the well-established association between mindfulness and mental health outcomes, it is also necessary to consider the impact of these variables on suicidality. For instance, research examining the association between greater PTSD symptom severity and elevated suicide risk found that higher levels of mindfulness (specifically facets of acting with awareness and nonjudging of inner experience) reduce the strength of this association (Stanley et al., 2019). Therefore, interventions that explicitly target mindfulness may serve to reduce suicidality among firefighters, which is a salient and growing concern for many fire departments across the USA.

Treatments and Interventions

Recent literature has extended these findings by applying and evaluating mindfulness-based intervention frameworks among firefighters (Kuehl et al., 2013; Matto & Sullivan, 2021), which have demonstrated promising results. For instance, Joyce et al. (2019) examined the efficacy of a mindfulness-based program (versus a program that only included education on health and well-being topics) to teach resilience exercises and skills through six, 20–25-min online training sessions in Australian firefighters and found that firefighters who received the intervention demonstrated significantly greater resilience skills compared to the control group. However, not all resilience-based interventions have similar effects. Indeed, Skeffington et al. (2016) were unable to demonstrate significant treatment effects for a 4-h resilience training intervention (four 1-h weekly sessions) designed for the primary prevention of PTSD that was comprised of (1) psychoeducation on stress, trauma, PTSD, and mental health, generally, as well as coping strategies; (2) review and practice of the mental agility and psychological strength (MAPS) skills, which include cognitive restructuring, support seeking, and self-soothing; and (3) self-care skills. Mental health professionals who are considering implementing similar programs may thus need to consider how the format (e.g., online versus in-person) and the length of the intervention may impact its potential to improve mental health, social support, and/or coping strategies among firefighters. These considerations can also be addressed via surveys or focus groups that can shed light on department- and personnel-specific challenges and needs.

Another program that is important to consider is the Disaster Worker Resiliency Training Program (DWRT) which seeks to address and improve resilience among first responders (Mahaffey et al., 2021). DWRT is a 4-h single-session program designed to (1) provide psychoeducation about disasters and traumatic events, PTSD, and resilience; (2) review traumatic stress and its impact on self and others and identifying PTSD-related risk and resilience factors; (3) identify self-care and stress management strategies; and (4) establish personal and professional goals and develop a plan to incorporate self-care and resilience-promoting behaviors. Compared to a waitlist control condition, DWRT was found to be efficacious in improving healthier lifestyle behaviors, stress management, and spiritual growth at follow-up. Additionally, among participants who experienced a traumatic event after the workshop, waitlist control participants were more likely to endorse increases in perceived stress, PTSD, and depressive symptoms when compared to DWRT participants (Mahaffey et al., 2021), highlighting DWRT's efficacy in improving resilience and preventing psychopathology.

Researchers have sought to disentangle whether mindfulness-based training evinces a different or greater effect compared to other wellness training approaches. Denkova et al. (2020) administered mindfulness and relaxation training, which included four 2-h sessions delivered over 4 weeks by the same trainer, as well as 10–15 min of daily skill practice for homework, to two distinct groups of firefighters. Results indicated that firefighters who completed the mindfulness training demonstrated greater increases in psychological resilience and positive affect compared to firefighters who completed the relaxation training or who did not receive either training (Denkova et al., 2020). Mental health professionals who are interested in addressing and improving resilience among first responder personnel should therefore focus on disentangling whether mindfulness-based training or other potentially attractive wellness initiatives, such as relaxation training, are most effective in promoting resilience and well-being.

Emergency Medical Services

The line between fire and EMS is not as clear as it is between LEOs and firefighters since many (63%) fire departments in the USA also run medical calls (Fahey et al., 2021). Some departments run their own EMS (i.e., staff ambulances), while others serve as support for a third-party EMS agency. On certain types of medical calls (e.g., cardiac arrest, central wound hemorrhage), the first-due engine is dispatched along with an ambulance since many engine companies have EMTs and paramedics on board and the truck may beat the ambulance to the scene. Additionally, most fire departments run more medical and rescue calls than working fires; 66% of 2019 US fire department calls were medical or rescue (Fahey et al., 2021); thus, firefighters are dispatched routinely for medical-related calls. It is important to note that for all of these reasons, firefighters are exposed repeatedly to traumatic scenes and life-threatening medical calls. Stanley et al. (2015) found that firefighters in departments that ran medical calls were six times more likely to have attempted suicide than those in non-EMS departments.

There is a paucity of research examining wellness and mindfulness among non-firefighter EMTs and paramedics who work in third-party EMS agencies. Nonetheless, Mitmansgruber et al. (2008) found that experiential avoidance (i.e., avoiding and/or suppressing unwanted emotions, thoughts, and/or bodily sensations) remained largely stable, while mindful attention increased and then declined with more years of experience among Austrian paramedics. Some studies indicate that low levels of mindfulness, specifically non-acceptance of thoughts and emotions, may not necessarily be detrimental to paramedics (Mitmansgruber et al., 2008). Indeed, maintaining focus and a healthy detachment from the patient in order to do the job can potentially support resilience. However, interventions that target mindfulness may benefit EMS personnel when they are off-duty or between calls and aid in their transition from work to home life. For instance, mindful breathing exercises may help EMS personnel after a particularly challenging call and improve their ability to "bounce back."

Emergency Dispatch

Similar to EMS providers, there is a notable dearth of studies on mindfulness and wellness among emergency dispatch operators. In a longitudinal study of dispatchers (n = 149), a web-based mindfulness intervention (no control or comparison group) demonstrated improved coping self-efficacy and greater empathy toward callers (Kerr et al., 2019). Participants reported barriers to practicing mindfulness, with the most common barriers being work-related, primarily having insufficient time to practice the intervention during work shifts (Kerr et al., 2019). A similar, but smaller, pilot study among emergency dispatchers in the Southeastern USA also evinced promising results (Anshel et al., 2012). As such, mental health professionals who are interested in tailoring existing RTP or MBRT interventions for emergency dispatchers may need to address logistical concerns. For instance, an intervention may be more successful if trainers/facilitators encourage emergency dispatchers to practice mindfulness-based exercises outside of their work shift or during work breaks and highlight the value of this practice, even when it is not during the most stressful moments of their work. Interventions available online or via apps also might enhance uptake and traverse pragmatic barriers (e.g., cost, scheduling).

Large-Scale Implementation

There is no standardized, evidence-based best-practice formula for the implementation of programs designed to enhance mindfulness, wellness, and resilience in first-responder organizations. Based on the current literature, departments and/or organizations can use the below steps to implement a peer-supported approach that allows for iterative and periodic program evaluation. Specifically, the following steps outline how to implement a model program that is focused on building mindfulness and resilience among a fire department.

Assess Department Needs

Approval and "buy-in" from command staff is required for the initiation of any successful initiative. Prior to implementing any program, the assessment of specific challenges faced by department personnel is necessary. This can be conducted through anonymous surveys (e.g., administered via online platforms), focus groups (e.g., members from multiple stations across the county or city), and/or interviews with first responders across ranks and volunteer/career status. Additionally, available research on first responders-specific mental health and occupational stress should be reviewed to inform the types of questions that need to be asked or avoided. This process can be bolstered by consulting with mental health professionals who have experience working with first responders. This can be facilitated by relying on extant work among other departments and/or by national organizations devoted to improving the mental health and well-being of first responders (e.g., First Responder Center of Excellence). A preliminary cost-benefit analysis may also be included (see the *Promote sustainability* subsection below for additional information).

Develop a Curriculum

A curriculum can be developed that is tailored to the specific challenges faced by department personnel identified in the assessment stage. For instance, poor sleep and/or difficulties in transitioning from work to home after a shift may be salient challenges endorsed by personnel. A curriculum can be developed that (1) highlights the current rates of sleep difficulties and occupational stress among first responders to normalize these challenges and (2) introduces psychoeducation on mindfulness and its effects on sleep, stress, and resilience. The curriculum can also include (3) opportunities to learn and practice mindfulness-based experiences (e.g., breathing exercises, guided meditations, and body scans) in individual and/or small group sessions and (4) discussion of experiences with exercises, reviewing methods on how to implement these techniques during a shift, after a shift, or at home and encouraging first responders to practice these exercises on a daily and/or weekly basis. This process may also be supported by consulting with mental health professionals who have experience working with first responders.

Train Program Facilitators

Facilitators can include (1) personnel from the department trained by a mental health professional (i.e., peer-support specialists), (2) mental health professionals, or (3) a combination of these two groups. Facilitators should be experienced in the practice and the delivery of mindfulness-based exercises, be familiar with the curriculum and program, and have foundational and applied knowledge of the needs of first responders in the department. Formal training of the facilitators can be achieved via courses/workshops led by mental health professionals who have experience working with first responders. Alternatively, departments could invest in the development of online programming that is available 24/7 via websites or apps, should such feedback be observed among their personnel.

Program Launch

RTP or MBRT programs can be launched through a variety of methods. Depending on the format of the program, a series of in-person or virtual workshops, training sessions, or retreats can be advertised throughout the department via email distribution lists, departmental web-sites, paper flyers posted in stations or apparatus, and/or direct messages from specific department chiefs or station captains. QR codes can be posted on paper flyers for easy scanning and access to content for first responders with smartphones. Raffle prizes and/or compensation can used to incentivize feedback about the programs (e.g., survey responses, focus groups), particularly in the early stages of implementation. See the *Promote sustainability* subsection below for additional information on financial support.

Program Evaluation and Feedback

Evaluating the effectiveness of the program on a routine basis (e.g., posttraining and/or 1-month follow-up), via brief surveys and group/individual feedback interviews with first responders, is essential. Specifically, program evaluation can help identify areas for improvement and ensure that the program is meeting its goals. It can also serve to quantify its utility and generate data that will support its longevity in the department. This may be important data to provide to command staff and emergency services district (ESD) boards, which may solidify their support of the program. Such program evaluation surveys can be presented after each curriculum component is delivered or after an entire program is completed by first responders. The surveys should take no more than 5 min to complete and might be comprised of quantitative (e.g., rating scales for key pieces of feedback) and qualitative (e.g., open-ended prompts) components. Program evaluation is most successful if it is brief and presented as *necessary and essential* for the continual improvement of the program and the prioritization of the behavioral health of first responders.

Promote Sustainability

Finally, the RTP and MBRT program should be designed to be sustainable, with ongoing support and training for facilitators, as well as regular opportunities for first responders to engage and reengage with the program (e.g., refresher courses or workshops; online or app-based learning; teletherapy/video conferencing options). Sustainability may also be maintained via financial support for the program. Specifically, applying for city-, state-, and/or federal-level grants that aim to improve access to mental health-related resources for first responders can assist with financially supporting RTP and MBRT programs. For instance, the Federal Emergency Management Agency "Preparedness Grants" can be used to fund non-disaster projects to support first-responder populations. These grants can be used for research-related initiatives to develop, implement, and evaluate a RTP or MBRT program and provide crucial funding for compensating personnel who are leading the program. City- or state-level internal funding may also be available to support programming. Finally, partnerships with a national first-responder organization or a university-based department or center with specialized experience in working with first responders can offer low-cost frameworks and mutually rewarding community partnerships for supporting the development and evaluation of RTP or MBRT programs.

Client-Focused Implementation

Mental health professionals may also be interested in using mindfulness-based and resilience-building skills in a therapy session with a first-responder client. Below is a sample dialogue between a therapist who is interested in introducing mindfulness-based skills (e.g., mindful attention) with a first-responder client who is experiencing increased stress and burnout.

First Responder: I've been really stressed out lately. I can't focus and I keep going over things in my head, especially after a long shift. It's getting in the way of work and I'm constantly on edge at home. My coworkers and family are always on my case.

Therapist: It sounds like you have a lot going on. A lot of first responders have similar experiences. Sometimes, not enough is said about how stressful and demanding the job can be. Transitions from that level of stress to home life can also be especially challenging. What you are experiencing, while difficult, is common among the first responder community. We have found that training the mind to be anchored in the present can be helpful. It's called mindful attention training. It has been used by the military for years, and they have found it to be effective in reducing stress and improving mental wellness among our service members. Would you like to learn more about mindful attention training?

First Responder: I've heard of it, but I'm not really sure what it means and how to use it.

Therapist: Mindful attention is about being present in the moment and paying attention to what's going on in your mind and body without judgment. It can be helpful for reducing stress and anxiety, particularly after a challenging shift or conflict at home. What do you think? Are you up to giving mindful attention training a shot?

First Responder: Sure.

Therapist: OK. Let's start by focusing on your breath. Learning to regulate our breathing and infuse our body with oxygen is the most reliable way to take the edge off of stress or anxiety – the same technique you use to conserve your air. It might not make it go away completely – it probably won't – but oxygen should take stress and anxiety down a notch. Ready to try?

First Responder: OK. Right now?

Therapist: We can try together right now, if you would like to go for it. It should only take a few minutes.

First Responder: OK.

Therapist: First, find a comfortable position, close your eyes or focus on an object, and take a few deep breaths through your nose. As you inhale, imagine the air filling your lungs and expanding your belly. As you exhale, imagine the air leaving your body. Now we'll try an exercise called "box breathing." Each breath interval will be 4 s long. Take in air for 4 s, hold it in for 4 s, breathe out for 4 s, and hold for 4 s. And then start again. This can help reduce your body's fight-or-flight response.

[Therapist demonstrates and first responder follows. They breathe together for a few minutes]

First Responder: Okay, I'm doing that now.

Therapist: Great. Now, as you continue to breathe, notice any thoughts that come up. You don't need to judge them or try to change them. Just observe them and let them go, like clouds passing in the sky or a leaf floating down a river.

First Responder: I'm having a hard time not getting distracted by my thoughts.

Therapist: That is normal. Our minds tend to wander! When you notice your mind wandering, gently bring your attention back to your breath; focus on counting the seconds that pass. Remember that thoughts are just thoughts. They are not truths or reality; they come and go. We can train our mind to let them pass and not get "stuck" in them by believing them as facts.

First Responder: Okay, I'll try that now.

Therapist: Great. It's important to remember that mindful attention is like trying out any new skill, it takes time and practice to develop. You can start by practicing for just a few minutes a day and gradually increase the time as you feel more comfortable.

First Responder: That makes sense. How else can I do mindful attention training?

Therapist: The cool thing about it is that you can practice anywhere, without people knowing that you're doing anything. For example, you can try mindful walking, where you coordinate breathing by number of steps. You can take a deep breath in for five steps and then exhale for ten steps. You can also try a body scan, where you focus on different parts of your body and notice any sensations or tension. There are many different mindful attention strategies to try, and we can explore them together. Most are super brief and you can really practice anywhere. Remember, the goal of mindful attention training is not to get rid of your thoughts or feelings but to be more aware of them and to gain some distance from them. Instead of experiencing your thoughts and feelings up close and getting stuck in them, mindful attention helps you create a bit of distance from them so you can observe them and let them go in the moment.

Considerations for Implementation

The most-cited obstacles for the successful implementation of RTPs and/or MBRTs are similar to those of first responders seeking mental wellness resources in general – culture, stigma, program cost, and hectic schedules (Crane et al., 2021; Papazoglou & Andersen, 2014; Taylor, 2022). While fire and law enforcement cultures share some similarities (e.g., "us vs. them" mentality, humor as coping), there are significant differences. In the fire service, the work is team-based (Papazoglou & Andersen, 2014; Van Scotter & Leonard, 2022); career firefighters normally operate as part of an engine or truck company of four personnel (minimum standard established by NFPA 1710 for safety; Moore-Merrell et al., 2021). Shifts vary by department but can be up to 48 h in duration; common shifts are 24 on/48 off and 48 on/96 off (Billings & Focht, 2016). Firefighters live at the station, share meals, perform station duties (e.g., apparatus and equipment checks, cleaning), exercise, participate in training, and engage in public relations activities (e.g., station tours and fire education for children, installing residential smoke detectors) in addition to running calls.

In contrast, the LEO culture is focused more on the individual (e.g., Paoline, 2003; Van Scotter & Leonard, 2022). Police are focused on protecting self (and patrol partner) and maintaining situational awareness of a variety of threats in the environment (Van Scotter & Leonard, 2022). The shiftwork schedule is also different from that in fire, with patrol officers normally assigned to 8–10-h shifts (Peterson et al., 2019). LEOs do not live at the station like firefighters do; however, overtime and changing shifts can be problematic. Moreover, shift duration and changing schedules may put more time constraints on LEOs for completing RTP training at their stations while on duty (Eddy et al., 2021).

First-responder populations are historically predominantly male, with self-induced (and culturally induced) pressure to be a "tough guy" and not exhibit weakness. In the USA, women represent only 8% of firefighters (4% in career departments; Fahey et al., 2021) and 13% of LEOs (National Institute of Justice, 2019). Research has suggested that men are less likely than women to acknowledge and seek help for mental health issues (e.g., O'Toole & Brown, 2021; Taylor, 2022). As such, this predominantly male environment may have implications for acceptance of RTPs.

Stigma is a significant barrier to first responders seeking help for mental health services (Johnson et al., 2020; Vujanovic & Tran, 2021), which may also translate to the acceptance (or lack thereof) of RTPs. First responders may exhibit concern about seeming weak, have anxiety about confidentiality, and experience fear of being deemed unfit for duty (Taylor, 2022). Supportive leadership that demonstrates empathy rather than judgment (Taylor, 2022) and actively supports resilience training (Crane et al., 2021) can help combat this stigma. Encouraging first responders experiencing distress at any level to participate in mental health services may also serve to reduce stigma for those who seek it in times of severe distress/crisis. In addition to acceptability, scalability and cost-effectiveness are important criteria by which to judge whether specific RTPs are feasible for specific departments (Crane et al., 2021). However, large group training can feel less personalized to the participants; a compromise is incorporating individual-based self-reflection activities (e.g., journaling; Papazoglou & Andersen, 2014) within the larger group training format (Crane et al., 2021) or delivering training online or via an app so that individuals can participate when they have time, confidentially and anonymously, and without pressure or worry about others' perceptions.

Ideally, resilience training should begin in the academy and continue throughout a career (Crane et al., 2021; Papazoglou & Andersen, 2014), or at the very least, first responders should be provided information on community-based providers and resources to encourage engagement. Beyond the academy, there is debate whether RTPs should be mandatory. Mandatory programs avoid singling out personnel with mental health issues since everyone has to attend training (Taylor, 2022); however, making training mandatory may decrease employee engagement and motivation (Crane et al., 2021). A middle-ground might be to tie such training to continuing education credits for career departments so that choice rests within each first responder or to incorporate such training into a menu of regular required training. Following a trauma-informed model, first responders should maintain choice about participating. It is up to departments to encourage, support, and provide access so that programming is available for those who choose to pursue it. Embedding resilience training into regular operational training may be more effective than having standalone "mental health" training (Papazoglou & Andersen, 2014; Wild et al.,

2020). Furthermore, using a strengths-based approach to resilience as a way to improve performance and cognitive ability, rather than focusing on weaknesses or mental health problems, can help combat stigma (Crane et al., 2021; Papazoglou & Andersen, 2014).

Since RTP acceptability can be such an issue for first responders, resilience and mindfulness smartphone application development may be an important area for future work. O'Toole and Brown (2021) discuss apps developed for Canadian military and public safety personnel and suggest that apps are more accessible and confidential than other modes of mental health care, thereby improving stigma. Indeed, many apps are free to use and are currently available via the US Department of Veterans Affairs. Moreover, other online trainings or apps might be developed by first-responder departments; while there may be more upfront financial costs, this approach may lead to greater longevity and sustainability over time.

Limitations and Future Directions

Research on RTPs, mindfulness, and wellness programs is in early stages of development in first responders. Extant RCTs have used a variety of methodological approaches. A systematic review of 13 studies examining the effectiveness of RTPs on resilience and well-being among first responders found larger effects for interventions that targeted modifiable risk factors for psychopathology compared to those that did not (Wild et al., 2020). Therefore, despite some promising results that suggest first responders may benefit from these interventions, a consolidated review of the literature underscores the pressing need for further research.

Future research should focus on developing and evaluating the most effective content and modes of delivery and implementation for these types of programs. A push toward developing first-responder-specific as well as online and/or mobile app-based RTPs and wellness programs may increase participant engagement and reduce barriers to services, including both pragmatic barriers (e.g., travel) and stigma (Scheuch et al., 2021). The ongoing demands and burdens of the COVID-19 pandemic, including mandated self-isolation and quarantine, have reshaped the landscape for virtual delivery of health-related services and enhanced uptake of virtual meeting formats and teletherapy. Furthermore, blended/hybrid approaches to delivery (e.g., a combination of online and face-to-face formats) may be promising (Scheuch et al., 2021). For instance, an RCT examining a single-session, group-based, virtual (video-conferencing format) mindfulness-based intervention for firefighters, as compared to a waitlist control condition, is currently underway to evaluate its potential efficacy in reducing mental health symptoms and improve resilience (Vujanovic et al., 2022). Overall, a greater emphasis on developing initiatives and programs that cater to the needs and culture of first responders and specific first-responder groups may be vital to increasing efficacy and effectiveness.

Conclusions

First responders are essential to the health and wellness of our communities. Increasing attention in recent years has been directed toward enhancing the resilience and wellness of first responders. However, these initiatives are largely in nascent stages at empirical, clinical, and public policy levels. With increasing attention to the inherent occupational stressors and demands of first responder occupations, we can continue to build awareness, reduce mental health stigma, and support the health and well-being of first responders through innovative programming that is evidence-based, specialized, and pragmatically tailored to meet the unique needs of first-responder populations.

References

Anshel, M. H., Umscheid, D., & Brinthaupt, T. M. (2012). Effect of a combined coping skills and wellness program on perceived stress and physical energy among police emergency dispatchers: An exploratory study. *Journal of Police and Criminal Psychology, 28*(1), 1–14. https://doi.org/10.1007/s11896-012-9110-x

Baer, R. A., Smith, G. T., Hopkins, J., Krietemeyer, J., & Toney, L. (2006). Using self-report assessment methods to explore facets of mindfulness. *Assessment, 13*(1), 27–45. https://doi.org/10.1177/1073191105283504

Billings, J., & Focht, W. (2016). Firefighter shift schedules affect sleep quality. *Journal of Occupational and Environmental Medicine, 58*(3), 294–298. https://doi.org/10.1097/JOM.0000000000000624

Bravo, A. J., Pearson, M. R., & Kelley, M. L. (2018). Mindfulness and psychological health outcomes: A latent profile analysis among military personnel and college students. *Mindfulness (New York), 9*(1), 258–270. https://doi.org/10.1007/s12671-017-0771-5

Carleton, R. N., Afifi, T. O., Taillieu, T., Turner, S., El-Gabalawy, R., Sareen, J., & Asmundson, G. J. G. (2018). Anxiety-related psychopathology and chronic pain comorbidity among public safety personnel. *Journal of Anxiety Disorders, 55*, 48–55. https://doi.org/10.1016/j.janxdis.2018.03.006

Christopher, M. S., Goerling, R. J., Rogers, B. S., Hunsinger, M., Baron, G., Bergman, A. L., & Zava, D. T. (2016). A pilot study evaluating the effectiveness of a mindfulness-based intervention on cortisol awakening response and health outcomes among law enforcement officers. *Journal of Police and Criminal Psychology, 31*(1), 15–28. https://doi.org/10.1007/s11896-015-9161-x

Congress, H. R. (2018). *Law enforcement mental health and wellness act of 2017*, H.R. 2228, 115th Congress (2018). Retrieved from https://www.congress.gov/115/plaws/publ113/PLAW-115publ113.pdf

Counson, I., Hosemans, D., Lal, T. J., Mott, B., Harvey, S. B., & Joyce, S. (2019). Mental health and mindfulness amongst Australian fire fighters. *BMC Psychology, 7*(1), 34. https://doi.org/10.1186/s40359-019-0311-2

Crane, M. F., Falon, S. L., Kho, M., Moss, A., & Adler, A. B. (2021). Developing resilience in first responders: Strategies for enhancing psychoeducational service delivery. *Psychological Services*. https://doi.org/10.1037/ser0000439

Denkova, E., Zanesco, A. P., Rogers, S. L., & Jha, A. P. (2020). Is resilience trainable? An initial study comparing mindfulness and relaxation training in firefighters. *Psychiatry Research, 285*, 112794. https://doi.org/10.1016/j.psychres.2020.112794

DOJ. (2021). *Justice department announces funding to promote law enforcement mental health and wellness*. Department of Justice, Office of Public Affairs. https://www.justice.gov/opa/pr/justice-department-announces-funding-promote-law-enforcement-mental-health-and-wellness.

Eddy, A., Bergman, A. L., Kaplan, J. B., Goerling, R. J., & Christopher, M. S. (2021). A qualitative investigation of the experience of mindfulness training among police officers. *Journal of Police and Criminal Psychology, 36*(1), 63–71. https://doi.org/10.1007/s11896-019-09340-7

Fahey, R., Evarts, B., & Stein, G. P. (2021). *US fire department profile 2019*. N. F. P. Association. https://www.nfpa.org/-/media/files/News-and-Research/Fire-statistics-and-reports/Emergency-responders/osfdprofile.pdf

Floyd, R., Rackelmann, S., McQuaide, S., Hartogensis, W., & Mehling, W. (2022). Yoga for firefighters: Evaluation of a quality improvement program in California fire departments. *Journal of Bodywork and Movement Therapies*. https://doi.org/10.1016/j.jbmt.2022.05.019

Grupe, D. W., McGehee, C., Smith, C., Francis, A. D., Mumford, J. A., & Davidson, R. J. (2021). Mindfulness training reduces PTSD symptoms and improves stress-related health outcomes in police officers. *Journal of Police and Criminal Psychology, 36*(1), 72–85. https://doi.org/10.1007/s11896-019-09351-4

Hartley, T. A., Burchfiel, C. M., Fekedulegn, D., Andrew, M. E., & Violanti, J. M. (2011). Health disparities in police officers: Comparisons to the U.S. general population. *International Journal of Emergency Mental Health, 13*(4), 211–220.

Huang, Q., Zhang, Q., An, Y., & Xu, W. (2019). The relationship between dispositional mindfulness and PTSD/PTG among firefighters: The mediating role of emotion regulation. *Personality and Individual Differences, 151*. https://doi.org/10.1016/j.paid.2019.07.002

IAFF. (2018). *The fire service joint labor management wellness-fitness initiative*. https://www.iafc.org/topics-and-tools/safety-health/wellness-fitness-task-force/wellness-fitness-program-summary

Jahnke, S. A., Poston, W. S., Haddock, C. K., & Murphy, B. (2016). Firefighting and mental health: Experiences of repeated exposure to trauma. *Work, 53*(4), 737–744. https://doi.org/10.3233/wor-162255

Johnson, C. C., Vega, L., Kohalmi, A. L., Roth, J. C., Howell, B. R., & Van Hasselt, V. B. (2020). Enhancing mental health treatment for the firefighter population: Understanding fire culture, treatment barriers, practice implications, and research directions. *Professional Psychology: Research and Practice, 51*(3), 304–311. https://doi.org/10.1037/pro0000266

Jones, S. (2017). Describing the mental health profile of first responders: A systematic review. *Journal of the American Psychiatric Nurses Association, 23*(3), 200–214. https://doi.org/10.1177/1078390317695266

Jones, S., Nagel, C., McSweeney, J., & Curran, G. (2018). Prevalence and correlates of psychiatric symptoms among first responders in a Southern State. *Archives of Psychiatric Nursing, 32*(6), 828–835. https://doi.org/10.1016/j.apnu.2018.06.007

Joyce, S., Shand, F., Tighe, J., Laurent, S. J., Bryant, R. A., & Harvey, S. B. (2018). Road to resilience: A systematic review and meta-analysis of resilience training programmes and interventions. *BMJ Open, 8*(6), e017858. https://doi.org/10.1136/bmjopen-2017-017858

Joyce, S., Shand, F., Lal, T. J., Mott, B., Bryant, R. A., & Harvey, S. B. (2019). Resilience@work mindfulness program: Results from a cluster randomized controlled trial with first responders. *Journal of Medical Internet Research, 21*(2), e12894. https://doi.org/10.2196/12894

Kahn, J. R., Collinge, W., & Soltysik, R. (2016). Post-9/11 veterans and their partners improve mental health outcomes with a self-directed mobile and web-based wellness training program: A randomized controlled trial. *Journal of Medical Internet Research, 18*(9), e255. https://doi.org/10.2196/jmir.5800

Kaplan, J. B., Bergman, A. L., Christopher, M., Bowen, S., & Hunsinger, M. (2017). Role of resilience in mindfulness training for first responders. *Mindfulness (N Y), 8*(5), 1373–1380. https://doi.org/10.1007/s12671-017-0713-2

Kaplan, J. B., Christopher, M., & Bowen, S. (2018). Dispositional mindfulness moderates the relationship between occupational stressors and perceived stress among law enforcement personnel. *Journal of Police and Criminal Psychology, 33*(3), 227–232. https://doi.org/10.1007/s11896-017-9246-9

Kaplan, J. B., Bergman, A. L., Green, K., Dapolonia, E., & Christopher, M. (2020). Relative impact of mindfulness, self-compassion, and psychological flexibility on alcohol use and burnout among law enforcement officers. *Journal of Alternative and Complementary Medicine, 26*(12), 1190–1194. https://doi.org/10.1089/acm.2020.0178

Kerr, D. C., Ornelas, I. J., Lilly, M. M., Calhoun, R., & Meischke, H. (2019). Participant engagement in and perspectives on a web-based mindfulness intervention for 9-1-1 telecommunicators: Multimethod study. *Journal of Medical Internet Research, 21*(6), e13449. https://doi.org/10.2196/13449

Kuehl, H., Mabry, L., Elliot, D. L., Kuehl, K. S., & Favorite, K. C. (2013). Factors in adoption of a fire department wellness program: Champ-and-chief model. *Journal of Occupational and Environmental Medicine, 55*(4), 424–429. https://doi.org/10.1097/JOM.0b013e31827dba3f

Lapum, D. (2020). *The maintenance of police officer health through a mandatory wellness program.* https://www.nationalpublicsafetypartnership.org/Clearinghouse/Resource/378/The-Maintenance-of-Police-Officer-Health-Through-A-Mandatory-Wellness-Program

Lebeaut, A., Zegel, M., Leonard, S. J., Bartlett, B. A., & Vujanovic, A. A. (2021). Examining transdiagnostic factors among firefighters in relation to trauma exposure, probable PTSD, and probable Alcohol Use Disorder. *Journal of Dual Diagnosis, 17*(1), 52–63. https://doi.org/10.1080/15504263.2020.1854411

Luthar, S. S., & Cicchetti, D. (2000). The construct of resilience: A critical evaluation and guidelines for future work. *Child Development, 71*(3), 543. https://doi.org/10.1111/1467-8624.00164

Mahaffey, B. L., Mackin, D. M., Rosen, J., Schwartz, R. M., Taioli, E., & Gonzalez, A. (2021). The disaster worker resiliency training program: A randomized clinical trial. *International Archives of Occupational and Environmental Health, 94*(1), 9–21. https://doi.org/10.1007/s00420-020-01552-3

Matto, H. C., & Sullivan, K. (2021). Ashes2Art: Mitigation strategies for short-and long-term distress in emergency services personnel during COVID-19. *Clinical Social Work Journal, 49*(4), 437–444. https://doi.org/10.1007/s10615-021-00797-w

Mitmansgruber, H., Beck, T. N., & Schüßler, G. (2008). "Mindful helpers": Experiential avoidance, meta-emotions, and emotion regulation in paramedics. *Journal of Research in Personality, 42*(5), 1358–1363. https://doi.org/10.1016/j.jrp.2008.03.012

Moore-Merrell, L., Kerber, S., Horn, G. P., & Smith, D. L. (2021). Effects of crew size on firefighter health and safety. *International Fire Service Journal of Leadership and Management, 15*, 7–25.

Nazari, G., Osifeso, T. A., & MacDermid, J. C. (2020). Distribution of number, location of pain and comorbidities, and determinants of work limitations among firefighters. *Rehabilitation Research and Practice, 2020*, 1942513. https://doi.org/10.1155/2020/1942513

National Institute of Justice. (2019). *Special Report: Women in Policing: Breaking Barriers and Blazing a Path. U.S.* Department of Justice, Office of Justice Programs. https://www.ojp.gov/pdffiles1/nij/252963.pdf.

National Fire Protection Association (2022). NFPA 1582 standard on comprehensive occupational medical program for fire departments. In *Codes & Standards*. National Fire Protection Association.

O'Toole, K., & Brown, C. A. (2021). Evaluating the quality of resilience apps for military members and public safety personnel. *Journal of Military, Veteran and Family Health, 7*(1), 87–101. https://doi.org/10.3138/jmvfh-2020-0002

Paoline, E. A. (2003). Taking stock: Toward a richer understanding of police culture. *Journal of Criminal Justice, 31*(3), 199–214. https://doi.org/10.1016/s0047-2352(03)00002-3

Papazoglou, K., & Andersen, J. P. (2014). A guide to utilizing police training as a tool to promote resilience and improve health outcomes among police officers. *Traumatology: An International Journal, 20*(2), 103–111. https://doi.org/10.1037/h0099394

Peterson, S. A., Wolkow, A. P., Lockley, S. W., O'Brien, C. S., Qadri, S., Sullivan, J. P., Czeisler, C. A., Rajaratnam, S. M. W., & Barger, L. K. (2019). Associations between shift work characteristics, shift work schedules, sleep and burnout in North American police officers: A cross-sectional study. *BMJ Open, 9*(11), e030302. https://doi.org/10.1136/bmjopen-2019-030302

Rachele, J. N., Heesch, K. C., & Washington, T. L. (2014). Wellness programs at firefighter and police workplaces: A systematic review. *Health Behavior and Policy Review, 1*(4), 302–312. https://doi.org/10.14485/HBPR.1.4.5

Reffi, A. N., Pinciotti, C. M., Darnell, B. C., & Orcutt, H. K. (2019). Trait mindfulness and PTSD symptom clusters: Considering the influence of emotion dysregulation. *Personality and Individual Differences, 137*, 62–70. https://doi.org/10.1016/j.paid.2018.08.010

Reichard, A. A., & Jackson, L. L. (2010). Occupational injuries among emergency responders. *American Journal of Industrial Medicine, 53*(1), 1–11. https://doi.org/10.1002/ajim.20772

Scheuch, I., Peters, N., Lohner, M. S., Muss, C., Aprea, C., & Furstenau, B. (2021). Resilience training programs in organizational contexts: A scoping review. *Frontiers in Psychology, 12*, 733036. https://doi.org/10.3389/fpsyg.2021.733036

Setti, I., & Argentero, P. (2014). The role of mindfulness in protecting firefighters from psychosomatic malaise. *Traumatology: An International Journal, 20*(2), 134–141. https://doi.org/10.1037/h0099398

Skeffington, P. M., Rees, C. S., Mazzucchelli, T. G., & Kane, R. T. (2016). The primary prevention of PTSD in firefighters: Preliminary results of an RCT with 12-month follow-up. *PLoS One, 11*(7), e0155873. https://doi.org/10.1371/journal.pone.0155873

Smith, B. W., Ortiz, J. A., Steffen, L. E., Tooley, E. M., Wiggins, K. T., Yeater, E. A., Montoya, J. D., & Bernard, M. L. (2011). Mindfulness is associated with fewer PTSD symptoms, depressive symptoms, physical symptoms, and alcohol problems in urban firefighters. *Journal of Consulting and Clinical Psychology, 79*(5), 613–617. https://doi.org/10.1037/a0025189

Stanley, I. H., Hom, M. A., Hagan, C. R., & Joiner, T. E. (2015). Career prevalence and correlates of suicidal thoughts and behaviors among firefighters. *Journal of Affective Disorders, 187*, 163–171. https://doi.org/10.1016/j.jad.2015.08.007

Stanley, I. H., Hom, M. A., & Joiner, T. E. (2016). A systematic review of suicidal thoughts and behaviors among police officers, firefighters, EMTs, and paramedics. *Clinical Psychology Review, 44*, 25–44. https://doi.org/10.1016/j.cpr.2015.12.002

Stanley, I. H., Boffa, J. W., Tran, J. K., Schmidt, N. B., Joiner, T. E., & Vujanovic, A. A. (2019). Posttraumatic stress disorder symptoms and mindfulness facets in relation to suicide risk among firefighters. *Journal of Clinical Psychology, 75*(4), 696–709. https://doi.org/10.1002/jclp.22748

Syed, S., Ashwick, R., Schlosser, M., Jones, R. E., Rowe, S., & Billings, J. (2020). Global prevalence and risk factors for mental health problems in police personnel: A systematic review and meta-analysis. *Occupational and Environmental Medicine, 77*(11), 737–747. https://doi.org/10.1136/oemed-2020-106498

Taylor, M. A. (2022). Building resilience in law enforcement through a mental wellness program. *Journal of Police and Criminal Psychology, 37*(1), 155–161. https://doi.org/10.1007/s11896-021-09479-2

Thoen, M. A., Dodson, L. E., Manzo, G., Pina-Watson, B., & Trejos-Castillo, E. (2020). Agency-offered and officer-utilized suicide prevention and wellness programs: A national study. *Psychological Services, 17*(2), 129–140. https://doi.org/10.1037/ser0000355

Van Scotter, J. R., & Leonard, K. M. (2022). Clashes of cultures during crises: Coordinating firefighter, police and paramedic interactions. *Disaster Prevention and Management: An International Journal*. https://doi.org/10.1108/dpm-09-2021-0273

Vujanovic, A. A., & Tran, J. K. (2021). Providing psychological services to firefighters. *Journal of Health Service Psychology, 47*(3), 137–148. https://doi.org/10.1007/s42843-021-00041-6

Vujanovic, A. A., Lebeaut, A., Zegel, M., & Buser, S. J. (2022). Mindful attention training workshop for firefighters: Design and methodology of a pilot randomized clinical trial. *Contemporary Clinical Trials Communications, 27*. https://doi.org/10.1016/j.conctc.2022.100905

Wild, J., El-Salahi, S., Degli Esposti, M., & Thew, G. R. (2020). Evaluating the effectiveness of a group-based resilience intervention versus psychoeducation for emergency responders in England: A randomised controlled trial. *PLoS One, 15*(11), e0241704. https://doi.org/10.1371/journal.pone.0241704

Williams, V., Ciarrochi, J., & Patrick Deane, F. (2010). On being mindful, emotionally aware, and more resilient: Longitudinal pilot study of police recruits. *Australian Psychologist, 45*(4), 274–282. https://doi.org/10.1080/00050060903573197

Critical Incident Stress Management (CISM)

Jeffrey T. Mitchell and George S. Everly Jr

Part I. A Sensible Staff Support System

> The ambulance was silent. Mark and I did not speak a word. I kept my eyes on the road. His were on the floor. We just dropped off a massively injured 6-year-old auto accident victim at the hospital. She didn't make it.
>
> Mark and I had become good friends in EMT school 6 months earlier. But I wasn't prepared for what would happen to our friendship in the next few minutes.
>
> At the station, he got out of the ambulance and walked over to the rack that held the fire turnout gear. He picked up his coat, helmet, and boots, gave them to the chief, and walked out of the station. I never saw him again. His pregnant wife called me a few days later and said that Mark was very sorry, but he was so badly shaken by the death of the child that he did not want any reminders of the fire service and EMS and, unfortunately, those reminders included my friendship. – Jeffrey T. Mitchell, Ph.D.

That summary of an event that happened over 50 years ago is just one sample of numerous tragedies and trauma exposures that have occurred in the experience of law enforcement, fire service, emergency medical, search and rescue, corrections, communications, disaster response, hospital emergency department, critical care, and military personnel. Traumatic events certainly laid the foundation for the development of the field of critical incident stress management (CISM).

In 50 years, much has happened in the CISM field. Its services have expanded far beyond anything that was envisioned when it began. Its primary focus remains on

J. T. Mitchell (✉)
Department of Emergency Health Services, University of Maryland, Baltimore County, Baltimore, MD, USA

International Critical Incident Stress Foundation, Ellicott City, MD, USA
e-mail: jmitch@umbc.edu

G. S. Everly Jr
International Critical Incident Stress Foundation, Ellicott City, MD, USA

School of Public Health, Johns Hopkins University, Baltimore, MD, USA

M. L. Bourke et al. (eds.), *First Responder Mental Health*,
https://doi.org/10.1007/978-3-031-38149-2_10

frontline emergency service and military personnel mentioned above, who experience the almost daily horrors associated with their work. CISM services are also utilized by people in a wide range of professions including, but not limited to, medicine, education, business, aviation, railroads and other forms of public transportation, utilities, a broad spectrum of manufacturing and construction industries, religious institutions, service organizations, and a wide range of governmental entities at the local, state, and federal levels. It should be noted that CISM services have been used by the significant others, families, and friends of frontline personnel in countries around the world (Mitchell, 2007).

The International Critical Incident Stress Foundation (ICISF), which provides training, consultation, and education for the many organizations listed above, is recognized by numerous educational institutions such as the University of Maryland, Baltimore County. It has also been recognized as a nongovernmental organization in special consultative status with the Department of Safety and Security of the United Nations, which has utilized CISM services many thousands of times in over 100 countries (United Nations Department of Safety and Security, 2007a, b, c).

This chapter contains extensive coverage of the critical incident stress management (CISM) field. There is a great deal of material for a single chapter. The chapter, therefore, has been split into two parts to enhance the organization of the material for the benefit of the reader. Both parts contain essential information on CISM. Both parts are critical for a full understanding the CISM field and how and why it works. Part one covers the history and key concepts that have been derived from its history. It ends with the signs and symptoms of critical incident stress.

Part two contains vital information on the components of CISM, their applications, and the research that supports the entire field. Skipping any aspects of parts one and two jeopardizes the reader's thorough understanding of the field and its applications.

No chapter, even one that is organized into two parts to provide a comprehensive review of the CISM field, can substitute for specialized training in the field. Readers who wish to apply CISM components and applications must take proper training from instructors who are approved by the International Critical Incident Stress Foundation (ICISF).

CISM History

CISM Defined

Before presenting a brief history of critical incident stress management (CISM), it is important to have a working definition of CISM. It is a comprehensive, integrated, systematic, and multicomponent "package" of crisis intervention tools. Some of the crisis intervention tools are used to support individuals who have critical incident stress or who are in a state of crisis. Other tools are used to assist groups. These terms and tools will become clear as you read further in the chapter.

CISM and crisis intervention have a shared history (Mitchell & Everly, 2001; Mitchell, 2007).

CISM is literally over 50 years old. The year 1972 marks the time when the first CISM services and interventions were developed and provided to people in the emergency services. CISM does not, however, mark the beginning of crisis intervention. That occurred a hundred years earlier. CISM is a subset of crisis intervention. A subset is a smaller part of a bigger field. A subset shares in the history, research, theories, tactics, principles, and practices of the larger field. It also shares in the research that was performed to ensure that the processes within the field are safe and effective.

Early Crisis Intervention History

In 1870–1871, the French nation was embroiled in a short but deadly and destructive war with Prussia which had the largest, most well-equipped, best-trained, and most combat-ready military force in the world at that time. French soldiers were fleeing the front lines in droves. The French were on the verge of a catastrophic loss and the destruction of Paris (Crocq, 1999; Crocq et al., 2007).

French medical officers decided to try an experiment. Instead of punishing fleeing soldiers as deserters, they provided an opportunity for rest, food, fluid, reduction of war stimuli, regrouping with their units, and a chance to discuss their fears and concerns with medical officers. After these interventions, enough soldiers returned to the frontlines, and they fought well enough to allow the French government and its military commanders to come to a negotiated settlement of the war. Paris was not destroyed, and many lives were saved. Crisis intervention was born out of that conflict. It was the first time in history that the rudimentary concepts of crisis intervention (CI) were used in a formal, structured manner (Crocq, 1999; Crocq et al., 2007; Mitchell and Resnik, 1981; Freeman, 1979; Lindemann, 1944; Roberts, 2005). Those concepts are still used today. They include (a) reduction of disturbing stimuli; (b) rest; (c) food; (d) hydration; (e) regrouping with colleagues, friends, and family members; and (f) opportunity to discuss their fear and other physical and emotional reactions with medical or psychological support personnel.

Crisis Intervention in Disasters

These interventions are not only helpful during a war. They are also quite useful when assisting survivors of large-scale events like disasters. Out of the wars and disasters over the last 150 years, many support services were introduced to form, what is today, the CISM program (APA, 1964; Artiss, 1963; Caplan, 1961, 1964, 1969; Crocq, 1999; Crocq et al., 2007; Freeman, 1979; Lindemann, 1944; Roberts, 2005; Salmon, 1919; Stierlin, 1909).

For instance, Eduard Stierlin, a psychiatrist in the early 1900s, used crisis intervention techniques like those used in the Franco-Prussian War when he was working with the anxious families of miners in a 1906 French mining catastrophe. He also used the interventions with the courageous rescue teams that tried to save the miners who were victims of a massive explosion that collapsed a large coal mine. For 1100 miners, the damage was extreme, and the interventions were too late. The miners were killed in a methane gas explosion in one of history's worst mining disasters (Stierlin, 1909).

That event set the stage for the very earliest research studies on traumatic loss involving the families and colleagues of those killed in the Courrières mining disaster. It is encouraging to know that research concerning the effectiveness of crisis intervention and, subsequently, the critical incident stress management system was put in place in the earliest stages of the development of formal crisis intervention services (Stierlin, 1909).

The two world wars sparked the development of considerably improved crisis intervention techniques. Those wars and numerous disasters in the early 1900s through the 1960s laid the foundations for the development of critical incident stress management (CISM) in the early 1970s. One study after another demonstrated the positive effects of crisis intervention on soldiers, sailors, airmen, survivors, communities, and later the emergency services personnel. As more was learned about crisis intervention, the support services for emergency services and military personnel as well as civilian populations continued to improve manner (APA, 1964; Appel et al., 1946; Artiss, 1963; Caplan, 1961, 1964; Forstenzer, 1980; Frederick, 1981; Hassling, 2000; Kardiner & Spiegel, 1947; Lindy, 1985; Salmon, 1919).

Another term for Crisis Intervention is "psychological first aid." It was first used before the Second World War (Dewey, 1933) and appeared in both civilian and military circles; it meant a variety of support services. "Emotional first aid" is another term that has frequently been used throughout the history of crisis intervention (Neil et al., 1974).

Crisis Intervention Specifically for Emergency Services Personnel

The first crisis intervention services specifically for emergency services personnel were provided to firefighters who fought massive fires in London during the blitzkrieg by the German Luftwaffe in 1940. As in the Franco-Prussian War and disasters of the early 1900s, simple and short interventions had the best results. Feeding people and making sure they were hydrated, reducing distressing stimuli, letting them rest, and reconnecting them with their colleagues were very effective. One WWII London rescuer later wrote:

> Every night, from dusk to dawn, the German bombs fell upon them. Woolton suggested that I might go down about six o'clock when the 'all clear' sounded and see what I could do to help. I found that, as they came out of the shelters, what comforted them was a kiss and a cup of tea. (Boothby, 1978)

Those support services were followed by similar crisis services in a series of civilian disasters during and after the war. For several decades, from the early 1900s until 1972, crisis intervention for military and civilian populations was intertwined (Lifton, 1970, 1973, 1993). Lessons learned in one population applied to the other. Gradually, the two fields separated, to some extent, from each other (Mitchell, 1982a, b). Now there are crisis intervention programs within categories such as military psychology, disaster psychology, and emergency services.

Drs. Gerald Caplan and Eric Lindemann provided crisis intervention services for many people who had experienced a range of traumatic events. They opened a crisis clinic in Boston in the late 1930s. Their clinic provided crisis intervention to the survivors and grieving families and friends of the 494 people who were killed in the horrific Cocoanut Grove fire in November 1942. They also used crisis intervention to support the first responders who worked that tragic fire. Thirty years later, CISM services were introduced to first responders in a comprehensive package of supportive crisis intervention services (Lindemann, 1944; Mitchell, 1983).

Police Psychological Services Contribute to CISM Development

There were other developments along the way to CISM. Police psychologists were brought into the law enforcement field in the 1960s (Bard, 1970; Reese & Goldstein, 1986). Some went beyond psychological assessments for recruits and general support services for operational personnel. They provided a limited amount of psychological education and psychotherapy for law enforcement individuals and their spouses. Crisis intervention, at that time, consisted of field consultations for difficult crisis situations and brief interventions for distressed officers. It would be the 1970s before structured crisis intervention services like CISM were offered to law enforcement personnel and other first responders (Mitchell, 1983, 1991).

Psychological services for law enforcement personnel were limited by budgets and resistance from administrations and field supervisors who feared that having services from mental health resources would reflect badly on their own leadership skills. The most challenging problem for police departments and even federal law enforcement agencies, however, was that very few departments outside of large cities and heavily populated suburban areas had the trained personnel and financial resources necessary to institute police psychology programs. Those services were, in fact, rare. In 1977, only six agencies had a full-time psychologist (Reese & Goldstein, 1986).

In the mid-1960s and early 1970s, the Federal Bureau of Investigation (FBI), under the leadership of pioneers in the field of criminal profiling, was building its Behavioral Science Unit to assist communities in understanding criminal thinking and behaviors. The program was successful in assisting law enforcement across the USA in the apprehension and conviction of numerous criminals who might have otherwise gotten away with their horrible crimes.

Critical Incident Stress Management Arrives

After many contributions by dedicated individuals and forward-looking first-responder organizations, critical incident stress management (CISM) emerged in 1972. The primary stimulus for the development of CISM was the work of the author of this chapter, Dr. Jeffrey T. Mitchell of the Department of Emergency Health Services at the University of Maryland, Baltimore County. He believes:

> The primary concept that underlies the term Critical Incident Stress is that healthy, well-functioning people can undergo enormously stressful circumstances and have powerful reactions to those experiences, but not be inherently weak, or psychologically impaired prior to the traumatic event. In fact, because they are typically hardy or resilient people, they can usually resist the ill effects of stress, bounce back from the shock and disruption associated with the experience, recover from critical incident stress, and resume normal life functions within a relatively short time of their exposure to the traumatic event.
>
> In the majority of cases, early support lessens the duration of the symptoms. This is especially so when early psychological support is provided by peer support teams. Family, friends, and colleagues are also important in providing support. The signs and symptoms of Critical Incident Stress can lessen within a few days of the critical incident.... (Mitchell, 2020)

He provided crisis and stress management education and training for emergency services personnel as well as individual support services when needed. Although still experimental at that time, the first critical incident stress debriefing (CISD) was conducted in 1972 for a mixed group of firefighters, EMTs, paramedics, and police officers who worked on an incident involving multiple deaths of children in a horrific auto accident.

Every year since, there have been thousands of small tragedies, numerous terrible disasters, and devasting wars that have generated the development and implementation of increasingly more sophisticated crisis intervention and CISM strategies and tactics. Over 1,500 CISM teams now exist in 35 countries and in every one of the 50 states. The CISM field has come far in its expansion of services in the 150 years since rudimentary crisis intervention services were used during a major battle to save the city of Paris from destruction.

Critical Incidents, Stress, and Crisis

To provide efficient and effective peer support services, we first must understand basic crisis terminology and the principles and practices of crisis intervention. This section will lay the foundation for a sensible staff support program in the emergency services professions by presenting clear definitions and explanations of crisis support services.

Let us start with the term "critical incident." A *critical incident* is an event, situation, or circumstance that causes a strong physical and psychological reaction in an individual or a group. A critical incident is any event that has such a powerful stressful impact that it is sufficient to overwhelm the usually effective coping skills of an individual and, sometimes, even an entire group of emergency operations personnel.

A critical incident is sometimes called a *stressor* or, if it is a very serious or overwhelming event, it might be called a *trauma*. For instance, "This woman sustained a severe trauma when she went to visit her mother and found her dead in her home." The word *trauma* is borrowed from the field of medicine where it is used to describe damage to human tissue or organs. It often means the ripping, tearing, piercing, burning, or other destruction of skin, bones, and internal organs. From a psychological perspective, trauma means significant damage to the human mind (thinking processes) and emotions.

In summary, a critical incident is the stimulus that initiates a state of crisis. Here are some critical incidents that happen to emergency services personnel: (*the first five are usually considered the most stressful for first responders, but the list can change depending on the circumstances*) (a) work-related deaths of colleagues (known as line-of-duty deaths); (b) serious work-related injuries to coworkers; (c) suicide of a colleague; (d) accidental killing or wounding of any innocent person in the performance of one's duties; (e) disasters; (f) deaths to children, especially babies or toddlers; (g) seriously ill or injured children; (h) events involving a high degree of personnel threat; (i) "close calls" in which self or a colleague narrowly escaped being injured or killed; (j) officer-involved shootings; (k) worsening medical emergencies that occur while working on a patient; (l) entrapped victims in a fire; (m) handling the remains of the dead; (n) actively psychotic person in custody who is self-mutilating; (o) murder scenes (especially child victims); (p) threats of violence against emergency personnel; (q) terrorism, (r) violent subjects; (s) serious accidents involving emergency response vehicles; (t) hazardous materials incidents; (u) medical errors that injure or kill patients; (v) damaged or inoperable equipment that jeopardizes lifesaving; (w) fetal demise in labor and delivery; (x) witnessing a suicide in a prison cell block; and (y) listening to someone die on the phone while emergency units are being dispatched. There are innumerable others that could be added to the list.

A *crisis* is an acute emotional reaction to a powerful stimulus. It is a state of emotional turmoil. A crisis is not the same thing as a critical incident. A critical incident causes a crisis reaction. It is the event that starts the crisis. Some people use the term "crisis" to mean both the event and the reaction, but this is inaccurate. The event (critical incident) causes a significant psychological reaction called a "crisis." A psychological reaction is composed of two parts: what a person *thinks* (cognitive) and how a person *feels* (emotional). What someone thinks and how that person feels may trigger a third and then a fourth aspect of a crisis. That is to say, a *physical manifestation* in reaction to the critical incident and *changes in behavior* related to the traumatic experience. It may be helpful to think of a crisis reaction as a chaotic condition.

Characteristics of Crises

The characteristics of a crisis include (a) disruption to one's general state of psychological balance; (b) usual coping mechanisms fail; and (c) distress, impairment, or dysfunction (Caplan, 1964). There are two main types of crises: (1) *maturational* which is caused by circumstances that arise during one's life, e.g., adolescence, marriage, retirement, old age, etc., and (2) *situational* which is caused by events such as accidents, acts of violence, divorce, deaths of loved ones, loss of property, fires, floods, disasters, etc.

Stress Before we get too far along in this section, we need to consider the concept of stress. After all, we are dealing with a critical incident stress management program for a good part of this chapter. There is some overlap between these terms *crisis* and *stress.* For instance, they both are reactions to stimuli. However, there are some considerable differences too. A crisis is, from the start, a state of emotional turmoil. When a person is in turmoil, their ability to manage themselves, to think clearly, to make good decisions, or to take actions in their own best interests is impaired. Stress, on the other hand, is a range of typically normal reactions to stimuli from low levels to severe. In some cases, a stress response may turn into a state of crisis if stress becomes overwhelmingly severe and prolonged.

In the section above, a crisis is described as an *acute* state of emotional *turmoil* in reaction to a strong stimulus. Notice the words "acute" and "turmoil." They are a key to understanding the difference between a crisis and stress. You would not expect thoughtful, organized, and effective reactions from someone in an acute state of emotional turmoil. In most cases, people in a crisis are struggling to sort things out in the midst of a chaotic situation and their thoughts, decisions, and behaviors are usually haphazard and, sometimes, dangerous to themselves or others.

Stress is defined as a state of physical and mental arousal. It usually accompanies the crisis reaction. It is a cognitive, physical, emotional, and behavioral reaction to a stimulus. Initially *stress reactions*, unlike a state of crisis, are useful, adaptive, and lifesaving. Stress helps us to focus our attention and mobilize our physical and psychological capacities to save ourselves and others. We may run away or take direct actions to fight in order to counteract a threat. In a stress reaction, people are normally thinking clearly and taking actions that can help them protect themselves. Usually, they remain under control unless the stress reaction becomes overwhelming. Under extremely stressful conditions, a stress reaction can spiral into the chaotic state known as a crisis. Stress is always a reaction to a stimulus. A mild stimulus produces a low-level response to the stimuli. Low stress reactions are generally harmless. Moderate stimuli or stressors create a stronger reaction to the stimuli. A severe stressor generates a very powerful response that may, in some circumstances, cause a break down in mental and physical health and damage that is difficult to repair. Generally speaking, a stress reaction is a wide range of normal reactions to a stimulus. The range starts at a very low level and rises as the stimulus or threat becomes more severe. Some people can function at a very high, or even an extreme, level of stress without ever experiencing a crisis.

Stress is a low-to-extreme measure of our reactivity to the stimulus. Crisis means we have already reached our maximum stress tolerance level and we are overwhelmed and in turmoil (Kobasse, 1979, 1982; Mitchell & Bray, 1990). Perhaps this comment can help clarify this discussion: you can have stress without a crisis, but you cannot have a crisis without stress.

Crisis Intervention

Crisis intervention is an active, temporary, and supportive entry into a person's or group's life during a period of acute distress. Remember that stress always accompanies a crisis. Crises (plural of crisis) do not exist in a cognitive, emotional, physical, or behavioral vacuum. When we intervene in a crisis, we are also intervening in a stress reaction, and we are providing some stress management support to the person, or group, in a state of crisis (Caplan, 1964; Mitchell, 1991).

Goals of Crisis Intervention

1. Stabilize the situation. We work very hard to keep a bad situation from becoming worse.
2. Reduce emotional tension and distress.
3. Mobilize helping resources for the distraught person or group.
4. Lessen the impact of the event or circumstances surrounding the event.
5. Help people to understand that their reactions to the situation are normal.
6. Restore an individual's adaptive functions. In other words, the aim with emergency services personnel is to help them get back to work as well as to their normal lives as soon as they are able and ready.
7. Facilitate normal recovery processes, in normal people who are experiencing normal reactions to abnormal events.
8. Restore unit cohesion.
9. Restore unit performance in homogeneous groups.
10. Identify individuals who may need additional care and assist them in accessing appropriate support and/or professional referrals.

The Seven Principles of Crisis Intervention

1. *Simplicity* – Crisis interventions should be simple. People typically respond to simple, not complex, instructions during a crisis.
2. *Brevity* – Keep the contacts short. Most crisis contacts last from a few minutes up to about an hour maximum. It is typical to have 3–5 contacts to complete crisis intervention work. If crisis contacts are between 6 and 8, then a referral for professional care should be seriously considered and is most often necessary. If

the contacts number 9 or more, then a referral for professional assistance should occur.

3. *Innovation* – Not every solution is printed in a chapter or an article. Nor do all solutions to crisis intervention problems appear on a handout. Crisis intervention support personnel should be creative when developing novel solutions to difficult and emotionally painful situations. You should also be aware that what may work for the average citizen may not apply to emergency services personnel. They have different needs and issues than the civilian populations.
4. *Pragmatism* – Suggestions must be practical if they are to work in resolving a crisis. If you suggest a solution to a crisis and the person or people involved cannot possibly do what you suggest, your crisis intervention efforts will fail. An example would be for a person to sit down and relax when a fellow firefighter is under a pile of debris. It is not in their nature nor is it in the training of emergency personnel to stand by and do nothing when teammates are in trouble.
5. *Proximity* – Work within the person or group's operational area or comfort zone. In crisis intervention, we still make "house calls." That is to say, we go to where they need us to go, not to someplace where they are not comfortable like a chief's office.
6. *Immediacy* – A crisis response cannot be delayed. The crisis is a "right now" circumstance and it demands rapid intervention. Delays increase pain and generate complications.
7. *Expectancy* – Try to suggest, if the person or group appears to be open to your suggestions and if the timing appears right, that most people can work through a crisis and that you are there to help them do that. Sometimes setting up a positive outcome will not work. Such a case would be the death of a loved one or a coworker. Apply this crisis intervention principle judiciously (Solomon & Benbenishty, 1986).

A crisis remains a crisis until some resolution is found. – JTM

I have had the privilege of working with veterans of the Second World War, the Korean Conflict, Vietnam War, and the more recent wars in the Middle East. Likewise, it is a great privilege to work with many thousands of first-response personnel who have experienced spirit-crushing traumas. One thing stands out for me with trauma work and that is people recover when they come to terms with the devastating trauma they experienced. Their recovery is not from someone like me on the outside of themselves. Instead, it only comes from within and only when they can make some sense out of the tragedy and find something meaningful that allows a resolution to come about. That resolution can take hours or days, weeks, months, and even years. It is not unusual for people to have unresolved trauma experiences haunting them 50 years or more after a tragedy. For some, it is a lifetime. For others, their resolution might never come. The best we can do is to support struggling people and guide them as they make their way along life's path. The following section contains a helpful set of guidelines for providing crisis intervention to emergency services personnel.

The "ASIF" Approach to Crisis Intervention

The "A" stands for *assessment.* Before we do anything to assist people in a state of crisis, we have to start somewhere important. That start is assessment. It includes surveillance. Simply put, surveillance means "look and listen." When you encounter a person or people in a crisis, look at them. What are they doing? How do they appear to you? What behaviors are you seeing? Next, what are they saying and how are they saying it? Listen carefully. Can you sense their distress? What emotions are being expressed? Does what you see indicate anything about their thoughts? After "look and listen," there are three essential elements that are part of the assessment: (a) the nature of the incident (what happened); (b) the magnitude of the incident (how horrible or terrible it is), and (c) the impact on (reactions of) those involved in the incident. Next, check to make sure there are no physical or medical conditions present that may be causing or contributing to the crisis state. Always rule out medical conditions first before assuming that the crisis or the distress is emotionally based. If medical conditions are present, treat them or have someone with the proper medical credentials treat them immediately or as quickly as possible.

After surveillance and assessment, the next step in crisis intervention is to develop a strategy. The "S" in the ASIF model stands for *strategy.* Without a strategy, members of a CISM team are headed for failure in their efforts to help others. The people in a state of crisis may be facing emotional and possibly physical harm. Strategy in crisis intervention is based upon following these five key considerations:

1. *Theme*. The theme is the basic information regarding the incident. Besides assessment, it includes the circumstances of the event, the threats associated with the event, the personnel dispatched to or managing the incident, problems encountered under field conditions, and other concerns, considerations, problems, or issues that are connected to the incident.
2. *Target*. Who needs crisis intervention? Who does not? Crisis support personnel need to know who was involved in the incident and to what extent were they involved. They are the targets of CISM interventions.
3. *Types*. What types of interventions are most likely to be helpful? The right tools need to be selected to assist the people involved in the crisis. One type of support service does not always work.
4. *Timing*. The most appropriate timing is essential in intervening during a crisis. Certain interventions for operations personnel become less effective or even useless if they are delayed. Other interventions are more effective if they are held off for a relatively brief period until personnel are ready to receive those services and achieve the maximum benefits.
5. *Team*. It is important to send the right person or people from the critical incident stress management (CISM) team to provide crisis intervention services. Efforts should always be made to, first, match the responding team member(s) to the person or people who need the assistance and, second, to their specific needs in the situation. It is not always possible, but we try to send law enforcement per-

sonnel to assist law enforcement personnel and fire personnel to assist fire personnel and so on. The list of service organizations was mentioned at the very beginning of this chapter. Occasionally, we run into situations in which we simply do not have CISM people trained within their own profession to provide services to their colleagues, and we must then send support personnel from another profession to help them. If the response team members are respectful, thoughtful, and understanding of differences in the different professions, one profession can help another in a difficult situation. It has been successful on many occasions with police helping corrections or fire personnel or EMS helping nurses and so on.

The "I" in the ASIF crisis intervention approach stands for *interventions*. Note the plural in the word "interventions." Crisis intervention is best when it is a blend of several crisis intervention techniques. Standalone interventions are never appropriate. CISM, by its very nature, is a blend of many interventions. The research on the effects of blending the interventions is quite strong (Richards, 2001). At the very least, crisis intervention personnel always need to follow up with the people they assist. No assumptions should be made that everything is okay simply because one crisis intervention service was provided. There are many techniques or tools in the critical incident stress management toolbox. They include, but are not limited to, the following: (a) pre-incident planning and preparation; (b) team member selection; (c) team building/training; (d) CISM policy development; (e) stress education; (f) crisis education; (g) surveillance/assessment; (h) strategic planning; (i) individual contacts (one-on-one); (j) SAFER-R model for individuals; (k) informational group interventions (RITS and CMB); (l) interactive group interventions (defusing and CISD); (m) family support; (n) follow-up services; (o) organizational consultation; (p) pastoral crisis intervention; (q) referrals for additional care; and (r) post-incident lessons learned and education. More detail on some of these interventions will be presented later in this chapter.

The "F" in the ASIF model stands for *follow-up*. It is easy to get fooled into thinking that people are doing just fine because they looked and sounded good when we completed our first crisis intervention contact with them. However, failure to follow up is a critical error in crisis intervention. It is essential to ensure that people are on the road to recovery by checking on their welfare. This can be accomplished by means of phone calls, text messages (not always a reliable gauge of recovery), personal contacts, and visits to their worksites or homes. Hearing them and seeing them are much better measures of how they are doing. Follow-up services may also be achieved by referrals for additional care from a professional should such referrals be warranted. The steps to cover the "F" portion of this crisis intervention model are as follows: (1) inquire about the well-being of the individual, i.e., station or home visits, calls, texts or do all three; (2) determine if there are additional needs that must be addressed, ask questions, and listen to what they say; and (3) complete the peer-based crisis intervention work with the available CISM team members or refer, if necessary. In crisis intervention, treat people "as if" they were one of your own (Mitchell, 2017).

Characteristics of Sensible Staff Support Programs

Before discussing the specific critical incident stress management (CISM) program, we will address some general characteristics of the CISM teams. Every successful CISM crisis-oriented sensible staff support program is comprehensive. That is to say, it has elements in place before, during, and after traumatic events. Additionally, staff support systems must be programmatic. That is to say, administration must accept the staff support system as a somewhat independent entity that is endorsed by administration and built into the fabric of the organization.

Although they remain functionally independent units, staff support programs must communicate, coordinate, and link their efforts with the administration and leadership of the department or agency. All the while, they must be confidential sources of assistance for stressed personnel or those in a crisis state. There must be links to human resource services, employee assistance, and psychological resources when referrals are necessary. Although it is part of a comprehensive, integrated, systematic, and multi-tactic (CISM) approach, linkages to a wide range of resources are an important key characteristic of any staff support program. The magnitudes of some events are so severe, or the personal reactions of some emergency personnel are so intense, that additional assistance may be necessary. An emergency services staff support program must have mental health resources or other types of services within easy access for people who need more help beyond crisis intervention and, perhaps, beyond their department or agency. It is also common for staff support programs to "borrow" skilled professionals from those resources during crises. Obviously, referrals for additional care or psychotherapy are made to those professionals. However, staff support programs work best when the differences between "support" and "therapy" are clearly recognized by the department or agency and the professionals who staff the ancillary services. Staff support services function at peak performance when they function separately under the umbrella of "operations support." A crisis intervention and stress management program for staff is a support function, not a management function or a psychotherapeutic function. Well-developed staff support programs to manage crises are integrated. All the elements of a CISM program are interrelated and blended with one another. The combined effects of an integrated program are far more powerful than any single element.

Staff members are best sustained by a systematic program or "support package" that has phases, segments, or logical steps. Staff support programs should, therefore, take a few simple steps such as resting personnel and talking with them on an individual basis, before increasing the complexity, number, and duration of the available staff support functions after a distressing event. Effective crisis staff support programs must be multi-tactic in approach. Many different types of support services must be available since every person will have a somewhat different response to a highly stressful event. Each person will have different requirements ranging from information to group support to help them recover from their stress. Training is an absolute necessity for a CISM team. Team members must be trained to assist individuals with CIS and people experiencing a crisis. There are six courses that are essential for CISM team members. They are listed in the section below entitled "Fundamental Components of a CISM Program." Among emergency services organizations, crisis support and stress teams are most effective when they are run and staffed by peer support personnel and backed up by both mental health professionals and chaplains who are trained in critical incident stress management (Mitchell, 2004).

Critical Incident Stress

The term *critical incident stress* was developed in the early 1970s. It describes a normal, predictable, and fairly standard response of normal, psychologically healthy people after exposure to an extraordinary traumatic event known as a critical incident. The term critical incident was discussed in the section entitled "Critical Incidents, Stress, and Crisis" early in this chapter. Critical incident stress, of course, is the stress that arises from exposure to a critical incident. Since emergency services, military, and other frontline personnel regularly experience critical incidents, they can easily understand the association between critical incidents and stress.

Critical incident stress is the cognitive, physical, emotional, behavioral, and spiritual reactions of people who experience a shocking and disturbing event. Although critical incident stress is typically associated with military, emergency services, and other professions that have frequent exposures to traumatic events, anyone can experience critical incident stress under certain circumstances. The key factor in critical incident stress is the exposure to a critical incident. Without exposure to the traumatic event, the critical incident stress reaction would not be possible. Some people use critical incident stress as a synonym for posttraumatic stress. The two terms are, in fact, synonymous, but frontline personnel of all types prefer the less psychological-sounding term, critical incident stress (Mitchell, 1982a, b, 1983, Mitchell & Everly, 2001; Mitchell & Mitchell, 2006).

Signs and Symptoms of Critical Incident Stress

It is a given that if emergency people are in a crisis (an acute state of emotional turmoil), they will have some of the signs and symptoms of critical incident stress. Remember, stress always accompanies a crisis, but you do not have to have a crisis to have stress. Keep the following points in mind. It is normal for operations personnel to have some stress symptoms after involvement in a traumatic event. The main features of critical incident stress (CIS) are physical and emotional arousal. However, let us be clear, having stress arousal does not mean that a person is in a crisis. It also does not necessarily mean that personnel must be taken off the incident or the job.

CIS can range from mild to severe. Many people go through a traumatic event and do not develop significant stress. It depends on many factors such as past experiences, training, circumstances of the incident, level of activity during the mission, having direct contact with the victim, or working on a person who reminds you of someone you love. It is kind of a role-of-the-dice situation. Nothing guarantees you will have critical incident stress, and nothing guarantees you will not have it. In any case, it is okay if you do not get critical incident stress and it is okay if you do. There are ways it can be fixed especially if help is requested quickly.

CIS is a part of the job. In most cases, it is fairly easy to reduce or eliminate it. Experience indicates that if the CIS is severe and none of the right things are done to properly manage it, the outcomes can be quite negative. People who experienced a traumatic event and developed CIS have helped us to identify five characteristics of critical incident stress:

1. They perceive that the critical incident was threatening, powerful, or overwhelming.
2. They are unable to manage the disruptive impact of the critical incident with their usual coping skills.
3. They experience increased fear, tension, and mental confusion.
4. They experience considerable subjective discomfort.
5. When the impact of an event is severe and unresolved, they can proceed to an intense state of emotional crisis with many more disturbing and disruptive signs and symptoms of CIS.

Critical incident stress manifests itself differently in each person. The volume and intensity of stress signs and symptoms may vary considerably. A reaction to a disturbing situation is lessened or intensified by a person's subjective perception of the traumatic event. There are, however, relatively common patterns of stress reactions after critical incidents. People typically react with a combination of the following: (a) mental confusion and disorganization; (b) difficulties in decision-making and problem-solving; (c) intense anxiety, shock, denial, and disbelief; (d) anger, agitation, and rage; (e) feelings of helplessness; (f) lowered self-esteem; (g) loss of self-confidence; (h) fear/terror; (i) guilt feelings; (j) feeling emotionally subdued or depressed; (k) feelings of intense grief; (l) emotional numbness; (m) apathy; (n) withdrawal from others; (o) increase use of alcohol or other substances; (p) periods of excessive activity to avoid thinking of the traumatic experience; (q) loss of faith; (r) cessation of the practice of religion; and (s) physical reactions such as nausea, shakes, headaches, intestinal disturbance, chest pain, or difficulty breathing (Everly, 1989).

Caution A good rule of thumb is to always rule out medical conditions first. Never assume that people's reactions are caused solely by psychological trauma. Medical staff should evaluate chest pain, difficulty breathing, elevated blood pressure, or any other severe physical conditions as soon as possible. Then, mental health professionals should assess severe psychological symptoms as soon as possible after medical conditions have been ruled out or stabilized. The above list is, by no means, exhaustive. Since so many diverse symptoms can be associated, directly or indirectly, with critical incident stress, a complete list of symptoms would not be feasible or useful here. Any cognitive, physical, emotional, behavioral, or spiritual symptom can be caused by or made worse by stress.

If, despite the efforts of CISM team members, CIS symptoms remain unrelieved for 3 weeks or more, additional peer support interventions or professional care should be initiated. Mental health professionals who have been trained in CISM have a reputation of being very helpful to emergency personnel and other frontline responders like disaster personnel.

When people reach a state of intense emotional disturbance, they enter a state of crisis. Their thinking becomes disorganized and their focus on managing the situation becomes unclear. Exaggerated feelings dominate one's reactions. If a person's thinking ability is suppressed and one's feelings explode out of control, CISM peer support personnel should provide immediate intervention. They should be aware that a referral for professional care may be necessary to assist their colleague in regaining their psychological balance and facilitating a return to normal adaptive functions. We hope that CIS can be recognized and managed before it reaches the levels of distress described above.

The works of Gerald Caplan, Robert Jay Lifton, Richard S. Lazarus, and Suzanne C. Kobassa are the most pertinent resources if one wishes to learn more about the historical and theoretical underpinnings of critical incident stress (Caplan, 1961, 1964, 1969; Lifton, 1970, 1973, 1993; Lazarus, 1966, 1969; Kobassa, 1979, Kobassa et al., 1982).

Part II. Components, Applications, and Research

As previously covered in part one, CISM is a package of crisis intervention tactics or support services, not one single intervention. Critical incident stress management (CISM) is a *comprehensive, integrated, systematic, and multicomponent crisis intervention program.* It is interesting to note that the initials, CISM, can be used in two ways as it is in the previous sentence. First, the initials, CISM, represent the title of the program, *critical incident stress management.* Second, the same initials, CISM, can be viewed as a description of the program – comprehensive, integrated, systematic, and multicomponent (Everly & Mitchell, 1999).

CISM is adaptable and has proven itself agile in adjusting to rapidly changing circumstances in day-to-day emergency operations and in major disasters. It is practical and the research shows it to be effective. CISM is a commonsense stress management system. It can do much to alleviate distress and to help maintain healthy levels of function for first responders and many other populations (Mitchell & Mitchell, 2006). Since its development in the 1970s, CISM has spread rapidly into many different types of agencies, organizations, and services, and over 1500 CISM teams have been developed in 35 nations. The United Nations developed its own internal CISM program to assist UN workers throughout its multinational community (Everly & Mitchell, 2008; United Nations Department of Safety and Security, 2007a, b, c).

Important Note CISM is neither psychotherapy nor a substitute for psychotherapy. It is a support service.

Fundamental Components of a CISM Program

Appropriate stress management education is required for anyone who serves on a CISM including the mental health professionals who assist those teams. Peer support personnel who are active on critical incident response teams take nearly 100 hrs. in training in the following topics: (a) assisting individuals in crisis, (b) advanced individual crisis intervention, (c) group crisis support, (d) advanced group crisis intervention for complex situations, (e) suicide prevention, intervention, and recovery, and (f) strategic approaches to crisis intervention. The essential training is divided into modules so personnel can spread the training over several years. The research is very clear that trained personnel are far more effective in staff support programs than those without training (Everly & Mitchell, 2008).

Although most of the support services in the following charts were historically part of the CISM field (Mitchell, 1983), others were developed and incorporated into the field more recently (Mitchell & Everly, 2001; Mitchell, 2020). This list of CISM interventions, however, should not be viewed as static or "fixed" list. The CISM system is dynamic and quite flexible. Its techniques are most effective when the various interventions are appropriately combined and blended with other. Other innovative crisis interventions and stress control techniques are to be added to the list as the needs arise within the context of critical events such as disasters.

Trained emergency service personnel and other crisis workers should always select, from the following table, interventions that make sense under the circumstances and that match the needs of the people who require assistance.

Summary of Commonly Used Crisis Intervention Tactics

Intervention/tactic	Timing	Target group	Potential goals
Pre-event Planning/ preparation	Prior to exposures to traumatic events	Anticipated target or even victim populations	Resistance building. Enhance resiliency anticipatory guidance
Assessment	Pre-intervention	Those directly and indirectly exposed	Determine need for intervention
Strategic planning	Pre-event/early stages of event	Actual and anticipated exposed populations	Improve overall crisis response
Individual crisis intervention (includes "psychological first aid") SAFER-R model	Whenever needed	Individuals as needed	Assessment, screening, education, reduction of acute distress, triage, referral

(continue)

Intervention/tactic	Timing	Target group	Potential goals
Informational groups: (a) Rest Information Transition Services (RITS) {formerly known as "demobilization"} (b) Crisis Management Briefings Group "group Psychological First Aid"	(a) Operation shift disengagement (b) Ongoing large-scale events As needed During or after event	(a) Emergency operations personnel (b) Any size group needing information, guidance, instructions. Large heterogeneous groups	(a) Decompression, ease transition, screening, triage, guidance, meet basic needs Respite, refreshment preliminary support (b) Information, rumor control, increase group cohesion, lower tension, and anxiety in the group. Enhance appropriate behaviors, instructions, guidance
Informational session for small-sized group crisis intervention (conversational somewhat like a CMB but with only a few people (sitting with them) conversational	During and after the event May be repeated as needed May use the CMB format even though the group size is quite small	Community groups seeking information and resources. Usually nonemergency groups. Often heterogeneous 3–6 in attendance	Provide information, control rumors, reduce acute distress, increase cohesion, facilitate resilience, screening, and triage
Interactive groups: (a) Defusing (group "psychological first aid") (b) Critical incident stress debriefing (CISD)	(a) Up to about 8 hours after the event. Becomes less effect as their defenses come back up (b) Post-event 24–72 hours = ideal sometimes 5–10 days. Longer times after disaster (3–4 weeks)	*(a) Homogeneous groups only*; usually small unit-sized groups; same exposure to the traumatic event *(b) Homogeneous groups only* with equal trauma exposure (workgroups, teams)	Stabilization, ventilation, reduction of acute distress, screening, information, increase cohesion, and facilitate resilience Restore unit cohesion and unit performance
Family crisis intervention	Pre-event preparation Post-event support as needed	Families of victims as well as emergency personnel	Wide range of interventions Preparation CMB, individual, other as needed
Organizational/community intervention, consultation	Pre-event preparation Support post-event as needed	Organizations, businesses, agencies impacted by trauma	Improve preparedness and response Leadership guidance. Assist in recovery
Pastoral crisis intervention	Before, during, after as needed	Individual, RITS, defusing, CMB, faith-based crisis intervention	Faith-based support
Follow-up/referral	Some follow-up is always necessary; referrals as needed	Intervention recipients, other exposed individuals, and groups	Assure continuity of care. Refer as necessary

Mitchell (2017, 2020)

Steps in Individual Crisis Support

CISM services, for the most part, utilize easy to remember and easy to apply formulas and guidelines that assist team members in supporting people in distress. The recommended procedures facilitate the individual and group work of the peer support personnel, clergy, chaplains, and mental health professionals who make up CISM teams.

Individual crisis intervention support services are the most common form of support offered by CISM team members. The following are some valuable guidelines that can make a positive difference in providing support services. All the tactics and techniques are taught in the *Assisting Individuals in Crisis* course offered by the International Critical Incident Stress Foundation (www.icisf.org).

1. Initiate contact – introduce yourself (and your team). Introductions are important to the people we are trying to help. It reduces their tension and encourages them to open up and discuss their situation and the distress they feel. It helps them to put their needs into words.
2. Let the person know why you are in contact with him or her. Did they call for assistance? Did you notice their distress yourself, or did someone send you to assist?
3. Ask about what is happening now or what had transpired shortly before your arrival. If you are uncertain, confirm if the person called for assistance or if someone else did so.
4. Ask, "How can I (we) assist you right now?" Offer support, direct assistance, information, and guidance as required. Sometimes a person may be mentally confused, and they do not know what they need. Have patience with them. Getting frustrated with the person is not helpful.
5. Gather additional information and background facts from the people involved (these are listed in a relative degree of order from most important to least important): (a) the distressed person (most important); (b) any emergency response personnel already on scene; (c) family members in the vicinity; (d) friends; (e) neighbors; (f) bystanders; and (g) people passing by who witnessed anything (usually least important).
6. Always use effective human communications with the subject such as (a) para-communications (silence, gestures, body language); (b) mirror statements (restatement, reflection of emotion, paraphrase); (c) questions (closed-ended, open-ended, multiple choice); and (d) action directives (specific instructions to the person) if you need them to do something to assist in their own care.
7. Gather information about the history of the person and the development of the main problem.
8. Ask many of your questions in the following order (closed, open, then paraphrase (COP): (a) closed-ended question (Did the red car strike you?); (b) open-ended question (Can you describe the car that struck you?); (c) paraphrase (If I understand what you said correctly, you stated…?); and (d) there are variations

on the use of the COP format for exploring a crisis reaction (COOOP, COOP, etc.).

9. Ask directly about any suicidal ideation.
10. Determine if there is any other threat or risk present.
11. React immediately to suicide attempts, or threats, or risks. Call police and ambulance.
12. Use your questioning techniques and other crisis communication skills to develop a "crisis action plan" (CAP).
13. Implement the crisis action plan.
14. Review the CAP with the person needing assistance.
15. Maintain the CAP.
16. Alter the CAP.
17. Cease the CAP.
18. Reassess.
19. Refer if necessary.

The SAFER-R model is part of the training in the *Assisting Individuals in Crisis* course. It has the following components: stabilize, acknowledge, facilitate, encourage, recovery, refer (if necessary). It is an integral part of the Assisting Individuals in Crisis course taught by the International Critical Incident Stress Foundation (www.icisf.org). Since the use of the SAFER-R model requires training, further discussion of it here would be inappropriate (Everly, 2015).

Never exceed your training. Ask for assistance.

Group Support Services

The nature of a group may indicate what type of crisis intervention is used with the participants.

Gathering A collection of people who may or may not have a relationship with each other but who gather in the same location sometimes with the same purpose in mind.

Crowd A large gathering of people, whose total numbers are near or over 100.

Group Two or more people, who share a relationship with each other in such a manner or to such a degree, that they are usually thought of as if one.

Gatherings, crowds, and general groups would be given informational groups services only. Typically, the most applicable service would be the crisis management briefing (CMB). They lack the homogeneity that is required to provide group support services like the defusing and the critical incident stress debriefing (CISD).

Primary Group A primary group is sometimes referred to as a homogeneous group. It has two or more people, who are known to each other and who fulfill the following criteria:

a shared history, background, and experiences; spent sufficient time together to have bonded to one another; a relationship with one another.

Secondary Group A larger grouping of people in which there may be several primary groups. Overall, the secondary group has more heterogeneity (mixed personnel) than a primary group. For instance, a large business entity often has several subgroups (sales, research and development, administration, manufacturing, shipping, etc.). The business itself is the secondary group ("I work for Acme Electrical Resources"). However, the person will identify more strongly with the specific unit in which he or she works ("I am an electrical engineer with the research and development team"). Despite having some people in the group who know each other, a secondary group has too many people who do not. The groups fail to reach the criteria for a homogenous group. It is, therefore, only a general group and defusing and CISD is not used with them.

Random Groups A random group does not have the relationships that can be found in primary and secondary groups. More likely than not, a random group's participants do not know each other and share little in the way of common bonds. Shoppers in a mall, riders on a train, and passengers on a plane are good examples of random groups. Only informational group services, like the CMB, are provided.

Four CISM Group Interventions

Rest, Information, and Transition Services (RITS)

This informational group process was developed for use only with groups of operations personnel after a large-scale incident like a disaster. The process was known as "demobilization" for many years, but that term caused difficulties with organizations like the United Nations, the military, and police agencies. The term was changed in 2007 to "Rest, Information and Transition Services" (RITS). The process is the same; only the name has been changed. One CISM team member provides information that may be helpful to the operations personnel who worked the large-scale incident. It is provided immediately after personnel are released from the disaster after their first exposure to it.

There are two main parts to the RITS. The CISM team member introduces oneself and states why he or she is present and offers to be available privately to anyone who has questions or any issue they may wish to discuss the incident after the brief presentation. Next, the CISM team member provides the operations group with information regarding stress and the signs and symptoms the staff members may be experiencing or which they might experience soon. The RITS ends with a very brief opportunity for the participants to ask any questions publicly before the session breaks up. They almost never ask any questions. The RITS concludes and the personnel are sent to another room where refreshments have been arranged. Then, the personnel are assigned to other duties beyond the disaster, or they are sent home or to their stations for approximately 6 h of rest before being allowed to return to duty.

Crisis Management Briefing (CMB)

This is an informational group process for operations personnel for the work shifts following the first shift at the disaster. It serves another purpose; it is used to provide information, guidance, and directions for groups of community members who may have witnessed or who are shocked by news of the traumatic exposure that just occurred in their community. The CMB can be provided before people are exposed to a shocking scene. It may be repeated as often as it is required. New information, however, should be added each time a CMB session is conducted. The CMB has a good tolerance for heterogeneity in groups. That is to say, mixed groups may benefit from the information presented in the CMB process. There is a very short question and answer period at the end of the CMB. Citizens tend to ask lots of questions so the CISM team should announce in advance that there will only be time for a limited number of questions. The CMB can be provided to groups as large as 300 if that is necessary. Unlike the RITS, the CMB it may be applied on any event that impacts many people in the community. It is not reserved for disaster situations.

The CMB uses a CISM team of at least two people. One of those people must be trained in the CISM program. The other may be an administrator, a department chief or a designated person, a representative of a church or a school, a representative of the community, or a politically appointed leader. There is a brief introduction of the team. Information about the situation is shared with the attendees. Helpful guidelines are presented. The CISM team member then discusses stress and the common symptoms of stress that are likely in the aftermath of the event. Helpful stress management suggestions are made to assist people in dealing with the stress associated with the traumatic experience.

The Difference Between Informational and Interactive Groups Informational group processes are only informational in nature (provide instructions, information, and guidance) and are aimed at both homogeneous and heterogeneous (mixed) groups. Interactive groups, on the other hand, are an active discussion of the incident. Interactive group processes are aimed at homogenous (same) groups only. The criteria include shared history, time enough together to form a friendship or a working relationship. Homogenous groups also participated in the same traumatic event.

Defusing

This is one of the two main interactive group processes used in crisis intervention. It is only used with homogeneous groups. It is used within a few hours of a unit's exposure to a traumatic event that impacts an operations team within an organization. The effectiveness of this small group intervention declines as time passes. It is rarely helpful after about 8 h post-incident. Defusing requires special training.

The defusing is intended only for homogeneous groups. A trained CISM team, which is composed of two team members, must always conduct the defusing. Members of the homogenous group attending the defusing should have experienced the same traumatic event. The event must be over, or at least moved beyond, the most acute stages of the traumatic event. No one is pressured to speak; and, if they do speak about their experience in the incident, they should only discuss what they wish to regarding the event. A defusing usually only lasts about 20–30 min.

There are three parts to a defusing:

1. An introduction by the CISM team and an explanation of the guidelines regarding the defusing.
2. A brief exploration of the traumatic event.
3. A short informational phase in which the team members provide some practical suggestions about managing the stress associated with the event.

Critical Incident Stress Debriefing

The critical incident stress debriefing (CISD) is one tactic within the whole field of CISM. It is a tool for use only with homogeneous groups. It is a guided discussion of a traumatic event experienced by the entire group. It is not therapy nor is it a substitute for psychotherapy. Its primary role is to provide emotional support to distressed personnel and restore unit cohesion and unit performance. The CISD process is applied by a team of trained CISM personnel to a group of operations personnel from an organization with front-line responsibilities for spectrum of traumatic events and tragedies. CISD requires special training.

Details on Critical Incident Stress Debriefing The first publication on CISD appeared in 1983 in the *Journal of Emergency Medical Services* (Mitchell, 1983). Even in that first article, many types of interventions were presented as part of a broad, systematic approach to managing distress in emergency personnel now known as critical incident stress management (CISM). It was expected from its inception that CISD would not be a standalone process (Mitchell 2007; Mitchell & Everly, 2001; Mitchell, 2017).

The CISD should never be used in isolation from other interventions. Stress management education should occur before emergency personnel experience a traumatic event as part of their service. Follow-up is always required after a CISD. The CISD process has received a great deal of unnecessary attention during the last decade. Some of that undue attention may have generated misinformation and faulty applications of the model. The material in this chapter provides accurate information on the CISD process.

The critical incident stress debriefing was developed solely as a support service for homogeneous groups who had experienced a traumatic event. The word "support" means *to help keep a person or a group stable. Support also means to care for people, to sustain them, or to reinforce the individual or the group*. Other meanings for the word support are *to give active help and encouragement; to help in a crisis; to provide active assistance; to provide comfort; or to bear some of the weight.* The word support best describes what CISM teams do when they provide a CISD. As stated earlier, a CISD is neither psychotherapy nor is it a substitute for psychotherapy. It is a group crisis intervention procedure. It is really about unit cohesion and unit performance.

CISD is an interactive group support process designed specifically for application with homogeneous (primary) groups that have experienced roughly the same level of exposure to the same traumatic event. Although it has been used successfully with a wide range of homogeneous populations, such as school children, businesses, and industries, it should be kept in mind that it was originally developed for operational groups such as first responders who know each other and who share both a common history and positive relationships with one another. It is inappropriate to use the CISD group crisis intervention process with groups that are heterogeneous. Likewise, it is inappropriate to use the CISD model with individuals. The CISD process was never designed for individual primary victims such as those who are ill, injured, medicated, or psychotic or who are hospital patients, victims of violence, people with suicidal ideation, or people currently undergoing grave personal threat. It is an egregious violation of the standard principles and practices of CISD to apply this group crisis intervention process to individual women who had difficult pregnancies, complicated deliveries, miscarriages, or stillborn babies. It is also an egregious violation of the standards of practice to apply the CISD interactive group crisis intervention process to individual auto accident victims, sexual assault victims, burn victims, and dog bite victims. These misguided and horribly flawed applications of the CISD group crisis intervention model are unequivocally condemned. CISD should only be used with appropriate homogeneous groups.

Goals of CISD The main goals of a CISD are to support the primary group after a shared traumatic experience and to restore the unit's cohesion and performance. The CISD is a not a treatment or a cure for any form of mental disorder, including post-traumatic stress disorder (PTSD). Any possible preventative value against PTSD would be of a secondary nature, not primary. The prevention of PTSD is not listed as one of the primary goals of the CISD process. The actual goals of the CISD process are:

1. Mitigate the crisis response.
2. Assist in the restoration of the group's ability to function.
3. Identify individuals within the small homogeneous group who might need additional support or a referral for professional care.

The CISD interactive crisis intervention group process plays an important role in screening and referral.

Benefits of CISD There are many benefits of the interactive group CISD process. The benefits, however, can only be realized when the interactive group process is conducted by trained personnel. The benefits are:

1. Providing practical information that serves as a useful guide for the group members' recovery from a traumatic experience.
2. Helping group members understand that they are not alone in the trauma experience.
3. Informing group members that help is available if they want it. It is generally reassuring to the members of the group to know that they are not unique and that others may be experiencing the same physical and emotional effects.
4. Normalizing the reactions that the group members are experiencing after the critical incident (Mitchell, 2017).

Stages of the CISD Process There are seven steps or stages in the CISD process. Proper training in CISM is a necessity before attempting to utilize the CISD process.

1. Brief introduction by the crisis team members.
2. Fact phase or a brief situation review.
3. Thought phase or first impressions of the traumatic event.
4. Aspects of the event that produced the greatest personnel impact on the group members.
5. Signals of distress.
6. Teaching phase or stress information and guidelines for recovery.
7. Re-entry phase or summary.

The preponderance of the studies cited in the literature on CISD indicates a positive effect if two conditions are in place. The first is that people who conduct the CISD process are properly trained to do so. The second condition is that the providers of the service must adhere to the standards of practice for the CISD that have been established and promulgated since 1983 (Mitchell, 1983; Everly & Mitchell 2017; Everly, 2019).

Effectiveness of CISM

The literature to date suggests that crisis intervention, in the form of a critical incident stress management program, has positive effects on the reduction of stress symptoms. Flannery and Everly (2004) conducted a review of investigations of CISM and found the data generally supportive when the interventions were applied with psychiatric hospitals. The review consisted of "black box" data coming from pre-experimental and quasi-experimental research. The first published study known to investigate the multicomponent CISM intervention program in response to a disaster were the studies conducted by Mitchell and Resnik (1981) and Everly et al. (1995). CISM interventions were provided in response to the Coldenham School disaster in 1989. The CISM intervention consisted of surveillance, town hall meetings (electronic and in-person), small group discussions, individual crisis interventions (in-person and telephonically), and follow-up and referral for higher levels of care, if needed. The study was a within-subjects repeated measures design of 18 first responders. A significant number of the responders to this disaster experienced symptom reductions when assessed for posttraumatic stress 3 months post-intervention.

The largest study on the use of CISM in a mass disaster was conducted after the 2001 World Trade Center attack in New York City. Boscarino et al. (2005) and the New York Academy of Medicine conducted a methodologically robust investigation of workplace-based crisis intervention. The study represented a prospective, random sample of 1681 New York adults interviewed by telephone at 1 and 2 years after the attack. "This article provides the first rigorous scientific evidence to suggest that post-disaster crisis interventions in the workplace significantly reduced mental health disorders and symptoms up to two years after the initial intervention" (Boscarino et al., 2005, p. 9). Boscarino et al. (2011) conducted a further analysis of their World Trade Center data set. They concluded:

> Using propensity score matching to control for selection bias, brief mental health interventions appeared more effective than multisession interventions. These intervention findings held even after matching on demographic, stress exposure, mental health history, treatment history, access to care, other key variables. Our study suggested that community-level mental health service use increased in the follow-up period and that brief interventions were more effective than conventional multisession interventions. (Boscarino et al., 2011, p. 275)

The authors described the interventions as CISM.

There is substantial evidence that when the CISM interventions are utilized by properly trained providers who adhere to the standards of practice, CISM programs may play a preventative role against the development of long-range psychological problems (Adler et al. 2008, 2009; Amir et al., 1998; Bohl, 1991, 1995; Boscarino, 2005, 2011; Campfield & Hills, 2001; Castro & Adler 2011; Chemtob et al., 1997; Dealh et al., 2000; Dyregrov, 1998; Eid et al., 2001; Everly et al., 2000; Everly et al. 2001; Flannery, 2005; Jenkins, 1996; Leonhardt, 2006; National Air Traffic Controllers Association & Federal Aviation Administration, 2003; North et al., 2002; Nurmi, 1999; Regel, 2007, 2010; Richards, 2001; Roberts, 2005; Robinson & Mitchell, 1993; Tuckey, 2007; Vogt et al., 2004; Vogt et al., 2006; Vogt et al., 2007; Wee et al., 1999; Western Management Consultants, 1996; Everly, 2019).

In an aviation industry study, Vogt and his colleagues (2004, 2006, 2007) performed a cost-benefit analysis of the German Air Traffic Control Services' (Deutsche Flugsicherung, DFS) CISM program. CISM peers intervened with air traffic controllers after "loss of separation" incidents (when two radar blips merge into one on the screen). An unforeseen loss of separation between aircraft is a major threat to the professional self-image of an air traffic controller officer. Such incidents are generally distressing reminders to the controllers of the ever-present risk of life-threatening aviation accidents. Prior to the development of a CISM support program, German

Air Traffic Control Officers lost an average of 3 days from work per incident because of distress. About 30 of these loss of separation events occur per month in the crowded skies above Europe (Vogt et al., 2004, 2006, 2007).

A series of studies by Vogt and his colleagues (2004, 2006, 2007) indicated that, since the introduction of the CISM peer support program in 1997, no air traffic controller reported a single lost day for stress related to a loss of separation critical incident. The estimated fiscal benefits associated with the prevention of absenteeism or reported stress-related illness while at work exceeded the program's costs by several times. The study concluded that a combination of factors assures the effectiveness of peer provided crisis intervention. They include a clear model, well-trained providers, and adherence to the standards and protocols of good practice (Vogt et al., 2004, 2006, 2007).

Dr. George S. Everly, Jr., recently published a review of over 100 studies on crisis intervention and critical incident stress management that indicate positive effects of CISM. CISM is, therefore, in the realm of evidence-based interventions. Several of the investigations are randomized controlled trials (RCT) which are considered the "gold standard" of research designs (Adler et al., 2008; Campfield & Hills, 2001; Deahl et al., 2000; Everly, 2019; Richards, 2001; Tuckey & Scott, 2013).

Summary

Over a century and a half of research and experience in crisis intervention and CISM leads us to the conclusion that sensible staff support services must be available to emergency services in communities throughout the USA and in other nations as well. They are a commonsense approach to keeping frontline personnel healthy and functional in the face of extraordinary stressors. They must be strategically thought out, simple to access, and confidential. CISM peer support personnel must be well-trained, and they must adhere to the standards of practice that have been established by the International Critical Incident Stress Foundation. Only those peer support personnel who received proper critical incident stress management training and maintain their skills by periodic update training should provide these support services to their colleagues. They should be especially carefully to select the crisis interventions that best match the needs of the people in distress.

In many hundreds of thousands of small tragedies and hundreds of largescale disasters, peer support personnel have stepped up and made a huge difference in the lives of emergency services and frontline personnel. At times, they made considerable sacrifices to offer an understanding ear and a generous heart to their struggling colleagues. The debt owed them cannot be adequately calculated nor can it be repaid. Only the rising up of a now-healed brother or a sister who experienced soul-crushing trauma can serve as their payment-in-full.

References

Adler, A. B., Litz, B. T., Castro, C. A., Suvak, M., Thomas, J. L., Burrell, L., McGurk, D., Wright, K. M., & Bliese, P. D. (2008). A group randomized trial of critical incident stress debriefing provided to U.S. peacekeepers. *Journal of Traumatic Stress, 21*(3), 253–263.

Adler, A. B., Bliese, P. D., McGurk, D., Hoge, C. W., & Castro, C. A. (2009). Battlemind debriefing and battlemind training as early interventions with soldiers returning from Iraq: Randomization by platoon. *Journal of Consulting and Clinical Psychology, 77*, 928–940.

American Psychiatric Association. (1964). *First aid for psychological reactions in disasters.* American Psychiatric Association.

Amir, M., Weil, G., Kaplan, Z., Tocker, T., & Witzum, E. (1998). Debriefing with group psychotherapy in a homogenous group of non-injured victims of a terrorist attack: A prospective study. *Acta Psychiatriaca Scandinavica, 98*, 237–242.

Appel, J. W., Beebe, G. W., & Hilgardner, D. W. (1946). Comparative incidence of neuropsychiatric casualties in World War I and World War II. *American Journal of Psychiatry, 102*, 196–199.

Artiss, K. (1963). Human behavior under stress: From combat to social psychiatry. *Military Medicine, 128*, 1011–1015.

Bard, M. (1970). *Training police as specialists in family crisis intervention.* National Institute of Law Enforcement and Criminal Justice, U.S. Government Printing Office.

Bohl, N. (1991). The effectiveness of brief psychological interventions in police officers after critical incidents. In J. T. Reese, J. Horn, & C. Dunning (Eds.), *Critical incidents in policing* (Rev. ed., pp. 31–38). Department of Justice.

Bohl, N. (1995). Measuring the effectiveness of CISD. *Fire Engineering*, 125–126.

Boothby, R. J. G. (1978). *Boothby: Recollections of a rebel.* Hutchinson & Co.

Boscarino, J. A., Adams, R. E., & Figley, C. R. (2005). A prospective cohort study of the effectiveness of employer-sponsored crisis interventions after a major disaster. *International Journal of Emergency Mental Health, 7*(1), 31–44.

Boscarino, J. A., Adams, R. E., & Figley, C. R. (2011). Mental health service use after the world trade center disaster: Utilization trends and comparative effectiveness. *Journal of Nervous and Mental Disease, 199*, 91–99.

Campfield, K., & Hills, A. (2001). Effect of timing of Critical Incident Stress Debriefing (CISD) on posttraumatic symptoms. *Journal of Traumatic Stress, 14*, 327–340.

Caplan, G. (1961). *An approach to community mental health.* Grune and Stratton.

Caplan, G. (1964). *Principles of preventive psychiatry.* Basic Books.

Caplan, G. (1969). Opportunities for school psychologists in the primary prevention of mental health disorders in children. In A. Bindman & A. Spiegel (Eds.), *Perspectives in community mental health* (pp. 420–436). Aldine.

Castro, C. A., & Adler, A. B. (2011). Re-conceptualizing combat-related posttraumatic stress disorder as an occupational hazard. In A. B. Adler, P. B. Bliese, & C. A. Castro (Eds.), *Deployment psychology: Evidence-based strategies to promote mental health in the military* (pp. 217–242). American Psychological Association.

Chemtob, C., Tomas, S., Law, W., & Cremniter, D. (1997). Post disaster psychosocial intervention. *American Journal of Psychiatry, 134*, 415–417.

Crocq, L. (1999). *Les Traumatismes psychiques de guerre.* Odile Jacob.

Crocq, L., Dalligand, L., Villerbu, L., Tarquinio, C., Duchet, C., Coq, J. M., Chidiac, N., & Vitry, M. (2007). *Traumatismes psychiques: Prise en charge psychologique des victimes.* Elsevier-Masson.

Deahl, M., Srinivasan, M., Jones, N., Thomas, J., Neblett, C., & Jolly, A. (2000). Preventing psychological trauma in soldiers: The role of operational stress training and psychological debriefing. *British Journal of Medical Psychology, 73*, 77–85.

Dewey, R. (1933). First aid to the newly arriving patient in the public hospital for mental diseases. *American Journal of Psychiatry, 90*(2), 299–301.

Dyregrov, A. (1998). Psychological debriefing: An effective method? *Traumatology, 4*(2), 6–15.

Eid, J., Johnsen, B. H., & Weisaeth, L. (2001). The effects of group psychological debriefing on acute stress reactions following a traffic accident: A quasi-experimental approach. *International Journal of Emergency Mental Health, 3*, 145–154.

Everly, G. (1989). *A clinical guide to the treatment of the human stress response*. Plenum Press.

Everly, G. (2019). *Critical Incident Stress Management (CISM) and psychological crisis intervention: A practical review of research*. Resiliency Science Institutes International.

Everly, G. S., Jr., & Mitchell, J. T. (1999). *Critical Incident Stress Management (CISM): A new era and standard of care in crisis intervention*. Chevron Publishing Corporation.

Everly, G. S., Jr., & Mitchell, J. T. (2008). *Integrative crisis intervention and disaster mental health*. Chevron Publishing Corporation.

Everly, G. S., & Mitchell, J. T. (2017). *Critical Incident Stress Management: A practical review of CISM*. International Critical Incident Stress Foundation.

Everly, G. S., Jr., Mitchell, J. T., & Schiller, G. (1995). Coldenham: Traumatic stress intervention in a community fire service. In G. S. Everly Jr. (Ed.), *Innovations in disaster and trauma psychology: Applications in emergency services and disaster response* (Vol. 1). Chevron Publishing.

Everly, G. S., Jr., Flannery, R. B., & Mitchell, J. T. (2000). Critical Incident Stress Management (CISM): A review of the literature. *Aggression and Violent Behavior, 5*(1), 23–40.

Everly, G. S., Jr., Flannery, R. B., Jr., Eyler, V., & Mitchell, J. T. (2001). Sufficiency analysis of an integrated multi-component approach to crisis intervention: Critical Incident Stress Management. *Advances in Mind-Body Medicine, 17*, 174–183.

Everly, G. S., Jr. (2015). *Assisting individuals in crisis* (5th ed.). International Critical Incident Stress Foundation.

Flannery, R. B. (2005, February 16–20). *Assaulted Staff Action Program (ASAP): Fifteen years of empirical findings* [Paper presentation]. Eighth World Congress on Stress Trauma and Coping: Crisis Intervention: Best Practices in Prevention, Preparedness and Response. Baltimore, MD, United States.

Flannery, R. B., Jr., & Everly, G. S., Jr. (2004). Critical incident stress management: An updated review. *Aggression and Violent Behavior, 6*, 319–329.

Freeman, K. (1979). CMHC responses to the Chicago and San Diego airplane disasters. *Technical Assistance Center Report, 2*(1), 10–12.

Forstenzer, A. (1980, July). Stress, the psychological scarring of air crash rescue personnel. *Firehouse, 50–52*, 62.

Frederick, C. J. (Ed.). (1981). *Aircraft accidents: Emergency mental health problems*. National Institute of Mental Health, U.S. Department of Health and Human Services.

Hassling, P. (2000). Disaster management and the Gothenburg fire of 1998: When first responders are blamed. *International Journal of Emergency Mental Health, 2*(2), 267–273.

Jenkins, S. R. (1996). Social support and debriefing efficacy among emergency medical workers after a mass shooting incident. *Journal of Social Behavior and Personality, 11*, 447–492.

Kardiner, A., & Spiegel, H. (1947). *War, stress, and neurotic illness*. Hoeber.

Kobassa, S. C. (1979). Stressful life events, personality, and health: An inquiry into hardiness. *Journal of Personality and Social Psychology, 37*, 1–11.

Kobassa, S. C., Maddi, S. R., & Kahn, S. (1982). Hardiness and health: A prospective study. *Journal of Personality and Social Psychology, 42*, 168–177.

Lazarus, R. S. (1966). *Psychological stress and the coping process*. McGraw-Hill.

Lazarus, R. S. (1969). *Patterns of adjustment and human effectiveness*. McGraw-Hill.

Leonhardt, J. (2006). Critical Incident Stress Management (CISM) in Air Traffic Control (ATC). In J. Leonhardt & J. Vogt (Eds.), *Critical Incident Stress Management CISM in aviation* (pp. 81–91). Ashgate Publishing Company.

Lifton, R. J. (1970). *History and human survival: Essays on the young and the old, survivors and the dead, peace and war, and on contemporary psychohistory*. Random House.

Lifton, R. J. (1973). *Home from the war: Vietnam veterans: Neither victims nor executioners*. Simon & Schuster.

Lifton, R. J. (1993). *The protean self: Human resilience in an age of fragmentation*. Basic Books.

Lindy, J. (1985). The trauma membrane and other clinical concepts derived from psychotherapeutic work with survivors of natural disasters. *Psychiatric Annals, 15*, 153–160.

Lindemann, E. (1944). Symptomatology and management of acute grief. *American Journal of Psychiatry, 101*, 141–148.

Mitchell, J. T. (1982a, October). The psychological impact of the Air Florida 90 Disaster on fire-rescue, paramedic and police officer personnel. In R. A. Cowley, S. Edelstein, & M. Silverstein (Eds.), *Mass casualties: A lessons learned approach, accidents, civil disorders, natural disasters, terrorism*. Department of Transportation (DOT HS 806302).

Mitchell, J. T. (1982b, Fall). Recovery from rescue. *Response, the Magazine of Emergency Management*, 7–10.

Mitchell, J. T. (1983). When disaster strikes…the critical incident stress debriefing process. *Journal of Emergency Medical Services, 13*(11), 49–52.

Mitchell, J. T. (1991). Law enforcement applications for critical incident stress teams. In J. T. Reese, J. M. Horn, & C. Dunning (Eds.), *Critical incidents in policing* (Rev. ed.). U.S. Government Printing Office.

Mitchell, J. T. (2004). Characteristics of successful early intervention programs. *International Journal of Emergency Mental Health, 6*(4), 175–184.

Mitchell, J. T. (2007). *Group crisis support: Why it works, when and how to provide it*. Chevron Publishing.

Mitchell, J. T. (2017). *Critical Incident Stress Management: Group crisis intervention* (5th ed.) International Critical Incident Stress Foundation.

Mitchell, J. T. (2020). Critical Incident Stress Management: A comprehensive, integrative, systematic, and multicomponent program for supporting first responder psychological health. In C. A. Bowers, D. C. Beidel, & M. R. Marks (Eds.), *Mental health interventions and treatment of first responders and emergency workers*. IGI Global.

Mitchell, J. T., & Bray, G. (1990). *Emergency services stress: Guidelines for preserving the health and careers of emergency services personnel*. Prentice-Hall, Inc.

Mitchell, J. T., & Everly, G. S., Jr. (2001). *Critical Incident Stress Debriefing: An operations manual for CISD, defusing and other group crisis intervention services* (3rd ed.). Chevron.

Mitchell, S. G., & Mitchell, J. T. (2006). Caplan, community and Critical Incident Stress Management. *International Journal of Emergency Mental Health, 8*(1), 1–10.

Mitchell, J. T., & Resnik, H. L. P. (1981). *Emergency Response to Crisis*. Bowie, MD: Brady Publishing.

National Air Traffic Controllers Association & Federal Aviation Administration. (2003). *You are not alone: Critical incident stress management program*. National Air Traffic Controllers Association & Federal Aviation Administration.

Neil, T., Oney, J., DiFonso, L., Thacker, B., & Reichart, W. (1974). *Emotional first aid*. Kemper-Behavioral Science Associates.

North, C., Tivis, C., McMillen, J., Pfefferbaum, B., Cox, J., Spitznagel, E., Bunch, K., Schorr, J., & Smith, E. (2002). Coping, functioning, and adjustment of rescue workers after the Oklahoma City bombing. *Journal of Traumatic Stress, 15*, 171–175.

Nurmi, L. (1999). The sinking of the Estonia: The effects of Critical Incident Stress Debriefing on rescuers. *International Journal of Emergency Mental Health, 1*, 23–32.

Reese, J. T., & Goldstein, H. A. (Eds.). (1986). *Psychological services for law enforcement*. U.S. Government Printing Office.

Regel, S. (2007). Post-trauma support in the workplace: The current status and practice of Critical Incident Stress Management (CISM) and Psychological Debriefing (PD) within organizations in the UK. *Occupational Medicine, 57*, 411–416.

Regel, S. (2010). Does psychological debriefing work? *Healthcare Counseling and Psychotherapy Journal, 10*(2), 14–18.

Richards, D. (2001). A field study of critical incident stress debriefing versus critical incident stress management. *Journal of Mental Health, 10*, 351–362.

Roberts, A. (2005). Bridging the past and present to the future of crisis intervention and crisis management. In A. Roberts (Ed.), *Crisis intervention handbook: Assessment, treatment and research* (3rd ed.). Oxford University Press.
Robinson, R., & Mitchell, J. (1993). Evaluation of psychological debriefings. *Journal of Traumatic Stress, 6*, 367–382.
Salmon, T. S. (1919). War neuroses and their lesson. *New York Medical Journal, 108*, 993–994.
Solomon, Z., & Benbenishty, R. (1986). The role of proximity, immediacy, and expectancy in frontline treatment of combat stress reaction among Israelis in the Lebanon War. *American Journal of Psychiatry, 143*, 613–617.
Stierlin, E. (1909). *Psycho-neuropathology as a result of a mining disaster, March 10, 1906*. University of Zurich.
Tuckey, M. R. (2007). Issues in the debriefing debate for the emergency services. *Clinical Psychology: Science and Practice, 14*, 106–116.
Tuckey, M. R., & Scott, J. E. (2013). Group critical incident stress debriefing with emergency services personnel: A randomized controlled trial. *Anxiety, Stress, and Coping, 27*(1), 38–54.
United Nations Department of Safety and Security CISMU Staff. (2007a). UNDSS CISMU Certification Training For Counsellors. *DSS Newsletter.* United Nations Secretariat, Department of Safety and Security.
United Nations Department of Safety and Security CISMU Staff. (2007b). New crisis and stress management training program launched. *I Seek (May 2, 2007)*. United Nations Secretariat.
United Nations Department of Safety and Security CISMU Staff. (2007c). *Certification training in Crisis and Stress Management.* UN Department of Safety and Security, Consultative Working Group on Stress in Collaboration with the International Critical Incident Stress Foundation, the American Academy of Experts in Traumatic Stress and the Comite National de L'urgence Médico-Psychologique. United Nations, Department of Safety and Security.
Vogt, J., Leonhardt, J., Koper, B., & Pennig, S. (2004). Economic evaluation of CISM—A pilot study. *International Journal of Emergency Mental Health, 6*(4), 185–196.
Vogt, J., & Leonhardt, J. (Eds.). (2006). *Critical Incident Stress Management in aviation*. Ashgate Publishing Limited.
Vogt, J., Pennig, S., & Leonhardt, J. (2007). Critical Incident Stress Management in air traffic control and its benefits. *Air Traffic Control Quarterly, 15*(2), 127–156.
Wee, D. F., Mills, D. M., & Koelher, G. (1999). The effects of Critical Incident Stress Debriefing on emergency medical services personnel following the Los Angeles civil disturbance. *International Journal of Emergency Mental Health, 1*, 33–38.
Western Management Consultants. (1996). *The medical services branch CISM evaluation report*. WMC.

Part III
Treatment Strategies

Cognitive Behavioral Therapy (CBT)

Colleen E. Martin

First responders and public service personnel (e.g., firefighters, emergency medical services [EMS] personnel, police officers, etc.) encounter a variety of high-stress situations that can leave long-lasting effects on both their mental and physical health. Individuals in these roles are often asked to quickly return to work following exposure to a high-stress and/or traumatic situation. This type of occupation places these individuals at increased risk for a range of psychiatric outcomes, including, but not limited to, depressive symptoms, posttraumatic stress, problematic substance use, and sleep difficulties (Jones, 2017). In fact, rates of suicidal thoughts and behaviors are far greater in public service personnel than in the general population (SAMHSA, 2018). One study found that those in an EMS role were significantly more likely to die by suicide than those in the general population (Vigil et al., 2019). Many do not receive or even attempt to seek the support that may help them navigate these symptoms and learn healthy coping techniques following traumatic incidents. With the heightened severity and risk issues highlighted here, it is imperative that clinicians have as many tools as possible to address them in the most effective way.

While many may not have the time, ability, or motivation to seek intensive treatment outside of work, certain skills-based, time-limited interventions may be particularly effective in alleviating distress stemming from the strain of public service occupations. One therapeutic approach that clinicians may consider using, cognitive behavioral therapy (CBT; Beck, 1976), lends itself well to this type of intervention. When public service personnel can practice and implement targeted skills outside of therapy sessions, they can become more comfortable using them in real-time settings. Attitudes toward seeking professional support have been studied in public

C. E. Martin (✉)
Cincinnati VA Medical Center, Cincinnati, OH, USA
e-mail: Colleen.Martin4@va.gov

M. L. Bourke et al. (eds.), *First Responder Mental Health*,
https://doi.org/10.1007/978-3-031-38149-2_11

service personnel, and it was found that many would seek out professional services only as a final option, if at all (Carleton et al., 2020).

The purpose of this chapter is to identify ways that CBT can provide appropriate and effective interventions with public service personnel to address a wide range of symptoms that stem from the nature of their occupations. Through this chapter, clinicians treating public service personnel will become better able to flexibly apply components of CBT in a way that fits for the given occupational role. The chapter will present an overview of CBT and its components, a review of current literature on how CBT is already being implemented with public service personnel, suggestions for how to apply CBT to clinical practice with this population, a case example involving fire service, clinical and research implications, and, finally, a discussion of future directions.

Background on Cognitive Behavioral Therapy (CBT)

The term *cognitive behavioral therapy* (CBT) encompasses a variety of therapeutic and conceptual elements and can be implemented in different ways depending on the specific presenting concern(s). CBT is part of what is known as the "second wave" of behavioral therapy approaches and has its roots in both behaviorism (modifying behaviors) and cognitive therapy (modifying thoughts) (Brown et al., 2013). Whereas many historical approaches to psychotherapy placed an emphasis on childhood memories and interpersonal processes, CBT's focus is on the present moment in order to identify and make effective changes immediately. The core elements of CBT involve modifying one's perceptions of situations to become more realistic and modifying unhelpful behaviors to eventually lead to progress in desired mental health outcomes.

Individuals can develop negative beliefs about themselves, others, and the world from a young age that can interfere with one's quality of life, particularly if additional life stress confirms these beliefs. A large emphasis of treatment in CBT is on modifying these unhealthy or maladaptive cognitions that have developed to gain other, more realistic, perspectives. In doing this, therapists assist clients in identifying "automatic thoughts," which are the often negative interpretations of situations that lead to emotional distress. If one views themselves, others, and the world with a negative lens, they are likely to interpret situations more negatively and/or extremely than one who does not hold these beliefs. Therefore, identifying these beliefs that occur automatically is an initial step in treatment before creating any alternative ways of looking at a situation. Examples of cognitive distortions that lead to negative interpretations include, but are not limited to, catastrophizing (thinking the worst will happen), black or white thinking (rigidity), jumping to conclusions (predicting the future), overgeneralization (one instance becomes a never-ending pattern), and emotional reasoning (taking emotions as facts).

The second component of CBT involves behavioral changes that can accompany the process of challenging maladaptive beliefs. Behavioral strategies can include behavioral activation, gradual exposures to feared stimuli, participating in pleasant activities, relaxation exercises, problem-solving, social skills training, role-playing, and goal-setting. When used in combination with challenging unhelpful thoughts, individuals can come to function much better in their present life without being weighed down by emotional distress.

At the heart of CBT lies the collaborative nature of the relationship between a therapist and client. Ideally, they are working together toward common goals set forth by the client in a way that meets them where they are in order to improve their quality of life. CBT proposes that at the end of treatment, the client will have the ability to "be their own therapist" and use the cognitive and behavioral strategies as needed in future situations. Core elements of CBT typically involve an understanding of the five primary components that contribute to problems in a person's life: situations, thoughts, emotions, physical symptoms, and behaviors. By evaluating each of these components, one can begin to develop healthier ways of coping with stress. CBT has been applied to many emotional and mental health problems such as depression (Gautam et al., 2020), substance use disorders (Zamboni et al., 2021), trauma and anxiety disorders (Mendes et al., 2008), relationship issues (Fischer et al., 2016), and psychosis (Dunn et al., 2012). Various meta-analyses have demonstrated that CBT is an effective treatment in alleviating distress in a time-limited, focused manner.

Variations of CBT

There are two other widely used approaches that have since been developed as part of the "third wave" of behavioral therapies, one of which is acceptance and commitment therapy (ACT; Hayes et al., 1999) which primarily uses a mindfulness-based approach to treating mental health symptoms. ACT encompasses a wide variety of techniques (e.g., acceptance, cognitive defusion) to help the client find greater enjoyment and satisfaction in their life. The goal of ACT is to become aware of thoughts and feelings and to decrease the amount of struggle they put into "fighting" with symptoms such as depression and anxiety, rather than on symptom reduction. This therapeutic approach can be flexibly delivered depending on the presenting concerns, so it may prove useful with first-responder and public safety populations where anything from scheduling issues to location constraints (e.g., onsite, office) can affect how and when interventions are delivered.

Dialectical behavior therapy (DBT; Linehan, 1993) is another type of cognitive behavioral therapy that incorporates challenges to unhelpful thoughts and behaviors but is also focused on accepting one's current emotional and behavioral state. The balance of acceptance and change is the hallmark of the dialectics espoused by DBT. Interventions include mindfulness training, skills to regulate emotions and tolerate distress, as well as interpersonal effectiveness training. As with most CBT therapies, the focus on skills and psychoeducation may make this type of therapy more appealing to first-responder populations who need tools they can use in the line of duty and in moments of crisis in order to be effective.

Application of CBT

Cognitive behavioral therapy is currently used to treat a number of mental health symptoms that are commonly seen in first-responder populations. In 2017, public service personnel screened positive for some type of mental health disorder at a higher level than the general population (Carleton et al., 2018). It is imperative that many of these mental health issues receive early intervention, as the avoidance of these conditions may lead to much more impairment down the line, particularly with repeated exposure to traumatic and/or aversive situations in the line of first-responder work. The emotional cost of these mental health conditions can be seen time and time again in the high rates of suicidal thoughts and behaviors experienced in this group. Based on the current literature of first-responder samples (SAMHSA, 2018), the following psychiatric disorders are most commonly cited as prevalent among first responders; however, this is by no means an exhaustive list.

Stressor-Related Disorders

Posttraumatic Stress Disorder Posttraumatic stress disorder (PTSD) stems from experiencing a traumatic event and encompasses symptoms of re-experiencing the event, avoidance of internal and external reminders, having negative thoughts and emotions, and arousal symptoms (American Psychiatric Association [APA], 2013). When these symptoms develop and persist for longer than 1 month, it has met the criteria for PTSD, whereas when these symptoms last for less than 1 month, it is considered acute stress disorder (see description in next paragraph). There are two gold standard treatments for PTSD that are under the umbrella of CBT: cognitive processing therapy (CPT) and prolonged exposure (PE). CPT (Resick & Schnicke, 1993) is based on cognitive theory and information processing theory. It teaches the individual skills to challenge maladaptive beliefs that have developed in response to the trauma (e.g., "I should've done more," "I'm never safe"). By challenging their current thoughts and creating more balanced beliefs, the individual can decrease their emotional distress and engage in more logical thinking. The second type of treatment, PE (Foa & Rothbaum, 1998), primarily uses a behavioral approach that allows the individual to emotionally process the traumatic event through verbal repetitions of the memory, as well as engaging in out-of-session exercises to approach situations and trauma reminders that they have been avoiding. Through emotional processing and habituation to their feared situations, the individual reduces their re-experiencing symptoms of the trauma and increases their quality of life by engaging more in activities they have been avoiding.

Acute Stress Disorder Acute stress disorder (ASD) is defined as a set of fear-related behaviors and symptoms that occur within the first month of experiencing a traumatic event (APA, 2013). The symptoms of ASD are a result of any type of trauma (e.g., actual or threatened death, sexual assault, exposure to aversive details of trauma) and can result in significant impairment for the individual. Specifically, an individual may have extreme or distorted beliefs about their role in the trauma, and many CBT techniques can help in alleviating distress from these negative thought patterns. In a meta-analysis of CBT and anxiety disorders, those in the CBT condition made significantly larger gains in ASD symptom improvement than those in the placebo condition (Carpenter et al., 2018). As with PTSD, CPT can be used as a primary treatment for ASD as it assists the individual in challenging maladaptive beliefs that have developed because of the traumatic event.

Anxiety Disorders

Panic Disorder Cognitive behavioral techniques can be used to treat symptoms of panic, whether the individual is suffering from expected panic attacks during already uncomfortable situations (e.g., trauma-related triggers) or if they experience panic attacks unexpectedly and avoid situations because of this unpredictability. With regard to first responders and public safety personnel, panic attacks may occur as a result of the already high-stress nature of the occupation in combination with repeated exposure to trauma. When using CBT with this population, there are several interventions (i.e., psychoeducation, relaxation, and exposure) that should be employed to reduce the panic. With this, the individual can feel more confident in fulfilling their job duties knowing they have skills to address panic symptoms.

First, providing psychoeducation on the physical symptoms of panic can reframe any beliefs the individual might have on the symptoms meaning they are in danger. This discussion may show them that these physical symptoms are quite normal within the realm of anxiety and are nothing to be feared. For instance, when anxiety increases, the tendency to experience shallow and quick breaths actually signals to the body that they are in danger; therefore, it can be helpful to provide education about feeling in danger versus being in danger. This can also provide the space for the clinician to thoroughly answer any questions about the physical symptoms of anxiety and panic. Breathing and relaxation techniques can be taught to decrease any physical tension that can come with panic attacks. Finally, exposure is a primary component of CBT for panic, and there are two types of exposure that can be implemented: physical symptoms and activities. For physical symptoms exposure, the individual would engage in techniques that induce the symptom (e.g., shortness of breath, heart pounding, dizziness) such as repeatedly breathing through a straw, activities that increase heart rate, etc. in order to reduce the fear of these symptoms in moments of panic. The activity exposure approach to panic would also have the individual confront the situations they avoid due to perceptions of danger (e.g., crowds, tight spaces).

Specific Phobias As with panic disorder, the treatment for specific phobias using CBT relies heavily on exposure exercises to feared stimuli. The literature has shown that engaging in routine gradual exposure (least anxiety-provoking to most) leads to significant decreases in anxiety (Böhnlein et al., 2020). While this behavioral approach leads to habituation of the feared stimuli, other cognitive techniques can help with reducing anxiety in the moment as well. Interventions such as cognitive restructuring allow the person with the specific phobia to challenge extreme ways of thinking and lower their anxiety by creating more realistic outcomes and ways of thinking. This has been shown to lead to less anxiety during exposures when the individual is able to engage in more balanced thinking beforehand.

Generalized Anxiety Given the high-stress nature of first-responder and public safety occupations, it is no surprise that generalized anxiety can develop. Often within CBT, clients are encouraged to monitor their thoughts and mood as a way to increase awareness of the context of their emotions. With symptoms of generalized anxiety disorder, it can be difficult to know when the anxiety is triggered; therefore, CBT for generalized anxiety includes an analysis of triggers for the individual's anxiety (e.g., where, when, intensity, etc.) to increase the individual's insight and knowledge. As with other anxiety disorders, psychoeducation about anxiety in itself is another important intervention, as it is likely to increase compliance from the client for treatment if they understand the rationale behind various therapeutic techniques. Behavioral techniques can also be flexibly applied within CBT for generalized anxiety disorder, such as engaging in exposure exercises with specific emotions in order to habituate to them. In this way, clients can gain more control over emotions by accepting that they exist. An example of this is for the client to think of the worst-case scenario about something that produces anxiety, and by doing so, the client actually becomes less anxious in thinking about the plausibility of these scenarios.

Mood Disorders

Depressive Disorders Depressive symptoms are commonly seen in the form of major depressive disorder and persistent depressive disorders in first responders and public service personnel (Huang et al., 2022). In a meta-analysis of 115 studies, CBT was shown to be an effective treatment for depression in a variety of populations. In general, the improvements found in these studies remained for up to 2 years after treatment occurred (Cuijpers et al., 2013). The goal of CBT for depression is to use interventions that address the cognitive triangle of how thoughts, emotions, and behaviors are connected. Many of the following interventions can be used in a combination of ways to address what the client is in need of most. As previously stated, cognitive restructuring teaches the client to challenge unhelpful beliefs about the self, others, and the world that are contributing to depressive thinking. Additionally, many therapists can institute journals about the client's thoughts and emotions as a way to understand what types of depressive automatic thoughts arise in different contexts. One tool for the cognitive restructuring of such thoughts is an ABC sheet that allows the client to identify the activating event ("A"), the beliefs about the event ("B"), and emotional and behavioral consequences of the event ("C"). By examining whether the thoughts in "B" are realistically based on facts, rather than emotions, it can help the client better align their emotional response with reality, as opposed to the negative emotional biases that come with depression. Behaviorally, therapists can teach their clients to improve symptoms of depression by using behavioral activation interventions. This requires the use of planned activities to increase action and pleasure in the individual's life through an intentional focus on doing things that are active (e.g., taking a walk, calling a friend, exercising) versus passive (e.g., laying on the couch, sleeping, watching television). When clients can restructure negative thought patterns to make them more fact-based and engage in activities that elicit pleasure and mastery, depression symptoms tend to decrease.

Suicidal Thoughts and Behaviors A very prominent symptom of depression in first responders is that of suicidal thoughts and behaviors (Bond & Anestis, 2021). Many studies have shown the prevalence of suicidal ideation in first-responder populations to be higher than that found in the general population. The repeated exposure to trauma and limited coping resources can lead individuals in these occupations to feel overwhelmed and potentially experience suicidal thoughts and/or behaviors in response to this feeling. Cognitive therapy for suicide prevention (CT-SP; Brown et al., 2012) was developed specifically to address suicidal thoughts and behaviors. There are three phases to this treatment; the first phase is focused on risk assessment, as well as a conceptualization of how the suicidal thoughts and/or behavior began. The second phase of treatment involves psychoeducation and teaching coping skills (e.g., relaxation techniques, cognitive restructuring). The last phase focuses on relapse prevention strategies, which encourage the client to imagine how they might cope in future suicidal crises based on the skills learned in the second phase of treatment.

Substance Use Disorders

Alcohol and substance use disorders are very often seen in first-responder and public safety personnel due to their comorbidity with other diagnoses, such as PTSD and depression. Many turn to alcohol or other substances as methods to cope with unwanted thoughts and emotions, particularly when they have to return to work immediately following exposure to high-stress situations. Often, there are specific automatic thoughts, primarily based on negative emotions that lead individuals to drink or use (e.g., "I can't handle this pain," "I need to drink to feel better"). CBT for substance use disorders is a short-term treatment that can help address the underlying thoughts leading to use. An important intervention in this treatment is to identify triggering situations by recognizing, avoiding, and coping with them using many available CBT skills discussed thus far. As with many other psychiatric diagnoses, awareness of unhelpful or maladaptive thoughts is critical in knowing how to address them. An example of cognitive restructuring in this context would be if a client in the public safety profession had the unhelpful belief that, "It was my fault I couldn't save them," which led them to use substances, they would be guided to examine the facts of the situation and challenge this belief to become something more balanced such as, "I did everything I could, and I wish I could have saved them." Imagery rehearsal has also been used in CBT to address substance use disorders. This involves having the client imagine a triggering scenario, such as being around friends who drink or use substances, and then how they would cope with it differently instead of engaging in substance use. The more they are able to play this out in their minds and identify coping skills that will allow them to avoid using, the more confident they will feel in these situations in the future. Finally, helping clients create more positive and pleasant activities to engage in will also help structure their time so that they do not fall into patterns of using substances or drinking when they do not have anything else to do.

Relationship Distress

Exposure to potentially traumatic events, such as those frequently encountered by first responders (e.g., suicide, homicide, motor vehicle accidents, deaths of children), has been shown to have a significant negative impact on relationship satisfaction (Neff & Karney, 2004) and perceived relationship support (Regehr et al., 2003). The various emotional and behavioral experiences of first responders and public safety personnel in response to these potentially traumatic events can certainly influence how they interact with close loved ones and friends. For instance, if a client is experiencing depression, they may isolate or withdraw, which may lead to relationship dissatisfaction for their significant other. There are several types of CBT treatments for couples that can be applied to first responders and public safety personnel. Many components of individual CBT explained previously can be applied in couples work. Interventions are aimed at improving communication within the dyad and challenging unhelpful beliefs about one another and the relationship. In an empirical review of CBT for couples, it was shown to be more effective at times than individual CBT, as the partner's involvement can enhance treatment benefit (Fischer et al., 2016).

CBT with First Responders and Public Safety Personnel

CBT has demonstrated that it is highly effective in alleviating mental and emotional distress in individuals with high-stress occupations, as well as improving overall functioning. Given the time-sensitive nature of addressing many of these concerns among first responders and public safety personnel, CBT allows for individuals to engage in an effective, focused treatment in order to get back to their previous functioning as quickly as possible. For instance, one study examined the effectiveness of both a long and brief course of CBT in a sample of emergency service personnel (i.e., police officers, firefighters, and paramedics) who met diagnostic criteria for PTSD. The treatment included psychoeducation and skills training in commonly seen mental health issues in emergency service members, exposure exercises, and relapse prevention. Results showed that those in the CBT conditions experienced significant decreases in PTSD symptoms, depression, and maladaptive beliefs and made improvements in social quality of life (Bryant et al., 2018). In a follow-up study 2 years later, reductions in PTSD symptoms remained, highlighting the potential for long-lasting effects of a short-term treatment like CBT (Bryant et al., 2021). The literature is lacking in empirical research investigating the effects of CBT with many mental health diagnoses that are currently seen in the first-responder and public safety personnel professions. The research that currently exists is primarily focused on examining PTSD and traumatic stress; therefore, additional research is critical to understand the effectiveness as a whole of CBT in this specific population.

A key advantage to using CBT to address any of the aforementioned diagnoses is that many of the skills and techniques can be practiced outside of session. As opposed to other types of therapy, most of the skills practice happens in between sessions in a way that is flexible for the client, especially when shifts in public safety personnel can be quite variable. Additionally, the influx of telemedicine in recent years makes access to treatment much easier for individuals in this line of work who may not be able to keep consistent office appointments for therapy. First responders and public safety personnel are even able to use mobile devices to engage in therapy to develop the skills they need.

Another benefit to using CBT with this population is that its focus on building and practicing skills can be applied in real time through on-site practice. Interventions for anxiety-related disorders, such as graduated exposure to feared situations, can be implemented with approval from leadership. For instance, if a firefighter client is struggling with panic attacks when in closed spaces, therapists can take the opportunity to build an exposure hierarchy with them that includes practicing the exercises with the therapist in real-world settings (e.g., training buildings). Being in the real-world settings of this population can allow the client to better test any unhelpful beliefs through ABC worksheets or to approach situations they are avoiding to gather more accurate data. This is particularly useful when clinicians are part of the departmental staff in public safety settings, as interventions can be tailored to reflect the day-to-day routines of clients.

Case Example

A 35-year-old female EMS driver presents to therapy due to nightmares, intrusive thoughts, isolation, poor concentration, and panic attacks that happen when she is out with her family and when she is on duty. She discloses that she had "a really bad run" about 2 months ago that involved a car accident where a child was severely injured. She was tasked with attempting to save the child, who eventually died at the hospital. A diagnostic assessment shows that she meets criteria for PTSD, with panic attacks, with increased anxiety particularly in situations involving children and vehicles. She believes it is her fault the child died, that she should have done more to save the child, and that if she had only driven faster to the scene, the child would still be alive. She also believes being around children and vehicles is dangerous and cannot trust herself to save anyone in future accidents. This has led her to frequently call off from work when she feels especially anxious, limit her interactions with her friends and family outside of work, and avoid driving when she can. She enters therapy given the amount of interference her symptoms have had on her work performance.

Cognitive processing therapy (CPT) appears to be the best fit for this client to address the PTSD symptoms stemming from the motor vehicle accident, given the amount of blame-related beliefs she has about why the event occurred and how it has affected her beliefs about herself, other people, and the world. She is open to starting CPT but will only do so via telehealth (her iPhone) since she does not feel comfortable driving into an office to meet. She is aware this is a 12-session protocol, and out-of-session assignments are an integral part of the treatment. During the first few sessions, she uncovers unhelpful beliefs ("stuck points") about the trauma (e.g., "If I had only gotten to the scene faster, that little girl would still be alive"). By engaging in Socratic dialogue around the belief and how she came to know this belief to be true, she is able to challenge this thought and see that the injuries the child sustained were likely fatal from the moment the accident occurred. As she gets more clarity on her role in the event itself, she is able to effectively challenge her beliefs that have developed about herself, others, and the world today. For instance, using challenging questions and cognitive restructuring on the belief, "I can't trust myself to save anyone else again," can allow her to truly examine the facts and create a more realistic belief such as "my training and experience make it likely that I will continue to save others in the future" and "my abilities had nothing to do with the child's death; it was the accident that killed her." She continues to build more realistic beliefs throughout CPT and reports feeling less blame, guilt, fear, and anxiety; however, she continues to avoid driving even though she has challenged unhelpful beliefs behind this avoidance in CPT.

At the completion of CPT, it may be indicated to assist her in creating a graduated hierarchy to address her avoidance of driving. This is a particularly important focus of intervention, as her primary responsibility in her position is driving. From a CBT approach, it would be important to expose herself to the feared situation of driving for about 30–45 min at a time, until her anxiety begins to decrease. In collaboration with the client, items on this hierarchy could include imagining herself driving, sitting in her vehicle at home, driving around her neighborhood, and/or driving with a family member. When she becomes less anxious with the initial exposure exercises, she can move to the next. The last step will be for her to become more confident in driving in high-stress situations at work.

By targeting her cognitions through CPT and her behavioral avoidance through an exposure hierarchy, this helps the client contextualize the trauma and increase her quality of life both at work and at home. At the completion of therapy, it is critical for her to continue practicing the skills she has learned in treatment in order for her to maintain these improvements. When clients can understand and believe in the rationale behind out-of-session assignments and skills practice, they are more likely to continue seeing benefit from their engagement in any type of CBT.

Conclusion

First responders and public service personnel encounter trauma and highly distressing events on a much more frequent basis than many other professions; however, stigma often prevents this population from seeking therapeutic help. By providing evidence-based psychotherapy, such as CBT, for a variety of mental health conditions, first responders can receive flexible and skills-based tools that they can quickly use to regain confidence at work and in their personal lives. Many times, this population will not be presenting to therapy with just one concern that they want to address; therefore, CBT can offer a number of interventions to address multiple symptom presentations. As a clinician working with first responders and public safety personnel, it will be beneficial to consider ways to bring the skills from therapy into real-life scenarios and generalize them to the individual's specific job setting. Further research into the effectiveness of CBT with first responders and public safety personnel will increase understanding of the specific needs of this population and the effectiveness of specific CBT interventions for different disorders.

References

American Psychiatric Association. (2013). *Diagnostic and statistical manual of mental health disorders* (5th ed.). https://doi.org/10.1176/appi.books.9780890425596

Beck, A. T. (1976). *Cognitive therapy and the emotional disorders*. International Universities Press.

Böhnlein, J., Altegoer, L., Muck, N. K., Roesmann, K., Redlich, R., Dannlowski, U., & Leehr, E. J. (2020). Factors influencing the success of exposure therapy for specific phobia: A systematic review. *Neuroscience and Biobehavioral Reviews, 108*, 796–820. https://doi.org/10.1016/j.neubiorev.2019.12.009

Bond, A. E., & Anestis, M. D. (2021). Understanding capability and suicidal ideation among first responders. *Archives of Suicide Research*, 1–12. https://doi.org/10.1080/13811118.2021.1993397

Brown, G. K., Wright, J. H., Thase, M. E., & Beck, A. T. (2012). Cognitive therapy for suicide prevention. In R. I. Simon & R. E. Hales (Eds.), *The American Psychiatric Publishing textbook of suicide assessment and management* (pp. 233–249). American Psychiatric Publishing.

Brown, L. A., Gaudiano, B. A., & Miller, I. W. (2013). Investigating the similarities and differences between practitioners of second and third wave cognitive-behavioral therapies. *Behavior Modification, 35*(2), 187–200. https://doi.org/10.1177/0145445510393730

Bryant, R. A., Kenny, L., Rawson, N., Cahill, C., Joscelyne, A., Garber, B., Tockar, J., Dawson, K., & Nickerson, A. (2018). Efficacy of exposure-based cognitive behavior therapy for posttraumatic stress disorder in emergency service personnel: A randomized clinical trial. *Psychological Medicine, 49*(9), 1565–1573. https://doi.org/10.1017/S0033291718002234

Bryant, R. A., Kenny, L., Rawson, N., Cahill, C., Joscelyne, A., Garber, B., Tockar, J., Tran, J., & Dawson, K. (2021). Two-year follow-up of trauma-focused cognitive behavior therapy for posttraumatic stress disorder in emergency service personnel: A randomized clinical trial. *Anxiety and Depression, 38*(11), 1131–1137. https://doi.org/10.1002/da.23214

Carleton, R. N., Afifi, T. O., Turner, S., Taillieu, T., Duranceau, S., LeBouthillier, D. M., Sareen, J., Ricciardelli, R., MacPhee, R. S., Groll, D., Hozempa, K., Brunet, A., Weekes, J. R., Griffiths, C. T., Abrams, K. J., Jones, N. A., Beshai, S., Cramm, H. A., Dobson, K. S., et al. (2018). Mental disorder symptoms among public safety personnel in Canada. *The Canadian Journal of Psychiatry, 63*(1), 54–65. https://doi.org/10.1177/0706743717723825

Carleton, R. N., Afifi, T. O., Taillieu, T., Vaughan, A. D., Anderson, G. S., Ricciardelli, R., MacPhee, R. S., Cramm, H. A., Czarnuch, S., Hozempa, K., & Camp, R. D. (2020). Mental health training, attitudes toward support, and screening positive for mental disorders. *Cognitive Behaviour Therapy, 49*(1), 55–73. https://doi.org/10.1080/16506073.2019.1575900

Carpenter, J. K., Andrews, L. A., Witcraft, S. M., Powers, M. B., Smits, J. A. J., & Hofmann, S. G. (2018). Cognitive behavioral therapy for anxiety and related disorders: A meta-analysis of randomized placebo-controlled trials. *Depression and Anxiety, 35*(6), 502–514. https://doi.org/10.1002/da.22728

Cuijpers, P., Berking, M., Andersson, G., Quigley, L., Kleiboer, A., & Dobson, K. S. (2013). A meta-analysis of cognitive-behavioral therapy for adult depression, alone and in comparison with other treatments. *The Canadian Journal of Psychiatry, 58*(7), 376–385. https://doi.org/10.1177/070674371305800702

Dunn, G., Fowler, D., Rollinson, R., Freeman, D., Kuipers, E., Smith, B., Steele, C., Onwumere, J., Jolley, S., Garety, P., & Bebbington, P. (2012). Effective elements of cognitive behavior therapy for psychosis: results of a novel type of subgroup analysis based on principal stratification. *Psychological Medicine, 42*(5), 1057–1068. https://doi.org/10.1017/S0033291711001954

Fischer, M. S., Baucom, D. H., & Cohen, M. J. (2016). Cognitive-behavioral couple therapies: Review of the evidence for the treatment of relationship distress, psychopathology, and chronic health conditions. *Family Process, 55*(3), 423–429. https://doi.org/10.1111/famp.12227

Foa, E. B., & Rothbaum, B. O. (1998). *Treating the trauma of rape: Cognitive behavioral therapy for PTSD*. Guilford Press.

Gautam, M., Tripathi, A., Deshmukh, D., & Gaur, M. (2020). Cognitive behavioral therapy for depression. *Indian Journal of Psychiatry, 62*(2), 223–229. https://doi.org/10.4103/psychiatry.IndianJPsychiatry_772_19

Hayes, S. C., Strosahl, K., & Wilson, K. G. (1999). *Acceptance and commitment therapy: An experiential approach to behavior change*. Guilford Press.

Huang, G., Chu, H., Chen, R., Liu, D., Banda, K. J., O'Brien, A. P., Jen, H., Chiang, K., Chiou, J., & Chou, K. (2022). Prevalence of depression, anxiety, and stress among first responders for medical emergencies during COVID-19 pandemic: A meta-analysis. *Journal of Global Health, 12*(05028). https://doi.org/10.7189/jogh.12.05028

Jones, S. (2017). Describing the mental health profile of first responders: A systematic review. *Journal of the American Psychiatric Nurses Association, 23*(3), 200–214. https://doi.org/10.1177/1078390317695266

Linehan, M. (1993). *Cognitive-behavioral treatment of borderline personality disorder*. Guilford Press.

Mendes, D. D., Mello, M. F., Ventura, P., Passarela, C. D., & Mari, J. J. (2008). A systematic review on the effectiveness of cognitive behavioral therapy for posttraumatic stress disorder. *International Journal of Psychiatry Medicine, 38*(3), 241–259. https://doi.org/10.2190/PM.38.3.b

Neff, L. A., & Karney, B. R. (2004). How does context affect intimate relationships? Linking external stress and cognitive processes within marriage. *Personality and Social Psychology Bulletin, 30*(2), 134–148. https://doi.org/10.1177/0146167203255984

Regehr, C., Hill, J., Knott, T., & Sault, B. (2003). Social support, self-efficacy, and trauma in new recruits and experienced firefighters. *Stress and Health: Journal of the International Society for the Investigation of Stress, 19*(4), 189–193. https://doi.org/10.1002/smi.974

Resick, P. A., & Schnicke, M. K. (1993). *Cognitive processing therapy for rape victims: A treatment manual*. Sage.

Substance Abuse and Mental Health Services Administration. (2018, May). First responders: Behavioral health concerns, emergency response, and trauma. *Disaster Technical Assistance Center Supplemental Research Bulletin*, (7). https://www.samhsa.gov/sites/default/files/dtac/supplementalresearchbulletin-firstresponders-may2018.pdf

Vigil, N. H., Grant, A. R., Perez, O., Blust, R. N., Chikani, V., Vadeboncoeur, T. F., Spaite, D. W., & Bobrow, B. J. (2019). Death by suicide – The EMS profession compared to the general public. *Prehospital Emergency Care, 23*(3), 340–345. https://doi.org/10.1080/10903127.2018.1514090

Zamboni, L., Centoni, F., Fusina, F., Mantovani, E., Rubino, F., Lugoboni, F., & Federico, A. (2021). The effectiveness of cognitive behavioral therapy techniques for the treatment of substance use disorders: A narrative review of evidence. *The Journal of Nervous and Mental Disease, 209*(11), 835–845. https://doi.org/10.1097/NMD.0000000000001381

The Benefits of Eye Movement Desensitization Reprocessing in a Law Enforcement Population

Robert J. Cipriano Jr, Samantha Rodriguez, and Katherine Kuhlman

The job duties of a police officer can vary and often include responsibilities that the general population will never experience. Given the unique and potentially traumatic nature of these responsibilities, police officers report high levels of chronic stress, job burnout, and a lack of social support from those both within and outside their profession. Consequently, this can place law enforcement professionals at an increased risk for experiencing numerous adverse mental health conditions, including posttraumatic stress disorder (PTSD). Research supports law enforcement populations are at an elevated risk for developing PTSD given the high rate of exposure to critical incidents reported, with rates ranging from 46% to 92% on a yearly basis (Wagner et al., 2020). The law enforcement culture reinforces the use of avoidant coping strategies to mitigate the results of consistent exposure to potentially traumatic events, or "critical incidents," such as substance use or social isolation (Arble et al., 2018; Becker et al., 2009). While traditional stress management and other preventative techniques may be offered through in-service trainings within a police department, there is added benefit in offering evidence-based treatments for trauma, including eye movement desensitization and reprocessing (EMDR).

R. J. CiprianoJr (✉)
Fort Lauderdale Police Department, Fort Lauderdale, FL, USA
e-mail: rcipriano@simcipgroup.com

S. Rodriguez
Nova Southeastern University, Davie, FL, USA

K. Kuhlman
Kuhlman Psychology and Counseling, Scottsdale, AZ, USA

M. L. Bourke et al. (eds.), *First Responder Mental Health*,
https://doi.org/10.1007/978-3-031-38149-2_12

Trauma Exposure in Law Enforcement

Public safety professionals, in particular police officers, are exposed to a variety of traumatic-based incidents that are of varying degrees of intensity, duration, and frequency. These events may include line of duty deaths, school or workplace shootings, familial violence, coming in contact with dead bodies, child drownings, and police-involved shootings (Violanti et al., 2006). Such trauma exposures can affect police and public safety professionals in a variety of ways. For example, catastrophic thoughts, or thoughts that can drastically turn negative and spin out of control into worst case scenarios (e.g., driving in the rain will result in a deadly car accident, going to the doctor will lead to the discovery of cancer), may be commonly reported.

Given the elevated frequency in which police officers experience critical incidents, it is estimated they are at an increased risk for developing PTSD symptoms. Within the general population, the prevalence of PTSD symptoms is estimated to be 4.7% within a 12-month period (Kilpatrick et al., 2013). However, Violanti et al. (2006) reported close to 30% of a random stratified officer sample from an urban police department endorsed moderate to severe PTSD symptoms. Wagner et al. (2020) utilized a best-evidence, systemic review to evaluate the prevalence of PTSD in police officers compared to the general population. Through this review, they found consistent predictive factors of PTSD reported among police officer samples, including incident-specific factors (e.g., type of critical incident, severity of exposure) and posttraumatic factors (e.g., presence of other mental health disorders). Additionally, they contended the impact of organizational factors, such as lack of support and perceived work stress, on officers' risk of PTSD was understudied considering the majority of traumatic experiences are work-related. Further, Huddleston et al. (2007) found organizational stressors further exacerbated reported PTSD symptoms in a sample of 512 police recruits.

In addition to organizational stressors, officers experience heightened stress following critical incidents that generate media attention. For example, an officer who uses appropriate lethal use of force may find their name and incident being discussed on the evening news or in a social media post. This can generate fear for them and their family's safety, or lead to feelings of dehumanization, especially with social media commentary. Media stories that are unrelated to the officer's own department can also elicit stress. Following the shooting of George Floyd in Minneapolis in 2020, and subsequent calls for defunding of police, many police departments saw increased rates of resignations and retirements, with many officers citing the stress of the job, lack of morale, and lack of feeling respected. Not only must officers manage their own stress and fears, but many have spouses and family members who also communicate their fears, causing additional stress.

Given the frequency with which police officers can experience traumatic events lends support and rationalization for providing EMDR treatment for police officers.

History and Mechanisms of EMDR Treatment

In 1987, Francine Shapiro was taking a walk in a park when she became aware that eye movements appeared to decrease the negative emotion connected with her own stressful memories. She hypothesized that eye movements had a lessening emotional effect, and when she tested this, she found that other people experienced similar responses to eye movements. Dr. Shapiro's hypothesis evolved to include other treatment mechanisms, including a cognitive method, and she developed a standard procedure that she called eye movement desensitization (EMD) (Shapiro, 1989).

Dr. Shapiro conducted studies utilizing EMD, and the results showed significant decreases in distress reported by the participants. In the early 1990s, she changed the name to eye movement desensitization and reprocessing (EMDR) to (1) emphasize the cognitive changes that occurred during treatment and (2) identify the adaptive information processing (AIP) model, which she developed to describe the treatment effects. This concept outlines that mental health disorders, including PTSD, are a result of unprocessed memories of earlier adverse life experiences that contain perceptions experienced at the time of the event and were maladaptively stored in the brain, leading to undesirable emotional, cognitive, and somatic symptoms (Hill, 2020; Shapiro, 2014). Thus, the AIP model supports the need to process the multiple elements of human experiences in order to store memories connected through related thoughts, images, emotions, and sensations in an accessible and useful way. As a result, EMDR can help an individual process their emotional response to a distressing event, as well as mitigate and/or lessen the emotional disruption the event may have caused that individual. New learning occurs when the new associations are formed with material already stored in memory, leading to less distressing memories (Shapiro, 2014; Shapiro, 1991). Further, EMDR research outcomes support the following: sleep improvement, a reduction in nightmares and flashbacks, a reduction in intrusive thoughts, and an overall improvement in sense of wellbeing (Shapiro, 1989). Its effectiveness has been evaluated in at least 16 randomized control studies; and 3 meta-analyses noted its effectiveness in decreasing subjects' symptoms following exposure to adverse events (Solomon et al., 2009).

There are three primary explanations concerning the mechanism of action of EMDR therapy: the orienting response, working memory, and the rapid eye movement hypotheses. The orienting response eye movements or other dual-attention stimuli produce an orienting response with associated physiological de-arousal that improves processing of trauma material (Söndergaard & Elofsson, 2008). Research supporting the working memory explanation has shown that performance is reduced when participants engage in two simultaneous tasks that require the same working memory resources (Baddeley, 2000). Related studies have found that eye movements impair the ability to hold a visual image in conscious awareness, resulting in reductions in clarity (Andrade et al., 1997; Kavanagh et al., 2001). Working memory theory rationalizes that both tasks require the same limited working memory resource and that competition for this resource impairs performance. The REM explanation in EMDR proposed by Stickgold (2002) shifts the brain into a memory processing mode similar to that of REM sleep.

Phases of EMDR

The intent of EMDR therapy is to assist a client in processing traumatic memories and distressing emotions to then develop a new meaning and understanding of that event (EMDR Institute, Inc., 2020). EMDR utilizes an eight-phase approach to identify memories of a traumatic event, address present distressing factors, and teach skills for future positive learning. During the first phase, a provider and client will collaborate to discuss "targets" in the client's treatment, meaning identifying memories and current situations that are causing the client emotional distress. Following this, the provider will assist the client in learning new skills to help them gain insight and process the adverse events. Moving into the second phase, treatment will focus on providing the client with imagery skills and stress reduction techniques to reduce and manage their emotional distress between sessions.

Phases three to six involve moving through the distressing "targets" previously identified at the beginning of treatment. First, the client will identify (1) a vivid image of the memory, (2) a negative belief about the self with a rating of that belief, (3) a positive belief about the self, and (4) related emotions and body sensations. The therapist will instruct the client to focus on the vivid image while concurrently participating in EMDR processing using bilateral stimulation, such as eye movements, taps, or tones. These sets of stimulation occur multiple times throughout the session, and following each set, the client is encouraged to take note of any thoughts, feelings, images, or sensations that may appear. When the thoughts, feelings, images, or sensations tied to that memory are no longer seen as distressing to the client, they are asked to think of the positive belief of self they previously acknowledged.

Moving forward into phase seven of treatment, the client will be instructed to keep a log of stressful activities or events they encounter throughout the week so the client can utilize the emotional distress techniques originally taught in phase one. Finally, phase eight will encompass the client's progress in treatment and review of the relevant historical events, current distressing situations, and potentially future distressing events (EMDR Institute, Inc., 2020).

Impact of Trauma on Memory

In one of the first meta-analyses, Günak et al. (2020) quantified the association between PTSD and the risk of dementia. The meta-analysis showed that PTSD is a strong and potentially modifiable risk factor for all-cause dementia. In this investigation, there was a thorough search of almost 8000 records including studies across a range of populations and countries. Meta-analyses showed that the risk of being diagnosed with dementia in individuals with a diagnosis of PTSD is 1.61 to nearly two times the risk compared to those without a PTSD diagnosis. Desmarais et al. (2020) conducted a systematic review of 25 articles pertaining to both dementia and PTSD. PTSD in mid-life was reported to increase the risk for late-life dementia of all types. Late-onset Alzheimer's disease and vascular dementia were reported to increase the risk for delayed emergence, re-emergence, or worsening of post-traumatic stress disorder. More rigorous longitudinal studies that include neuroimaging and biomarkers are needed to corroborate the association between the two conditions as well as to better understand the underlying pathological mechanisms (Desmarais et al., 2020).

The Officer-Involved Shooting (OIS; IACP Police Psychological Services Section, 2018) guidelines provide recommendations to public safety agencies and the mental health providers who provide the service, prepare, and respond to the health and well-being of law enforcement personnel following such an officer-involved shooting. The guidelines were developed to offer information and recommendations to public safety agencies and their mental health providers that can be flexibly applied in response to the complexity of demands that may vary across jurisdictions following such incidents. Many of these recommendations apply to officer-involved shootings and other potentially distressing critical incidents (e.g., severe motor vehicle accidents, crime scenes, child fatalities, drownings). The OIS guidelines help to identify and assist those individuals at higher risk for experiencing and/or developing subsequent mental health problems.

The impact on memory following an officer-involved shooting can present in a variety of ways. During a shooting, for example, officers often experience tunnel vision; that is, they are solely focused on the elimination of the threat. Other factors, such as the number of other officers around them, amount of rounds they fire, and even some physical characteristics of the suspect, may not be present in the moment (Hartman et al., 2017). One example involves an officer who was involved in a vehicle pursuit that resulted in the suspect vehicle in a ditch and the suspect in the vehicle pointing a firearm at officers. The incident resulted in 4 officers firing their guns at the suspect, with about 30 additional officers as backup in the vicinity. In a debriefing about 2 days after the shooting with one officer, the officer commented, "In the moment, all I saw was a silhouette and their gun. I couldn't have told you what they were wearing, their race, anything." About a week after the shooting, after being able to sleep and process the incident more, the officer could recall more details.

Additionally, the inability to recall specific details of a traumatic incident is one symptom of PTSD. While some details may be recalled in vivid detail, others may be vague at best. Below is one of the author's detailed experiences with the impact of EMDR regarding an officer's ability to recall details of their involvement in a traumatic incident:

> During a debrief, an officer was asked to recall the details of a scene involving a double fatal motor vehicle accident. While the officer was able to explain some details vividly, such as the way the victim's eyes appeared or the smell of gas leaking from the vehicles, the officer was not able to recall parts of his involvement on scene or even the images of the other

> vehicles that had stopped to assist. The officer was later told that he had attempted to resuscitate one of the victims, an important piece of the officer's involvement that could not be recalled. Two years following the incident, the officer voluntarily participated in mental health treatment to address some of the challenges experienced. After engaging in EMDR treatment, the officer was able to report a more detailed encounter of on-scene involvement in that motor vehicle accident.

In another research study evaluating the benefits of EMDR on memory and concurrent treatment of PTSD, data suggested there is memory dysfunction with PTSD, particularly involving specific functions such as encoding and recall. Individuals with PTSD present less activity in the prefrontal cortex triggered by a decrease in encoding and recall capacities. EMDR through bilateral eye movements can facilitate a fast relief of PTSD symptoms that, in turn, can potentially increase the brain's prefrontal, ventromedial, amygdala, and thalamic regions during the desensitization phase. After comparing cerebral activity before and after the therapy, research on EMDR has shown that a reduction of stressful symptoms had some sensitive link to PTSD (in the prevention of dementia) (Vieira et al., 2017).

Dr. Francine Shapiro hypothesized that EMDR therapy facilitates the accessing of the traumatic memory network, so that information processing is enhanced with new associations paralleled between the traumatic memory and more adaptive memories or information. The new associations are thought to result in complete information processing, new learning, elimination of emotional turmoil, and the development of cognitive understanding (EMDR Institute Inc., 2020).

Efficacy of EMDR for PTSD Symptoms in Law Enforcement

Following its introduction in 1989, more than 30 randomized controlled trials (RCTs) have been published looking at the efficacy of EMDR in comparison to other modalities for the treatment of PTSD (de Jongh et al., 2019). The effectiveness of EMDR for PTSD symptoms has commonly been compared to cognitive behavioral therapies (e.g., Jaberghaderi et al., 2004; Lee et al., 2002; Power et al., 2002). Additionally, other studies have evaluated the use of psychopharmacology (e.g., van der Kolk et al., 2007), exposure therapy (e.g., Ironson et al., 2002; Rothbaum et al., 2005; Taylor et al., 2003; Vaughan et al., 1994), and a wait-list condition (e.g., Acarturk et al., 2016; Högberg et al., 2007).

When evaluating its effectiveness in the reduction of PTSD symptoms, several of these studies reported results ranging from 36% to 95% (de Jongh et al., 2019). Other studies reported a reduction in other psychological presentations outside of PTSD (e.g., Van den Berg, et al., 2015). In fact, several organizations, including the American Psychiatric Association, Department of Defense, and World Health Organization, now endorse EMDR as an efficacious intervention for trauma survivors (Shapiro, 2014).

The majority of EMDR studies that assessed PTSD treatment utilized adult civilian participants. Nonetheless, recent investigations have expanded their sample populations to include military combatants, disaster survivors, traumatized children, and adult survivors of childhood trauma (Maxfield, 2007). In looking specifically at a police officer sample, Wilson et al. (2001) implemented an EMDR stress management program (three, 2-h standard EMDR sessions for each participant) and a traditional stress management program (six, 1-h session video course focusing on tools for stress reduction) within a local police department to evaluate each program's ability to help participants manage their stress related to the nature of their profession. The authors found participants in the EMDR condition reported lower ratings of PTSD symptoms, subjective distress, job stress, and higher marital satisfaction than those in the traditional stress management program condition. Additionally, these results were maintained at a 6-month follow-up. While this study does not exclusively focus on the reduction of PTSD symptoms, its results suggest EMDR can also be utilized for stress management in this population. Nonetheless, future research on the direct effect of EMDR on PTSD symptoms in a police officer sample would be beneficial in determining effective treatment options.

Lansing et al. (2005) examined the effectiveness and physiological effects of EMDR in six police officers diagnosed with PTSD. Participants had been involved with on-duty shootings and were diagnosed with subsequent delayed-onset PTSD. The researchers utilized standardized treatment measures, the Posttraumatic Stress Diagnostic Scale (PDS), and high-resolution brain single-photon emission computed tomography (SPECT) imaging before and after treatment. All officers showed clinical improvement and marked reductions in the PDS. There were also decreases in the left and right occipital lobe, left parietal lobe, and right precentral frontal lobe as well as significant increased perfusion in the left inferior frontal gyrus. It was concluded that EMDR was an effective treatment for PTSD in this police officer group, showing both clinical and brain imaging changes.

Other Psychological and Medical Concerns for Law Enforcement Officers

The cumulative stress of the profession, coupled with the consistent exposure to critical incidents, places law enforcement at an increased risk for experiencing a range of other mental and physical health conditions. For instance, unmanaged stress may increase the risk of gastrointestinal disorders, high blood pressure, and coronary heart disease in police officers (Sheehan & Van Hasselt, 2003). In addition, officers must respond to unpredictable emergency calls that require bursts of intense and strenuous activity, which may also add stress to the cardiovascular system (Hartley et al., 2011). Consequently, this population is known to have a higher mortality rate compared to the civilian population. Indeed, Violanti et al. (2013) found that white male police officers are at an increased risk of dying at an earlier age compared to white male civilians. Specifically, the average difference in life expectancy between the two populations was 21.9 years. Nonetheless, research supports that EMDR can also provide relief from the physiological consequences of experiencing adverse or traumatic events (Shapiro, 2014).

Numerous investigations highlight the maladaptive coping mechanisms (e.g., substance use, avoidance) and personality characteristics (e.g., cynicism, suspiciousness, emotional detachment, depersonalization) that develop in police officers over the course of their careers (Gershon et al., 2009; Ménard & Arter, 2013; Patterson, 1999; Soomro & Yanos, 2019). Thus, it is important to note that EMDR can also factor in avoidance behaviors that, consequently, can also lead to the accumulation of negative emotional responses (Shapiro, 1991). Alcohol use, in particular, has historically been a concern in law enforcement. Many studies have concluded that alcohol consumption in police officers is reinforced by law enforcement culture and used as a way to socialize and cope with the stressors of the profession (Violanti, 2004; Violanti et al., 2013). Consequently, it is estimated that approximately 25% of police officers abuse alcohol at detrimental levels (Ballenger et al., 2011; Ménard & Arter, 2013). Alcohol use can also be classified as a risk factor for other psychological consequences in this population. For example, Violanti (2004) carried out self-report assessments of critical incident trauma, trauma symptomatology, substance abuse, and suicidal ideation in 115 police officers. He found that with increased exposure to traumatic events and PTSD symptoms, there were also higher rates of alcohol use and suicidal ideation. Moreover, Arble et al. (2018) also reported that substance use as an avoidant coping strategy resulted in diminished well-being when compared to other non-military first responder groups. This further underscores the need to address avoidant behaviors, including alcohol use, in police officers, as it has been shown to be an ineffective coping strategy (Ménard & Arter, 2013). Elevated cortisol levels from critical incident exposures, sleep deprivation, shift work, and cumulative stress within the profession can lead to a number of medical ailments over time. Findings from a study of more than 300 members of the Buffalo Police Department suggested police events or conditions considered to be highly stressful by the officers may be associated with disturbances of the normal awakening cortisol pattern. This may leave the officers vulnerable to disease, particularly cardiovascular disease, which already affects a large number of officers (Violanti et al., 2017).

Occupational and Organizational Stressors

It is also important to consider the integration of occupational and organizational factors in trauma treatment for police officers. An occupational stressor is regarded as any critical incident that police officers are at risk for encountering, including officer-involved shootings, failed rescues, murder/suicides, or line of duty deaths. On the other hand, organizational stressors encompass the day-to-day factors of the job, such as administrative challenges, inadequate training/supervision, lack of recognition/organizational support, or inadequate pay (Soomro & Yanos, 2019). Patterson (1999) investigated the frequency police officers are exposed to stressful occupational and organizational events, as well as which type of event would be classified as more stressful to the officer. The officers' reported psychological distress to the stressful situation(s) was also measured. A sample of 223 police officers from every unit in a department located in a mid-sized city in the USA was recruited. After receiving a 67% response rate, results showed that officers ranked organizational events as more stressful, while operational (field) events were seen as "less meaningful" (Patterson, 1999). These results are consistent with those of similar studies (e.g., Huddleston et al., 2007) that evaluated the impact of organizational stressors on officers' well-being. In fact, Huddleston et al. (2007) concluded that organizational stress further exacerbated PTSD symptoms. This indicates that both traumatic and organizational stress are predictive of psychological distress.

Additonal stressors could include: stigma for seeking confidential mental health services, fear for being perceived as "unfit" for work by departmental colleagues and supervisors, beliefs and feelings surrounding vulnerability, interactions with the criminal justice system and the public, now more than ever given the negative view of law enforcement through the media (Clark-Miller & Brady, 2013). Nonetheless, studies have found that it is the frequency of routine stressors, not the severity, that leads to greater stress in police officers (Berg et al., 2006; Clark-Miller & Brady, 2013). In addition to the array of occupational stressors police officers experience, there are also personal stressors, such as financial concerns, familial issues, or coping styles, that can contribute to their physiological and psychological difficulties (Habersaat et al., 2015).

Integrating Law Enforcement Culture and Mental Health

Law enforcement culture often stigmatizes mental health, making it difficult for officers to openly discuss these difficulties for fear of being seen as "weak" or incapable of performing their responsibilities by their peers (Soomro & Yanos, 2019). Throughout their rigorous training, police officers learn to value self-reliance, toughness, independence, and suppressing weakness. They further come to understand that deviating from these characteristics can be consequential (Wester & Lyubelsky, 2005). Consequently, discussing mental health and seeking outside resources has become taboo. Law enforcement culture further fosters suspicion and mistrust of "outsiders" (Soomro & Yanos, 2019). As a result, mental health providers find it difficult to integrate themselves within this population, unless they have a background or previous experience in the profession. Thus, when considering offering trauma treatment, such as EMDR, it is equally as important for mental health providers to be familiar with law enforcement culture as it is for them to have received formal training to practice EMDR. This way, providers can integrate formal EMDR training and relevant aspects of law enforcement culture to inform their treatment of officers with trauma symptoms.

In instances during which police officers have sought mental health treatment from providers who did not have a foundational understanding of law enforcement culture, it is common for police psychologists or other clinicians who regularly work with this population to hear "horror stories" of their clients' experiences with previous therapists. These complaints typically include the officer feeling misunderstood or judged, or that they needed to care for the therapist when exposing them to their personal trauma. Due to the "mistrust of outsiders," one officer's negative experience with a mental health provider can discredit that provider's reputation and result in a feeling of hesitancy or reluctance in other officers interested in seeking treatment. Consider the following examples provided by one of the authors from their clinical experience with law enforcement:

> One police officer working in a specialized unit recounted previous details of the child abuse and traumatic cases that were handled by an external mental health provider; this resulted in the external mental health provider being shocked, becoming tearful, and asking the police officer to stop talking. The police officer waited two years before seeking treatment again, feeling shamed by his previous mental health provider and experiencing guilt-based emotions that the issues attempted to be addressed in treatment were "too big" for any external mental health provider to handle.

> In another case, a patrol officer involved in a fatal shooting decided to seek counseling to be proactive in the event of experiencing an adverse reaction, post-shooting. The external mental health provider immediately began conducting a risk assessment of violence toward others due to learning that the client had shot and killed another person. The officer refused to see the external mental health provider again and felt judged for using appropriate force.

Clinicians may find it difficult to gain competency in working with law enforcement, and few former police officers will decide to become mental health providers. However, gaining cultural competency in working with this population is paramount to preventing examples like the ones outlined above that will inhibit the development of therapeutic rapport, and, therefore, positive treatment outcomes. In a 2018 survey conducted by the National Fraternal Order of Police, over half of surveyed officers worried that mental health providers would not understand their job, creating a barrier for them to seek help. Further, research suggests that the perception of a provider's competency is one component in developing rapport (Okiishi et al., 2003). In fact, it is commonplace for officers to have a negative perception of mental health-related services following knowledge gleaned from another peer's negative experience from utilizing their agency's Employee Assistance Program (EAP), licensed clinicians, peer support professionals, or clergy members.

Below is one of the authors' experiences implementing EMDR with a law enforcement population, which highlights the importance of cultural competence:

> Historically, rumors, punitive actions for seeking services both on and off duty, demotions, and passing up candidates for utilization of mental health services have been barriers for officers to seek services from a mental health provider or continue in ongoing mental health treatment. For providers to be unaware of these barriers, can mean that they lack the cultural competence needed to effectively implement a treatment modality, such as EMDR, within this population. Without an understanding of police culture, mental health providers may find it frustrating and difficult to understand why officers are reluctant to speak with them or take advantage of their expertise. Mental health treatment, especially utilizing EMDR, requires a level of vulnerability from officers that they may not be willing to divulge to an

> "outsider," which only further emphasizes the importance of building trust with this population. Developing trust with police officers may invoke: going on ride alongs, spending time together on scenes, adapting to their sense of humor and language, experiencing adversity together, and being authentic in order to build genuine rapport. Police officers are taught to not trust in the "short-term encounter" on the job as this dynamic will help them survive in an uncontrolled environment within the community. Sound mental health for an individual is predicated on trust that is also commensurate with effective mental health treatment to manage an array of mental health challenges that police officers may face throughout a 25- to 30-year career (i.e., depression, anxiety, marital distress, work stress). So, initiating EMDR too fast, too soon could potentially lead to a one visit and quick treatment termination initiated by the police officer, thus feeding the narrative of mistrust. When introducing EMDR, it may be helpful to take extra time with the police officer to provide psychoeducation surrounding how EMDR can help, and explain more in depth over time each step of each EMDR phase to help the police officer to cultivate insight for the target behavior/theme to address. In addition, utilizing relevant law enforcement analogies and metaphors from past and/or current experiences can cultivate such insight with police officers that will not only facilitate trust, but lead to building behavioral momentum for continued treatment where police officers know that the clinician does not just know the "words, but the music" of the profession.

With few formal post-graduate educational programs specializing in the psychology or mental health treatment of law enforcement or other first responders, clinicians often seek continuing education or certifications in working with law enforcement. Professional organizations, such as the International Association of Chiefs of Police (IACP) Psychological Services Section, the Society for Police and Criminal Psychology (SPCP), and the American Psychological Association (APA), Division 18- Psychologists in Public Service offer such continuing education. Psychologists can also seek board certification in Police and Public Safety Psychology through the American Board of Professional Psychology (ABPP). While certifications and memberships are not inclusive of all mental health providers competent in treating law enforcement officers, they can assist officers who are searching for a clinician with cultural competence. Cultural competence is important on many levels. For police officers to trust a clinician during the therapeutic process, informed consent of what is confidential and what is not confidential (from the inception of contact and from a state reporting mandate process) is key. Some examples of cultural competence in police psychology can be a clinician's comfort level regarding an officer attending session in full uniform with his/her firearm, having patience for officers testing the environment as it relates to trust (i.e., late arrivals, flexibility and stress tolerance and reactions of the clinician to name a few), responsiveness to critical incidents, and follow-up contact, dependability, utilization of a non-judgmental approach, use of humor, and having a quick response time, to name a few.

A significant cultural competence variable is understanding the administrative nature of decision-making within a police department/agency. One example would be understanding the chain of command and some of the unique differences between civilian personnel and sworn personnel. Another is a civilian being supervised by a sworn supervisor who may not have the same educational background as the supervisee, but may have experience supervising personnel. Having an understanding of changing shifts and the challenges that go along with such shifts for family, stress levels, health, and sleep are also significant. Other examples would be "shift pick(s)," an understanding of the "in basket" assessment process for promotions, an appreciation and understanding for navigating the political arena between local government and the police department/agency, understanding specialized divisions and mobility within the unit/division, hardships, the use of discipline, and having an overall understanding and appreciation for the command staff structure, both functions and capabilities. Some of the additional challenges a civilian clinician may be faced with include navigating potential barriers upon hire with police department/agency and maintaining a goal-oriented approach when encountering resistance to change as an "outsider" due to the territorial nature of some personnel who may display rigidity and suspiciousness early on.

Resilience

Balmer et al. (2014) found resilience was negatively affected by increased rank, age, and years of service in a sample of 285 police officers from Western Australia. Specifically, they reported resilience levels were significantly higher in officers with up to 10 years of service compared to officers with 11–20 years of service and 21 years or more. The decline of officers' resiliency with greater years of service is consistent with previous research findings regarding the impact of coping styles on resilience levels. Studies have found that cumulative exposure to stressful and traumatic incidents may influence an officer's coping abilities, often leading to more maladaptive strategies (e.g., alcohol use, avoidance, isolation) (Ménard & Arter, 2013; Pasillas et al., 2006). However, police officers with less reliance on distancing and avoidant coping strategies during times of stress or adversity are likely to be more resilient (Balmer et al., 2014).

Posttraumatic Growth (PTG), a term coined by Calhoun and Tedeschi (1999, 2014), is the theory that positive psychological change can result from experiencing trauma or other significant life challenges. This growth occurs as the result of making sense or finding purpose from a traumatic experience. Following trauma, individuals' comfort zones are shattered, and they are left to rebuild and refocus their world and themselves. For some, this means greater appreciation of life, what they have, and strengthening relationships. Some officers, following a trauma and a long healing process, decide to become ad hoc spokespeople for mental health and trauma in law enforcement. Clinicians can further facilitate healing by incorporating the theory of PTG into treatment.

Research has shown an array of personal and collective benefits for maintaining a culture of resilience, which can lead to a healthy police organization and employee retention (Hill & Giles, 2019). Significant outcomes include a sense of organizational pride, a feeling of inclusiveness, an increase in psychological and relational health and organizational satisfaction, improved self-esteem, an enhanced ability to achieve goals, and an elevated sense of personal control having overcome negative, and, sometimes, volatile emotions (e.g., consider an officer's emotional state during the use of force) (Buzzanell & Houston, 2018).

EMDR can help facilitate resilience by lessening the emotional intensity of the stressor(s) or traumatic event(s) that have potentially impacted the individual from an approach avoidance/freeze perspective. EMDR allows the new, adaptive information to become the primary approach, as opposed to the past trauma response that can lead to dysfunction and avoidance behaviors.

Conclusion

Law enforcement officers are at great risk for exposure to significantly stressful, dangerous, and traumatic situations throughout their careers. Consequently, the possibility of developing symptoms of PTSD and co-occurring mental health disorders also increases (Wagner et al., 2020). In recognizing this, many law enforcement agencies have provided, and encouraged the use of, necessary mental health resources for their officers. With more licensed mental health providers approaching and familiarizing themselves with the law enforcement culture, there is a new opportunity to promote effective trauma treatment tailored to this population. EMDR can be a significant positive therapeutic modality of mental health treatment for law enforcement that can impact the profession through normalization of seeking mental health treatment without ridicule, punitive measures, stigma, demotion, or loss of one's job. EMDR has been an established evidence-based therapeutic approach in trauma treatment for over 30 years (de Jongh et al., 2019). Utilizing an eight-step approach, this treatment modality intends to assist trauma survivors in accessing and successfully processing traumatic memories. EMDR has helped a number of individuals with extreme stress-based reactions, such as PTSD, acute stress disorder, and adjustment disorder, including police officers (Lansing et al., 2005; Solomon et al., 2009; Wilson et al., 2001). If implemented with standardized practices (inclusive of factoring in law enforcement culture competence), EMDR can have a significant positive impact in assisting police officers and others in the public safety profession. EMDR has the potential to manage trauma-based symptoms police officers can experience over time, not only related to their exposure to critical incidents on the job but also traumatic events that they experienced prior to joining this profession.

It is important to note that in order for this therapeutic approach to be effectively implemented in a law enforcement population, mental health providers must become certified in the EMDR modality. Mental health providers must also integrate, familiarize, and possess cultural competence with the law enforcement culture, language, rank system, etc. prior to implementing EMDR with the police and public safety population.

First responders, in general, would benefit from further investigations of the effectiveness of EMDR in addressing trauma symptoms related to the current challenges including the COVID-19 pandemic, unwavering public scrutiny, and challenges with various forms of violence across the USA. Public safety professionals can greatly benefit from normalization and having the availability of efficacious evidence-based, consistent mental health treatments to address the mental and physical health challenges of their profession. This is a significant, and attainable goal to strive for, not only for the here and now but for the future of the profession.

References

Acarturk, C., Konuk, E., Cetinkaya, M., Senay, I., Sijbrandij, M., Gulen, B., & Cuijpers, P. (2016). The efficacy of eye movement desensitization and reprocessing for post-traumatic stress disorder and depression among Syrian refugees: Results of a randomized controlled trial. *Psychological Medicine, 46*(12), 2583–2593.

Andrade, J., Kavanagh, D., & Baddeley, A. (1997). Eye-movements and visual imagery: A working memory approach to the treatment of post-traumatic stress disorder. *British Journal of Clinical Psychology, 36*(2), 209–223.

Arble, E., Daugherty, A. M., & Arnetz, B. B. (2018). Models of first responder coping: Police officers as a unique population. *Stress and Health, 34*(5), 612–621.

Baddeley, A. (2000). The episodic buffer: A new component of working memory? *Trends in Cognitive Sciences, 4*(11), 417–423.

Ballenger, J. F., Best, S. R., Metzler, T. J., Wasserman, D. A., Mohr, D. C., Liberman, A., Delucchi, K., Weiss, D. S., Fagan, J. A., Waldrop, A. E., & Marmar, C. R. (2011). Patterns and predictors of alcohol use in male and female urban police officers. *The American Journal on Addictions, 20*(1), 21–29.

Balmer, G. M., Pooley, J. A., & Cohen, L. (2014). Psychological resilience of Western Australian police officers: Relationship between resilience, coping style, psychological functioning and demographics. *Police Practice and Research, 15*(4), 270–282.

Becker, C. B., Meyer, G., Price, J. S., Graham, M. M., Arsena, A., Armstrong, D. A., & Ramon, E. (2009). Law enforcement preferences for PTSD treatment and crisis management alternatives. *Behaviour Research and Therapy, 47*(3), 245–253.

Berg, A. M., Hem, E., Lau, B., & Ekeberg, Ø. (2006). An exploration of job stress and health in the Norwegian police service: A cross sectional study. *Journal of Occupational Medicine and Toxicology, 1*(1), 1–9.

Buzzanell, P. M., & Houston, J. B. (2018). Communication and resilience: Multilevel applications and insights – A journal of applied communication research forum. *Journal of Applied Communication Research, 46*(1), 1–4.

Calhoun, L. G., & Tedeschi, R. G. (1999). *Facilitating posttraumatic growth: A clinician's guide*. Routledge.

Calhoun, L. G., & Tedeschi, R. G. (2014). The foundations of posttraumatic growth: An expanded framework. In *Handbook of posttraumatic growth* (pp. 3–23). Routledge.

Clark-Miller, J., & Brady, H. C. (2013). Critical stress: Police officer religiosity and coping with critical stress incidents. *Journal of Police and Criminal Psychology, 28*(1), 26–34.

de Jongh, A., Amann, B. L., Hofmann, A., Farrell, D., & Lee, C. W. (2019). The status of EMDR therapy in the treatment of posttraumatic stress disorder 30 years after its introduction. *Journal of EMDR Practice and Research, 13*(4), 261–269.

Desmarais, P., Weidman, D., Wassef, A., Bruneau, M. A., Friedland, J., Bajsarowicz, P., Thibodeau, M. P., Hermann, N., & Nguyen, Q. D. (2020). The interplay between post-traumatic stress disorder and dementia: A systematic review. *The American Journal of Geriatric Psychiatry, 28*(1), 48–60.

EMDR Institute, Inc. (2020). *What is EMDR?* https://www.emdr.com/what-is-emdr/

Gershon, R. R., Barocas, B., Canton, A. N., Li, X., & Vlahov, D. (2009). Mental, physical, and behavioral outcomes associated with perceived work stress in police officers. *Criminal Justice and Behavior, 36*(3), 275–289.

Günak, M. M., Billings, J., Carratu, E., Marchant, N. L., Favarato, G., & Orgeta, V. (2020). Post-traumatic stress disorder as a risk factor for dementia: Systematic review and meta-analysis. *The British Journal of Psychiatry, 217*(5), 600–608.

Habersaat, S. A., Geiger, A. M., Abdellaoui, S., & Wolf, J. M. (2015). Health in police officers: Role of risk factor clusters and police divisions. *Social Science & Medicine, 143*, 213–222.

Hartman, M., O'Neill, D. A., O'Neill, J., & Lewinski, W. (2017). Law enforcement memory of stressful events: Recall accuracy as a function of detail type. *Law Enforcement Executive Forum, 17*(3), 21–41.

Hartley, T. A., Burchfiel, C. M., Fekedulegn, D., Andrew, M. E., & Violanti, J. M. (2011). Health disparities in police officers: Comparisons to the US general population. *International Journal of Emergency Mental Health, 13*(4), 211.

Hill, M. D. (2020). Adaptive information processing theory: Origins, principles, applications, and evidence. *Journal of Evidence-Based Social Work, 17*(3), 317–331.

Hill, S., & Giles, H. (2019, May 29). Resilience as a department cultural initiative. *Police Chief.* https://www.policechiefmagazine.org/resilience-as-a-department-cultural-initiative

Högberg, G., Pagani, M., Sundin, Ö., Soares, J., Åberg-Wistedt, A., Tärnell, B., & Hällström, T. (2007). On treatment with eye movement desensitization and reprocessing of chronic post-traumatic stress disorder in public transportation workers – A randomized controlled trial. *Nordic Journal of Psychiatry, 61*(1), 54–61.

Huddleston, L., Stephens, C., & Paton, D. (2007). An evaluation of traumatic and organizational experiences on the psychological health of New Zealand police recruits. *Work, 28*(3), 199–207.

Jaberghaderi, N., Greenwald, R., Rubin, A., Zand, S. O., & Dolatabadi, S. (2004). A comparison of CBT and EMDR for sexually-abused Iranian girls. *Clinical Psychology & Psychotherapy, 11*(5), 358–368.

IACP Police Psychological Services Section. (2018). *Officer-involved shooting guidelines.* https://www.theiacp.org/sites/default/files/2019-05/Officer%20Involved%20Shooting%20Guidelines%202018.pdf

Ironson, G., Freund, B., Strauss, J. L., & Williams, J. (2002). Comparison of two treatments for traumatic stress: A community-based study of EMDR and prolonged exposure. *Journal of Clinical Psychology, 58*(1), 113–128.

Kavanagh, D. J., Freese, S., Andrade, J., & May, J. (2001). Effects of visuospatial tasks on desensitization to emotive memories. *British Journal of Clinical Psychology, 40*(3), 267–280.

Kilpatrick, D. G., Resnick, H. S., Milanak, M. E., Miller, M. W., Keyes, K. M., & Friedman, M. J. (2013). National estimates of exposure to traumatic events and PTSD prevalence using *DSM-IV* and *DSM-5* criteria. *Journal of Traumatic Stress, 26*(5), 537–547.

Lansing, K., Amen, D. G., Hanks, C., & Rudy, L. (2005). High–resolution brain SPECT imaging and eye movement desensitization and reprocessing in police officers with PTSD. *The Journal of Neuropsychiatry and Clinical Neurosciences, 17*(4), 526–532.

Lee, C., Gavriel, H., Drummond, P., Richards, J., & Greenwald, R. (2002). Treatment of PTSD: Stress inoculation training with prolonged exposure compared to EMDR. *Journal of Clinical Psychology, 58*(9), 1071–1089.

Maxfield, L. (2007). Current status and future directions for EMDR research. *Journal of EMDR Practice and Research, 1*(1), 6–14.

Ménard, K. S., & Arter, M. L. (2013). Police officer alcohol use and trauma symptoms: Associations with critical incidents, coping, and social stressors. *International Journal of Stress Management, 20*(1), 37.

Okiishi, J., Lambert, M. J., Nielsen, S. L., & Ogles, B. M. (2003). Waiting for supershrink: An empirical analysis of therapist effects. *Clinical Psychology & Psychotherapy: An International Journal of Theory & Practice, 10*(6), 361–373.

Pasillas, R. M., Follette, V. M., & Perumean-Chaney, S. E. (2006). Occupational stress and psychological functioning in law enforcement officers. *Journal of Police and Criminal Psychology, 21*(1), 41–53.

Patterson, G. T. (1999). Coping effectiveness and occupational stress in police officers. In J. M. Violanti & D. Paton (Eds.), *Police trauma: Psychological aftermath of civilian combat* (pp. 214–226). Charles C Thomas Publisher.

Power, K., McGoldrick, T., Brown, K., Buchanan, R., Sharp, D., Swanson, V., & Karatzias, A. (2002). A controlled comparison of eye movement desensitization and reprocessing versus exposure plus cognitive restructuring versus waiting list in the treatment of post-traumatic stress disorder. *Clinical Psychology & Psychotherapy, 9*(5), 299–318.

Rothbaum, B. O., Astin, M. C., & Marsteller, F. (2005). Prolonged exposure versus eye movement desensitization and reprocessing (EMDR) for PTSD rape victims. *Journal of Traumatic Stress: Official Publication of The International Society for Traumatic Stress Studies, 18*(6), 607–616.

Shapiro, F. (1989). Eye movement desensitization: A new treatment for post-traumatic stress disorder. *Journal of Behavior Therapy and Experimental Psychiatry, 20*(3), 211–217.

Shapiro, F. (2014). The role of eye movement desensitization and reprocessing (EMDR) therapy in medicine: Addressing the psychological and physical symptoms stemming from adverse life experiences. *The Permanente Journal, 18*(1), 71.

Shapiro, M. A. (1991). Memory and decision processes in the construction of social reality. *Communication Research, 18*(1), 3–24.

Sheehan, D. C., & Van Hasselt, V. B. (2003). Identifying law enforcement stress reactions, early. *FBI Law Enforcement Bulletin, 72*, 12–17.

Solomon, E. P., Solomon, R. M., & Heide, K. M. (2009). EMDR: An evidence-based treatment for victims of trauma. *Victims and Offenders, 4*(4), 391–397.

Söndergaard, H. P., & Elofsson, U. (2008). Psychophysiological studies of EMDR. *Journal of EMDR Practice and Research, 2*(4), 282–288.

Soomro, S., & Yanos, P. T. (2019). Predictors of mental health stigma among police officers: The role of trauma and PTSD. *Journal of Police and Criminal Psychology, 34*(2), 175–183.

Stickgold, R. (2002). EMDR: A putative neurobiological mechanism of action. *Journal of Clinical Psychology, 58*(1), 61–75.

Taylor, S., Thordarson, D. S., Maxfield, L., Fedoroff, I. C., Lovell, K., & Ogrodniczuk, J. (2003). Comparative efficacy, speed, and adverse effects of three PTSD treatments: Exposure therapy, EMDR, and relaxation training. *Journal of Consulting and Clinical Psychology, 71*(2), 330.

van den Berg, D. P., de Bont, P. A., van der Vleugel, B. M., de Roos, C., de Jongh, A., Van Minnen, A., & van der Gaag, M. (2015). Prolonged exposure vs eye movement desensitization and reprocessing vs waiting list for posttraumatic stress disorder in patients with a psychotic disorder: A randomized clinical trial. *JAMA Psychiatry, 72*(3), 259–267.

Van der Kolk, B. A., Spinazzola, J., Blaustein, M. E., Hopper, J. W., Hopper, E. K., Korn, D. L., & Simpson, W. B. (2007). A randomized clinical trial of eye movement desensitization and reprocessing (EMDR), fluoxetine, and pill placebo in the treatment of posttraumatic stress disorder: Treatment effects and long-term maintenance. *Journal of Clinical Psychiatry, 68*(1), 37.

Vaughan, K., Armstrong, M. S., Gold, R., O'Connor, N., Jenneke, W., & Tarrier, N. (1994). A trial of eye movement desensitization compared to image habituation training and applied muscle relaxation in post-traumatic stress disorder. *Journal of Behavior Therapy and Experimental Psychiatry, 25*(4), 283–291.

Vieira, S. S. A., Di Giorgio, M., Cohen, E., Caurand, M., Manchon, A., Quaderi, A., & Palazzolo, J. (2017). Benefits of EMDR therapy on the memory in the treatment of PTSD. *European Psychiatry, 41*(S1), S359–S359.

Violanti, J. M. (2004). Predictors of police suicide ideation. *Suicide and Life-threatening Behavior, 34*(3), 277–283.

Violanti, J. M., Andrew, M. E., Burchfiel, C. M., Dorn, J., Hartley, T., & Miller, D. B. (2006). Posttraumatic stress symptoms and subclinical cardiovascular disease in police officers. *International Journal of Stress Management, 13*(4), 541–554.

Violanti, J. M., Hartley, T. A., Gu, J. K., Fekedulegn, D., Andrew, M. E., & Burchfiel, C. M. (2013). Life expectancy in police officers: A comparison with the US general population. *International Journal of Emergency Mental Health, 15*(4), 217.

Violanti, J. M., Fekedulegn, D., Andrew, M. E., Hartley, T. A., Charles, L. E., Miller, D. B., & Burchfiel, C. M. (2017). The impact of perceived intensity and frequency of police work occupational stressors on the cortisol awakening response (CAR): Findings from the BCOPS study. *Psychoneuroendocrinology, 75*, 124–131.

Wagner, S. L., White, N., Fyfe, T., Matthews, L. R., Randall, C., Regehr, C., White, M., Alden, L. E., Buys, N., Carey, M. G., Corneil, W., Fraess-Phillips, A., Krutop, E., & Fleischmann, M. H. (2020). Systematic review of posttraumatic stress disorder in police officers following routine work-related critical incident exposure. *American Journal of Industrial Medicine, 63*(7), 600–615.

Wester, S. R., & Lyubelsky, J. (2005). Supporting the thin blue line: Gender sensitive therapy with male police officers. *Professional Psychology: Research and Practice, 36*(1), 51.

Wilson, S. A., Tinker, R. H., Becker, L. A., & Logan, C. R. (2001). Stress management with law enforcement personnel: A controlled outcome study of EMDR versus a traditional stress management program. *International Journal of Stress Management, 8*(3), 179–200.

Exposure Treatments and First Responders: An Embedded Behavioral Health Perspective

Keith Cox, Rick Baker, Crystal Joudry, and Ron Acierno

Clinical Vignette: PTSD Treatment with a Sheriff's Deputy[1]

"Max" was a field investigator in a sheriff's office and a former Marine with deployments in Iraq. I was an embedded behavioral health clinician in the sheriff's office where Max worked. In the first month of my embedded role at his agency, officers asked me to encourage Max to try treatment, as they felt he had a clear case of Posttraumatic Stress Disorder (PTSD). I visited his office area to introduce myself to his division and explain the embedded program. Max and his colleagues were sitting in their cubicles. He appeared overweight and spoke with a stutter. He quickly disclosed to me (in front of his colleagues) that he had been in Iraq, and the local Veterans Affairs (VA) hospital had diagnosed him with PTSD. I invited him to treatment as Max's colleagues suggested he take advantage of this "employee benefit."

[1] This vignette is written by the second author of this chapter and happens in the context of an embedded behavioral health program in a law enforcement agency. The nature of the embedded program is explained later. Client names have been changed in the three clinical vignettes for the sake of confidentiality.

K. Cox (✉)
University of North Carolina—Asheville, Asheville, NC, USA

Responder Support Services, Asheville, NC, USA
e-mail: kcox2@unca.edu

R. Baker · C. Joudry
Responder Support Services, Asheville, NC, USA

R. Acierno
University of Texas Health Science Center, Houston, TX, USA

Faillace Department of Psychiatry and Ralph H. Johnson VA Medical Center, Charleston, SC, USA

M. L. Bourke et al. (eds.), *First Responder Mental Health*,
https://doi.org/10.1007/978-3-031-38149-2_13

He declined saying, "My family is already afraid of me because I act out my nightmares. I'm not going into therapy and make things worse for them."

Over the next 3 years, I made regular visits to Max with invitations to treatment. His response was always "no." Then late one night I received a phone call from the chief deputy of the sheriff's office. Max, while on duty and in uniform with his gun, had driven himself to the local VA hospital and asked to be admitted for psychiatric reasons. The VA notified the sheriff's office, and the sheriff and chief deputy both went to the VA hospital. Ultimately, Max was not admitted, and the sheriff put Max on paid administrative leave and gave him two choices: (a) engage in treatment and return to his current role at the completion of treatment, or (b) resign from the agency. Max agreed to begin treatment. A diagnostic interview confirmed the PTSD diagnosis, including pronounced avoidance behaviors, significant re-experiencing symptoms, and constant emotional distress.

Max and I discussed a few treatment options including Cognitive Processing Therapy, the Acceptance and Commitment Therapy (ACT) Trauma Protocol, and Prolonged Exposure Therapy (PE). He was interested in PE due to the likelihood that treatment duration could be brief and action-oriented. (In my experience, first responders overwhelmingly choose PE over other treatment options.) Having come to know Max, and understanding the culture of law enforcement, I suspected that obtaining Max's full buy-in and consistent engagement with PE in-session activities and homework would be a challenge. My intuition told me a direct approach could be helpful. (I would not recommend this approach for every law enforcement officer struggling with PTSD, and I do not use it regularly.) As I gave a more in-depth description of PE, I could tell by his facial expression he was apprehensive. I leaned forward and looked directly at him, and said, "I'm happy to finally be working with you. You mentioned your desire to get back to work, and I think PE may help you get there. You're not going to like parts of the treatment and you're probably not going to like the homework I'm going to be assigning, at all. To have the best chance to get back to work, you're going to need to do what I ask you to do, even if it makes you anxious…in fact, that's the point. And you'll need to stay in treatment, even when it gets tough and dropping out seems like your best option. If you can't do that, you'll be wasting your time and mine. Don't know about you, I don't want my time wasted. Do you think you can do this, even when you really don't want to?" He quickly replied with "Yes."

Max showed up on time at my office for the first treatment session. He appeared nervous. We proceeded through the PE session 1 protocol, and when completing the trauma interview, he indicated his index (or focal) trauma was an incident he had experienced many years prior while deployed in Iraq. Max had followed direct orders from his superiors, and a civilian died as a result (experience indicates that these type of guilt/bereavement events are often perceived as more traumatic than personal threat events). Per the protocol, we practiced the breathing retraining exercise and afterward, he remarked that it helped him relax a little bit.

The treatment sessions proceeded better than I anticipated. Max attended twice a week for the first few sessions, and, as he was on mandatory leave, he used much of his daily time to do the imaginal and in vivo exposure assignments. With in vivo exposures, clients face situations from daily life they have been avoiding due to the fact that the situations remind them of the traumatic event. We typically take a reminder stimulus, like visiting a crowded department store, and break it down into "doable" parts, starting slowly, such as going to the parking lot of the crowded department store for the first few exposure homework trials. Max and I completed an in vivo hierarchy, a list of avoided situations ranked from least to most distressing. Max's hierarchy ranged from items eliciting lower levels of distress (e.g., attending family functions) to items eliciting high levels of distress (e.g., responding to calls with trauma cues). With imaginal exposures, or imaginals, clients go through the memory of their most intrusive trauma with their eyes closed, experiencing the memory in all five senses and narrating it to the therapist like they are describing the traumatic event to someone on a cell phone as it is happening.

Max's first imaginal exposure, in PE session 3, was difficult for him. By the protocol, his first retelling was self-directed and only contained as much detail as he was comfortable including. Approximately halfway through the first imaginal retelling, Max said, "I feel like I'm going to throw-up." I praised him for "attacking" this first imaginal retelling and assured him he was doing a great job. I let him know if he needed to throw-up, he could use the trash can next to him, and this meant he was on the right track. He never threw-up (but some patients do). In "processing" the imaginal exposure, which is an unstructured discussion of the imaginal experience, he said that since he had spent so many years not telling that story, he could not believe he had retold it repeatedly. Even though he felt physically sick, he admitted nothing bad happened to him outside of feeling uncomfortable. The first imaginal felt like a win to him.

His second imaginal exposure in the next session was also tough. I guided the imaginal by slowing it down and probing for the content he had avoided in the previous session. My approach was if there was a "blank spot" in the movie my mind was creating from his retelling, I asked him to include it. I also had him include the thoughts going through his mind, his emotional reactions, body sensations, and smells and sounds experienced during the traumatic event. I encouraged him to include the most horrific details of the experience, later realizing his most potent self-judgments stemmed from these aspects of the event. In processing this imaginal exposure, Max saw he did not feel like throwing-up even though this imaginal had much more detail than the first. He saw this as progress, which helped secure his buy-in for the rest of the treatment.

The remaining in-session imaginal exposures focused on his "hot spots," the parts of the trauma event to which he had the strongest reactions. He was highly engaged in treatment and did not hesitate to include additional, horrific details when prompted. He also started to approach his PE homework, listening to recordings of in-session imaginal and doing his in vivo exposures, spending considerable daily time on them.

PTSD symptom data were collected at each session using the Posttraumatic Stress Disorder Checklist for DSM-5 (PCL-5), a standardized PTSD symptom self-report scale. Max's PCL-5 scores declined steadily through treatment, starting in the PTSD diagnostic range with a score of 51 and ending at 2 – basically no symptoms.

His scores declined gradually each week, save 2 weeks where his scores did not change. Max completed PE in 10 sessions and has not needed follow-up sessions for PTSD.

Max was then referred by his command for a Fit for Duty Evaluation, which he passed. Max returned to his role as a field investigator and was excited to work. His stutter was so improved that 911 dispatchers did not recognize his voice on the radio and inquired as to who was using Max's call number. I had noticed the stutter improve during sessions with me and thought he was just becoming more comfortable with me. Max's stuttering had always increased with being "stressed," a less frequent state after treatment.

Max called several months later to check in and said he was doing well. He had been promoted to K9 Handler, a role he had always wanted. He reported he felt compelled to speak openly about his treatment experience and guide fellow deputies to treatment, something we have seen with other first responder clients. Max also reported that he lost 60 pounds and was sleeping through the night without nightmares. The weight loss was concurrent with Max seeking medical care for his diabetes during treatment and maintaining healthy behaviors after PE.

Max's transformation was so dramatic that his agency (with his consent) invited the local television news station to do a feature story on him and his treatment experience. During the interview with the reporter, Max said that my discussion about not wasting time "got under [his] skin" and motivated him to prove me wrong. He said the approach was exactly what he needed. To my relief, the news station did not include this detail in the broadcast story. Now 3 years after treatment, Max continues to do well. He is looking forward to retirement from law enforcement. He reports that what stands out to him the most now is that he enjoys the Christmas holiday season. After his traumatic event, which happened close to Christmas, his mood became much more dysregulated in December, and he "hated the holidays."

Being an embedded clinician in Max's agency was an advantage for treatment. Max said that having his therapist embedded made it easier for him to participate in treatment. He stated he did not have to wait "forever" for treatment as would be the case with his VA. He also related that, because I was embedded in his agency, "You had a grasp of who and what we [sheriff's deputies] are and what we do. You didn't make assumptions based on what you saw on TV."

Exposure and Common First Responder Mental Health Issues

While Max's case might be exceptional, a robust evidence base shows that PE and other exposure approaches are highly effective in treating a wide range of disorders. We put forth that exposure is one of the most powerful tools in the psychotherapist's toolbox and can be impactful in treatment with first responders.

First responders experience potentially traumatic events and stressors as a regular part of work. This heavy trauma and stressor load increases the risk for mental health problems, the most common of which are trauma and stressor-related disorders, such as PTSD, depression, anxiety disorders, suicidality, sleep problems, and substance use disorders (Jones, 2017; Kleim & Westphal, 2011; Syed et al., 2020). Exposure-based psychotherapy treatments have a strong evidence base for treating many of these clinical issues among the general population and military-related samples. Limited high-quality research exists on psychological interventions with first responders (Alden et al., 2021), including exposure-based treatments. Still, given the preponderance of evidence for the efficacy and effectiveness of exposure-based treatments with nonfirst responder samples, including veterans and active duty military personnel, we believe exposure therapies should be a first-line treatment in many instances when working with first responders. We also see a significant need for quality treatment research with first responders, as they are a distinct clinical population.

We use the term "exposure" to designate a wide range of clinical interventions, taking a "big tent" approach in conceptualizing it. The central component of exposure is using approach over avoidance to address dysfunctional and distressing responses to external and internal stimuli. That is, confronting feared objects and situations instead of avoiding them. Exposures are oftentimes graded (starting with less anxiety-provoking triggers), well-planned, repeated daily or multiple times per day, and discussed afterwards. The kind of action or the type of approach an exposure entails depends on the stimuli to be addressed. In vivo exposures target external stimuli from daily life. Imaginal exposures target autobiographical memories or feared future scenarios. Exposures can also target internal sensations such as physical aspects of panic attacks or the urge to use a substance (as in the third clinical vignette below). Exposures can also target internal experiences such as depressive cognitions or avoided emotions (e.g., shame). Thus, exposure is highly flexible. Subjective units of distress (SUDs) are commonly used in planning, completing, and discussing exposures. SUDs are an agreed upon 0–10 or 0–100 scale of subjective distress, where 0 is no anxiety and 100 is overwhelming, full-blown panic. SUDs provide the therapist and client with a quantitative and efficient way for the client to communicate their level of internal distress before, during, and after exposure. Grading exposures, moving from lower to higher distressing stimuli, is facilitated by using SUDs, but not all exposure approaches are graded or use SUDs.

Exposures are most commonly part of behavioral or cognitive behavioral treatments (CBT), although they can appear in treatments not typically classified in those ways. For example, we consider Eye Movement Desensitization and Reprocessing (EMDR), a PTSD treatment, to include a form of imaginal exposure, even though EMDR is not typically discussed with that frame. Moreover, there are different theoretical accounts of exposure, for example, exposure in ACT versus standard CBT or Emotional Processing Theory versus Inhibitory Learning Models. These theoretical debates point to the rich ways to understand and describe how exposure works.

Evidence for Exposure-Based Treatments for Common First Responder Diagnoses

PTSD The Departments of Veterans Affairs and Defense PTSD treatment guidelines (Card, 2017) designate PE as a first-line treatment for PTSD among military-related samples, including those with complex presentations and comorbidities. These guidelines also note that there is sufficient evidence to recommend other exposure-based treatments, i.e., Written Exposure Therapy (WET) and Narrative Exposure Therapy (NET). PE is also a first-line treatment in general population treatment guidelines (e.g., Forbes et al., 2020). These treatment guidelines are based on expert reviews, meta-analyses, and represent the summative knowledge derived from over 350 clinical trials. EMDR is designated as a first-line treatment in these treatment guidelines, which we take to indicate the effectiveness of another exposure-based treatment. In addition, PE is one of the few empirically supported treatments for any disorder that performed consistently well in a meta-scientific review (Sakaluk et al., 2019) investigating replication biases in psychotherapy trials, an issue arising with the recent replication crisis across sciences. EMDR performed less consistently in this meta-scientific review.

Depression Recent innovations in CBT suggest exposure can be part of an effective treatment package for depression. Two CBT treatments for depression include emotion exposures, with each showing promise in a single randomized clinical trial (RCT) (Grosse Holtforth et al., 2019; Sauer-Zavala et al., 2020). Depression is a common comorbidity with PTSD, and effective PTSD treatment often co-occurs with depression reductions (Acierno et al., 2021).

Anxiety Disorders Based on a large database, multiple international guidelines for the treatment of anxiety disorders foreground CBT with exposure components (e.g., Bandelow et al., 2015; National Institute for Health and Clinical Excellence, 2011). For example, the Royal Australian and New Zealand College of Psychiatrists clinical practice guidelines for Panic Disorder indicate that CBT with exposure elements, among other treatments, has the highest level of evidence of success (Andrews et al., 2018). Panic Disorder is a common sequala of trauma exposure and comorbidity with PTSD, as illustrated in the next clinical vignette.

Substance Use Disorders Exposure can also have a role in the treatment of substance use disorders (SUDs). While one meta-analysis found little support for the use of a specific form of exposure therapy (i.e., cue exposure therapy) in treating alcohol use disorder (Mellentin et al., 2017), another meta-analysis (Lee et al., 2015) and literature review (Osaji et al., 2020) supported using ACT in the treatment of SUDs. ACT for SUDs emphasizes, among other things, acceptance, rather than avoidance of urges to use (Hayes, 2019) and uses exposure techniques as one way to develop acceptance, as illustrated in the third clinical vignette. PTSD is a regular comorbidity with SUDs, as substance use can be a maladaptive method of coping with PTSD symptoms. In a meta-analysis of 28 RCTs for co-occurring

PTSD and SUDs (Simpson et al., 2021), several RCTs combined exposure treatments for PTSD and SUDs treatment elements. These treatments reduced both PTSD and SUDs symptoms, as did other types of treatments, e.g., SUDs-focused treatments. One recently developed treatment combines PE with SUDs treatment elements and has shown superior outcomes to a SUDs treatment on PTSD symptoms and on a substance use outcomes at follow-up but not during treatment (Back et al., 2019).

First Responders The RCTs discussed thus far have not typically had first responder samples, a clear concern given the unique stressor load experienced by first responders. A 2012 review of PTSD treatments among first responders identified two "bona fide" RCTs and described the literature as "startlingly sparse and…not sufficient for evidence-based recommendations for first responders" (Haugen et al., 2012, p. 370). Alden and colleagues (2021) reviewed psychological interventions with first responders with a focus on posttraumatic stress but also reviewed interventions for acute stress disorder, depression, and anxiety. They judged there to be ***one*** high-quality RCT across all disorders, a trial of exposure-based CBT for PTSD (Bryant et al., 2019), which found the treatment efficacious in reducing PTSD and depression with emergency personnel. Alden and colleagues judged that the results for treating anxiety disorders with first responders were too inconsistent to draw conclusions. Our review, using Clinicaltrials.gov and other search engines, did not find more recent RCTs with first responder samples, for any disorder, or any RCTs at any time for SUDs. There is also a lack of research on exposure-based treatments in the context of embedded behavioral health, the treatment context in the clinical vignettes in this chapter.

Embedded Behavioral Health

Embedded behavioral health (EBH),[2] locating mental health providers on-site and as part of an agency team, is an important aspect of Max's exposure treatment in the first vignette. EBH was developed over a decade ago in the U.S. Armed Forces to increase access and reduce the stigma around mental health services (Vergun, 2018). EBH is now widely used in the Army and, to a lesser extent, in other U.S. military branches, even as the form of EBH varies by context. Initial evidence from Army samples suggests EBH has a positive impact on fitness for duty and mental health outcomes (Russell et al., 2014; Srinivasan, 2017).

Mental health stigma is a major barrier to first responder treatment usage (Haugen et al., 2017). EBH with first responder agencies might mitigate this barrier, resulting in more first responders like Max obtaining treatment. Moreover, it is our experience that EBH is an excellent platform for the delivery of exposure-based therapies, as described in the vignettes in this chapter.

[2] The military uses the term behavioral health instead of mental health.

Responder Support Services (RSS) was founded in 2017, adapting the military EBH model for civilian first responders. RSS provides EBH to 15 first responder agencies in North and South Carolina. As described in the case of Max's exposure therapy, RSS clinicians have offices inside police stations, sheriff's offices, fire stations, emergency medical services bases, etc. Typical behavioral health services are provided on location at the agency. Clinicians also engage in other supportive services, most commonly "riding along" on first responder calls for service. Ride-alongs accomplish two objectives: (1) they allow clinicians to build rapport and connect to responders "in their office," and (2) they give clinicians a clearer perspective of what it is like to be a first responder. This serves as a bridge to responders seeking services as they know the embedded clinician understands their job and will not be shocked by what the responder will describe in treatment. A dilemma for the embedded clinician is possible exposure to the same potentially traumatic scenes as the responders.

RSS also provides services through a first responder-only outpatient behavioral health clinic. The outpatient clinic is available when treatment in the agency-based office is not appropriate such as when there is no agency-based office, as with detention/corrections or emergency room staff, or when seeing a first responder spouse. First responder-only clinics give first responders access to community-based behavioral health counseling in a space dedicated to them. First responders find this appealing, as they can be confident they will not share the waiting room with a community member they have transported or arrested.

The first responder-only outpatient clinic has unique physical features with first responders in mind. The chairs in the waiting room are extra wide to accommodate law enforcement clients who show up before or after duty in full gear, i.e., chairs are wide enough so a handgun and other equipment can be worn comfortably while sitting. Unlike other outpatient behavioral health clinics in our communities, weapons are accepted, so that clients are not required to leave their weapons in their vehicle. Other unique physical features of the clinics include artwork on the walls specific to various emergency services disciplines, and there is no signage on the building or roadside to increase confidentiality when entering and exiting the building.

Clinical Vignette: PTSD Treatment and Panic with a Paramedic[3]

"Sarah" was a community paramedic for a county department. She self-referred for treatment to a community-based first responder-only clinic. At intake, she reported she was on family and medical leave (FMLA) due to stress. She had recently gone to an urgent care clinic with complaints of high heart rate, dizziness, chest tightness, and had passed out at the clinic. The doctor explained this was a panic attack. She

[3] This vignette is written by the third author and was her first PE case.

said she did not plan to return to work because of a paramedic call about 6 months prior that involved the death of children, what she called "the peds call." She presented as abrupt and guarded during the intake interview and stated she would not engage in therapy if I did not understand her profession or was not educated about excited delirium (something I would not understand until later). She reported she had engaged in a debriefing following "the peds call" as well as individual therapy, which she said worsened her psychological state. After a lengthy conversation about her profession and assuring her I would be knowledgeable about excited delirium at the next session, she agreed to enter treatment. She met the criteria for PTSD, Panic Disorder, and Generalized Anxiety Disorder and indicated she most wanted relief from panic and anxiety. In addition, I noted that her responses on the PCL-5 were not consistent with her interview responses. She appeared to underreport her symptoms on the questionnaire, a seemingly common response style for first responders. Her PCL-5 score suggested a possible PTSD diagnosis, while her interview responses and behavior clearly supported this diagnosis, among others.

At that time, I was an embedded clinician with firefighters and law enforcement but knew less about paramedic work. Before the next session, I learned that excited delirium is a state of agitation, aggression, and distress, typically associated with drug use, which is most often seen in prehospital care settings. We spent the second session talking about excited delirium, her distaste for therapy, and her severe panic symptoms. She expressed prior to "the peds call" she was experiencing feelings of career burnout. She explained community paramedics commonly treated highly acute patients that were seen repeatedly, so-called "frequent flyers." She was overwhelmed by the work and was becoming emotionally numb and detached.

Further assessment identified specific anxiety-based avoidance patterns in her daily life, including avoiding going to the store and showering when no one was home. She no longer did outdoor recreational activities and feared being around the elderly, children, and crowds, as with each, she might be expected to perform paramedic duties in an emergency. She felt shame that she did not feel competent to perform medical procedures. Given these symptoms, I judged that PE could relieve Sarah's PTSD and thereby reduce her panic and anxiety. I saw her PTSD as the driver of much of her panic and anxiety. We discussed PE in the third session, and she reluctantly agreed to try it but was hesitant about doing homework. I challenged her on this point in a therapeutic manner, informing her the treatment would not be nearly as effective if she did not do homework. Sarah and I had built a small amount of rapport by now, and she was willing to try treatment with homework. Typically, it is preferable to start PE right after the assessment session, as it involves an active, behaviorally focused approach to therapy, and engaging in "talk therapy" first often makes the shift toward action-oriented treatment difficult. However, our initial sessions were necessary to convince Sarah to try such a behaviorally focused intervention.

Our fourth session together was protocol PE session 1, psychoeducation and the trauma interview. Sarah described her index (most intrusive or focal) trauma as "the peds call." She stated a male was driving erratically with his young children in the car, and, while rounding a curve, he lost control of the car and crashed into a tree.

Three children died in the accident. She reported she experienced tunnel vision at the scene, a first for her. After, she struggled to sleep and carried anger toward the father. The three children who died were the same age as Sarah's children, which was an important part of her distress. She fully engaged in all aspects of the session despite having feelings of panic and pacing the room throughout the session.

At the start of the next session, Sarah explained she was not being truthful about what incident was causing her the most distress. She had not felt comfortable or ready to share the event that was likely the primary cause of her symptoms. She stated that after "the peds call" and this other call (the actual index trauma), she lost trust in anyone outside her family and began feeling paranoid. She paced my office as she shared the second narrative, the trauma that she saw as causing her breakdown and desire to not return to work. She described a medical call with a male patient experiencing excited delirium. He was erratic and aggressive and fought law enforcement. She needed to administer a shot as the patient was at risk of heart failure. She had to give the shot as the officers were struggling with the man and feared for her life, the officers' lives, and the patient's life. No one was seriously harmed, and the patient received the care he needed. This did not change her feelings about the call. We decided to switch our focus in PE to this event and completed PE session 2. She learned how to use subjective units of distress, and we developed an in vivo exposure hierarchy, including items such as going out to restaurants, showering alone, and driving by scenes where past calls had occurred. Her first in vivo homework assignment was in the moderate distress SUDs range of 35–65.

Coming into the next session, Sarah was agitated, reporting she did an in vivo exposure and had a highly distressing reaction. She expressed that if she was going to have bad weeks like this repeatedly, she would refuse to continue therapy. She was pacing in my office, saying she felt like she was going to pass out. I challenged Sarah to push through these uncomfortable experiences and said we could handle it together if she passed out. She expressed some openness to leaning into the discomfort. We worked on cognitively reframing some of the threat assessments that fueled her distress during the in vivo. She was able to reframe her week and stated she felt accomplished in the work rather than overwhelmed. I saw this as a turning point.

Sarah engaged in imaginal exposure during the next session, telling the narrative of the excited delirium incident repeatedly. She paced the entire session with visible signs of anxiety, reporting a sense of panic and the desire to stop. She reported the fear she would pass out, and I again reassured her we could deal with that if it happened. I encouraged her to continue with the imaginal, which she did. The pacing required some adjustment to manualized PE, as the imaginal exposure instructions are for the client to have their eyes closed. Sarah progressed toward eyes-closed imaginals in later sessions. Her symptoms dropped steadily through PE, with her PCL-5 scores decreasing accordingly. By PE session 5, her symptoms had reduced a significant amount, with her PCL-5 scores dropping by 64%. In PE session 7, Sarah described herself as a "poster child for therapy" given the progress she saw. I saw she could talk about her focal and other traumas with greatly reduced distress from baseline. She was now sitting for the entire session. She was expanding her daily life activities, like showering at home alone. Still, in PE session 8, Sarah reported she had avoided her homework and that symptoms of panic were starting to appear again. We discussed her avoidance. I challenged Sarah, stating she would not be able to complete PE, an important goal for her, until she finished her homework. Sarah committed to returning to homework.

Sarah reported zero PTSD symptoms on the PCL-5 in sessions 9 and 10, possibly influenced by her underreporting response style. Overall, she had gone from presenting as irritable and cagey to pleasant and hopeful. She stated she had gained clarity in her understanding of the excited delirium event. During postimaginal processing, she was able to identify what was in her control during the event and what was not. She also now saw how she had acted competently in the call. (Trying to control uncontrollable aspects of situations had been a source of her anxiety.) These insights helped her view herself as competent again, which reduced her panic about being in public. She now believed she could provide medical attention in a crisis, and so was not fearful of interacting with children or the elderly. She stated she was proud of herself for taking showers when she was alone without panic symptoms. She stated she had "found herself again." Addressing Sarah's PTSD symptoms with PE resolved her panic symptoms, even as no interoceptive exposures were done. After completing PE, Sarah wanted to focus on the idea of going back to work. We continued therapy using ACT, with a focus on values, to help her decide what to do with her career. After a few sessions, Sarah returned to work.

Underutilization of Exposure Therapy

The clinical vignettes of Max and Sarah point to the power of exposure-based treatments but also include some of the challenges, e.g., trauma-based avoidance patterns contributing to treatment avoidance. Such client factors are one part, we think a smaller one, of a substantive issue in psychotherapy provision—the underutilization of exposure resulting in missed opportunities for high-quality care.

Psychotherapist-reported utilization rates of exposure vary by disorder, exposure technique, and population. A large study of North American psychotherapists (N = 2200) found 13% of participants reported using exposure regularly (Cook et al., 2010), but results were not broken down by disorder, making this study more difficult to interpret. In a study of 91 providers treating PTSD among U.S. active duty military personal, 3% of participants reported using exposure-based treatment, i.e., PE (Borah et al., 2017). In a study of 207 psychologists drawn from three U.S. states (Becker et al., 2004), 17% of participants reported using imaginal exposure, and 11% reported using in vivo exposure with PTSD cases. A study of 490 members of the Dutch Association for Behavioral and Cognitive Therapy found that 98% endorsed using exposure to anxiety disorders (Sars & van Minnen, 2015). A study of 51 Wyoming psychologists (Hipol & Deacon, 2013) found self-reported usage of imaginal exposure with PTSD and Panic Disorder to hover just above 60%, while usage of therapist-assisted in vivo exposure ranged from 19% to 27%. Given the strong evidence base for exposure treatments for PTSD and anxiety disorders, many researchers, including the authors of this chapter, interpret the above results as indications of exposure underutilization.

Many studies attempt to understand barriers to exposure utilization (e.g., Finch et al., 2020), typically focusing on system-level barriers (e.g., third-party nonreimbursement for additional clinician time with exposures or agency scheduling blocks that do not allow for longer session times) or therapist level barriers (lack of training with or negative attitudes about exposure). Large-scale efforts, like the VA Rollout of PE (Eftekhari et al., 2013) have shown promise in addressing psychotherapist training gaps with exposure, while some efforts attempt to change psychotherapist attitudes by addressing misconceptions (Murray et al., 2022).

Our review did not find studies empirically studying exposure utilization rates among psychotherapists treating first responders. Consistent with the underutilization interpretation, two reviews of mental healthcare for first responders judged that evidence-based care was not widely accessible (Kleim & Westphal, 2011; Lanza et al., 2018). We believe psychotherapist exposure usage with first responders is likely similar to the usage rates above, i.e., underutilized, resulting in missed opportunities for high-quality care.

Two commonly expressed concerns regarding exposure therapy, especially with PTSD, are client dropout and fear of symptom worsening. These concerns likely contribute to therapist underutilization of exposure even as there is substantive evidence contrary to each of these concerns. In a meta-analysis of dropout in RCTs of PTSD psychotherapies, Lewis et al. (2020) found that the average dropout rate was 16% overall. The average dropout rate among the three treatments with the best evidence was 22% for PE (across 22 studies), 18% for EMDR (across 21 studies), and 30% for a cognitively focused intervention (across 8 studies). Given overlapping 95% confidence intervals, these rates are considered statistically indistinguishable. The only RCT data on dropout in exposure therapy with first responder samples comes from the Bryant et al. (2019) PTSD trial using exposure-based CBT, which found dropout was like other RCTs for PTSD. Beyond RCTs, there is data from standard clinical contexts. Kehle-Forbes et al. (2016) found among 427 veterans offered PE or a cognitively focused treatment during standard care that 82% attended session 1, with 39% overall dropping out of treatment. There were slightly higher dropout rates for PE than cognitively focused treatment in later sessions. Two other studies with samples drawn from standard care yielded differing results, as PE had lower dropout rates in one and higher in another, when compared to the cognitively focused treatment (Jeffreys et al., 2014; Mott et al., 2014). Further study is needed on dropout in standard care settings, but two further points are noteworthy: (1) dropout estimates across all psychotherapies range from 20% to 47% (Swift & Greenberg, 2012; Wierzbicki & Pekarik, 1993), and (2) a large percentage of patients who dropout might still obtain significant symptom improvement (Szafranski et al., 2017).

Fear of symptom worsening is hypothesized to contribute to exposure underutilization. In two PTSD RCTs, Larsen et al. (2016) found that 20% in the PE condition experienced symptom worsening, while 29% and 15% did so in two cognitively focused treatments. Across treatments, symptom worsening did not predict dropout, and those who experienced worsening symptoms also achieved clinically significant improvements by the end of treatment. Symptom worsening thus appears to be a temporary state experienced by a small percentage of clients, which does not mean the treatment will be ineffective, and it is present in multiple treatments, not just exposure. To that last point, in the trial discussed above, in which a modified version of PE was compared with a standard substance use treatment for comorbid PTSD/SUD, symptom worsening was minimal and similar in both treatments (Lancaster et al., 2020).

Therapist exposure utilization rates do not matter if first responders do not engage in psychotherapy. Stigma surrounding mental illness is well known to be a major barrier to first responders engaging in mental healthcare (Haugen et al., 2017). To circumvent stigma as a barrier to care, Arble and Arnetz (2019) suggest agency-level training practices that could prevent work-related mental health disorders like PTSD. They offer initial evidence for the benefits of a police cadet training program that includes imaginal exposures to future, potentially stressful on-the-job incidents. Preliminary evidence from a sample of 75 Swedish police officer trainees and 32 police officer trainees in Detroit, MI suggests the psychological benefits of the program. The second and third authors of this chapter are developing a training program with law enforcement trainees, which makes behavioral health part of the law enforcement experience from the start and thereby possibly reducing stigma. In addition, embedded behavioral health in first responder agencies is a promising route to address stigma-based barriers to treatment.

Clinical Vignette: Treating Cannabis Use Disorder with a Firefighter[4]

"Scott" was a firefighter from a paid (vs. volunteer) city fire department who self-referred for treatment. He was seen at an outpatient clinic instead of at an embedded office location as he had been recently fired for violating the department's drug policy. He had crashed the fire truck he was driving into a building while responding to a call for service. During the accident investigation, he tested positive for marijuana on a drug screen. At intake, he was discouraged and remorseful. He met criteria for Cannabis Use Disorder, and anxiety symptoms were also present. Scott's goal was to be re-hired at his fire department. In the meantime, he was delivering home appliances, a job he hated. Discouraged, he reported increasing his marijuana use.

I felt Scott would be a good candidate for ACT because of his remorse and shame. We discussed this treatment model, and he agreed to weekly ACT sessions, especially focused on marijuana use. Prior to doing ACT exposure, we spent time exploring other ACT components, such as creative hopelessness, cognitive fusion,

[4] This vignette was written by second author.

and values work. He was fully engaged in session, did his homework assignments, and never missed a session. During the first half of treatment, he reported reducing his marijuana use, although his usage was not formally tracked. He admitted that when having a "bad day" he would cope by smoking more than otherwise.

When treatment reached the point of doing exposure, we discussed that the objective would be to help him become the "Zen-master" of having the urge to smoke marijuana and NOT smoking, instead of eliminating or avoiding the urge to smoke. For imaginal exposure, I had Scott close his eyes and reflect on the last time he had a really bad day. He described the worst moment of that day in the present tense, as if it were happening at that moment. He identified unwanted private experiences such as negative thoughts and emotions. We worked on developing his ability to accept these experiences without resistance. He returned to the target experience repeatedly until he identified the urge to smoke marijuana. He then worked on simply sitting with the urge to smoke marijuana for 2 minutes without judgment or resistance. This same exposure was repeated, extending the time to up to 5 minutes. During processing, he said he was surprised that the urge did not increase in intensity during the imaginal. His homework was to look for the urge to smoke marijuana and do independent exposures to the urge working up to sitting with the urge, without judgment or resistance, for up to 5–7 minutes.

At the start of the following session, Scott reported that his exposure to the urge to smoke marijuana was not as effective as it had been in the previous session. I normalized that experience and worked with him to let himself "off the hook" with that homework experience. We repeated the imaginal ACT exposure to the urge to smoke using his most recent lapse, where he smoked marijuana. We worked on his accepting his unwanted experiences, including the urge to smoke marijuana, without judgment or resistance and without doing anything about the urge. This second ACT exposure session was similar to the first. Scott reported very little change in the intensity of the urge. I reinforced his willingness to sit peacefully with something he would rather not have. His homework assignment was to have or welcome a bad day or two, something which amused him, and to be looking for the urge to smoke marijuana.

At the follow-up session, Scott reported that though he had not had a bad day since the last session, he had encountered the urge to smoke. He used this as an exposure practice, which he felt was successful. He claimed he had not smoked marijuana since the previous week. Imaginal ACT exposure to the urge to smoke marijuana was facilitated again. He reported a decrease in the intensity of the urge to smoke during this imaginal. We processed the imaginal exposure, and I directed questions in a way that he was able to point out to himself that the goal of the exposure was NOT to reduce the intensity of the urge. The goal was simply to get good at having the urge to marijuana and accept it. His homework was more independent ACT exposures to the urge to smoke. Planning for valued living was also part of this session.

Sessions proceeded to focus on ACT exposure and valued living for several weeks. Scott continued to report abstinence from smoking marijuana. At one point, late in treatment, he reported he had acquired a position as a firefighter at a nearby volunteer fire department. He had successfully passed the drug screen for that department. He saw this as the first step in returning to his former agency. He continued treatment with monthly maintenance sessions for 3 months, until he felt he was able to maintain sobriety and live for his values.

Sometime later, Scott telephoned me to report he had been hired back at his former agency. He had lost seniority and would need to rebuild his reputation at the agency. Over time, Scott became an advocate for mental health at his fire department, talking to other firefighters about his marijuana use and participation in therapy. Several years later, he is still at his agency. He has been promoted and is an active member of his department's internal peer support team.

Conclusions, Limitations, and Future Directions

The clinical vignettes of Max, Sarah, and Scott illustrate the impact that exposure-based treatments can have on individual first responders as they address issues with PTSD, depression, suicidality, panic, anxiety, and substance use disorders. Admittedly, anecdotes are not data, but the database is strong: exposure has large, positive effects on the treatment of the disorders most commonly faced by first responders. Based on this, we put forth that exposure approaches should be a first-line treatment for many clinical issues experienced by first responders. We make this recommendation while recognizing that there are few high-quality studies and possibly only one high-quality RCT of mental health interventions, specifically with first responder samples. We recognize that first responders face unique mental health challenges given the consistent and ongoing experience of potentially traumatic events and stressors. In addition, first responders typically live in and around the communities where they experience stressor events. This makes first responders relevantly different than many of the samples described in the clinical studies in this chapter and thereby points out the significant need for high-quality treatment research with first responders. While the unique risk profile of first responders might dampen treatment effect sizes, including for exposure treatments, research is needed to clarify this issue.

Moreover, as stigma and other barriers result in low treatment engagement among first responders, we believe innovative approaches like embedded behavioral health and the incorporation of mental health modules into the standard training of first responders could be promising paths forward. As illustrated in the clinical vignettes and discussed more broadly in this chapter, exposure can pair well with these kinds of innovations, i.e., using imaginal exposures in the first responder training curriculum (Arble & Arnetz, 2019) or as part of an embedded behavioral health program. These innovations are largely untested, and therefore rigorous study designs with replicated findings are needed to understand their possible benefits.

References

Acierno, R., Jaffe, A. E., Gilmore, A. K., Birks, A., Denier, C., Muzzy, W., Lopez, C. M., Tuerk, P., & Grubaugh, A. L. (2021). A randomized clinical trial of in-person vs. home-based telemedicine delivery of Prolonged Exposure for PTSD in military sexual trauma survivors. *Journal of Anxiety Disorders, 83*, 102461. https://doi.org/10.1016/j.janxdis.2021.102461

Alden, L. E., Matthews, L. R., Wagner, S. L., Fyfe, T., Randall, C., Regehr, C., White, M., Buys, N., Carey, M. G., Corneil, W., White, N., Fraess-Phillips, A., & Krutop, E. (2021). Systematic literature review of psychological interventions for first responders. *Work & Stress, 35*(2), 193–215. https://doi.org/10.1080/02678373.2020.1758833

Andrews, G., Bell, C., Boyce, P., Gale, C., Lampe, L., Marwat, O., Rapee, R., & Wilkins, G. (2018). Royal Australian and New Zealand College of Psychiatrists clinical practice guidelines for the treatment of panic disorder, social anxiety disorder and generalised anxiety disorder. *Australian & New Zealand Journal of Psychiatry, 52*(12), 1109–1172. https://doi.org/10.1177/0004867418799453

Arble, E. P., & Arnetz, B. B. (2019). Evidence-based practices to enhance first responder well-being and performance. In C. A. Bowers, D. C. Beidel, & M. R. Marks (Eds.), *Mental health intervention and treatment of first responders and emergency workers* (pp. 205–228). IGI Global. https://doi.org/10.4018/978-1-5225-9803-9

Back, S. E., Killeen, T., Badour, C. L., Flanagan, J. C., Allan, N. P., Ana, E. S., Lozano, B., Korte, K. J., Foa, E. B., & Brady, K. T. (2019). Concurrent treatment of substance use disorders and PTSD using prolonged exposure: A randomized clinical trial in military veterans. *Addictive Behaviors, 90*, 369–377. https://doi.org/10.1016/j.addbeh.2018.11.032

Bandelow, B., Lichte, T., Rudolf, S., Wiltink, J., & Beutel, M. E. (2015). The German guidelines for the treatment of anxiety disorders. *European Archives of Psychiatry and Clinical Neuroscience, 265*(5), 363–373. https://doi.org/10.1007/s00406-014-0563-z

Becker, C. B., Zayfert, C., & Anderson, E. (2004). A survey of psychologists' attitudes towards and utilization of exposure therapy for PTSD. *Behaviour Research and Therapy, 42*(3), 277–292. https://doi.org/10.1016/S0005-7967(03)00138-4

Borah, E. V., Holder, N., & Chen, K. (2017). Providers' use of evidence-based treatments for posttraumatic stress disorder: The influence of training, attitudes, and barriers in military and private treatment settings. *Best Practices in Mental Health: An International Journal, 13*(1), 34–46.

Bryant, R. A., Kenny, L., Rawson, N., Cahill, C., Joscelyne, A., Garber, B., Tockar, J., Dawson, K., & Nickerson, A. (2019). Efficacy of exposure-based cognitive behaviour therapy for post-traumatic stress disorder in emergency service personnel: A randomised clinical trial. *Psychological Medicine, 49*(9), 1565–1573. https://doi.org/10.1017/S0033291718002234

Card, P. (2017). *VA/DoD clinical practice guideline for the management of posttraumatic stress disorder and acute stress disorder*. Department of Veterans Affairs & Department of Defense. https://www.healthquality.va.gov/guidelines/MH/ptsd/VADoDPTSDCPGFinal012418.pdf

Cook, J. M., Biyanova, T., Elhai, J., Schnurr, P. P., & Coyne, J. C. (2010). What do psychotherapists really do in practice? An Internet study of over 2,000 practitioners. *Psychotherapy: Theory, Research, Practice, Training, 47*(2), 260–267. https://doi.org/10.1037/a0019788

Eftekhari, A., Ruzek, J. I., Crowley, J. J., Rosen, C. S., Greenbaum, M. A., & Karlin, B. E. (2013). Effectiveness of national implementation of prolonged exposure therapy in Veterans Affairs care. *JAMA Psychiatry, 70*(9), 949–955. https://doi.org/10.1001/jamapsychiatry.2013.36

Finch, J., Ford, C., Grainger, L., & Meiser-Stedman, R. (2020). A systematic review of the clinician related barriers and facilitators to the use of evidence-informed interventions for posttraumatic stress. *Journal of Affective Disorders, 263*, 175–186. https://doi.org/10.1016/j.jad.2019.11.143

Forbes, D., Bisson, J. I., Monson, C. M., & Berliner, L. (Eds.). (2020). *Effective treatments for PTSD*. Guilford Publications.

Grosse Holtforth, M., Krieger, T., Zimmermann, J., Altenstein-Yamanaka, D., Dörig, N., Meisch, L., & Hayes, A. M. (2019). A randomized-controlled trial of cognitive–behavioral therapy for depression with integrated techniques from emotion-focused and exposure therapies. *Psychotherapy Research, 29*(1), 30–44. https://doi.org/10.1080/10503307.2017.1397796

Haugen, P. T., Evces, M., & Weiss, D. S. (2012). Treating posttraumatic stress disorder in first responders: A systematic review. *Clinical Psychology Review, 32*(5), 370–380. https://doi.org/10.1016/j.cpr.2012.04.001

Haugen, P. T., McCrillis, A. M., Smid, G. E., & Nijdam, M. J. (2017). Mental health stigma and barriers to mental health care for first responders: A systematic review and meta-analysis. *Journal of Psychiatric Research, 94*, 218–229. https://doi.org/10.1016/j.jpsychires.2017.08.001

Hayes, S. (2019). *A liberated mind: The essential guide to ACT*. Random House.

Hipol, L. J., & Deacon, B. J. (2013). Dissemination of evidence-based practices for anxiety disorders in Wyoming: A survey of practicing psychotherapists. *Behavior Modification, 37*(2), 170–188. https://doi.org/10.1177/0145445512458794

Jeffreys, M. D., Reinfeld, C., Nair, P. V., Garcia, H. A., Mata-Galan, E., & Rentz, T. O. (2014). Evaluating treatment of posttraumatic stress disorder with cognitive processing therapy and prolonged exposure therapy in a VHA specialty clinic. *Journal of Anxiety Disorders, 28*(1), 108–114. https://doi.org/10.1016/j.janxdis.2013.04.010

Jones, S. (2017). Describing the mental health profile of first responders: A systematic review. *Journal of the American Psychiatric Nurses Association, 23*(3), 200–214. https://doi.org/10.1177/1078390317695266

Kehle-Forbes, S. M., Meis, L. A., Spoont, M. R., & Polusny, M. A. (2016). Treatment initiation and dropout from prolonged exposure and cognitive processing therapy in a VA outpatient clinic. *Psychological Trauma: Theory, Research, Practice, and Policy, 8*(1), 107–114. https://doi.org/10.1037/tra0000065

Kleim, B., & Westphal, M. (2011). Mental health in first responders: A review and recommendation for prevention and intervention strategies. *Traumatology, 17*(4), 17–24. https://doi.org/10.1177/1534765611429079

Lancaster, C. L., Gros, D. F., Mullarkey, M. C., Badour, C. L., Killeen, T. K., Brady, K. T., & Back, S. E. (2020). Does trauma-focused exposure therapy exacerbate symptoms among patients with comorbid PTSD and substance use disorders? *Behavioural and Cognitive Psychotherapy, 48*(1), 38–53. https://doi.org/10.1017/S1352465819000304

Lanza, A., Roysircar, G., & Rodgers, S. (2018). First responder mental healthcare: Evidence-based prevention, postvention, and treatment. *Professional Psychology: Research and Practice, 49*(3), 193–204. https://doi.org/10.1037/pro0000192

Larsen, S. E., Stirman, S. W., Smith, B. N., & Resick, P. A. (2016). Symptom exacerbations in trauma-focused treatments: Associations with treatment outcome and non-completion. *Behaviour Research and Therapy, 77*, 68–77. https://doi.org/10.1016/j.brat.2015.12.009

Lee, E. B., An, W., Levin, M. E., & Twohig, M. P. (2015). An initial meta-analysis of Acceptance and Commitment Therapy for treating substance use disorders. *Drug and Alcohol Dependence, 155*, 1–7. https://doi.org/10.1016/j.drugalcdep.2015.08.004

Lewis, C., Roberts, N. P., Gibson, S., & Bisson, J. I. (2020). Dropout from psychological therapies for post-traumatic stress disorder (PTSD) in adults: Systematic review and meta-analysis. *European Journal of Psychotraumatology, 11*(1), 1709709. https://doi.org/10.1080/20008198.2019.1709709

Mellentin, A. I., Skøt, L., Nielsen, B., Schippers, G. M., Nielsen, A. S., Stenager, E., & Juhl, C. (2017). Cue exposure therapy for the treatment of alcohol use disorders: A meta-analytic review. *Clinical Psychology Review, 57*, 195–207. https://doi.org/10.1016/j.cpr.2017.07.006

Mott, J. M., Mondragon, S., Hundt, N. E., Beason-Smith, M., Grady, R. H., & Teng, E. J. (2014). Characteristics of US veterans who begin and complete prolonged exposure and cognitive processing therapy for PTSD. *Journal of Traumatic Stress, 27*(3), 265–273. https://doi.org/10.1002/jts.21927

Murray, H., Grey, N., Warnock-Parkes, E., Kerr, A., Wild, J., Clark, D., & Ehlers, A. (2022). Ten misconceptions about trauma-focused CBT for PTSD. *Cognitive Behaviour Therapist, 15*. https://doi.org/10.1017/S1754470X22000307

National Institute for Health and Clinical Excellence. (2011). *Generalised anxiety disorder and panic disorder (with or without agoraphobia) in adults: Management in primary, secondary and community care*. NICE. https://www.nice.org.uk/guidance/cg113

Osaji, J., Ojimba, C., & Ahmed, S. (2020). The use of acceptance and commitment therapy in substance use disorders: A review of literature. *Journal of Clinical Medicine Research, 12*(10), 629–633. https://doi.org/10.14740/jocmr4311

Russell, D. W., Whalen, R. J., Riviere, L. A., Clarke-Walper, K., Bliese, P. D., Keller, D. D., Pangelian, S. I., & Thomas, J. L. (2014). Embedded behavioral health providers: An assessment with the Army National Guard. *Psychological Services, 11*(3), 265–272. https://doi.org/10.1037/a0037005

Sakaluk, J. K., Williams, A. J., Kilshaw, R. E., & Rhyner, K. T. (2019). Evaluating the evidential value of empirically supported psychological treatments (ESTs): A meta-scientific review. *Journal of Abnormal Psychology, 128*(6), 500–509. https://doi.org/10.1037/abn0000421

Sars, D., & van Minnen, A. (2015). On the use of exposure therapy in the treatment of anxiety disorders: A survey among cognitive behavioural therapists in the Netherlands. *BMC Psychology, 3*(1), 26. https://doi.org/10.1186/s40359-015-0083-2

Sauer-Zavala, S., Bentley, K. H., Steele, S. J., Tirpak, J. W., Ametaj, A. A., Nauphal, M., Cardona, N., Wang, M., Farchione, T. J., & Barlow, D. H. (2020). Treating depressive disorders with the Unified Protocol: A preliminary randomized evaluation. *Journal of Affective Disorders, 264*, 438–445. https://doi.org/10.1016/j.jad.2019.11.072

Simpson, T. L., Goldberg, S. B., Louden, D. K., Blakey, S. M., Hawn, S. E., Lott, A., ... & Kaysen, D. (2021). Efficacy and acceptability of interventions for co-occurring PTSD and SUD: A meta-analysis. *Journal of Anxiety Disorders, 84*, 102490.

Srinivasan, J. (2017, June 25–27). *Embedded behavioral health: A novel mental health care delivery model to reduce stigma and improve outcomes* [Conference session]. Academy Health Annual Research Meeting, New Orleans, LA, United States.

Swift, J. K., & Greenberg, R. P. (2012). Premature discontinuation in adult psychotherapy: A meta-analysis. *Journal of Consulting and Clinical Psychology, 80*(4), 547–559. https://doi.org/10.1037/a0028226

Syed, S., Ashwick, R., Schlosser, M., Jones, R., Rowe, S., & Billings, J. (2020). Global prevalence and risk factors for mental health problems in police personnel: A systematic review and meta-analysis. *Occupational and Environmental Medicine, 77*(11), 737–747. https://doi.org/10.1136/oemed-2020-106498

Szafranski, D. D., Smith, B. N., Gros, D. F., & Resick, P. A. (2017). High rates of PTSD treatment dropout: A possible red herring? *Journal of Anxiety Disorders, 47*, 91–98. https://doi.org/10.1016/j.janxdis.2017.01.002

Vergun, D. (2018, April 6). *Army behavioral health sees dramatic improvements, says Surgeon General's Office*. U.S. Army News Service. https://www.army.mil/article/203416/army_behavioral_health_care_sees_dramatic_improvements_says_surgeon_generals_office

Wierzbicki, M., & Pekarik, G. (1993). A meta-analysis of psychotherapy dropout. *Professional Psychology: Research and Practice, 24*(2), 190–195. https://doi.org/10.1037/0735-7028.24.2.190

Psychopharmacologic Treatment of Psychiatric Disorders in First Responders

Leonard M. Gralnik and Jose A. Rey

First responders are vulnerable to the same psychiatric conditions and symptoms that affect the general population. However, they are particularly vulnerable to certain conditions by virtue of the stressful, often traumatic nature of their work environment. This includes disorders such as posttraumatic stress disorder and acute stress disorder, as defined in the Diagnostic and Statistical Manual of Mental Disorders, Fifth edition, Text Revision (DSM-5-TR) (American Psychiatric Association [APA], 2022). This chapter will address the treatment of the most common disorders and symptoms that first responders are likely to experience. We will focus on the treatment of first responders who, despite their symptoms, are continuing to work. In some cases, the symptoms may cause so much distress or impairment that the first responders may need to take a leave of absence for treatment. A common thread in this chapter will be the importance of choosing medications that are safe to use in this population. For example, wherever possible, the use of a controlled substance that could lead to, or exacerbate, addictions will be avoided, or recommended with great caution. Second, medications that could cause intolerable side effects and interfere with the first responder's work will also be avoided or used sparingly. Sedation occurring during the work shift hours is an example of such a side effect. We will not address the treatment of psychotic disorders, such as schizophrenia or schizoaffective disorder, in this chapter, since the presence of these disorders is thought to be uncommon in high-functioning individuals such as first responders and other professionals. While it is possible that an actively working first

L. M. Gralnik (✉)
Department of Psychiatry and Behavioral Health, Herbert Wertheim College of Medicine, Florida International University, Miami, FL, USA
e-mail: gralnikl@fiu.edu

J. A. Rey
Department of Pharmacy Practice, College of Pharmacy, Nova Southeastern University, Fort Lauderdale, FL, USA

M. L. Bourke et al. (eds.), *First Responder Mental Health*,
https://doi.org/10.1007/978-3-031-38149-2_14

responder could develop a psychotic illness that would later interfere with their work and require treatment, we will not address these disorders due to their relative rarity in this population. We will, however, touch upon the use of antipsychotics in other conditions, for example, as augmenting agents in depressive disorders, or for the treatment of severe anxiety, usually in combination with other medications, or their use as mood stabilizers. We will not go into depth in this chapter on the diagnostic criteria for the various disorders, focusing more on a practical approach to pharmacologic treatment once the diagnoses have been established. For diagnostic criteria, we refer the reader to DSM-5-TR (APA, 2022) and the *Comprehensive Textbook of Psychiatry* (10th ed.) (Sadock et al., 2017).

The treatment of substance use disorders in first responders is a vitally important topic and should always involve a multimodal approach, including psychotherapeutic approaches, and, in some cases, pharmacologic treatment. In this chapter, we will address the treatment of alcohol and opioid use disorders, since they are common in the population of first responders (Beauchamp et al., 2022; Harvey et al., 2016; Vargas de Barros et al., 2013), and are often amenable to psychopharmacological interventions. We will also address the addiction potentials of some of the psychopharmacologic treatments we recommend, including benzodiazepines.

In some instances, we will define our recommended treatments based on diagnoses, and in others, based on symptoms. There is often a significant overlap between these two approaches. It is always desirable to establish a psychiatric diagnosis before prescribing psychopharmacologic treatment. A thorough medical history is a necessary part of this evaluation, and referral to a primary care physician, such as a family medicine physician or internist, for a medical evaluation, is almost always recommended before initiating psychopharmacologic treatment. This is especially important in first responders, who, by the nature of their jobs and lifestyles, may be particularly vulnerable to medical conditions such as heart disease, diabetes mellitus, chronic pain syndromes, and cerebrovascular accidents. Because of their busy schedules and multiple, often overwhelming, demands on their time, first responders may neglect seeking routine medical care, and may, therefore, suffer from undiagnosed medical conditions. This should always be considered by prescribers considering treatment with psychotropic medications and will sometimes influence the choice of medication (e.g., avoiding older medications such as tricyclic antidepressants, which have significant cardiac side effects).

While this chapter focuses on psychopharmacology, we wish to emphasize the importance of psychotherapy in the treatment of psychiatric disorders and symptoms in first responders, often in combination with medication. It is sometimes naïve to think that therapy alone will be sufficient for severe symptoms, just as it would be naïve to think that prescription medications can work alone when the combination of therapy with medication may work synergistically and be able to address the etiology of the trauma and the symptoms. We often conceptualize this as the medications providing symptom reduction and functional improvement that allows the first responder to more fully and effectively participate in psychotherapy, thus leading to significant alleviation of symptoms, reduced distress, and improved functioning. The frequent visits for psychotherapy also allow for closer monitoring of the first responder's response to treatment. Therapists may also delve into, and help to address, any reluctance or misconception about medications that could lead to nonadherence with treatment, and, therefore, prevent effective and positive outcomes. A close collaboration between psychotherapists and prescribers is crucial to achieving the optimal response to treatment with the least adverse effects or negative outcomes. The busy schedule and time demands of first responders make attendance to psychotherapy visits challenging; we must recognize this and put measures in place to help make attendance easier and less demanding. Medication management visits are also sometimes difficult to work into the first responder's daily routine. Recent work with the general public has shown that telehealth visits are often easier to schedule and can sometimes increase attendance rates at follow-up appointments (Pruitt et al., 2014). Some of this work was begun during the COVID-19 pandemic. However, the convenience of telehealth visits for providers and patients has continued to be useful in increasing attendance rates at follow-up visits (Lipschitz et al., 2022).

Psychopharmacological treatment of the following conditions and/or symptoms will be addressed in this chapter: posttraumatic stress disorder, major depressive disorder, bipolar disorders, generalized anxiety disorder, panic disorder, social anxiety disorder, and insomnia. Pharmacologic treatments for the following substance use disorders will also be addressed: alcohol use disorder; opioid use disorder; and sedative, hypnotic, or anxiolytic use disorder. The reader will realize that many of the recommended medications are helpful for more than one disorder or symptom, which simplifies the armamentarium of medications that the provider will need to use.

Posttraumatic Stress Disorder

Posttraumatic Stress Disorder (PTSD) is described in DSM-5-TR as one of the trauma- and stressor-related disorders. For the diagnosis of PTSD, there must be exposure to actual or threatened death, serious injury, or sexual violence (Roberts, 2019). The following types of symptoms occur: intrusion symptoms including recurrent memories, nightmares, and flashbacks; avoidance symptoms, including efforts to avoid distressing thoughts or feelings or external reminders; negative changes in cognition and mood, including blaming oneself, detachment from others, and inability to experience positive emotions; and altered arousal and reactivity, including hyperarousal, increased startle response, decreased concentration, and disturbed sleep. The disturbance lasts more than 1 month, causes clinically significant distress or impairment, and is not attributable to the effect of a substance or another medical condition (Roberts, 2019).

It is apparent that first responders are often exposed to stressors that include actual or threatened death, or serious injury, either of themselves or others. Responders who deal with the aftermath of accidents or homicides may be particularly vulnerable. Police officers, paramedics, and firefighters often deal with trauma of this level in the line of duty. In addition to the symptom clusters outlined above, PTSD is often accompanied by significant symptoms of depression, anxiety, and insomnia, which also require treatment.

The first-line treatment of choice for PTSD is psychotherapy. The second-line treatment is pharmacotherapy, usually given in combination with psychotherapy, despite a relative lack of evidence for the combination being superior to individual treatments (Guideline Development Panel for the Treatment of PTSD in Adults, American Psychological Association, 2019; Hetrick et al., 2010). The treatment of PTSD with psychotropic medications, once begun, should usually be continued for at least 1 year. The most well-studied medications for the treatment of PTSD are antidepressants, particularly selective serotonin reuptake inhibitors (SSRIs). In the United States, the Food and Drug Administration (FDA) has approved the SSRIs sertraline and paroxetine for the treatment of PTSD based on clinical research trials (Brady et al., 2000; Tucker et al., 2001). Therefore, these two antidepressants are described as being indicated for the treatment of PTSD. However, evidence shows that other SSRIs are also effective, especially fluoxetine (Davidson, 2000; The Department of Veterans Affairs/Department of Defense Evidence-Based Practice Working Group (EBPWG), 2018; van der Kolk et al., 1994). The serotonin-norepinephrine reuptake inhibitor (SNRI) venlafaxine also has considerable evidence of efficacy for PTSD (Charney et al., 2018; Davidson, 2006; Davidson et al., 2006; The Department of Veterans Affairs/Department of Defense EBPWG, 2018; Wright et al., 2019).

As a group, antidepressants have the best evidence of efficacy for the treatment of PTSD. Since many antidepressants have been shown to be effective for PTSD, the choice should be made primarily on the side effect profile and previous response to the medication. Response in first-degree relatives may also be helpful. The antihypertensive medication prazosin (alpha-1 antagonist) has been shown to reduce the frequency and intensity of nightmares in PTSD (Hudson et al., 2012). Blood pressure must be monitored regularly when prazosin is prescribed. Many medications such as mood stabilizers (lithium, valproic acid, lamotrigine), antipsychotics (risperidone, aripiprazole, quetiapine, and others), and anxiolytic medications (benzodiazepines) have been tried and studied in the treatment of PTSD. There is little evidence for their effectiveness in this disorder (Guideline Development Panel, 2019; Department of Veterans Affairs/Department of Defense EBPWG, 2018). Despite the relative lack of specific efficacy in PTSD and recommendations against their use in the guidelines, they may sometimes be used effectively to treat comorbid conditions. For example, quetiapine may be used to augment the antidepressant effect of an SSRI in the treatment of a patient with PTSD and major depressive disorder. Quetiapine and other medications with sedative qualities may also help with insomnia, as will be described below. Benzodiazepines may be used with caution in some PTSD patients to treat associated anxiety and insomnia. However, the high potential for dependence and/or addiction with these medications makes their use in this disorder problematic, especially given the high rate of comorbidity of substance use disorders and PTSD. The use of benzodiazepines in PTSD patients who are actively misusing substances, such as alcohol, should be avoided. They should only be used with great caution in PTSD patients with a history of a substance use disorder that is now controlled with treatment or in remission.

Some new medications are showing promise for the treatment of PTSD: D-cycloserine has sporadically shown some promise as an enhancer of fear extinction/exposure therapy when administered along with psychotherapy. This is thought to act through an NMDA receptor partial agonist effect (Baker et al., 2018). The NMDA receptor agonist ketamine has shown some promise in the treatment of PTSD. Severe, treatment-resistant depression often co-occurs with PTSD, since the latter symptoms complicate the treatment of depression. Recent studies with intranasal esketamine have been promising in this group of patients. Administration of esketamine in severely depressed PTSD patients was shown to significantly reduce depressive symptoms and to reduce the percentage of patients who were suicidal from 64% at baseline to 27% after 1 month of intranasal esketamine treatment, with no serious adverse effects (Rothärmel et al., 2022).

Since depression very commonly co-occurs with PTSD, the treatment of depression, as described in the next section, will be particularly relevant to first responders with PTSD (as will the section on substance use disorders, which also co-occur very commonly). Transcranial Magnetic Stimulation (TMS) which will be described more fully below as it applies to the treatment of treatment-resistant depression, has also shown promise as a treatment for PTSD, particularly when combined with psychotherapy such as Cognitive Processing Therapy (CPT) (Petrosino et al., 2021; Trevizol et al., 2016).

Depression

Major depressive disorder is characterized by depressed mood, loss of interest in pleasurable activities (anhedonia), and neurovegetative signs including low energy, disturbed sleep, poor concentration, weight loss or weight gain, slowed movements, and suicidal thoughts or behaviors. The symptoms must be present for at least 2 weeks, and cause significant distress or impairment. Highlighting the importance of a thorough medical evaluation, the symptoms must not be better explained by another medical condition such as hypothyroidism. Highlighting the importance of evaluating the first responder for the presence of a substance use disorder, the depressive symptoms must not be better explained by the effects of a substance such as alcohol or illicit drugs. Major depressive disorder is very often diagnosed concurrently with PTSD, making these conditions commonly comorbid. Comorbidity is the rule in psychiatric diagnosis and treatment. Many patients who require treatment with psychotropic medications meet the criteria for more than one diagnosis, such as major depressive disorder co-occurring with PTSD or generalized anxiety disorder, or both. The treatment provider must be diligent in looking for comorbid diagnoses that may be present. In some instances, multiple comorbid diagnoses can be treated with a single medication because some medications are effective for multiple disorders and have more than one indication. A good example of this is the SSRI antidepressants, which are effective for both depression and anxiety.

Given their safety profile, efficacy, usefulness in comorbid conditions such as PTSD or anxiety, and favorable side effect profile, SSRIs are the medications of first choice for the treatment of depression (major depressive disorder) in first responders and in the general population. How do we know when medications are necessary for depression? Generally, the evidence shows that moderate or severe major depressive disorder benefits significantly from antidepressant medication treatment, either alone, or preferably, in combination with psychotherapy; mild depression may often be treated with psychotherapy alone. The choice to treat with medication, psychotherapy, or both, also depends on the first responder's wishes and the availability of psychotherapy. If a first responder meets the criteria for mild major depressive disorder, which is causing a significant degree of distress, treatment with antidepressants alone would be appropriate if that is the preference of the first responder, or if psychotherapy is not readily available.

The SSRIs listed in Table 1 are all indicated and useful for the treatment of major depressive disorder in adults. These are the medications of first choice for the treatment of depression in first responders. Of note, many of the older antidepressants such as tricyclic antidepressants are lethal in overdose. Since suicidal ideation is commonly a symptom of depression, it is particularly important to prescribe medications that are relatively safe if taken in overdose. The SSRIs fit this description and safety need.

Other medications that are useful and safe in the treatment of depression in first responders include Serotonin-Norepinephrine Reuptake Inhibitors (SNRIs), such as venlafaxine and duloxetine. Similar to the SSRIs, these medications have a relatively good side effect profile and relative safety in overdose compared to older medications. Like the SSRIs, the SNRIs are also effective for treating symptoms of PTSD and for treating anxiety. Due to a relatively short half-life, SNRIs can have a significant discontinuation syndrome if stopped abruptly, which can include body aches, headaches, and other flu-like symptoms. Patients sometimes describe sensations akin to electric shocks, described as "zaps," when SNRIs are discontinued abruptly. Slow, gradual tapering is important when discontinuing these medications or when switching to a different antidepressant. SSRIs with short half-lives, such as paroxetine, are also associated with a higher incidence of discontinuation syndromes. An advantage of the SSRI fluoxetine is that its long half-life, along with the long half-life of its active metabolite, nor-fluoxetine, greatly reduces the chances of a discontinuation syndrome when this medication is discontinued.

The possibility of a discontinuation syndrome is important to consider in a population, such as first responders, who, for various reasons, including the stigma associated with psychiatric medications, may not be adherent to treatment and may abruptly stop the medication on their own. If a discontinuation syndrome occurs when the first responder stops taking the medication, this could reinforce the stigma they associate with psychotropic medications, and make future trials of antidepressant treatments difficult or impossible. Thus, choosing a medication, such as fluoxetine, may have advantages in this regard, given its long half-life and reduced chance of discontinuation syndrome.

Table 1 Antidepressants used as first-line treatments for major depressive disorder, anxiety, and PTSD

Antidepressant	Brand name	Usual dosage range	Sedation	Clinical considerations
Tricyclic agents or TCAs (FwO)				
Amitriptyline	Elavil	25–300 mg/day	PLUS_SPI PLUS_SPI PLUS_SPI PLUS_SPI	Also commonly used as an off-label treatment for chronic pain syndromes
Doxepin	Adapin/ Sinequan	25–300 mg/day	PLUS_SPI PLUS_SPI PLUS_SPI PLUS_SPI	Silenor at 3–6 mg at bedtime for insomnia
Imipramine	Tofranil	25–300 mg/day	+++	Very anticholinergic
Trimipramine	Surmontil	25–300 mg/day	+++	
Nortriptyline	Pamelor/ Aventyl	25–200 mg/day	+++	Lower SE incidence than amitriptyline
Desipramine	Norpramin	25–300 mg/day	++	Lower SE incidence than imipramine
Protriptyline	Vivactil	10–60 mg/day	++	Can be activating
Clomipramine	Anafranil	25–250 mg/day	PLUS_SPI PLUS_SPI PLUS_SPI PLUS_SPI	Only FDA-approved for OCD in US
Tetracyclic agents (FwO)				
Amoxapine	Asendin	25–600 mg/day	+++	Possible EPS
SSRIs				Class effects: Sexual dysfunction, insomnia, anxiety, gastrointestinal discomfort; Take all SSRIs w/food
Fluoxetine	Prozac	10–80 mg/day	−/+	*Evidence for efficacy for the treatment of PTSD*
Sertraline	Zoloft	25–200 mg/day	−/+	*FDA-Approved for the treatment of PTSD*
Paroxetine	Paxil and Paxil CR Pexeva	10–60 mg/day	+	*FDA-Approved for the treatment of PTSD* shorter t1/2 than FLX or SERT, and higher risk for discontinuation syndrome (DS)
Fluvoxamine	Luvox (CR)	100–300 mg/day	+	FDA-approved for OCD and social anxiety disorder
Citalopram	Celexa	10–40 mg/day	+	Higher risk for QTc prolongation among the SSRIs low risk for drug-drug interactions

(continued)

Table 1 (continued)

Antidepressant	Brand name	Usual dosage range	Sedation	Clinical considerations
Escitalopram	Lexapro	10–20 mg/day	+	Low risk for drug-drug interactions
Others				
Trazodone	Desyrel/ Oleptro	50–600 mg/day	+++	Sedation, Orthostasis, and Priapism
Nefazodone	–	10–600 mg/day	++	BW: Hepatotoxicity
Vilazodone	Viibryd	10–40 mg/day	+	SSRI-side effect profile & 5HT-1a partial agonist
Bupropion	Wellbutrin IR/SR/XL Zyban*	200–450 mg/day 150–300 mg/day	+	Can be activating/ insomnia provoking; Also used for smoking cessation
Venlafaxine	Effexor Effexor XR	25–375 mg/day 37.5–225 mg/day	+	SNRI/GI side effects/ HTN risk *Evidence for efficacy for the treatment of PTSD*
Desvenlafaxine	Pristiq	50–400 mg/day	+	SNRI/HTN risk
Mirtazapine	Remeron	15–45 mg/day	+++	Sedation & weight gain as SEs
Duloxetine	Cymbalta	20–120 mg/day	+	SNRI/HTN risk FDA-approved for chronic pain management
Vortioxetine	Trintellix	10–20 mg/day	+	Serotonin reuptake and receptor agonist/ antagonist
Levomilnacipran	Fetzima	40–120 mg/day	+	SNRI (GI and cardiac side effects)
Brexanolone*	Zulresso	*** IV/60 h		Postpartum Depression
Esketamine*	Spravato	56–84 mg/dose*	++	Multiple BWs; controlled substance; Only for Treatment-Resistant Depression in addition to another antidepressant
Dextromethorphan PLUS_SPI Bupropion	Aulvelity	90 mg/210 mg/day in divided dosing	++	NMDA receptor antagonist/sigma-1 receptor agonist/NDRI ADRs: dizziness, headache, diarrhea, somnolence, dry mouth, sexual dysfunction, and hyperhidrosis

Note. Table Key: *FwO* possibly fatal with overdose, *HTN* hypertension, *OCD* obsessive-compulsive disorder, *TCA* tricyclic antidepressant, *SS* serotonin syndrome, *Anticholinergic side effects commonly include* dry mouth, constipation, urinary retention, tachycardia, blurred vision, confusion, *BW* boxed warning, *SE* side effects, *DS* Discontinuation Syndrome, *t1/2* half-life

Other antidepressants that are useful in treating depression in first responders include bupropion, a medication that enhances the activity of dopamine and norepinephrine in the brain, rather than serotonin. Bupropion also has particular efficacy in improving concentration, which helps improve functioning in first responders who experience the symptoms of poor concentration as part of their depression. It is also a second-line and off-label, treatment of attention-deficit/hyperactivity disorder (ADHD). Therefore, it is particularly effective in first responders who have a comorbid major depressive disorder and ADHD, which can also commonly co-occur. One disadvantage of bupropion is that it is not an effective treatment for anxiety, and may sometimes exacerbate anxiety symptoms. It also must be given early in the day, to avoid exacerbating or causing insomnia. Bupropion is contraindicated in individuals with a history of seizures or an eating disorder. Consequently, thorough history-taking is of paramount importance before prescribing bupropion. Since patients who are actively drinking alcohol may experience an increased likelihood of seizures due to alcohol withdrawal, bupropion should be used only with caution, or not at all, in this population.

Combining medications with different mechanisms of action, such as SSRIs plus bupropion, or SNRIs plus bupropion, is often effective when a single medication alone has not been effective. If a first responder is tolerating an adequate trial of one antidepressant but not achieving the desired response, adding another medication is often helpful and well-tolerated instead of switching medications. (Refer to Table 1 regarding some common side effects associated with antidepressants.)

Another issue with SSRIs that can contribute to problems with adherence in relatively healthy and sexually active persons, is an increased risk for sexual dysfunction, in both men and women, often expressed as delayed orgasm or anorgasmia. The prescriber should inquire regarding sexual functioning at baseline and during follow-up assessments because some sexual dysfunction may be preexisting as a symptom of depression (e.g., low libido). Many persons cite sexual dysfunction as a reason for nonadherence, especially when they were not informed of this possible side effect when initiating treatment. Further, all antidepressants have a boxed warning (BW) for an increased risk of suicidal thoughts and behaviors in younger persons aged less than 25 years old. This may affect some first responders as they are entering the workforce at these young ages. Anyone being prescribed an antidepressant for any indication should be screened at baseline for suicidal ideation and/or plans/behaviors and monitored closely with safety plans, especially if suicidal ideation preexists the use of the antidepressant and is part of the clinical presentation.

With appropriate monitoring, the use of an antidepressant is preferred over the fear of a boxed warning that keeps the prescriber from utilizing an antidepressant. If the concern is present, especially if the first responder patient has a history of suicidal behaviors with an overdose of medications/drugs, then a safety plan should be formulated as a suicide prevention measure with resources for the patient to utilize including emergency contact numbers. Medication treatment, and adherence to follow-up appointments with the prescriber, can all be part of the safety plan. Indeed, referral for evaluation at the beginning of medication treatment can be part of a safety plan that a therapist sets up with a first responder patient they see for evaluation and treatment. Safety plans have been shown to be effective in reducing suicidal thoughts and behaviors, and in preventing suicide deaths. Safety plans are, therefore, a crucial part of the treatment plan for a first responder being treated with antidepressants for depression (Rogers et al., 2022).

Some commonly used medications to augment the effectiveness of an antidepressant, such as an SSRI, may include: aripiprazole, brexpiprazole, and quetiapine, which are second-generation antipsychotics. Some of these antipsychotics are also used as "mood stabilizers" in various aspects of bipolar disorder and will be described more fully below. The anticonvulsant mood-stabilizing agent lamotrigine may also be used off-label as an augmenting agent for antidepressants with mixed results in research (Fleurence et al., 2009; Solmi et al., 2016). Other treatment alternatives for individuals who do not respond to trials of two or more antidepressants, even with augmentation, include Transcranial Magnetic Stimulation (TMS) and Electroconvulsive Therapy (ECT). Of the two, TMS is less invasive and does not require anesthesia. It is becoming more widely available and would be a good choice for first responders who do not respond adequately to pharmacotherapy, with or without psychotherapy. Individuals who have a partial response to antidepressant therapy, with or without augmenting medications, such as aripiprazole, can continue these medications during and after TMS treatment. And, the combination therapy is often significantly more effective than the medication alone. While TMS has the advantage of being very safe and effective, and also noninvasive, a disadvantage that could be particularly relevant for first responders is the necessity for a 6-week course of treatment, with attendance 5 days per week. While each TMS treatment is usually brief (less than 20 minutes), the necessity for attendance every weekday for 6 weeks could be inconvenient or impractical to a first responder and would have to be discussed and considered prior to initiating treatment.

A common question that arises in patients when antidepressants are prescribed is, "Do I have to take this for the rest of my life?" This question is related to the stigma associated with the treatment of depression, and with the use of psychotropic medications in general. Stigma and misunderstanding are strong impediments to accepting treatments that can be beneficial, and even lifesaving. First responders work in a culture that values strength and self-reliance. Seeking help, especially in the form of medication, may be seen as a weakness. Indeed, depression itself is often seen as a sign of weakness, an indication that the person who needs treatment is weak because they cannot "tough it out" on their own. Taking medication for the rest of one's life may be perceived as a sign of profound weakness. To avoid this misunderstanding, it is important for prescribers to fully discuss the usual recommendations for the treatment of major depressive disorder with antidepressant medications. For the first episode of depression (i.e., the patient has never had a previous episode), treatment is usually given to bring the symptoms of depression into remission, and then continuing the antidepressant medication for at least 6–12 months before tapering and discontinuing the medication would be considered.

For the second episode of depression, it is usually recommended that the antidepressant be continued for at least 1–2 years. And, if there is a third episode, it is usually recommended that the treatment be continued indefinitely. Patient preference and severity of the episodes also play a strong role in the decision-making process. For example, if the first episode was particularly severe, especially if it included a strong component of suicidal behavior, continuation for longer than 1 year might be recommended. If the patient preferred to continue the medication indefinitely to avoid or minimize the chance of relapse, this would also be appropriate (see APA, 2000). Gradual tapering is always recommended whenever an attempt is made to discontinue the antidepressant treatment.

Anxiety Disorders

Generalized Anxiety Disorder (GAD) is characterized by multiple worries about multiple different topics, occurring for 6 months or more, and accompanied by somatic symptoms such as muscle tension, fatigue, and insomnia. The reader will note that there is some overlap between the symptoms of depression and GAD. These two disorders often co-occur, so treatment of both conditions concomitantly is often the rule. The mainstay of the pharmacological treatment of GAD is antidepressant treatment. While there is some variation in official FDA indications, the preponderance of evidence shows that all SSRIs are effective in the treatment of GAD. Thus, the clinician can choose from sertraline, fluoxetine, paroxetine, citalopram, escitalopram, or fluvoxamine, based on side effect profile, family history of response, clinician experience, and patient preference.

The SNRIs, such as venlafaxine and duloxetine are also effective in the treatment of GAD. It should be noted that SSRIs and SNRIs are effective in the treatment of other anxiety disorders as well, including panic disorder and social anxiety disorder. Nonantidepressant treatment of GAD includes buspirone, a 5-HT-1a receptor partial agonist. Buspirone is only useful and effective for GAD, and not for other anxiety disorders, in contrast with the SSRIs and SNRIs (see Table 2 for other medications for anxiety and their dosing). Buspirone may also be used as an augmenting agent when combined with SSRIs for the treatment of depression and/or anxiety. When antidepressants or buspirone are ineffective, benzodiazepines may be used to treat GAD. However, this should usually be avoided in first responders because of the risk of dependence and addiction, and the potential for side effects such as sedation or cognitive blunting, that could impair their job performance. The danger of withdrawal symptoms with benzodiazepines is also real and can include a dangerous withdrawal state that includes the risk of seizures, as will be described in more detail below.

As with depression, the treatment of anxiety can also be accomplished with psychotherapy, either alone or with medication. Generalized anxiety disorder, and indeed other anxiety disorders, such as panic disorder and social anxiety disorder, are often chronic and tend to require ongoing maintenance medication therapy to keep the symptoms in remission. This is important to discuss at the outset of treatment with the first responder so the expectations of the need for ongoing treatment

Table 2 Anxiolytic medications other than antidepressants

Benzodiazepine (C-IV)	Brand	Usual dosage range	Approx. Equivalent
Long-Acting			
Chlordiazepoxide	Librium	15–100 mg/day (200 mg)	10
Diazepam	Valium	2–60 mg/day	5
Clonazepam	Klonopin	1.5–10 mg/day (20 mg)	0.25
Clorazepate	Tranxene	7.5–60 mg/day	7.5
Shorter-Acting			
Alprazolam	Xanax	0.75–4 mg/day (8 mg)	0.5
Lorazepam	Ativan	2–6 mg/day (10 mg)	1
Oxazepam	Serax	30–120 mg/day	15
Other anxiolytics	Brand	Usual dosage range	Clinical considerations
Buspirone	Buspar	15–60 mg/day	Only FDA-approved for GAD May help as an adjunctive tx. Nonaddicting
Diphenhydramine	Benadryl	25–200 mg/day	SEs (sedation, anticholinergic)
Hydroxyzine	Vistaril	50–400 mg/day	Mild SEs (sedation, mild anticholinergic)
Propranolol (antihypertensive)	Inderal	40–160 mg/day	Used for Performance Anxiety (dec. cardiac/physical response) May have use in therapy when processing trauma memories

are openly discussed and explored. The doses of antidepressants required for the treatment of anxiety disorders and maintenance treatment are often equal to, or larger, than the doses required for depression.

Panic Disorder

Panic disorder is characterized by recurrent, unexpected panic attacks (Roberts, 2019). In a panic attack, the individual experiences a sudden onset of extreme anxiety, along with physical symptoms that usually include palpitations, sweating, dizziness, nausea, tingling sensations, and chest pressure. In panic disorder, the individual exhibits excessive worry about having another panic attack and avoidant behavior to minimize exposure to anxiety-provoking situations or environments. The effects of a panic attack usually peak within minutes. Panic attacks may occur in many contexts, such as phobias or other anxiety disorders, and are not themselves an anxiety disorder per se. When they occur unexpectedly ("out of the blue"), and are accompanied by a month or more of the fear of having another panic attack, then the criteria for panic disorder are met.

As with many of the conditions that we treat in first responders, SSRIs are the mainstay of the treatment of panic disorder. Only the SSRIs (fluoxetine, paroxetine, and sertraline) are FDA-approved for panic disorder, but all SSRIs have been shown to be efficacious. The SNRI venlafaxine is also FDA-approved for the treatment of panic disorder. A potential disadvantage to some patients is that there is a delay in the onset of effectiveness of the SSRI for anxiety disorders for several weeks. Indeed, at the beginning of treatment, SSRIs may exacerbate anxiety and trigger panic attacks. Thus, the rule of thumb is that the treatment of anxiety disorders needs to be started with a low dose and titrated slowly. For example, a 5 mg daily dose of escitalopram may be prescribed for the first week or so, and, if well-tolerated, may then be increased to 10 mg per day (and higher if needed over time). While anxiety disorders may require doses as high or higher than those needed for depression, the dosages must be started lower and titrated more slowly when treating anxiety disorders. If the anxiety is exacerbated due to starting with too high a dose or raising the dose too rapidly, this may lead to a lack of adherence to the treatment regimen, and the first responder may become frustrated with the treatment and not continue.

During the initial weeks while the SSRI is being titrated to a therapeutic dosage (see Table 1 for SSRI usual dosage ranges), the anxiety may be controlled by prescribing a benzodiazepine for the short term to reduce and/or prevent the panic attacks, or their early worsening with the SSRI. The benzodiazepines alprazolam and clonazepam are FDA-approved for panic disorder, although, like the SSRIs, benzodiazepines as a class can manage anxiety. Clonazepam may be preferable due to its longer half-life and resulting slightly lower potential for misuse. After a few weeks of treatment with the benzodiazepine, and once the SSRI has reached therapeutic dosage levels and a reduction in anxiety has been observed, a gradual tapering of the benzodiazepine can be undertaken. Usually, the patient is able to maintain good control of the panic disorder with an SSRI or SNRI alone, without the need for an ongoing routine/daily dose of benzodiazepine. After the benzodiazepine has been tapered and discontinued, patients often find it reassuring to have on hand a very small number of benzodiazepine (usually alprazolam or clonazepam) tablets to take on an as-needed (PRN) basis at the earliest signs of a panic attack. At the beginning of treatment, it is preferable to prevent panic attacks from occurring; however, once they are well controlled, having a backup medication to take as needed is reassuring. Many patients use this PRN medication very sparingly, keeping a backup tablet for weeks or months to take if needed. As with other anxiety disorders, the use of benzodiazepines should be avoided in a first responder who is actively drinking alcohol or misusing other addictive substances. They may be used in caution in individuals with a history of difficulties with alcohol or drugs that are currently in remission.

Bipolar Disorder

The development of bipolar disorder is not expected as a consequence of being a first responder. Nevertheless, bipolar disorder may present, or be exacerbated while working as a first responder, and thus its management is important. The medications to manage bipolar disorder, both acutely, and for maintenance and prevention of relapse of the mood episodes of mania or depression include the four classic mood stabilizers: lithium, valproate, carbamazepine, and lamotrigine, along with some antipsychotic medications that have FDA-approval to manage acute manic or mixed episodes, or acute depressive episodes associated with either bipolar type I or type II. Extensive medical work-ups, including laboratories, such as electrolytes/glucose, liver function tests, renal function tests, complete blood counts, and thyroid function tests, are required before initiating these medications and for the proper monitoring of changes and side effects of these psychotropics. Serum plasma levels may also be drawn at a laboratory to target the dosing of medications such as lithium, carbamazepine (400–1600 mg/day), and valproate, when used to treat bipolar disorder. When considering an antidepressant (e.g., SSRI) to manage a comorbid PTSD or anxiety disorder, in addition to bipolar disorder, the prescriber should exercise caution and increased monitoring to avoid or be able to detect early, the onset or switch to a manic episode, which is a concern when prescribing antidepressants to a person with bipolar disorder. Other unique issues with some mood stabilizers, such as lamotrigine and carbamazepine, are the risk for significant dermatological reactions, including the rare but potentially deadly Stevens-Johnson Syndrome.

As there is no rule against a person with bipolar disorder becoming a first responder, or if they became a first responder before the onset of their bipolar disorder, the clinician should discuss the clinical issues of both bipolar I and bipolar II with the patient, as some treatments are similar, and the presentation and risk of depression and suicide are significant.

Bipolar I disorder is characterized by the presence of manic episodes, consisting of at least 1 week of an elevated and expansive (or irritable) mood, accompanied by increased energy or activity, grandiosity, rapid thoughts and speech, distractibility, increase in goal-directed activity, and excessive involvement in activities with negative consequences (loss of judgment). Bipolar I disorder may or may not also include major depressive episodes. The presence of one manic episode is sufficient for the diagnosis of bipolar I disorder. This is a chronic, persistent disorder that requires ongoing treatment, almost always with medication, to prevent relapse. The manic episodes of bipolar I disorder are characterized by marked impairment in functioning, the need for hospitalization to prevent harm to self or others, or the presence of psychotic symptoms (APA, 2022).

Bipolar II disorder is characterized by the presence of hypomanic episodes and major depressive episodes. The depressive episodes of bipolar II disorder may be quite severe, and the overall suicide risk in bipolar II disorder is thought to be greater than that of bipolar I disorder (usually attributable to the severity of the depressive episodes). The hypomanic episodes of bipolar II disorder are characterized by the same symptoms as bipolar I disorder, but the duration of the episodes is only required to be at least four consecutive days, and the level of impairment is not marked. The change in functioning in a hypomanic episode is described as an observable change in mood and behavior that does not cause marked impairment. It also does not include psychotic symptoms and does not require hospitalization.

Thus, the hypomanic episodes of bipolar II disorder are less severe than the manic episodes of bipolar I disorder. Most individuals with bipolar I disorder also experience major depressive episodes during the course of their illness, but this is not a requirement for the diagnosis. The presence of at least one major depressive episode is a requirement for the diagnosis of bipolar II disorder. These depressive episodes may be quite severe, with a greatly elevated risk of suicide for the individual. Between episodes, individuals with bipolar I or bipolar II disorder may function quite well. They may be able to work as a first responder during these periods of stability, and the importance of maintaining their stability with adequate mood-stabilizing medication is paramount. While there may be some differences in FDA indications, for the most part, the treatment of bipolar I and bipolar II disorders are quite similar in practice. In the description below, we will combine bipolar I and bipolar II disorders and call them bipolar disorders.

Lithium is the gold standard of treatment for bipolar disorders. Lithium is indicated for the treatment of acute manic episodes, as well as maintenance to prevent relapse. This section will focus, for the most part, on maintenance treatment. First responders experiencing acute manic episodes leading to impaired judgment, as described above, may require hospitalization to achieve stability. Of course, the stigma involved with psychiatric hospitalization must be kept in mind as the treatment plan is developed and discussed with the patient. Lithium (600–2400 mg/day) maintenance treatment requires monitoring of blood tests, including lithium blood levels, thyroid function tests, and renal function tests. Lithium toxicity can occur even at slightly elevated levels and may consist of excessive thirst, frequent urination, tremor, nausea, vomiting, and cognitive changes, although some patients may experience these side effects with normal dosing. The treatment of severe lithium toxicity is hemodialysis. Lithium is quite dangerous in overdose, and this must be taken into consideration for patients who are experiencing suicidal ideation.

Some anticonvulsants have also been shown in many studies to function as mood stabilizers (Roberts, 2019). Divalproex is primarily used for the acute treatment of manic episodes and the prevention of relapse of manic episodes, but it also has been shown to have some efficacy against depressive episodes as well. Blood levels should be monitored, and liver function tests need to be checked periodically as well. Side effects of divalproex include nausea and vomiting, tremor, sedation, pancreatitis, hepatotoxicity, and hematologic effects, making the monitoring of complete blood counts important. Divalproex is often combined with other mood-stabilizing medications for the treatment of bipolar disorders.

Lamotrigine is another anticonvulsant that plays an important role in the treatment of bipolar disorders. It is indicated for maintenance treatment to prevent relapse of mood episodes and has more efficacy for the prevention of depressive episodes than manic or hypomanic episodes. Lamotrigine (50–400 mg/day) is often combined with lithium and may be combined with divalproex (valproate PLUS_SPI valproic acid = divalproex [Depakote] at 500–3000 mg/day); however, an interaction between valproic acid and lamotrigine requires lowering the lamotrigine dose when combined. The most serious side effect of lamotrigine is Stevens-Johnson Syndrome (FDA-approved labeling), a severe, life-threatening rash that requires discontinuation of the lamotrigine. Patients must be instructed to discontinue lamotrigine at the onset of any rash, and should be evaluated by a dermatologist.

Many of the second-generation antipsychotics are useful in the treatment of bipolar disorders, either alone or in combination with other mood-stabilizing medications. Many individuals with bipolar disorders require combinations of two or three medications to ensure adequate mood stability; this can be done safely with appropriate monitoring of clinical parameters and blood tests.

Table 3 shows the second-generation antipsychotics and their indications for the treatment of bipolar disorders. Note that these antipsychotics are beneficial for bipolar disorders even in the absence of psychotic symptoms; however, they do play an important role in managing an acutely manic patient who is also psychotic. One particular advantage of the use of second-generation antipsychotics in the treatment of bipolar disorders is in the management of acute depressive episodes that occur in an otherwise stable patient who is being maintained on mood-stabilizing medications. For example, a patient with bipolar I disorder may be prescribed therapeutic doses of lithium in combination with divalproex and may present after several years of mood stability with a major depressive episode. Interestingly, SSRIs and SNRIs are *not* indicated in this situation. They have not been shown to be effective for acute bipolar depression, and they have the added liability that they may precipitate a manic episode in these patients, even in the presence of mood-stabilizing medication. There are, however, several second-generation antipsychotics that are indicated for acute bipolar depression. These include quetiapine, lusrasidone, cariprazine, lumateperone, and the combination of olanzapine with fluoxetine (known as Symbyax). These medications may be added to a mood stabilizer to effectively treat a depressive episode in a patient with bipolar disorder, with little or no chance of precipitating a manic episode. (See Table 3 for the indications of second-generation antipsychotics in the treatment of bipolar disorders.)

When prescribing second-generation antipsychotics, patients must be monitored for the development of abnormal movements (referred to as extrapyramidal symptoms or EPS) and for tardive dyskinesia (TD). While the chances of developing TD are much lower with second-generation antipsychotics than with first-generation antipsychotics, such as haloperidol or chlorpromazine, there is still a possible incidence of 0.8%, or higher, per year, depending on other factors, such as age, substance use, and the presence of mood disorder (Correll et al., 2004).

Patients should be examined for abnormal movements at baseline and again at least once a year, using the AIMS (Abnormal Involuntary Movement Scale), and the presence or absence of abnormal movements should be documented in the medical record. Patients receiving second-generation antipsychotics should also be monitored for the development of metabolic syndrome, which includes weight gain, increased abdominal girth, hyperlipidemia, and elevated fasting blood sugar. This monitoring can also help to monitor the general health of first responders who are taking psychotropic medications; and, referrals should be made for control of blood lipids, and blood pressure, when indicated.

When choosing a mood stabilizer to treat a first responder who has been diagnosed with bipolar disorder, several considerations should be taken into account.

Table 3 Antipsychotic agents (used as mood stabilizers and to augment antidepressants)

Generic	Brand	Dose	Sedation	EPS	Notes
Phenothiazines (FwO)					
Chlorpromazine	Thorazine	50–2000 mg/day	+++	+++	1st marketed AP, EPS
Thioridazine	Mellaril	50–800 mg/day	PLUS_SPI PLUS_SPI PLUS_SPI PLUS_SPI	++	Pigmentary retinopathy, QT changes, sedation, very anticholinergic
Perphenazine	Trilafon	8–64 mg/day	++	+++	Tx. for Intractable hiccups CATIE trial arm
Trifluoperazine	Stelazine	2–40 mg/day	++	+++	
Fluphenazine	Prolixin	2–40 mg/day	+	PLUS_SPI PLUS_SPI PLUS_SPI PLUS_SPI	Depot LAI/high EPS
Other					
Thiothixene	Navane	5–60 mg/day	++	+++	
Haloperidol	Haldol (Depot)	1–100 mg/day (50–450 mg/month)	+	PLUS_SPI PLUS_SPI PLUS_SPI PLUS_SPI	Depot LAI/high EPS
Loxapine*	Loxitane Adasuve	20–250 mg/day 10 mg PRN inhaled	++	++	Met. = amoxapine BW: bronchospasm
Molindone*	Moban	15–225 mg/day	++	++	Weight loss/no longer available in US
Atypical APs					
Clozapine	Clozaril	75–900 mg/day	PLUS_SPI PLUS_SPI PLUS_SPI PLUS_SPI	−/+	Low EPS, agranulocytosis, seizures, anticholinergic, sialorrhea, orthostasis, wt. gain
Risperidone	Risperdal (Consta LAI)	1–16 mg/day* (25–50 mg/2 weeks)	−/+	+*	Dose-related EPS, orthostatic hypotension, inc. PRL; **LAI**

(continued)

Table 3 (continued)

Generic	Brand	Dose	Sedation	EPS	Notes
Olanzapine	Zyprexa (Zydis & Inj.) (Relprevv LAI)	5–20 mg/day (150–300 mg/2–4 weeks)	+++	+	Low EPS, **weight gain**, sedation, anticholinergic; **LAI**
Quetiapine	Seroquel (XR)	200–800 mg/day	+++	−/+	Low EPS, sedation, orthostatic hypotension, BPD
Ziprasidone	Geodon	40–160 mg/day	+	+	Low EPS, GI distress, QT warnings, low wt. gain
Aripiprazole	Abilify (Maintena LAI) (Aristada LAI)	10–30 mg/day 300–400 mg/month 441-882-1064 mg/month (6w/8w)	−/+	+	Low EPS, N&V, HA, insomnia agitation, low wt. gain
Paliperidone	Invega (Sustenna LAI)	3–12 mg/day 39–234 mg/month	−/+	+	Low EPS, low wt. gain **LAI** available. / PP3M = Trinza*
Iloperidone	Fanapt	2–24 mg/day	+	+	Low EPS, low wt. gain, QT warnings
Asenapine	Saphris Secuado	5–20 mg/day SL 3.8–7.6 mg/day TD	++	+	Low EPS, low wt. gain, sublingual form/flavored/ daily patch
Lurasidone	Latuda	40–160 mg/day	+	+	Low EPS, low metabolic SEs Also for Bipolar Depression
Brexpiprazole	Rexulti	1–4 mg/day	+	+	Also approved as adjunct for MDD
Cariprazine	Vraylar	1.5–6 mg/day	+	PLUS_SPI / PLUS_ SPI PLUS_SPI	D2/D3 Partial agonist Also approved for Mania & BPD
Lumateperone	Caplyta	42 mg/day	++	+	5-HT/DA antagonist/modulator, sedation, dry mouth
Olanzapine PLUS_SPI Samidorphan	Lybalvi	5, 10, 15, 20 mg of olanzapine PLUS_SPI 10 mg samidorphan	+++	+	Indicated for schizophrenia and bipolar I disorder (acute and maintenance) Reduced risk of significant weight gain

The need for frequent blood monitoring is more present with medications, such as lithium and divalproex, and this may discourage adherence to these regimens. Lithium is the only mood-stabilizing medication that has been shown to reduce suicidal ideation and behavior in bipolar disorders (Baldessarini et al., 2001). This may be important in choosing the mood-stabilizing regimen for a first responder who has experienced frequent recurrences of suicidal ideation. There is some evidence that augmenting antidepressants with lithium in patients with major depressive disorder may also reduce suicidal thoughts and behaviors in these individuals (APA, 2000; Cipriani et al., 2005).

Substance Use Disorders

Alcohol detoxification is done by tapering doses of benzodiazepines. For safety, detoxification is best done in an inpatient setting, either a dedicated detoxification unit; or, for more serious cases of alcohol use disorder, in a hospital setting. Close medical monitoring is necessary. Traditionally, lorazepam and chlordiazepoxide are the most commonly used benzodiazepines for alcohol detoxification, but others, such as diazepam or clonazepam, may be used. Lorazepam has the advantage of one-step metabolism in the liver and is also available in oral, intramuscular, and intravenous forms. The latter may be used in the medical setting (medical ward or intensive care unit) for severe cases of withdrawal. The goal of treating withdrawal is to prevent serious, life-threatening complications such as delirium tremens (Shuckit, 2014) or withdrawal seizures. Once the patient is stable enough for outpatient treatment, detoxification may be continued using long-acting oral benzodiazepines such as chlordiazepoxide. Close outpatient monitoring, usually in a partial hospitalization program dedicated to the detoxification of alcohol, is indicated.

Treatment of benzodiazepine withdrawal is very similar to alcohol withdrawal. Alcohol and benzodiazepines both potentiate inhibitory GABA receptors in the brain, and their withdrawal precipitates the hyperexcitable states that lead to seizures and delirium. Benzodiazepine detoxification consists of gradual tapering doses of benzodiazepines, similar to alcohol withdrawal treatment. Particular attention must be paid during alcohol detoxification to the patient's overall physical health and to the administration of adequate fluids, as well as B Vitamins, particularly thiamine. Thiamine deficiency can lead to severe neurological sequelae including Wernicke's encephalopathy and Korsakoff Syndrome (Isenberg-Grzeda et al., 2012). These can lead to irreversible memory deficits and are avoided by administering adequate dosages of thiamine during the detoxification period.

Once the first responder has completed a detoxification program, aftercare should include psychotherapy and often support programs such as alcoholics anonymous (AA) to help maintain sobriety. Medications also play a role in maintaining sobriety. The following medications have been shown to be effective in reducing the chance of relapse in alcohol use disorder: Disulfiram, a medication that blocks the metabolism of alcohol by inhibiting the enzyme aldehyde dehydrogenase (Mutschler et al., 2016). Aversive symptoms, such as flushing, nausea, vomiting, and headache, occur if an individual drinks while taking disulfiram. Because of the associated medical risks of the disulfiram/alcohol interaction, its use should be reserved for individuals who are in relatively good health, are highly motivated to maintain abstinence, and are closely supervised. Naltrexone is available in oral form and a long-acting injectable form. It has shown great promise as a medication to help prevent relapse in alcohol use disorder. Side effects include nausea and sedation, and its use requires monitoring of liver function tests. Overall, it is very well-tolerated and effective. It reduces the craving for alcohol and helps prevent the progression of alcohol use from mild to severe. The long-acting injectable form of naltrexone is useful in individuals who are not adherent to daily oral medications and may be helpful in the treatment of first responders who are reluctant to take medication every day. Acamprosate is another medication that is useful in maintaining abstinence from alcohol and is metabolized by the kidney, so it can be used in individuals with liver disease. Of these three medications, the current state of evidence favors the use of naltrexone as a medication to prevent relapse of alcohol use in patients with alcohol use disorder.

Opioid Use Disorder (Medication-Assisted Treatment)

Opioid use disorder is a serious, life-threatening disorder. Overdose deaths from opioids, including prescription opioids, heroin, and synthetic opioids, like fentanyl, have increased more than eightfold since 1999 (Centers for Disease Control and Prevention, 2021). Almost 69,000 people died from opioid overdoses in 2020, and more than 82% of those deaths involved synthetic opioids (Hedegaard et al., 2021). Opioid use disorder is associated with increased criminality, violence, HIV, hepatitis C, poor quality of life, and mortality (Hulse et al., 1999).

Opioid withdrawal is not life-threatening unless the patient is frail due to age, physical illness, or both. This is in contrast to the withdrawal from alcohol or benzodiazepines, which is life-threatening, primarily due to the association of seizures and delirium with severe withdrawal states. While not life-threatening, opioid withdrawal is uncomfortable, to say the least. Patients develop symptoms such as muscle and bone pain, nausea, vomiting, diarrhea, piloerection (gooseflesh), yawning, agitation, and insomnia. These withdrawal symptoms can be quantified using the Clinical Opiate Withdrawal Scale (COWS) (Wesson & Ling, 2003). Opioid withdrawal is treated symptomatically, by prescribing anti-nausea and anti-diarrheal medications, nonaddictive medications for insomnia and anxiety (e.g., hydroxyzine), and medications such as clonidine to treat autonomic hyperarousal (Gold et al., 1980). A young, healthy person may choose to go "cold turkey," and withdraw from opiates with no medical treatment or observation. This should be discouraged, even in physically healthy first responders who may feel this is the best approach.

Maintenance of abstinence in opioid use disorder can be achieved with several approaches. Methadone is a full opioid agonist at the opioid mu receptor, with a long half-life. It is generally safe, but must be closely monitored because there is a risk of fatal overdose. Methadone may be used for the maintenance of sobriety and also plays a role in detoxification therapy.

Naltrexone, an opioid receptor antagonist, has been show to block the euphoric effects of opioids and may be used for relapse prevention. Extended-release injectable naltrexone is also useful. This is similar to the use described above for the maintenance of alcohol abstinence. There is a danger that patients taking naltrexone may lose the tolerance they had built up to opioids. Therefore, if they stop taking naltrexone and relapse to previous levels of opioid use, they could develop a fatal overdose (Saucier et al., 2018).

The combination of buprenorphine with naloxone (Suboxone) is currently used frequently to maintain abstinence from opioids (Soyka, 2015). The combination is usually administered sublingually. Buprenorphine is a partial opioid agonist, and it exhibits a ceiling effect, so it is less dangerous than methadone in overdose. It is absorbed orally and is usually given sublingually. Naloxone is not absorbed orally or sublingually but is a potent blocker of opioid activity (antagonist) if injected. Including naloxone with the preparation of buprenorphine serves to help prevent the diversion and injection of buprenorphine by the individual who is addicted to opioids. The combination treatment of buprenorphine with naloxone (known as Suboxone) has become widely available and useful in the treatment of opioid use disorder. Special training and licensing for physicians prescribing so-called Medically Assisted Therapies (MAT) for opioid use disorder are widely available. Policies regarding such training are being liberalized to help make it easier for patients to obtain MAT. First responders who have achieved abstinence from opioid use could benefit greatly from continued treatment with MAT, such as Suboxone, along with appropriate therapy and support groups such as Narcotics Anonymous. Naloxone is a potent antagonist of opioid receptors and can provide a lifesaving reversal of the effects of opioid overdose, particularly respiratory suppression. The widespread availability of naloxone with fewer restrictions has been a lifesaving development. First responders, such as paramedics and police officers, are very familiar with its use, and if they are struggling with opioid addiction themselves, it could be lifesaving. It is possible in the near future that naloxone will be widely available as an over-the-counter medication without the requirement of a doctor's prescription. Any individual struggling with opioid addiction should be given access to naloxone to keep on hand in the event of an overdose. Particularly dangerous are overdoses with opioid preparations that are laced with extremely potent opioids, such as fentanyl, which is 100 times as potent as morphine. Overdoses involving fentanyl are often fatal and can only be reversed by the rapid administration of the opioid antagonist naloxone (also known by the brand name Narcan). (See Table 4 for medications used in the treatment of opioid use disorder and alcohol use disorder.)

Table 4 Medications used for alcohol use disorder and opioid use disorder (MAT)

Generic	Brand	Dose	Notes
Disulfiram	Antabuse	125–500 mg po once per day	Significant and dangerous reaction if consume alcohol while taking disulfiram
Acamprosate	Campral	666 mg po three times per day	Well-tolerated; not punitive if consume alcohol
Naltrexone	Revia Vivitrol	50–100 mg po once per day 380 mg as LAI every month	Well-tolerated; not punitive if consume alcohol. Monitor liver function tests Indicated for both alcohol and opioid dependence
Burprenorphine	Subutex	2–24* mg/day SL	Sublingual film; dose is the amount of buprenorphine
Buprenorphine (with naloxone)	Suboxone	2–24* mg/day SL	
Methadone		10–120 mg/day po per day at clinic as liquid	Dispensed only by Opioid Treatment Programs (OTPs) certified by the Federal Substance Abuse and Mental Health Services Administration (SAMHSA) and registered by the Drug Enforcement Administration (DEA)

Insomnia

Medications used to treat insomnia are outlined in Table 5. Medications from several different classes have been shown to be effective and safe. This section will summarize recommendations from recent practice guidelines for treating insomnia in adults (Qaseem et al., 2016; Sateia et al., 2017). Low-dose doxepin, a tricyclic antidepressant, has been found to be safe and effective, and is not addictive. Dosages of 10 mg or less have a very good side effect profile and are, therefore, well-tolerated. The antidepressant mirtazapine is very effective for insomnia and is recommended for treating insomnia in depressed patients. This would be particularly useful in a first responder suffering from insomnia related to PTSD and depression. Ramelteion, a melatonin receptor agonist, has good safety and efficacy and is not addictive. Benzodiazepines, such as clonazepam, diazepam, or alprazolam, are generally not recommended due to their potential for addiction and dependence. "Z-drugs" (GABA receptor agonists similar to benzodiazepines), such as solpidem, zaleplon, and eszopiclone are recommended by the American Academy of Sleep Medicine and American College of Physicians for treating insomnia in adults. However, they carry some potential for addiction and dependence, although not as much as benzodiazepines. Nonaddictive medications, such as doxepin, mirtazapine, and ramelteon, should be strongly considered when treating insomnia in first responders, due to their efficacy, good side effect profile, and low potential for addiction.

Table 5 Medications used to treat insomnia

Sedative-Hypnotics (C-II-IV)	Brand	Usual dosage range	Clinical considerations
Zolpidem (C-IV)	Ambien	2.5–10 mg/HS	For insomnia only Cases of amnesia and odd behaviors*
Zaleplon (C-IV)	Sonata	5–20 mg/HS	"
Eszopiclone (C-IV)	Lunesta	1–3 mg/HS	"
Barbiturates (C-II-IV)	Various (Nembutal, Mysoline, Seconal, Phenobarbital)	Various	Fatal with OD Popular with patients seeking suicide, often obtained illegally
Ramelteon	Rozerem	8 mg/HS	Melatonin receptor agonist, not a controlled substance
Tasimelteon	Hetlioz	20 mg/HS	Melatonin receptor agonist FDA-approved for Non-24 sleep-wake disorder
Doxepin	Silenor	3–6 mg/HS	Old TCA, the strongest antihistamine, is not a controlled substance
Trazodone	Desyrel	25–150 mg/HS	Very common off-label use of low-doses of Trazodone for insomnia
Mirtazapine	Remeron	7.5–15 mg/HS	Common off-label use of low doses of mirtazapine For insomnia (higher doses are less sedating)
Suvorexant (C-IV)	Belsomra	5–20 mg/HS	Orexin receptor antagonist Possible cataplexy, sleep paralysis, hallucinations
Lemborexant (C-IV)	Dayvigo	5–10 mg/HS	Orexin receptor antagonist
Daridorexant	Quviviq	25–50 mg/HS	Orexin receptor antagonist
Flurazepam	Dalmane	7.5–30 mg/HS	Controlled substances; risk for dependency/addiction
Temazepam	Restoril	7.5–30 mg/HS	
Triazolam	Halcion	0.125–0.25 mg/HS	
Estazolam	Prosom	1–2 mg/HS	
Quazepam	Doral	7.5–15 mg/HS	
Prazosin		1–15 mg/HS	May reduce nightmares in PTSD

Summary

We have outlined in this chapter an approach to treating disorders and symptoms that commonly occur in first responders. Due to the stressful and often traumatic nature of their work, first responders are particularly vulnerable to PTSD,

Table 6 FDA-approved indications of the 'antipsychotics' in adults, other than schizophrenia

Generic	Brand	Bipolar I – Mania as Monotherapy	Bipolar I – Mania as Adjunct to Lithium or Valproate	Bipolar I – Depression Monotherapy	Bipolar I – Depression as Adjunct with Lithium or Valproate	Bipolar II – Depression	Maintenance Monotherapy for Bipolar I Disorder	Maintenance as Adjunct with Lithium or Valproate for Bipolar I Disorder	Adjunct for Refractory Depression with an Antidepressant	Generalized, Nonpsychotic Anxiety	Agitation Associated with Bipolar I Disorder or Schizophrenia
Aripiprazole	Abilify	✓					✓	✓	✓		
	Abilify Inj.										✓
	Abilify Maintena LAI						✓				
Asenapine	Saphris	✓	✓				✓				
Brexpiprazole	Rexulti								✓		
Cariprazine	Vraylar	✓		✓					✓		
Loxapine	Adasuve Inhalation										✓
Lumateperone	Caplyta			✓	✓	✓					
Lurasidone	Latuda			✓	✓						
Olanzapine	Zyprexa	✓	✓				✓				
	Zyprexa Inj.										✓
Olanzapine PLUS_SPI Fluoxetine	Symbyax			✓					For Resistant Depression		
Olanzapine PLUS_SPI Samidorphan	Lybalvi	✓	✓				✓				

Prochlorperazine	Compazine									✓	
Quetiapine	Seroquel (XR)	✓	✓	✓		✓		✓	✓		
Risperidone	Risperdal	✓	✓								
Risperidone	Risperdal Consta – LAI						✓	✓			
Trifluoperazine	Stelazine									✓	
Ziprasidone	Geodon	✓						✓			

Table 7 FDA-approved indications, other than major depression, of the orally available 'antidepressants' in adults

Generic	Brand	Posttraumatic Stress Disorder	Panic Disorder	Generalized Anxiety Disorder	Social Anxiety Disorder	Chronic Pain (Diabetic Peripheral Neuropathy, Fibromyalgia, Musculoskeletal)	Insomnia	Obsessive – Compulsive Disorder	Premenstrual Dysphoric Disorder (PMDD)	Bulimia Nervosa	Smoking Cessation	Seasonal Affective Disorder
Bupropion	Wellbutrin										as Zyban	✓ M
Clomipramine	Anafranil							✓				
Doxepin	Silenor						✓					
Duloxetine	Cymbalta			✓		✓						
Escitalopram	Lexapro			✓								
Fluoxetine	Prozac		✓					✓	✓*	✓		
Fluvoxamine	Luvox				✓			✓				
Paroxetine	Paxil (CR)	✓	✓	✓	✓			✓	✓			
Sertraline	Zoloft	✓	✓		✓			✓	✓			
Venlafaxine	Effexor (XR)		✓	✓	✓							

depression, anxiety, and insomnia. A pharmacologic approach may be very helpful for these individuals when their symptoms are severe enough to cause significant impairment in their functioning, or significant distress in their everyday lives. A multimodal approach that includes psychotherapy is usually preferable, but not always available, due to a lack of available therapy resources or due to a reluctance on the part of the first responder to participate in therapy. When prescribing medication for first responders, the prescriber should be aware of the many factors that might interfere with the treatment, including misunderstandings about the goals of treatment, preconceived notions about side effects, and, most importantly, about the stigma involved in taking psychotropic medications.

First responders are, by the nature of their occupations, focused on helping others and seeing themselves as strong and invulnerable. Seeking help, particularly medication, may be perceived by them or their peers as a sign of weakness. Awareness of these factors by the prescriber, and a frank, open, and ongoing discussion with the first responder prior to beginning treatment, and on an ongoing basis as treatment continues, can be a very important factor in increasing the chances of adherence to the treatment plan. If the first responder is willing and able to adhere to the prescribed treatment regimen, the chances of successful treatment are greatly improved. Please refer to Tables 6 and 7 for further information regarding the FDA approved indications of selected medications. First responders deserve nothing less than the best we can give them in our approach to their treatment. As treatment providers, our approach should be evidence-based, empathic, and compassionate. Overcoming the stigma associated with medication treatment should be paramount.

References

American Psychiatric Association. (2000). Practice guideline for the treatment of patients with major depressive disorder (Rev.). *The American Journal of Psychiatry, 157*(4), 1–45.

American Psychiatric Association. (2022). *Diagnostic and statistical manual of mental disorders* (5th ed., text rev.). https://doi.org/10.1176/appi.books.9780890425787

Baker, J. F., Cates, M. E., & Luthin, D. R. (2018, March). D-cycloserine in the treatment of posttraumatic stress disorder. *Mental Health Clinician, 7*(2), 88–94.

Baldessarini, R. J., Tondo, L., & Hennen, J. (2001). Treating the suicidal patient with bipolar disorder: Reducing suicide risk with lithium. *Annals of the New York Academy of Sciences, 932*, 24–43.

Beauchamp, A. M., Weerakoon, S. M., Ponder, W. N., & Jetelina, K. K. (2022). Possible substance use disorders among first responders during the COVID-19 era: A quasi-experimental study of personal and residential vulnerability. *The American Journal of Drug and Alcohol Abuse, 48*(6), 724–733. https://doi.org/10.1080/00952990.2022.2088376

Brady, K., Pearlstein, T., Asnis, G. M., Baker, D., Rothbaum, B., Sikes, C. R., & Farfel, G. M. (2000). Efficacy and safety of sertraline treatment of posttraumatic stress disorder: A randomized controlled trial. *Journal of the American Medical Association, 283*(14), 1837–1844.

Centers for Disease Control and Prevention. (2021). *Wide-ranging online data for epidemiologic research (WONDER)*. National Center for Health Statistics. http://wonder.cdc.gov

Charney, M. E., Hellberg, S. N., Bui, E., & Simon, N. M. (2018). Evidenced-based treatment of posttraumatic stress disorder: An updated review of validated psychotherapeutic and pharmacological approaches. *Harvard Review of Psychiatry, 26*(3), 99–115.

Cipriani, A., Pretty, H., Hawton, K., & Geddes, J. R. (2005, October). Lithium in the prevention of suicidal behavior and all-cause mortality in patients with mood disorders: A systematic review of randomized trials. *American Journal of Psychiatry, 162*(10), 1805–1819.

Correll, C. U., Leucht, S., & Kane, J. M. (2004). Lower risk for tardive dyskinesia associated with second-generation antipsychotics: A systematic review of 1-year studies. *The American Journal of Psychiatry, 161*(3), 414–425.

Davidson, J. R. (2000). Pharmacotherapy of posttraumatic stress disorder: Treatment options, long-term follow-up, and predictors of outcome. *The Journal of Clinical Psychiatry, 61*(5), 52–59.

Davidson, J. R. (2006). Pharmacologic treatment of acute and chronic stress following trauma: 2006. *The Journal of Clinical Psychiatry, 67*(2), 34–39.

Davidson, J., Baldwin, D., Stein, D. J., Kuper, E., Benattia, I., Ahmed, S., Pedersen, R., & Musgnung, J. (2006). Treatment of posttraumatic stress disorder with venlafaxine extended release: A 6-month randomized controlled trial. *Archives of General Psychiatry, 63*(10), 1158–1165.

Fleurence, R., Williamson, R., Jing, Y., Kim, E., Quynh-Van, T., Pikalov, A. S., & Thase, M. E. (2009). A systematic review of augmentation strategies for patients with major depressive disorder. *Psychopharmacology Bulletin, 42*(3), 57–90.

Gold, M. S., Pottash, A. C., Sweeney, D. R., & Kleber, H. D. (1980). Opiate withdrawal using clonidine: A safe, effective, and rapid non opiate treatment. *Journal of the American Medical Association, 243*(4), 343–346.

Guideline Development Panel for the Treatment of PTSD in Adults, American Psychological Association. (2019). Summary of the clinical practice guideline for the treatment of posttraumatic stress disorder (PTSD) in adults. *American Psychology, 74*(5), 596–607.

Harvey, S. B., Milligan-Saville, J. S., Paterson, H. M., Harkness, E. L., Marsh, A. M., Dobson, M., Kemp, R., & Bryant, R. A. (2016). The mental health of fire-fighters: An examination of the impact of repeated trauma exposure. *The Australian and New Zealand Journal of Psychiatry, 50*(7), 649–658. https://doi.org/10.1177/0004867415615217

Hedegaard, H., Miniño, A. M., Spencer, M. R., & Warner, M. (2021, December). *Drug overdose deaths in the United States, 1999–2020.* National Center for Health Statistics Data Brief No. 428. Centers for Disease Control and Prevention. https://www.cdc.gov/nchs/data/databriefs/db428.pdf

Hetrick, S. E., Purcell, R., Garner, B., & Parslow, R. (2010, July). Combined pharmacotherapy and psychological therapies for post traumatic stress disorder (PTSD). *The Cochrane Database of Systematic Reviews*, (7), CD007316.

Hudson, S. M., Whiteside, T. E., Lorenz, R. A., & Wargo, K. A. (2012). Prazosin for the treatment of nightmares related to posttraumatic stress disorder: A review of the literature. *Primary Care Companion for CNS Disorders, 14*(2), PCC.11r01222.

Hulse, G. K., English, D. R., Milne, E., & Holman, C. D. J. (1999). The quantification of mortality resulting from the regular use of illicit opiates. *Addiction, 94*(2), 221–229.

Isenberg-Grzeda, E., Kutner, H., & Nicolson, S. (2012). Wernicke-Korsakoff-Syndrome: Under-recognized and under-treated. *Psychosomatics, 53*(6), 507–516.

Lipschitz, J. M., Connolly, S. L., Van Boxtel, R., Potter, J. R., Nixon, N., & Bidargaddi, N. (2022). Provider perspectives on telemental health implementation: Lessons learned during the COVID-19 pandemic and paths forward. *Psychological Services*. https://doi.org/10.1037/ser0000625. Advance online publication.

Mutschler, J., Grosshans, M., Soyka, M., & Rosner, S. (2016). Current findings and mechanisms of action of disulfiram in the treatment of alcohol dependence. *Pharmacopsychiatry, 49*(4), 137–141.

Petrosino, N. J., Cosmo, C., Berlow, Y. A., Zandvakili, A., van't Wout-Frank, M., & Philip, N. S. (2021). Transcranial magnetic stimulation for post-traumatic stress disorder. *Therapeutic Advances in Psychopharmacology, 11*, 20451253211049921. https://doi.org/10.1177/20451253211049921

Pruitt, L. D., Luxton, D. D., & Shore, P. (2014). Additional clinical benefits of home-based telemental health treatments. *Professional Psychology: Research and Practice, 45*(5), 340–346.

Qaseem, A., Kansagara, D., Forciea, M. A., Cooke, M., & Denberg, T. (2016). Management of chronic insomnia disorder in adults: A clinical practice guideline from the American College of Physicians. *Annals of Internal Medicine, 165*(2), 125–133.

Roberts, L. W. (2019). *Textbook of psychiatry* (7th ed.). The American Psychiatric Association Publishing.

Rogers, M. L., Gai, A. R., Lieberman, A., Musacchio Schafer, K., & Joiner, T. E. (2022). Why does safety planning prevent suicidal behavior? *Professional Psychology Research and Practice, 53*(1), 33–41.

Rothärmel, M., Benosman, C., El-Hage, W., Berjamin, C., Ribayrol, D., Guillin, O., Gaillard, R., Berkovitch, L., & Moulier, V. (2022). Efficacy and safety of intranasal esketamine in patients with treatment-resistant depression and comorbid chronic post-traumatic stress disorder: Open-label single-arm pilot study. *Frontiers in Psychiatry, 13*, 865466. https://doi.org/10.3389/fpsyt.2022.865466

Sadock, B. J., Sadock, V. A., Ruiz, P., & Kaplan, H. I. (2017). *Kaplan and Sadock's comprehensive textbook of psychiatry* (10th ed.). Wolters Kluwer.

Sateia, M. J., Buysse, D. J., Krystal, A. D., Neubauer, D. N., & Heald, J. L. (2017). Clinical practice guideline for the pharmacologic treatment of chronic insomnia in adults: As American Academy of Sleep Medicine clinical practice guideline. *Journal of Clinical Sleep Medicine, 13*(2), 307–349.

Saucier, R., Wolfe, D., & Dasgupta, N. (2018). Review of case narratives from fatal overdoses associated with injectable naltrexone for opioid dependence. *Drug Safety, 41*(10), 981–988.

Shuckit, M. (2014). Recognition and management of withdrawal delirium (delirium tremens). *New England Journal of Medicine, 371*(22), 2109–2013.

Solmi, M., Veronese, N., Zaninotto, L., Van der Loos, M., Gao, K., Schaffer, A., Reis, C., Normann, C., Anghelescu, I. G., & Correll, C. U. (2016). Lamotrigine compared to placebo and other agents with antidepressant activity in patients with unipolar and bipolar depression: A comprehensive meta-analysis of efficacy and safety outcomes in short-term trials. *CNS Spectrums, 21*(5), 403–418.

Soyka, M. (2015). New developments in the management of opioid dependence, focus on sublingual buprenorphine-naloxone. *Substance Abuse and Rehabilitation, 6*, 1–14.

The Department of Veterans Affairs/Department of Defense Evidence-Based Practice Working Group (EBPWG). (2018). VA/DOD clinical practice guideline for the management of posttraumatic stress disorder and acute stress disorder: Clinician summary. *Focus, 16*(4), 430–448.

Trevizol, A. P., Barros, M. D., Silva, P. O., Osuch, E., Cordeiro, Q., & Shiozawa, P. (2016). Transcranial magnetic stimulation for posttraumatic stress disorder: An updated systematic review and meta-analysis. *Trends in Psychiatry and Psychotherapy, 38*(1), 50–55.

Tucker, P., Zaninelli, R., Yehuda, R., Ruggiero, L., Dillingham, K., & Pitts, C. D. (2001). Paroxetine in the treatment of chronic posttraumatic stress disorder: Results of a placebo-controlled, flexible-dosage trial. *Journal of Clinical Psychiatry, 62*(11), 860–868.

van der Kolk, B. A., Dreyfuss, D., Michaels, M., Shera, D., Berkowitz, R., Fisler, R., & Saxe, G. (1994). Fluoxetine in posttraumatic stress disorder. *The Journal of Clinical Psychiatry, 55*(12), 517–522.

Vargas de Barros, V., Martins, L. F., Saitz, R., Bastos, R. R., & Ronzani, T. M. (2013). Mental health conditions, individual and job characteristics, and sleep disturbances among firefighters. *Journal of Health Psychology, 18*(3), 350–358.

Wesson, D. R., & Ling, W. (2003). The clinical opiate withdrawal scale (COWS*). Journal of Psychoactive Drugs, 35*(2), 253–259.

Wright, L. A., Sijbrandij, M., Sinnerton, R., Lewis, C., Roberts, N. P., & Bisson, J. I. (2019). Pharmacological prevention and early treatment of post-traumatic stress disorder and acute stress disorder: A systematic review and meta-analysis. *Translational Psychiatry, 9*(1), 334.

Virtual Reality Treatments

Deborah C. Beidel, Kathryn D. Sunderman, Ashley T. Winch, and Clint A. Bowers

Traumatic events are ubiquitous. In one worldwide sample, the reported prevalence of exposure to trauma ranged from 55% to 83.1% of the general population. In the United States, an estimated 82.7% of the population has been exposed to a traumatic event (Benjet et al., 2016). Although it appears that the entire population of the United States is at risk of exposure to trauma, as demonstrated in the previous sections of this book, certain groups, including first responders, experience traumatic events at a much higher rate. Given their repeated exposure, first responders are at higher risk for the development of negative mental health consequences. Three interventions, trauma-focused CBT, eye movement desensitization and reprocessing (EMDR), and brief eclectic psychotherapy, have been used to treat first responders with posttraumatic stress disorder (PTSD). However, the number of randomized controlled trials is limited, and results are unclear (Alden et al., 2021). In this chapter, we present the rationale for the use of virtual reality (VR) to enhance psychological treatment for first responders, review the extant literature, present some preliminary data from our center, and consider some future directions.

Psychological Disorders Following Exposure to Traumatic Events in First Responders

Individuals who are most likely to be directly affected by traumatic events are those who have direct exposure to the sights and sounds of the event and those who experience direct injury or threat of injury. Certainly, first responders fit into this high-risk category, with studies suggesting that more than 87,000 law enforcement

D. C. Beidel (✉) · K. D. Sunderman · A. T. Winch · C. A. Bowers
Department of Psychology, University of Central Florida, Orlando, FL, USA
e-mail: Deborah.Beidel@ucf.edu

M. L. Bourke et al. (eds.), *First Responder Mental Health*,
https://doi.org/10.1007/978-3-031-38149-2_15

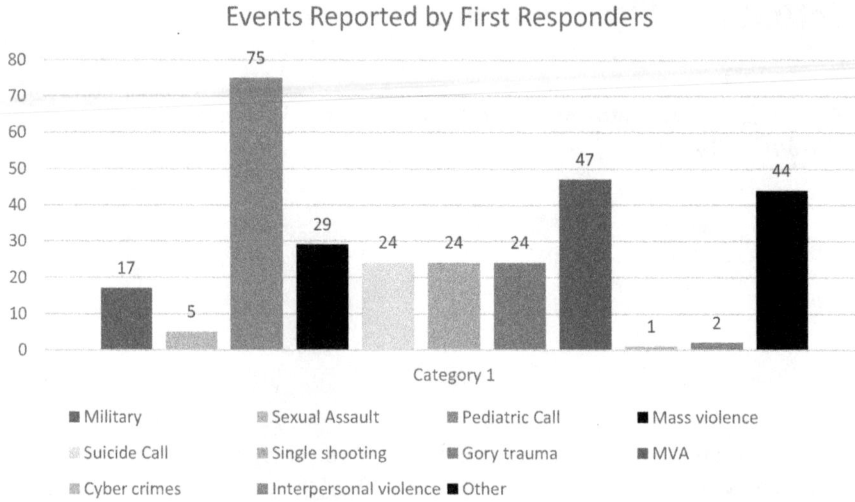

Fig. 1 Traumatic events that lead first responders to seek mental health treatment

officers, 21,000 EMT/paramedics, and 804,000 firefighters may suffer from PTSD (Lewis-Schroeder et al., 2018). Other research indicates that between 10% and 15% of first responders (Klimley et al., 2018), or perhaps as many as approximately one in three first responders, will develop PTSD (SAMHSA, 2018). Traumatic stress and PTSD are unfortunate byproducts of the first responder occupation that can negatively impact a first responder in multiple areas of their life.

Over the last 6 years, our clinical research center has been providing treatment to first responders who developed negative mental health consequences following exposure to a traumatic event. In Fig. 1, we provide an overview of the types of traumatic events experienced by first responders (n = 344) who sought services at our clinic. As illustrated, the most common event precipitating traumatic stress is pediatric calls resulting in severe injury or death. These events account for 26% of all traumatic events represented in our patient population. Motor vehicle accidents (MVA), typically involving horrific injury to the human body, represent 16% of the events that preceded first responders seeking services. It is important to note that while sexual assaults (2%), mass violence (10%), single shootings (8%), etc., are represented as individual categories, there is still a broad range of other types of traumatic events that could not be captured in our categorizations (15%).

It is critical to understand that experiencing a traumatic event may result in many different mental health outcomes. In Fig. 2 (n = 410), we present the diagnoses assigned to first responders seeking treatment at our clinic for trauma-related emotional distress. Our results are slightly skewed as, per our location in Orlando, Florida, we were the site of one of the largest mass shootings and have provided services for many of the first responders involved in that event. As represented in our clinical sample, first responders seeking treatment following exposure to traumatic events have a range of mental health consequences. While 49% of the first

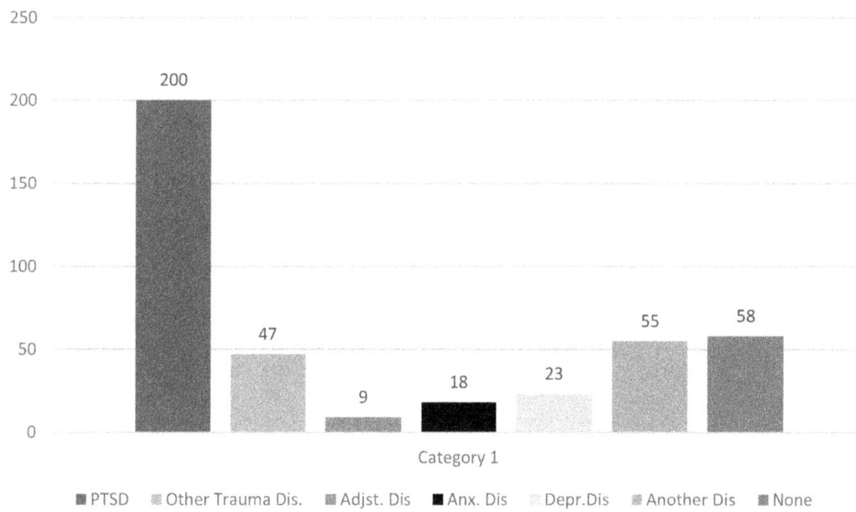

Fig. 2 Diagnoses assigned after seeking treatment for exposure to traumatic events

responders seeking treatment met the criteria for PTSD, it is important to note that 14% of first responders who sought out mental health services did not meet the criteria for a mental health disorder.

Of those who did not meet the criteria for a mental health disorder, a number were required by their command to seek an evaluation because they responded to the Orlando mass shooting or they worked on sensitive topic areas such as sex crimes units. This illustrates the point that not everyone exposed to traumatic events develops a psychological disorder. Nevertheless, and consistent with other reviews of this area (Alden et al., 2021), the predominant disorder for our sample was PTSD, representing 49% of the overall sample, and 57% of those who met the criteria for a mental health disorder. Finally, when restricting the sample to only those individuals with a diagnosis of PTSD, Fig. 3 depicts the traumatic events that precipitated that diagnosis, with pediatric calls representing the largest category (24.5%).

Figures 1, 2, and 3 illustrate the scope of events that can impact first responders and the varying disorders, or lack of disorders that can result from exposure to these events. Understanding (a) the types of events that lead first responders to seek treatment and (b) the various psychological disorders that can result from these traumatic events is necessary for accurate diagnosis, case conceptualization, and treatment planning.

With respect to treatment, exposure therapy remains one of the most efficacious interventions for anxiety-related disorders, including PTSD (American Psychological Association [APA], 2017). A review of the use and efficacy of exposure therapy for PTSD, or even exposure therapy within the first responder group, is not within the scope of this chapter. However, in order to understand the role of virtual reality and how it augments traditional exposure therapy, a brief review of the foundation of exposure therapy is necessary.

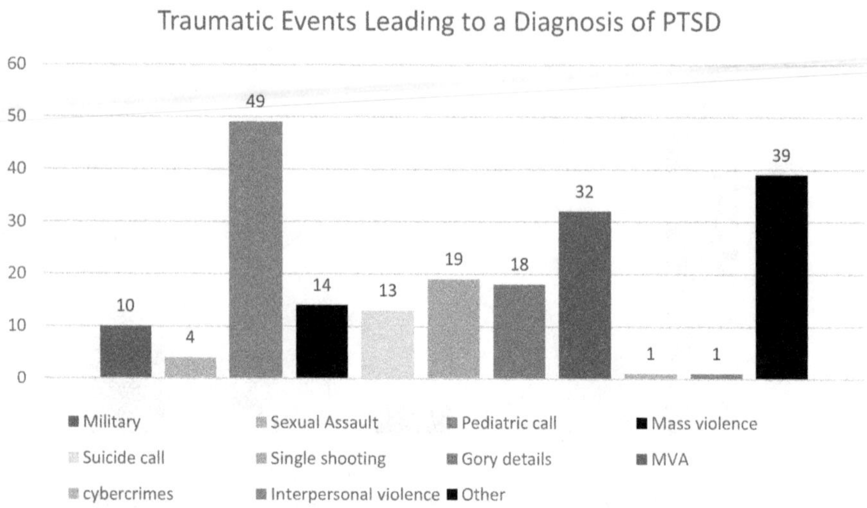

Fig. 3 Traumatic events reported by first responders leading to a diagnosis of PTSD

The emotion underlying anxiety disorders and PTSD is fear/anxiety. According to one model (Foa & Kozak, 1986), people feel anxiety or fear when they encounter a situation, event, or object that activates a fear structure in the brain. In the case of PTSD, this cognitive representation has been learned as a result of a traumatic event (e.g., the person is the victim of an armed robbery). All aspects of the event (what the perpetrator was wearing, the sight of the weapon, perhaps traffic sounds if the event occurred outside, and even any smells) now become part of the encoded memory. Even though that particular event does not occur again, when a person encounters an aspect of the event (a person who looks like the perpetrator, the sound of traffic, etc.), the fear structure in the brain is activated, producing emotional distress (Foa & Kozak, 1986). The aspects of the event that can activate a fear response are specific to each individual. Exposure therapy involves having the person repeatedly come in contact with the cues that elicit their distress *but in the absence of the actual negative event* – the person is not robbed at gunpoint. Through repeated presentations of the cues, without the negative outcome, the fear response is extinguished. On a neurological level, new neuronal connections are made within the brain, resulting in new learning (Davis et al., 2006) that is stronger than the original conditioning (traumatic) event. At the emotional level, the repeated exposure results in a diminished anxiety response, until even immediate contact with the cues does not elicit anxious distress (Foa & Hearst-Ikeda, 1996).

As noted above, exposure therapy is one of the most efficacious treatments for PTSD (APA, 2017). It is important to note that even among the overall positive outcomes, not everyone responds positively to traditional exposure therapy. Particularly with respect to combat-related PTSD, the effect of exposure therapy has been less than optimal (Hoge et al., 2017). Specifically, there are high rates of treatment attrition, with a range of 28–40% of veterans dropping out of treatment. Further, although many studies report a statistically significant decrease in symptoms, 55–60% of veterans still retain their PTSD diagnosis after a full course of treatment (Steenkamp, 2016). This has led to attempts to find ways to augment exposure therapy's effectiveness. One successful augmentation has been incorporating the use of virtual reality.

Virtual Reality to Enhance the Efficacy of Exposure Therapy

Prior to the introduction of virtual reality, exposure therapy was conducted in one of two ways. In vivo (in real life) exposure therapy means that the individual is exposed to the actual cues that precipitate their distress. This may be appropriate for fears such as heights or dogs, but it is not possible when the cues are combat scenarios, motor vehicle accidents involving life-threatening and gruesome injuries, or mass violence. The alternative was to use imaginal exposure, which required the patient, with guidance from the therapist, to imagine the traumatic event. The challenge for this approach is that the therapist does not actually have control over the patient's mental processes. The patient is responsible for imagining the event (including the cues) as they are presented by the therapist. However, the therapist is dependent upon the patient to envision the cues accurately, and if they do not, the therapy will not be effective. As a result of the deficits that are inherent to imaginal exposure, alternative methods were developed to increase the efficacy of exposure therapy.

Why Virtual Reality?

Any form of exposure therapy will be ineffective if the appropriate cues are not presented. As noted above, in the case of imaginal exposure therapy, one challenge for effective implementation is that the therapist is dependent upon the patient to imagine the cues appropriately – the therapist cannot control or force the patient to imagine something. In the case of PTSD, many patients spend significant time trying *not* to imagine the horrific event and will go out of their way to avoid any encounter with a cue that creates distress. It is counterintuitive to many patients that imagining the traumatic event will lead to a positive treatment outcome and they express reluctance in therapy sessions to do so (Difede & Hoffman, 2002). Even if they agree to try, they may not do it appropriately, leaving out or modifying cues that are necessary for the most effective treatment outcome. A second challenge is that some individuals just have difficulty imagining anything. Although in the case of PTSD the event is typically easy to recall, certain elements that may be cues precipitating emotional distress – such as sounds or smells – are not that easy to imagine.

Table 1 Barriers identified by first responders for not seeking treatment

Barriers	Percent (#) of agencies ($n = 145$)
Stigma associated with seeking/receiving mental health care	59% (85)
Availability of culturally competent resources	23% (31)
Fear of lack of confidentiality	17% (24)
Lack of knowledge of available resources	14% (21)
Funding for mental health resources	13% (19)
Fear of retaliation of employer	12% (18)
Availability of mental health resources	12% (18)
Denial of needing mental health care	12% (17)
Time required to identify and access resources	9% (13)
Ease of access to resources	7% (10)
Lack of first responder use of available resources	6% (9)
Leadership issues	6% (9)
Mental health services are reactive rather than proactive	4% (6)

Note: State of Florida Department of Children and Families (2021)

The implementation of virtual reality into exposure therapy has allowed for the mitigation of some of the challenges faced with imaginal exposure. By utilizing virtual reality, the therapist has better control of the relevant cues, therefore removing a barrier to treatment that can result from a patient's engagement in avoidance strategies. Further, the use of virtual reality mitigates the problems related to a patient's inability to engage in imagery of sufficient detail and affective magnitude. In short, virtual reality is not a stand-alone treatment; however, it makes exposure therapy for PTSD more potent.

Another reason to consider the use of virtual reality to augment exposure therapy for PTSD has to do with the nature of first responders. For many years, there was a reluctance for first responders to speak openly about the traumatic events that they experienced and the psychological toll that it exerted upon them (Lewis-Schroeder et al., 2018). This stigma not only extends to their reluctance to speak about the impact of the traumatic events but also affects their decision to seek treatment. Table 1 lists the results of one survey regarding reasons first responders were reluctant to seek mental health treatment.

By far the most common reason for not seeking treatment for mental health issues is the stigma associated with psychological distress. We have found that discussing a psychological treatment program that included virtual reality broke down some of the stigma surrounding what mental health treatment might entail. Once they heard about the use of the technology, many first responders would start the conversation by showing us pictures of traumatic events to which they had responded, suggesting that we "needed" to build such a scenario. We found that first responders were willing to consider a treatment that used VR because it was different than traditional "talk therapy." Once engaged with our clinic, they were willing to discuss their traumatic experiences and the impact on their daily functioning.

Breaking through this stigma about seeking treatment for mental health is particularly important as interventions cannot be considered effective if patients will not engage in them.

Why Olfaction?

As noted above, efficacious exposure therapy requires confronting all the cues that can precipitate distress, bring on flashbacks, or contribute to behavioral avoidance. Sights and sounds are the most common sensory cues. In the aftermath of the Pulse nightclub shooting, many first responders reported that the sounds of cell phones ringing triggered flashbacks of being in the nightclub searching for the shooter – that night the cell phones of the deceased and wounded kept ringing, but no one could answer.

Much less attention has been given to olfactory cues, even though first responders, like other individuals with PTSD, often describe certain scents as eliciting distress. One Pulse first responder who was involved in collecting evidence from the crime scene told us that the smell of a permanent marker now triggered emotional distress and flashbacks to the crime scene. A responder to the Uvalde school shooting described the smell of blood when they were processing the scene, stating "Even weeks later, on occasion, I will actually still smell it." From a neuroanatomical, experimental, and clinical perspective, the impact of odors on emotional status is quite clear. Neuroanatomically, the olfactory system is a straight "run" from the olfactory bulb to the amygdala and the hippocampus, which are within the limbic system, the emotional center of the brain (Krusemark et al., 2013). Because the signal does not go through other parts of the brain on its way to the limbic system, the odor does not degrade, but retains its "potency," creating very powerful and emotional memories.

Experimentally, when olfactory cues are paired with aversive stimuli, they produce conditioned fearful behavior in rats, not only to the situational context but also to the odor itself (Kroon & Carobrez, 2009). Data gathered from our clinic demonstrated findings consistent with the animal literature. Studies of combat veterans with and without PTSD (Gramlich et al., 2019) suggest that when presented with an odor that was part of a traumatic event, patients with PTSD exhibited increased activation in the left ventrolateral prefrontal cortex when compared to veterans who had experienced the same traumatic events but did not have a diagnosis of PTSD. The left ventrolateral prefrontal cortex is associated with facilitating the regulation of memory and emotional processes, suggesting that this area of the brain becomes activated when combat veterans with PTSD smell an odor associated with their trauma. Taken together, these data suggest that including olfactory cues (when appropriate) may enhance exposure therapy's treatment efficacy.

Initial Development of Virtual Reality for the Treatment of PTSD

As noted by Rizzo and Shilling (2017), there are two types of virtual reality (VR). Non-immersive VR uses a flat-screen display, whereas immersive VR uses a head-mounted display (HMD), earphones (which may or may not be integrated into the HMD), and an olfaction delivery system. The latter system is preferred for use in exposure therapy as it allows a truly immersive experience. The image below illustrates the equipment needed to conduct exposure therapy using virtual reality (BRAVEMIND system, Institute of Creative Technologies [ICT], University of Southern California). The needed equipment fits easily within standard therapy spaces, and systems are designed for clinicians with no prior experience with virtual reality.

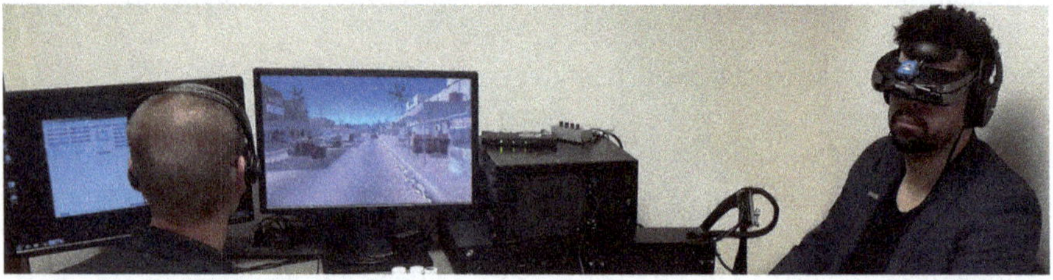

Initially, virtual reality was used for anxiety disorders such as fear of flying (Price et al., 2008). Treatment software for fear of heights and fear of public speaking soon followed. For another review of this literature, see Maples-Keller et al. (2017).

The most widely recognized VR system used for the treatment of PTSD is the work of Rizzo and his colleagues at the University of Southern California's Institute for Creative Technologies. Motivated by the continued findings that even the most powerful cognitive-behavioral treatments for PTSD (including exposure therapy) were far less effective in treating combat-related PTSD relative to civilian PTSD (Beidel et al., 2017), Rizzo and colleagues developed Virtual Iraq/Afghanistan, a four-scenario clinical system designed to treat combat-related PTSD. We incorporated the use of this VR system into our comprehensive behavioral treatment program for veterans with PTSD. The treatment protocol, known as Trauma Management Therapy (TMT), includes 14 sessions of daily individual VR augmented exposure therapy coupled with 14 group therapy sessions that included sleep hygiene, brief behavioral activation for depression, anger management, and social reintegration (Beidel et al., 2017). Initial investigations documented significantly improved treatment outcomes for individuals with combat-related PTSD, and changes in PTSD symptoms were unrelated to the group therapy, as our comparison condition consisted of VR exposure therapy alone (Beidel et al., 2017, Beidel et al., 2019; Rizzo & Schilling, 2017). An expanded VR system, called BRAVEMIND, consists of a larger number of military scenarios (combat, medic, and sexual assault), allowing VR to be used with various types of military trauma.

Despite the (a) initial success of VR in enhancing treatment outcomes of exposure therapy for combat-related PTSD and (b) the prevalence of trauma and PTSD in first responders, the use of VR for the treatment of PTSD in first responders has received limited attention. One preliminary study (Difede et al., 2007) examined the use of virtual reality exposure therapy (VRET) for the treatment of PTSD in first responders and civilian disaster workers who responded to September 11, 2001. Among the 13 people enrolled in this treatment protocol, 5 participants were firefighters, 4 were non-rescue disaster workers, and 4 were civilians. The VR was an immersive system, which used a graduated, hierarchical approach to treatment. The hierarchy focused on the crash of the jets into the buildings and the collapse of the twin towers. Of note, a subset of the participants had been treated with non-VR treatments previously with no positive effect. When compared to a waitlist control group, the participants treated with VR exposure had a significant decrease in their PTSD symptoms, and treatment effects were maintained at 6-month follow-up. Despite the success of this initial trial, we were unable to find any other published trials where virtual reality was used to treat PTSD in first responders.

Our work with first responders emerged after the mass shooting at the Pulse nightclub in Orlando, FL, on June 12, 2016. Having already conducted peer support trainings for a number of fire departments in the Central Florida area, we were called to provide psychological first aid to first responders in the immediate aftermath of the event. From there, requests for treatment emerged. We reasoned that TMT, developed for the treatment of combat trauma, might be an appropriate place to start treatment for first responders, particularly those who had been exposed to a mass shooting. There were no VR scenarios for first responders available at that time, but in some cases, scenarios from BRAVEMIND closely resembled some of the visual cues, allowing us to use those scenarios. When the VR system did not have the correct visuals, we used the non-immersive approach, incorporating videos of the event from YouTube, which was also the source of sounds needed to recreate the needed trauma cues. Triggering smells consisted mostly of alcohol or gunpowder, which were easily accessible.

The outcome of first responders seeking treatment in the aftermath of the Pulse nightclub shooting is presented in Fig. 4. Two measures were used to assess the outcome. The Posttraumatic Stress Disorder Checklist-5 (PCL-5; Blevins et al., 2015) is a self-report measure of PTSD severity. A score of 33 or higher is considered indicative of a PTSD diagnosis. The Clinician Administered PTSD Scale-5 (CAPS-5; Weathers et al., 2018) is an interview administered by a trained clinician and is considered the gold standard for the diagnosis of PTSD. These two measures were administered at pretreatment and posttreatment. All first responders were treated in an intensive outpatient setting using TMT as described above. A paired sample t-test indicated a significant decrease in CAPS-5 scores at posttreatment ($M = 6.50$, $SD = 7.59$) compared to pretreatment ($M = 36.1$, $SD = 4.03$, t(9) = 11.24, $p < 0.001$). Additionally, there was also a significant decrease in PCL-5 scores at posttreatment ($M = 12.90$, $SD = 3.36$) compared to pretreatment ($M = 47.70$, $SD = 2.47$, $t(9) = 9.33$, $p < 0.001$). Although the data provided cannot parse out the specific effects of virtual reality, none of the participants resisted the use of this

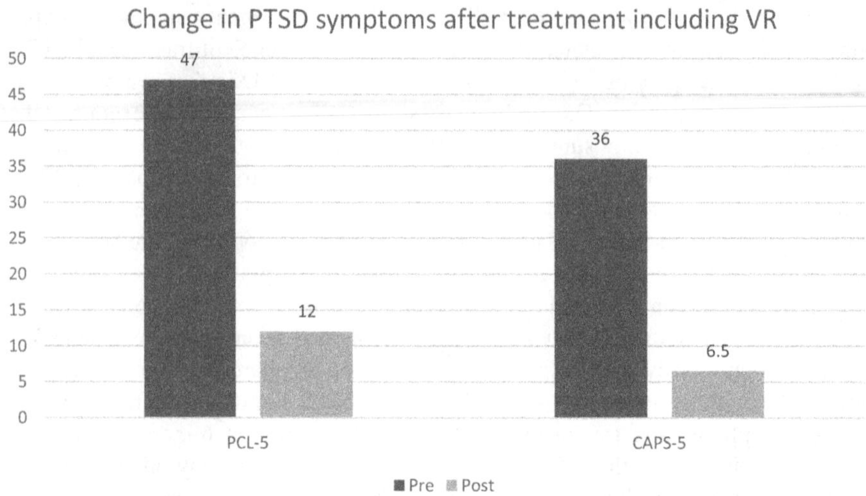

Fig. 4 PCL-5 and CAPS-5 scores at pre and posttreatment (Trauma Management Therapy)

technology; they were often the ones to suggest particular sounds and smells that needed to be included in their treatment. In summary, these results suggest that the multimodal behavioral treatment, which includes exposure therapy augmented by VR, holds significant promise in treating PTSD symptoms that develop after a mass violence event.

Development and Validation of a VR System Specifically Addressing the Traumas of First Responders

As the number of first responders and mass violence survivors seeking treatment in our clinic increased, we realized that exposure therapy augmented with VR appeared to be efficacious, but there were no systems that contained the trauma scenarios reported by first responders, as illustrated in Fig. 1. Therefore, we developed an immersive system that would contain a robust number of pre-scripted scenarios, including those commonly identified by first responders. We currently have more than 40 different scenarios. Each scenario is modifiable, in order to better match the specific aspects of the individual's trauma. For example, if the traumatic event was a traffic accident with fatalities or severe injuries, the therapist could change the color of the car, and/or the people injured, including hair color and skin tone. We continue to design new scenarios for unusual/unique events, such as the Champlain Towers condominium collapse (Surfside, Florida). For that mass casualty event, we built a VR scenario based on the rubble and the remains of the collapsed tower and the activities of the rescue crew. In Fig. 5, on the left is a photograph of the collapsed tower that search and rescue teams worked under every day, with the constant threat

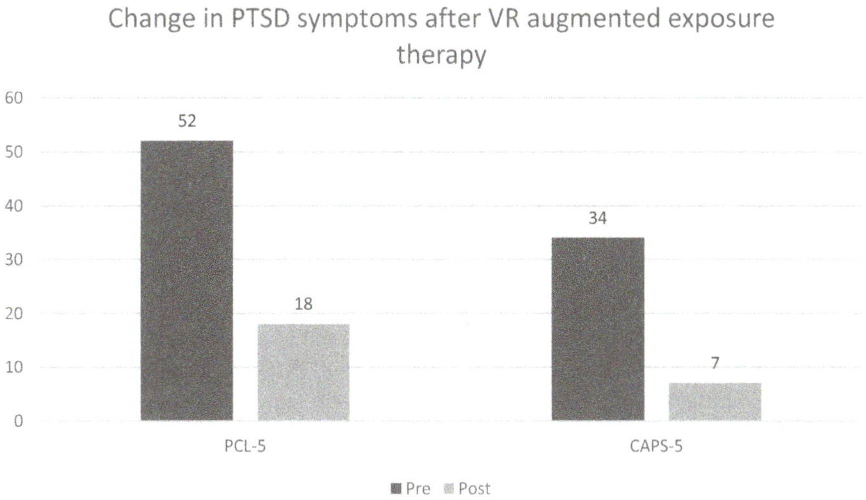

Fig. 5 PCL-5 and CAPS-5 scores at pre- and posttreatment (VR Augmented Exposure Therapy Alone)

that the rest of the tower would suddenly collapse. On the right is the VR model that mimics that site, including one specific element that several first responders identified as creating distress – the bunk bed up in the right-hand corner. To first responders, that meant the possibility that children had been sleeping there at the time of the collapse and had perished in the rubble (recall Fig. 1, in which pediatric calls were the most reported traumatic event). Although it was determined later that the condominium had been unoccupied at the time of the collapse, the sight of bunk beds continued to produce some emotional arousal in several first responders who were working on the recovery teams during the initial days of the search.

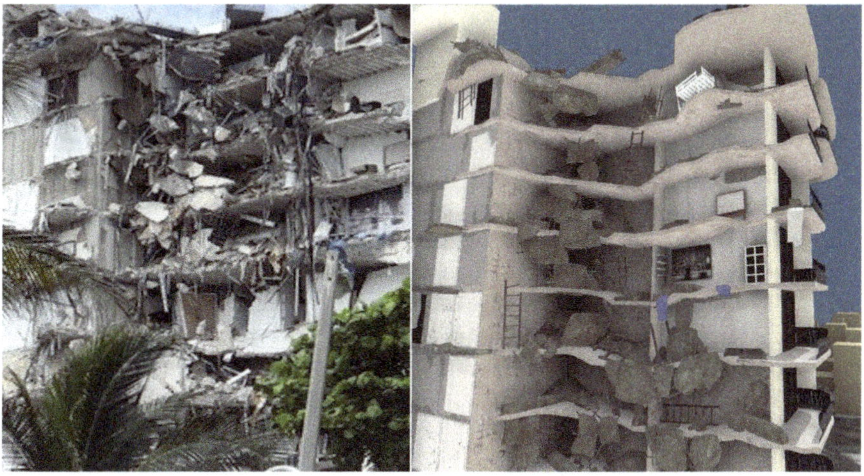

In the pilot testing of this new VR system, 13 first responders were treated with exposure therapy only, augmented by VR. Prior research from our clinic determined that most first responders needed about ten exposure therapy sessions for their anxiety to be extinguished. Therefore, the treatment was delivered daily over 10 consecutive weekdays. Among the 13 first responders who participated in the pilot study, 7 were firefighters and 6 were law enforcement officers. Not all were seeking treatment as a result of the Champlain Towers event, but all had a diagnosis of PTSD as a result of a traumatic event they experienced in their work as a first responder. The severity of PTSD symptoms was assessed with the PCL-5 and CAPS-5 (as described above).

Using paired sample t-tests, the results indicated statistically significant decreases in CAPS-5 scores ($t(11) = 11.91$, $p < 0.001$) and PCL-5 scores ($t(11) = 8.24$, $p < 0.001$), and again, the means were well below the cut-off scores for a probable PTSD diagnosis.

Is VR Necessary for Positive Treatment Outcome?

Exposure therapy often (a) is perceived negatively by therapists and patients alike, (b) has high treatment attrition, (c) has a substantial number of patients who retain their diagnosis after a full course of treatment (Hoge et al., 2017), and (d) suffers from the fallacy that its use in people with PTSD will produce iatrogenic effects such as psychosis, suicidal intent, or increased substance use (Beidel et al., 2017). Although iatrogenic effects have not been reported, it is correct that when exposure therapy is delivered in the traditional fashion, positive outcomes for combat-related PTSD have not been optimal. The other concerns, even if unfounded, decrease the likelihood that people will be willing to engage in exposure therapy.

As discussed above, there are theoretical as well as practical reasons to consider using VR to augment exposure therapy (better control of the necessary cues, no need to rely on patient's imaginal abilities – some people are just not good at imagining situations – and additionally, breaking through the stigma of what therapy entails). Only one study has directly compared one form of exposure therapy, prolonged exposure (PE) to PE plus VR (Reger et al., 2016). That study, conducted with a sample of active-duty military personnel, did not find that PE plus VR was more effective than PE alone, although both were more effective than a waitlist control group. However, this study had significant limitations including dropout rates of 40% or higher, and an average of only seven treatment sessions, suggesting that neither group received an optimal dose of therapy. Further, the mean scores for both groups at posttreatment were still indicative of the continued presence of PTSD. Therefore, the actual additional value of VR for the treatment of PTSD in military personnel remains unclear.

In contrast to the outcome of that study, the data gathered from our clinic suggest that VR with exposure therapy is highly effective, with better treatment outcomes for both military personnel (Beidel et al., 2017; Beidel et al., 2019) and first responders (as presented above). Although the specific additive effect of VR on our version of exposure therapy (which is different from PE) remains unknown, it is the subject of ongoing investigation.

Future Directions

For clinicians interested in incorporating VR into their treatment armamentarium, there are several factors to consider. On the positive side, systems that originally cost $35,000 can now be purchased for less than $5000, making them more accessible to a larger number of clinicians.

One challenge is the continuously changing technology. As the hardware continues to improve, what is currently available will eventually be rendered obsolete. New hardware often does not work with the existing software, and it can become difficult to find compatible replacement parts. However, as the technology continues to improve, these compatibility problems may be more easily addressed.

Another consideration is the recent change in how mental health services are delivered. Although telehealth has been in existence for some time, COVID-19 propelled this modality to the forefront of mental health treatment. Even after the pandemic eased, many individuals still prefer to meet with their therapists over the internet. Current systems using VR for the treatment of PTSD are "wired," requiring the first responder to travel to the therapist's office for treatment. Some VR headsets are wireless and deliver scenarios for relaxation and mindfulness. However, these headsets do not include scenarios that are most typically associated with trauma, and the scenarios typically cannot be modified. Ultimately, with some improvements to functionality, wireless systems could allow for the expanded delivery of VR-augmented exposure therapy for first responders.

Summary

When considering how to effectively treat PTSD in high-risk populations, we asked the question: do we need to develop *different* treatments, or do we need to develop evidence-based treatments *differently*? Beginning with a therapy demonstrated to be efficacious in other populations and with other anxiety-based disorders, we set out to determine the rate-limiting factors of exposure therapy and to address them. One of the limitations was that, when a traumatic event could not be recreated in real life, therapy rested upon the person's ability to imagine the traumatic event. But how effective could that be for cues such as sounds and smells, which are not as easily recreated in our imagination, which is primarily visual? VR bridges that gap, allowing the therapist to present the sights, sounds, and smells that serve as cues to trigger emotional distress, flashbacks, nightmares, sleep disturbance, and other symptoms of PTSD. It is important to emphasize again that VR is not the treatment. In the hands of an inexperienced therapist, or one that is not familiar with the learning theory that underlies exposure therapy, VR will not be effective. However, when used as a tool to ensure that the appropriate cues are presented, this treatment modality holds significant promise for first responders as indicated by the outcome data presented above.

As noted above, incorporating VR into psychological treatment also could function to decrease the stigma associated with seeking psychological help. First responders are the rescuers, the ones who save others. Asking for help is difficult, and until recently, the culture did not allow discussing the emotional distress associated with their occupation. Instead, they were told to "stuff it." When there was no more room in the trash can, many first responders resorted to drastic measures such as suicide, in order to end their distress. Thankfully, there is increasing recognition that this profession is exposed repeatedly to traumatic events and in some cases to events that no one can be expected to be unaffected. There is also increasing recognition that therapy may be effective at getting back to the job at an optimal level of performance. VR appears to be a significant component of a comprehensive treatment program, encouraging treatment access and providing positive treatment outcomes.

References

Alden, L. E., Matthews, L. R., Wagner, S., Fyfe, T., Randall, C., Regehr, C., White, M., Buys, N., Carey, M. G., Corneil, W., White, N., Fraess-Phillips, A., & Krutop, E. (2021). Systematic literature review of psychological interventions for first responders. *Work & Stress, 35*(2), 193–215. https://doi.org/10.1080/02678373.2020.1758833

American Psychological Association. (2017). *Clinical practice guidelines for the treatment of posttraumatic stress disorder (PTSD) in adults*. American Psychological Association.

Beidel, D. C., Frueh, B. C., Neer, S. M., & Lejuez, C. W. (2017). The efficacy of Trauma Management Therapy: A controlled pilot investigation of a three-week intensive outpatient program for combat-related PTSD. *Journal of Anxiety Disorders, 50*, 23–32. https://doi.org/10.1016/j.janxdis.2017.05.001

Beidel, D. C., Frueh, B. C., Neer, S. M., Bowers, C. A., Trachik, B., Uhde, T. W., & Grubaugh, A. (2019). Trauma Management Therapy with virtual-reality augmented exposure therapy for combat-related PTSD: A randomized controlled trial. *Journal of Anxiety Disorders, 61*, 64–74. https://doi.org/10.1016/j.janxdis.2017.08.005

Benjet, C., Bromet, E., Karam, E. G., Kessler, R. C., McLaughlin, K. A., Ruscio, A. M., Shahly, V., Stein, D. J., Petukhova, M., Hill, E., Alonso, J., Atwoli, L., Bunting, B., Bruffaerts, R., Caldas-de-Almeida, J. M., de Girolamo, G., Florescu, S., Gureje, O., Huang, Y., Lepine, J. P., et al. (2016). The epidemiology of traumatic event exposure worldwide: Results from the World Mental Health Survey Consortium. *Psychological Medicine, 46*, 327–343. https://doi.org/10.1017/S0033291715001981

Blevins, C. A., Weathers, F. W., Davis, M. T., Witte, T. K., & Domino, J. L. (2015). The Posttraumatic Stress Disorder Checklist for *DSM-5* (PCL-5): Development and initial psychometric evaluation. *Journal of Traumatic Stress, 28*(6), 489–498. https://doi.org/10.1002/jts.22059

Davis, M., Ressler, K., Rothbaum, B. O., & Richardson, R. (2006). Effects of d-cycloserine on extinction: Translation from preclinical to clinical work. *Biological Psychiatry, 60*, 369–375.

Department of Children and Families. (2021, July 1). *First Responder Suicide Deterrence Task Force 2021 Annual Report*. Department of Children and Families Office of Substance Abuse and Mental Health. https://www.myflfamilies.com/sites/default/files/2022-11/First%20Responder%20Task%20Force%202021%20Report%20-%20Final%20-%208-4-21.pdf

Difede, J., & Hoffman, H. G. (2002). Virtual reality exposure therapy for World Trade Center post-traumatic stress disorder: A case report. *Cyberpsychology & Behavior: The Impact of the Internet, Multimedia and Virtual Reality on Behavior and Society, 5*, 529–535. https://doi.org/10.1089/109493102321018169

Difede, J., Cukor, J., Jayasinghe, N., Patt, I., Jedel, S., Spielman, L., Giosan, C., & Hoffman, H. G. (2007). Virtual reality exposure therapy for the treatment of posttraumatic stress disorder following September 11, 2001. *Journal of Clinical Psychiatry, 68*, 1639–1647.

Foa, E. B., & Hearst-Ikeda, D. (1996). Emotional dissociation in response to trauma: An information-processing approach. In L. K. Michelson & W. J. Ray (Eds.), *Handbook of dissociation: Theoretical and clinical perspectives* (pp. 207–222). Plenum Press.

Foa, E. B., & Kozak, M. J. (1986). Emotional processing of fear: Exposure to corrective information. *Psychological Bulletin, 99*, 20–35.

Gramlich, M. A., Neer, S. M., Trachik, B., Bohil, C. J., Batien, B., & Beidel, D. C. (2019). *Neurological reactivity to personalized odors and sounds in combat-related posttraumatic stress disorder [Unpublished doctoral dissertation]*. University of Central Florida.

Hoge, C. W., Lee, D. J., & Castro, C. A. (2017). Refining trauma-focused treatments for service members and veterans with posttraumatic stress disorder. *JAMA Psychiatry, 74*, 13–14.

Klimley, K. E., Van Hasselt, V. B., & Stripling, A. M. (2018). Posttraumatic stress disorder in police, firefighters, and emergency dispatchers. *Aggression and Violent Behavior, 43*, 33–44. https://doi.org/10.1016/j.avb.2018.08.005

Kroon, J. A. V., & Carobrez, A. P. (2009). Olfactory fear conditioning paradigm in rats: Effects of midazolam, propranolol or scopolamine. *Neurobiology of Learning and Memory, 91*, 32–40.

Krusemark, E. A., Novak, L. R., Gitelman, D. R., & Li, W. (2013). When the sense of smell meets emotion: Anxiety-state-dependent olfactory processing and neuronal circuitry adaptation. *Journal of Neuroscience, 33*, 15324–15332. https://doi.org/10.1523/JNEUROSCI.1835-13.2013

Lewis-Schroeder, N. F., Keran, K., Murphy, B. L., Wolff, J. D., Robinson, M. A., & Kaufman, M. L. (2018). Conceptualization, assessment and treatment of traumatic stress in first responders: A review of critical issues. *Harvard Review of Psychiatry, 26*(4), 216–227. https://doi.org/10.1097/HRP0000000000000176

Maples-Keller, J. L., Bunnell, B. E., Kim, S.-J., & Rothbaum, B. O. (2017). Harvard. *Review of Psychiatry, 25*(3), 103–113. https://doi.org/10.1097/HRP.0000000000000138

Price, M., Anderson, P., & Rothbaum, B. O. (2008). Virtual reality as treatment for fear of flying: A review of recent research. *International Journal of Behavioral Consultation and Therapy, 4*, 340–347.

Reger, G. M., Koenen-Woods, P., Zetocha, K., Smolenski, D. J., Holloway, K. M., Rothbaum, B. O., Difede, J., Rizzo, A. A., Edwards-Stewart, A., Skopp, N. A., Mishkind, M., Reger, M. A., & Gahm, G. A. (2016). Randomized controlled trial of prolonged exposure using imaginal exposure vs. virtual reality exposure in active duty soldiers with deployment-related posttraumatic stress disorder (PTSD). *Journal of Consulting and Clinical Psychology, 84*(11), 946–959. https://doi.org/10.1037/ccp0000134

Rizzo, A., & Shilling, R. (2017). Clinical virtual reality tools to advance the prevention, assessment, and treatment of PTSD. *European Journal of Psychotraumatology, 8*(sup 5), 1414560. https://doi.org/10.1080/20008198.2017.1414560

Steenkamp, M. M. (2016). True evidence-based care for posttraumatic stress disorder in military personnel and veterans. *JAMA Psychiatry, 73*, 431–432. https://doi.org/10.1001/jamapsychiatry.2015.2879

Substance Abuse and Mental Health Services Administration. (2018). *First responders: Behavioral health concerns, emergency response, and trauma*. https://www.samhsa.gov/sites/default/files/dtac/supplementalresearchbulletin-firstresponders-may2018.pdf

Weathers, F. W., Bovin, M. J., Lee, D. J., Sloan, D. M., Schnurr, P. P., Kaloupek, D. G., Keane, T. M., & Marx, B. P. (2018). The Clinician-Administered PTSD Scale for DSM-5 (CAPS-5): Development and initial psychometric evaluation in military Veterans. *Psychological Assessment, 30*(3), 383–395. https://doi.org/10.1037/pas0000486

Motivational Interviewing in Clinical Work with First Responders

Lori L. Eickleberry

Introduction to Motivational Interviewing

Dramatic changes over the past three decades have significantly affected the way mental health services are conceptualized and provided. An important aspect of this change has been the introduction of motivational interviewing (MI). It has been 40 years since the first article on MI for clients struggling with alcohol use was published by psychologist Dr. William Miller (1983). Since that time, MI has been effectively applied to improve outcomes in addiction (Miller & Rollnick, 1991) and health issues (Rollnick et al., 2008), such as weight loss (Simpson et al., 2015) and diabetes (Bilgin et al., 2022). There has been successful implementation within a wide variety of mental health treatments (Iarussi, 2020; Schumacher & Madson, 2015), and it has utility in individual as well as group and family work (O'Kane et al., 2019; Sobell & Sobell, 2011). This list is certainly not exhaustive. In fact, there are well over 100 books and book chapters in addition to the hundreds of peer-reviewed articles and randomized controlled trials showing the efficacy of MI.

This chapter aims to highlight how MI is best suited to address the unique needs of first responders. Specifically, first responders are vulnerable to occupational stressors that put them at risk for several mental health concerns. Further, cultural norms often reinforce stigma around help-seeking, particularly for mental health treatment. MI specifically acknowledges this ambivalence; therefore, much of this

L. L. Eickleberry (✉)
Motivational Institute for Behavioral Health, Fort Lauderdale, FL, USA

Institute for Life Renovation, LLC, Fort Lauderdale, FL, USA

College of Psychology, Nova Southeastern University, Davie, FL, USA
e-mail: DrLori@mifbh.com

M. L. Bourke et al. (eds.), *First Responder Mental Health*,
https://doi.org/10.1007/978-3-031-38149-2_16

chapter will showcase important aspects of MI and its application. While hopefully it provides insights and increased interest, it is by no means meant to cover the depth and breadth of MI, nor to take the place of formal training and feedback.

Occupational Stress and Mental Health Stigma

First responders are exposed to high levels of occupational stress. Many experience life-or-death situations and have the responsibility of keeping others alive, and many experience threats to their own lives because of their work. They are not only exposed to trauma of their own, but also the vicarious trauma of others. Despite exposure to stress and occupational demands, their culture often expects them to stay strong and heroic. Because of occupational stress, first responders are at a high risk of developing mental health issues, such as trauma symptoms, substance abuse, sleep difficulties, depression, and anxiety – all of which leave them at a greater risk of suicide than the general population (Henderson et al., 2016). To further complicate these issues, a meta-analysis of 14 articles revealed that over 33% of first responders endorsed items related to stigma associated with mental health (Haugen et al., 2017). They reported that their work culture often stigmatizes help-seeking and sees those who seek mental health services as weak (Corrigan, 2004), which influences their willingness to seek services when needed (Wheeler et al., 2021). There may also be fear associated with job loss (Miller, 2006), fear of mistrust by comrades or team members who may view them as unstable, and fear of being seen as a liability (Henderson et al., 2016).

While there has been a growing number of reported suicides among first responders (Bah, 2016; Firefighter Behavioral Health Alliance, 2022), the limited research on stigma and its impact on treatment is in stark contrast to the amount of existing literature that documents mental health prevalence and need for services (Haugen et al., 2017). In a culture where mental health is stigmatized and a sub-culture that may view those with mental health issues as weak, hesitancy to disclose mental health concerns poses an obstacle in the therapeutic environment. Royle et al. (2009) eloquently described the compounding challenges stigma brings to the therapeutic process. Premature termination of therapy and lack of engagement also serve as barriers to effective treatment. While little is known about the specific characteristics that predict drop-out rates, the numbers are higher among individuals with PSTD. Further, women first responders with PTSD symptoms have a greater likelihood of dropping out of treatment than do men (Hinton et al., 2022).

While many first responders seek treatment on their own accord, many may be referred by work or family. Thus, there may be reluctance to seek treatment or hesitancy to disclose information. Because MI has been used to improve attendance, retention rates, and successful outcomes (Jake-Schoffman et al., 2021), it is a natural strategy for use with first responders. In fact, researchers have found positive outcomes with MI among police officers and firefighters (Elliot et al., 2007; Kappler & Otterstetter, 2018), coerced clients (Miller & Rollnick, 2013), and military groups

(Seal et al., 2012). Because PTSD treatment outcomes for first responders were nearly identical to those obtained among military personnel, we can assume some similarities exist among groups (Marks et al., 2020).

What Is Motivational Interviewing?

The technical definition of MI is stated by Miller and Rollnick (2013) as "a collaborative, goal-oriented style of communication with particular attention to the language of change. It is designed to strengthen personal motivation for and commitment to a specific goal by eliciting and exploring the person's own reasons for change within an atmosphere of acceptance and compassion" (p. 29). It is also described as a style of engaging with people that blends well with other evidence-based therapies.

The Spirit of MI

There are two core aspects of MI–the techniques themselves (technical) and the spirit in which the techniques are delivered (relational). Often referred to as the "spirit of MI," practitioners are encouraged to view their role with the client as one that is equal in power and to create an environment that is conducive to change, but not coercive. The spirit of MI is thought to be a vital component in the effective practice of MI (Miller & Rollnick, 2013). Because first responders may be fearful of negative judgment or adverse consequences associated with seeking help, conveying empathy, respect, and equality is even more crucial.

The spirit of MI is easily remembered by the acronym PACE: Partnership, Acceptance, Compassion, and Evocation (Miller & Rollnick, 2013). The clinician and the client work as partners, examining the client's reasons for changing and not changing with a neutrality that conveys understanding and acceptance of a client's right to decide whether or not to make changes. MI is essentially a person-centered approach that accepts where a client is in terms of their decision to change or not change and joins with them accordingly. In this sense, it is truly collaborative. It can at times seem contradictory that the most effective manner to help people move toward change is to respect and accept with nonjudgment and compassion their right to maintain their current processes. Yet, acceptance has been identified as a key component of the change process in several therapies, including acceptance and commitment therapy (Hayes & Strosahl, 2005) and dialectical behavior therapy (Linehan, 1993). Fundamentally, a therapist's capacity to let go of pushing someone toward change creates the safest space for a person to engage in dialogue about change – a dialogue that is often necessary for change to occur.

The use of metaphors in MI is common, and a metaphor for practicing the spirit of MI is to view the process as one where you and the client are examining a map together – the destinations and the routes, as well as the detours, shortcuts, and roadblocks along the way. When clients feel judged regarding their destination or route, they may be more likely to shut down or defend themselves. When defensiveness arises, it becomes a diversion from the task; you are no longer talking about the path or change, but instead have detoured to dialogue about the client's character (i.e., whether or not they are good or bad, or right or wrong).

Triggering defensiveness can be avoided through the process of evocation, which is the notion of eliciting ideas from the client, rather than imposing your own. A clinical process that highlights symptoms and deficits can often be followed by swift emphasis on problem areas with clinical insights, expertise, advice, and problem-solving strategies to evoke change. In contrast, the MI model views clients as experts on themselves and focuses instead on their strengths and resources. MI techniques are tools for highlighting these aspects and evoking insights, reasons for change, and solutions from the client.

While Miller and Rollnick (2013) highlight the importance of the underlying "spirit of MI," they also recognize the challenge of its practice. They encourage practitioners by reminding us that the practice of MI techniques leads to increased development of the overall spirit of MI and over time becomes more internalized and automatic, with proficiency continuing to develop over years of practice. They jest that the difference between doing MI and being MI is "about 10 years."

The Processes of Motivational Interviewing

Engaging, Focusing, Evoking, and Planning are the four processes of MI, which flow, merge, and reoccur (Miller & Rollnick, 2013). Therapy is a vulnerable process, especially among first responders who may experience greater stigma associated with seeking mental health services. During initial sessions, clients may be hesitant due to uncertainty, doubt, and mistrust, and their initial impression of the clinician can impact subsequent engagement and outcomes (Rimondini et al., 2019). *Engaging* is the initial process meant to establish connection, trust, and a working relationship. It is fundamental not only in therapeutic relationships but also in providing any quality service. There are six "traps" that can serve as barriers during this engaging process (Miller & Rollnick, 2013). One is the *assessment trap*, where an excess of questions can lead to an increased power imbalance and misperception of the subsequent processes. The *expert trap* is the pitfall in which the clinician communicates that they have all the answers. This also highlights the power differential and sends the message that the clinician is an expert on the client's personal life. It can also be invalidating by insinuating that the answer is obvious and easy, which can leave the client feeling defeated or defensive.

A *premature focus* on a clinician-identified problem or solution takes away from the collaborative nature of problem identification and solutioning, which leaves the interaction more at risk of discord. Further, *labeling*, which emphasizes the client's connection to a particular label (e.g., addict, alcoholic, denial), can increase stigma and the fear associated with it. While stigma is likely unhelpful with any treatment population, it can be especially problematic for first responders. *Blaming* places the focus on who is at fault for the client's problems and is irrelevant for solving problems in therapy. Blaming the client can increase unproductive defensiveness, while focusing blame on others may decrease empowerment. A person need not be at fault for their problems in order to solve them.

Avoiding these "traps" through skillful listening is not only fundamental to good communication but is also a central premise in MI. Skillful listening conveys a willingness to understand and collaborate. Open-ended questions, affirmations, reflections, and summaries are used in MI to effectively engage throughout the therapeutic process, and OARS is the MI acronym used to remember these four core skills.

Engaging

Open-Ended Questions

Open-ended questions are less directive and allow for elaboration; they encourage clients to tell their stories and often yield more information without numerous successive questions. It is important to note that close-ended questions are not contraindicated in MI, but instead used sparingly and purposefully. Closed-ended questions ask specific information requiring little to no elaboration, while open-ended questions are an invitation for the client to bring in specifics that they find relevant or important.

When clinicians use open-ended questions, it shows interest and allows for a deeper and more natural flow of conversation. In contrast, too many closed-ended questions may feel like an interrogation (e.g., "Do you use cocaine?" "How often do you use it?" "When did you start using it?"). Open-ended questions encourage more client dialogue, which allows the clinician to practice skillful listening, accurate reflections, normalizing, and empathy skills with an underlying goal of promoting trust and open communication.

Examples of Open-Ended Questions*

"What is it like for you at the fire station?"
"How do you feel around your colleagues at the hospital?"
"Tell me what you like the most about your job."
"How were things different between you and your partner then?"
"What do you like about drinking?"

*Open-ended questions typically begin with What, How, and Tell. Closed-ended typically begin with Do, Which, and Who. The use of "why" is cautioned because it can insinuate disagreement, blame, accusation, or judgment and can trigger defensiveness (Evans et al., 2016).

Affirmations

Affirmations are positive statements made by clinicians in response to what clients have said or done that are used to highlight a client's strengths, successes, and efforts. Affirmative responses by clinicians verify and acknowledge first responders' abilities to make decisions, overcome adversity, and implement changes. Affirmations can increase openness (Li et al., 2022), result in a more positive therapeutic experience for the client (Jones et al., 2016), and result in greater treatment retention (Linehan et al., 2002). When providing an affirmation, clinicians should avoid statements that may sound overly ingratiating or condescending (e.g., "Wow, I'm so proud of you!" or "That's great, I knew you could do it!"); affirmations are statements about the client, not the clinician. While affirmations help to increase clients' confidence in their ability to change through acknowledgment of strengths and abilities, they are most effective when they are genuine.

Examples of Affirmations

"*Your commitment really shows* by coming here even though you don't feel it's necessary. That *says a lot about how important your job as a nurse is to you.*"
"*Being a good EMT is important* to you."
"You *showed a lot of determination* by doing that."
"It's clear that you're *really working hard to change* the way you express your anger."

Reflective Listening

Reflective listening is one of the fundamental ways of responding to clients that builds rapport and conveys empathy. Reflective listening involves listening carefully to clients and then paraphrasing their comments back to them (e.g., "It sounds like relaxing and spending time with friends is important to you, and having a drink or two together has been a big part of that"). Reflections show that the clinician is listening and communicates that the clinician understands what the client has said (i.e., "It sounds like it is upsetting for you that others think there is a problem when you honestly don't feel there is"). When stated with MI spirit in a neutral and nonjudgmental tone, it conveys empathy and understanding, which builds rapport. When clinicians' reflections are correct, clients usually respond in agreement, often by continuing the dialogue. If the guess is wrong (e.g., "It sounds like you aren't interested in making changes right now"), clients usually quickly disconfirm the hypothesis (e.g., "No, I do want to make changes, but I am worried that I will fail"). Reflections can range in depth, and aside from being less likely than a question to evoke defensiveness, they can convey empathy and help clients better understand their own narrative.

Examples of Reflective Listening

"You're fearful of letting your fellow police officers at work know how much the situation impacted you."
"I get the sense that you sometimes feel misunderstood at the station."
"It sounds like you feel lonely and would like to have more friendships."
"I get the feeling that you don't think the other EMTs would be supportive if you shared that information with them."

Summaries

Summaries are used to summarize larger chunks of information, to convey active listening, to link to what clients have previously expressed, or to move to a new topic. They also serve for the elaboration of a topic, to pivot the conversation in a new direction, or to end a session (i.e., wrap up at the end by offering a short summary of the session). A summary is one of the basic ways of responding to clients that not only conveys you are listening but also shows that you understand the big picture of how the specifics of their situation fit together.

Examples of Summaries

For elaboration: "It sounds like on the one hand you enjoy how alcohol makes you feel relaxed and you enjoy spending time with your friends at happy hour, but on the other hand, you are concerned about how your use of alcohol upsets your wife and that it may be negatively impacting your marriage. You feel like you are being pulled in two directions."
To pivot: "We have talked a lot about your life growing up in Virginia and how although it was hard with the discord in your family, you were able to get through it because you had a lot of supportive friendships. Tell me a bit about the friendships and support you have now."
For elaboration: "So, you've shared a lot about the intensity of your anger at times and how while the reasons for it feel valid, it often leaves you feeling guilty and worried about the impact on the relationship with your coworkers. You also mentioned that although your use of alcohol does not feel problematic, you notice that sometimes you feel more irritable the day after having a few drinks."

Normalizing

Validation has long been identified as an important component of empathy in therapy (Linehan, 1997). Where empathy is described as the understanding of another's perspective, validation is to communicate that their response makes sense by being relevant, meaningful, or effective (Linehan, 1997). Normalizing is a specific type of validation that goes beyond honoring the perspective of the client by helping them to understand that their experience, which may seem distressingly abnormal to them, is within the parameters of normal in that others experience it similarly (Knapp, 2015).

Validation and normalization are two essential ways to convey empathy, acceptance, and compassion. It is important to note that validation and normalization are not "agreeing with" or supportive of ineffective or problematic behavior, but instead conveyance of a nonjudgmental and radical understanding of the client's current perspective and experience.

Examples of Normalizing

"It makes sense that you may feel hesitant to share information regarding your experiences. It can feel very vulnerable to do so and many people worry about stigma or possible consequences."

"Many people feel discouraged after a relapse. Relapse, however, is often a normal part of the change process."

Focusing

Rather than a completed stage, engaging occurs throughout MI and lays a strong foundation for the other processes: focusing, evoking, and planning. Focusing is an ongoing practice of obtaining and maintaining direction in therapy. During focusing, the therapist uses engaging strategies in a more directive way to pivot sessions toward a specific area of focus in therapy. A client's goals may differ from those of their referrer or clinician, or there may be several areas of difficulty and the client may need help deciding where to focus. In these situations, agenda mapping on paper can prove useful. Structuring the session openly can bring attention to the possible topics for exploration with a general summary of each area, without addressing any particular topic(s) in depth. Once areas are identified, the conversation can move toward choosing a specific topic where the client is willing to pursue change. This provides a first step that can later link to other areas of change. In many circumstances, clients may be uncertain as to what they want to get out of therapy, if they want to change, and, if so, how to achieve it. Beneficial work can still be achieved, even when a client has low readiness for change. In fact, MI was initially developed specifically for individuals who were ambivalent about change (Miller & Rollnick, 2013).

In contrast, there are times when the focus is clear and the client is motivated for change. This alleviates a strong need for evoking, which focuses on increasing motivation and commitment for change, and the session can move into the planning phase. During this process, the exchange of information is important – asking questions, as well as providing information or advice. Asking permission and engaging by eliciting information remain respectful and collaborative ways to exchange information. They also allow the client to solicit information from the clinician prior to the clinician proceeding, which likely opens receptiveness to the questions or information to come. Once it is clear which information the client wants and needs, it is best to provide it in a clear manner and allow the client to interpret the information with time to ask questions – always emphasizing their autonomy and freedom to agree or disagree with the information provided.

Asking Permission

Some close-ended questions can be necessary and even helpful. One example is the MI strategy of asking permission. A simple strategy, used frequently, conveys a collaborative and respectful stance. Clinicians can become desensitized to broaching topics that elicit discomfort and, as a result, fail to use sensitivity in doing so. Asking for permission to discuss these topics communicates respect for clients. Once a client gives permission for questions to proceed, there is naturally less guardedness. Clients are more likely to discuss difficult areas when asked for permission ahead of time, in contrast to when difficult subjects are broached without permission. If a client has not asked for your advice, always ask permission before providing it. Although rare, a client may decline a permission request. In this case, asking permission may be of even greater value, as it presents an opportunity to convey respect for the client by respecting their freedom to choose.

Examples of Asking Permission

"Do you mind if I ask a few specific questions about your alcohol use?"

"I noticed on this questionnaire that you endorsed difficulties in your relationship, do you mind if I ask you a few specific questions about that?"

"May I provide you with some information on that topic?"

"I'm wondering if you are interested in hearing about some of the things that I have noticed with other people who were struggling similarly."

Evoking

The processes of engaging and focusing are common within many therapies; however, the process of evoking is where skills become more specific to MI. The goal of evoking is to work through ambivalence and increase change talk. This is artfully conducted through openly discussing ambivalence, examining goals and values, highlighting discrepancies, providing feedback, and evoking change talk. While the goal is to discuss sustain talk and change talk with neutrality, it is important to recognize change talk when you hear it. MI uses the acronym DARN for identifying different change talk: Desire (e.g., "I would like to have a better relationship with my husband"), Ability (e.g., "I have made some changes already"), Reasons (e.g., "I would probably feel better about myself if I made changes"), and Need (e.g., "I have to do something different or I will lose my job"). The following strategies are ways to elicit more of this change talk dialogue in order to highlight and work through ambivalence.

Evoking Change Talk

Change talk is associated with successful outcomes (Joramo et al., 2021). This strategy elicits need or reasons for changing from clients. Rather than the clinician telling clients why they should change, change talk is voiced by clients, and their responses typically contain reasons for change that are personally relevant for them.

Examples of Questions to Evoke Change Talk

"What would you like to see differently about your current situation?"
"If you did decide to change the relationship with your coworkers, how might your life be different?"
"Suppose you don't change, what is the worst thing that might happen?"

Evoking Statements of Self-Efficacy

The objective is to increase clients' confidence in their *ability* to change. Eliciting statements of self-efficacy is done by asking questions that nudge clients to give voice to the changes they have already made. Many clients see the end result as the only success and fail to recognize small steps along the way as success. This can be discouraging. Self-confidence statements can be sought from clients using some of the tools below (e.g., Readiness Ruler), but also can be done by asking clients how they were able to accomplish something difficult, or by asking them to elaborate on a small change.

Examples of Evoking Statements of Self-Efficacy

"So even though you have not been abstinent every day this past week, on Sunday you didn't drink at all. How were you able to do that?"
"Coming here sounds like it was very difficult for you. What does that tell you about your ability to do difficult things?"

Values and Goals

Discussion of values is used in a number of therapeutic approaches (Yadavaia & Hayes, 2009). Values and goals are discussed by Miller and Rollnick (2013) within the process of engaging, although are noted as also having powerful utility within the processes of focusing, evoking, and planning. Goals and values are noted as important areas to springboard appreciation for another person's working frame of reference and they highlight the *desire* for change. There are several ways to explore a person's values (LeJeune & Luoma, 2019), and the Values Card Sort exercise is a common technique (Miller & Rollnick, 2013). The process consists of sorting cards each labeled with a different value into piles from least important to most important. Discrepancies between values and behavior also create space for cognitive dissonance and change talk by highlighting a *need* for change. The Values Card Sort task is available for free as an online PDF file for printing or as a web-based tool.

Decisional Balance

Decisional balancing, which has clients look analytically at the costs and benefits of changing and not changing a specific behavior, can be used anytime throughout treatment, including during the initial stages of therapy when a client may be ambivalent about participating in treatment. The sigma associated with seeking mental health treatment may make this especially relevant for first responders. Clinicians can conduct a decisional balance exercise with clients by simply asking them in an open-ended way about the good and less good things regarding a particular behavior (e.g., engaging in therapy, quitting drinking, expressing anger). While examining the pros and cons of a situation is not a novel task, how it is presented and used is what makes the decisional balance exercise an effective MI tool.

Specifically, neutrality and empathy are again important. After all, ambivalence is a normal human occurrence; otherwise, each of us would have successfully mastered every New Year's resolution made. Additionally, it is important to ask about the benefits of the risky or unwanted behavior first. For example, the benefits of drinking, using drugs, acting out in anger, or avoiding therapy. This allows for an open, nonjudgmental, and validating conversation about the good things (benefits) of the risky or problem behavior, which not only conveys neutrality by the clinician but also provides an opportunity for the clinician to make reflective statements of empathy, understanding, and nonjudgment. The decisional balance creates a prime opportunity to develop trust and rapport by connecting through the client's truth. Once this happens, clients tend to feel less judged and defensive and thus more open to giving voice to the less good things (costs) of the risky or problematic behavior. This also allows for increased opportunity for change talk.

Example of Decisional Balancing

Clinician: What are some of the good things about drinking alcohol? What do you like about it?

Client: Well, it's relaxing.

Clinician: So, it has a calming effect for you (reflection). It makes sense with your stressful job that you would want a way to relax (normalizing). What else do you like about it? (open-ended question).

Client: It is a way of relaxing at the end of the day with my husband.

Clinician: Ok, so after a long day, it is a way of coming together with your husband and decompressing (reflection). So it sounds like it has a social element to it as well. Having rituals like that with your spouse can be bonding. It makes sense that having that time would be enjoyable for you (normalizing and conveying empathy).

Client: Yes, and I like the social aspect of it with my girlfriends as well. Sometimes we go to dinner or happy hour and have drinks together.

Clinician: Not only does drinking have relaxing effects, it is associated with multiple social benefits for you as well. Winding down from stress and spending time with social supports are both very important things and it sounds like alcohol plays a critical role in that (summary and conveyance of empathy and nonjudgment). On the flip side, what are some of the less good aspects to drinking?

Client: Well, sometimes when I have too much, I have regret and anxiety about some of what I said and did.

Clinician: Sometimes you reflect and feel embarrassed (reflection). That is an uncomfortable feeling and sounds stressful for you (empathy). Alcohol can certainly have that effect on people sometimes (normalizing). What else do you notice that is less good about it?

Client: I think it impacts my ability to get up in the morning feeling refreshed and sharp.

Clinician: That makes sense; that sluggish fogginess is common after drinking. You have a lot on your plate and it sounds like it makes morning responsibilities much more challenging for you. So, what I am hearing from you in summary is that while drinking is associated with some very positive aspects of your life like relaxing and socializing, it can also bring about feelings of remorse and can make mornings much more challenging (summary).

Providing Feedback

When clients are less ready to make changes and provide minimal change talk, providing feedback can be a particularly useful MI strategy because clients may either lack information or have misinformation about their behavior. Traditionally, therapists and other healthcare practitioners have encouraged clients to change their behavior by using simple advice (e.g., "You should be drinking less;" "You really need to lose weight;" "You may want to file a formal complaint;" "Therapy will benefit you"). Researchers show that by and large the effectiveness of simple advice is very limited. This may be due to feelings of judgment, that the advice is an infringement on freedom of choice, or that it invalidates the complexity of the situation (Anderson & Handelsman, 2010; Diller, 1986). This can result in a defense of the behavior rather than an open discussion of it. Most individuals respond more favorably when their freedom to choose is respected, particularly with behavior change (Rollnick et al., 2008).

What we have learned from MI is that how information is presented can affect how it is received. When relevant, new information should be presented in a neutral, nonjudgmental, and sensitive manner that empowers clients to make informed decisions about changing a risky/problem behavior. One way to do this is to provide feedback that allows clients to compare their behavior to norms (e.g., drinking norms or concerns about stigma). Another way to do this is to provide statistical/factual information that is incongruent with beliefs (e.g., effects of smoking cessation or effectiveness of therapy). Last, but certainly not least, is to supply the client with idiographic information regarding personal assessment measures.

Examples of Providing Feedback

For norms or personal assessment: "You were kind enough to provide information last week that enabled us to calculate your average drinks per week. Your score is at the bottom and you can see the norms for U.S. men on the sheet as well (summary with affirmation). [Hand the completed feedback/norms sheet to the client]. What stands out to you (open-ended question)?"

For information: "You feel discouraged about quitting because you worry that if you quit smoking now, it won't make a difference in your health (reflection). Would you mind if I provided you with information about the physical changes that occur after a person quits smoking (asking permission)? [Hand the Smoking Healing Timeline to the client]. What stands out to you?"

Scaling Questions

Scaling questions are used in a multitude of professions and therapies and are not exclusive to MI. They are most often used to assess a client's specific state (e.g., distress, pain, motivation); and MI utilizes them not only to assess but also to evoke DARN change talk previously discussed.

Readiness to Change

Assessing readiness to change is a very important task in MI. Motivation, which is considered a fluctuating state, not a stable personality trait, can change rapidly from moment to moment. Clients enter treatment at different levels of readiness to change (e.g., some may be very ready to change; others may feel no desire to change). A clinician's knowledge regarding a client's readiness for change will allow for greater congruency, which is critical for empathy and rapport building. The concept of readiness to change comes from the Stages of Change Model by Prochaska and DiClemente (1983) which conceptualizes individuals as being at different stages of change when entering treatment. The Readiness to Change Ruler is a scaling strategy that conceptualizes readiness to change along a continuum and asks clients to give voice to how ready they are to change using a 10-point scale that looks like a ruler, where 1 = not at all ready to change and 10 = very ready to change. A Readiness Ruler allows clinicians to immediately assess their client's state of readiness for change, allows clients to give affirmative voice to personal strengths, and allows clients to make statements in the area of change talk.

Example of Using the Readiness to Change Ruler

Clinician: On the following scale from 1 to 10, where 1 is not at all ready to change and 10 is very ready to change, what number best reflects how ready you are right now to engage in therapy?

Client: Five.

Clinician: A five. How did you arrive at that number?

Client: Well, part of me wants to, but I also have some reservations about it.

Clinician: I see; you feel conflicted (reflection). There are some aspects that make you want to do it, and some aspects that give you pause. That makes sense; it is a big decision with both pros and cons (empathy and nonjudgment). And on the same scale, where were you one year ago?

Client: Two.

Clinician: So it sounds like you went from not being ready to engage in this process to now contemplating engaging in the process (reflection). Curious, how did you get from a two, a year ago, to a five today (elicit change talk)?

Client: Well, it has become a more acceptable thing to do and I am a bit tired of feeling the way I do.

Clinician: So, you feel more favorable toward therapy because the world is more supportive of it, and you are exhausted (reflection). I am wondering how you were able to get yourself here today regardless of your conflict about it (elicit change talk).

Client: Well, I thought I could at least take this step to find out more about the process.

Clinician: Hmm, despite your hesitancy about this process, you were able to get yourself here anyway. That must have been hard. How were you able to do that (elicit change talk)?

Client: It was. I almost canceled this morning, but I am a person of my word and didn't want to cancel last minute.

Clinician: Being dependable is important to you (affirmation).

Client: Yes.

Clinician: What do you think it would take to move a bit higher on the scale, say from a 5 to a 6 (elicit change talk; focusing)?

Client: To have more information about what the process actually looks like and if it can help.

Exploring Confidence and Importance

Confidence and importance are also relevant variables in a person's decision to change (Miller & Rollnick, 2013). Using scaling questions to gauge how important change is to the client and how confident they are in their ability to change can be helpful tools. As with The Readiness Ruler, these scales can also be used to assess where clients are, how far they have come, and what they would need to move further along in the change process. While presented and explored in the same manner as the example above, confidence and importance ratings are queried using a scale of 0–100.

Use of Discrepancy

Use of discrepancy can be used to increase change talk by addressing incongruencies between clients' words and actions (e.g., saying that they want to become abstinent, but continuing to use) in a non-confrontational manner. The idea is to get clients who present with discrepancies to recognize them rather than being confronted by their clinician. It is important to have an empathic and inquisitive – not sarcastic – tone. Discussion regarding the discrepancy between a client's values, goals, thoughts, or beliefs and their behavior is at the heart of ambivalence and can lead to heightened conflict and discomfort that can fuel change. The way in which this conversation occurs is critical because it can lead to shame and defensiveness, or it can lead to an open discussion fostering desire and opportunity for change (Miller & Rollnick, 2013). The role of acceptance in the change process was highlighted earlier in the chapter and is a key component in using discrepancy effectively. To decrease defensiveness and open clients to hearing potentially painful information, a tone depicting a dialectical middle path between acceptance and confusion is recommended. Discrepancy can be found by examining values, exploring others' concerns, decisional balancing, highlighting the client's thoughts and feelings, and assessment feedback.

Example of the Use of Discrepancy

"It has been clear in our discussion how much you love your job, how good at it you are, and how big of a part of your identity it is; yet, on the other hand, you really enjoy the escape of using cocaine occasionally with your boyfriend. Since you've been worried lately about problems at work and are being randomly drug-screened, I am wondering what your thoughts are about how these fit together."

"What is it about the value of integrity that had you label it as very important?" [Client responds]. "It sounds like being impeccable with your word is something that has been instilled in you since a young age and it is important to you to practice it. Do you think that drinking fits with this value, conflicts with it in any way, or is completely irrelevant?"

Planning

The planning process in MI does not differ from the other processes in MI as far as skills are concerned, but rather deviates in focus. While the processes of engaging, focusing, and evoking are aimed at building a collaborative and respectful relationship, finding an agreed upon direction, and increasing motivation for change, the planning process is about how to reach the identified goal. Sometimes the path is clear, sometimes there are a number of existing options to choose from, and occasionally a unique plan needs to be developed. Whichever scenario, the same collaborative, respectful, and empathic MI spirit is used in conjunction with the other MI skills toward change. A client's willingness to change does not eliminate the need or utility of MI skills. The path through implementing change is often a difficult one, wrought with difficulty, setbacks, and reluctance. The use of MI to support clients through the change process can help them persist through these difficulties (Miller & Rollnick, 2013).

Development and Maintenance of MI Skills

A common misperception in MI is that once a clinician does a training in MI and gains information about what it is and how to do it, they obtain some level of proficiency. Knowledge alone rarely translates to skill. Even with practice, aptitude is unlikely without continued training and feedback. In fact, research shows that self-perception of MI proficiency is unreliable, making direct observation of skills with feedback an important part of not only learning MI skills but also maintaining the practice of them. This is important to know up front because Miller and Mount (2001) found that attending an initial workshop decreased interest in learning more about MI because of the belief that it had already been acquired. That said, a good place to start is an initial MI training workshop, but without continued training and feedback, skills tend to erode (Schwalbe et al., 2014). Understanding the underlying spirit of MI is important, as it is a foundational part of the MI practice and helps the specific skills within MI be practiced effectively. It helps to think of MI in an integrated way rather than a specific technique. When practicing, however, it can be beneficial to focus on practicing one MI skill at a time and then integrating them (Miller & Rollnick, 2013). And, practicing through role-playing has been shown to be an effective strategy (Lane et al., 2008). While attending subsequent trainings, listening to your own MI sessions, learning communities, and subjective feedback from an MI coach are good ways to improve MI skills, more objective and reliable feedback can come from coding systems (Moyers et al., 2016). Many MI resources can be found at www.motivationalinterviewing.org.

Conclusion

Given the challenges and stress that first responders face in their jobs, the impact that it has on their mental health, and the stigma that serves as a barrier to the help they need, MI is a natural tool for not only increasing willingness to engage in the therapeutic process but also increasing the willingness to explore making changes to improve their mental and physical health. Yet, the delivery of MI is done independently of the client's decision whether or not to make changes. Despite the best training and implementation of MI, there will be clients who ultimately decide that they are not interested in change. Part of the spirit of MI is accepting and honoring their autonomy in making that decision. Doing so leaves the door open to a compassionate and respectful space that can be revisited at a later date when and if the client chooses to do so. Not doing so may leave the client feeling frustrated or ashamed and decrease the likelihood of seeking services in the future. The irony is not lost in that this chapter seeks to increase the willingness to use MI with first responder clients. In alignment with the MI spirit, while it is hoped that MI will be a useful tool in working with first responders, at the very least, a seed has been planted and the door is open for future exploration.

Acknowledgments Lori L. Eickleberry, Ph.D., ABPP has no conflicts of interest to disclose. Correspondence concerning this chapter should be addressed to Dr. Lori L Eickleberry.

References

Anderson, S. K., & Handelsman, M. M. (2010). *Ethics for psychotherapists and counselors: A proactive approach*. Wiley-Blackwell.

Bah, A. (2016). *Amid culture of silence, more firefighters die of suicide than on the job*. Al Jazeera America.

Bilgin, A., Muz, G., & Yuce, G. E. (2022). The effect of motivational interviewing on metabolic control and psychosocial variables in individuals diagnosed with diabetes: Systematic review and meta-analysis. *Patient Education and Counseling, 105*(9), 2806–2823.

Corrigan, P. (2004). How stigma interferes with mental health care. *American Psychologist, 59*(7), 614–625.

Diller, L. H. (1986). On giving good advice successfully. *Family Systems Medicine, 4*(1), 78–90.

Elliot, D. L., Goldberg, L., Kuehl, K. S., Moe, E. L., Breger, R. K. R., & Pickering, M. A. (2007). The PHLAME firefighter study: Outcomes of two models of behavior change. *Journal of Occupational and Environmental Medicine, 49*(2), 204–213.

Evans, D. R., Hearn, M. T., Uhleman, M. R., & Ivey, A. E. (2016). Essential interviewing: A programmed approach to effective communication.. Cengage.

Firefighter Behavioral Health Alliance. (2022). *Suicide reports archive*. https://www.ffbha.org/

Haugen, P. T., McCrillis, A. M., Smid, G. E., & Nijdam, M. J. (2017). Mental health stigma and barriers to mental health care for first responders: A systematic review and meta-analysis. *Journal of Psychiatric Research, 94*, 218–229.

Hayes, S. C., & Strosahl, K. D. (Eds.). (2005). *A practical guide to acceptance and commitment therapy*. Springer Science PLUS_SPI Business Media.

Henderson, S. N., Van Hasselt, V. B., LeDuc, T. J., & Couwels, J. (2016). Firefighter suicide: Understanding challenges for mental health professionals. *Professional Psychology: Research and Practice, 47*, 224–230.

Hinton, E., Steel, Z., Hilbrink, D., & Berle, D. (2022). Anger and predictors of drop-out from PTSD treatment of veterans and first responders. *Behavioural and Cognitive Psychotherapy, 50*(2), 237–251.

Iarussi, M. M. (2020). *Integrating motivational interviewing and cognitive behavior therapy in clinical practice*. Routledge/Taylor & Francis Group.

Jake-Schoffman, D. E., Brown, S. D., Baiocchi, M., Bibeau, J. L., Daubenmier, J., Ferrara, A., Galarce, M. N., Hartogensis, W., Hecht, F. M., Hedderson, M. M., Moran, P. J., Pagoto, S. L., Tsai, A. L., Waring, M. E., & Kiernan, M. (2021). Methods-motivational interviewing approach for enhanced retention and attendance. *American Journal of Preventative Medicine, 61*(4), 606–617.

Jones, S. A., Latchford, G., & Tober, G. (2016). Client experiences of motivational interviewing: An interpersonal process recall study. *Psychology and Psychotherapy: Theory, Research and Practice, 89*(1), 97–114.

Joramo, I., Solem, S., Romundstad, B., & Nordahl, H. M. (2021). Change talk and sustain talk in treatment of generalized anxiety disorder: A secondary analysis of cognitive behavioral therapy and metacognitive therapy in adult outpatients. *Journal of Behavior Therapy and Experimental Psychiatry, 72*(4), 101650.

Kappler, R., & Otterstetter, R. (2018). Changes in physical activity using motivational interviewing in law enforcement officers. *Medicine & Science in Sports & Exercise, 50*, 205.

Knapp, H. (Ed.). (2015). *Therapeutic communication: Developing professional skills* (2nd ed.). Sage Publications, Inc.

Lane, C., Hood, K., & Rollnick, S. (2008). Teaching motivational interviewing: Using role play is as effective as using simulated patients. *Medical Education, 42*(6), 637–644.

LeJeune, J., & Luoma, J. B. (2019). *Values in therapy: A clinician's guide to helping clients develop psychological flexibility and live a more meaningful life*. Context Press.

Li, S., Xia, Y., Zhao, W., Miao, X., & Xu, Q. (2022). February, 8. In *Self-affirmation increases acceptance of information on covid-19 vaccines and promotes vaccination intention* (Vol. 46, p. 303). Journal of Behavioral Medicine.

Linehan, M. M. (1993). *Cognitive-behavioral treatment of borderline personality disorder*. Guilford Publications.

Linehan, M. M. (1997). Validation and psychotherapy. In A. C. Bohart & L. S. Greenberg (Eds.), *Empathy reconsidered: New directions in psychotherapy* (pp. 353–392). American Psychological Association.

Linehan, M. M., Dimeff, L. A., Reynolds, S. K., Comtois, K. A., Welch, S. S., Heagerty, P., & Kivlahan, D. R. (2002). Dialectical behavior therapy versus comprehensive validation therapy plus 12-step for the treatment of opioid dependent women meeting criteria for borderline personality disorder. *Drug and Alcohol Dependence, 67*(1), 13–26.

Marks, M., Cunningham, A., Bowers, C., & Beidel, D. (2020). Trauma management therapy for first responders. In C. A. Bowers, D. C. Beidel, & M. R. Marks (Eds.), *Mental health intervention and treatment of first responders and emergency workers* (pp. 230–242). Medical Information Science Reference/IGI Global.

Miller, W. (1983). Motivational interviewing with problem drinkers. *Behavioural Psychotherapy, 11*(2), 147–172.

Miller, L. (2006). *Practical police psychology: Stress management and crisis intervention for law enforcement* (6th ed.). Charles C. Thomas.

Miller, W. R., & Mount, K. A. (2001). A small study of training in motivational interviewing: Does one workshop change clinician and client behavior? *Behavioural and Cognitive Psychotherapy, 29*(4), 457–471.

Miller, W. R., & Rollnick, S. (1991). *Motivational interviewing: Preparing people to change addictive behavior*. The Guilford Press.

Miller, W. R., & Rollnick, S. (2013). *Motivational interviewing: Helping people change* (3rd ed.). Guilford Press.

Moyers, T. B., Rowell, L. N., Manuel, J. K., Ernst, D., & Houck, J. M. (2016). The motivational interviewing treatment integrity code (MITI 4): Rationale, preliminary reliability and validity. *Journal of Substance Abuse Treatment, 65*, 36–42.

O'Kane, C., Irwin, J. D., Morrow, D., Tang, L., Wong, S., Buchholz, A. C., Ma, D. W. L., & Haines, J. (2019). Motivational interviewing with families in the home environment. *Patient Education and Counseling, 102*(11), 2073–2080.

Prochaska, J. O., & DiClemente, C. C. (1983). Stages and processes of self-change of smoking: Toward an integrative model of change. *Journal of Consulting and Clinical Psychology, 51*(3), 390–395.

Rimondini, M., Mazzi, M. A., Busch, I. M., & Bensing, J. (2019). You only have one chance for a first impression! Impact of patients' first impression on the global quality assessment of doctors' communication approach. *Health Communication, 34*(12), 1413–1422.

Rollnick, S., Miller, W. R., & Butler, C. C. (2008). *Motivational interviewing in health care: Helping patients change behavior* (Vol. 5, p. 203). Guilford Publications.

Royle, L., Keenan, P., & Farrell, D. (2009). Issues of stigma for first responders accessing support for post traumatic stress. *International Journal of Emergency Mental Health, 11*(2), 79–85.

Schumacher, J. A., & Madson, M. B. (2015). *Fundamentals of motivational interviewing: Tips and strategies for addressing common clinical challenges*. Oxford University Press.

Schwalbe, C. S., Oh, H. Y., & Zweben, A. (2014). Sustaining motivational interviewing. *Addiction, 109*, 1287–1294.

Seal, K. H., Abadjian, L., McCamish, N., Shi, Y., Tarasovsky, G., & Weingardt, K. (2012). A randomized controlled trial of telephone motivational interviewing to enhance mental health treatment engagement in Iraq and Afghanistan veterans. *General Hospital Psychiatry, 34*(5), 450–459.

Simpson, S. A., McNamara, R., & Shaw, C. (2015). A feasibility randomised controlled trial of a motivational interviewing-based intervention for weight loss maintenance in adults. *Health Technology Assessment, 19*(50), 1.

Sobell, L. C., & Sobell, M. B. (2011). *Group therapy for substance use disorders: A motivational cognitive-behavioral approach*. Guilford Press.

Wheeler, C., Fisher, A., Jamiel, A., Lynn, T. J., & Hill, W. T. (2021). Stigmatizing attitudes toward police officers seeking psychological services. *Journal of Police and Criminal Psychology, 36*(1), 1–7.

Yadavaia, J. E., & Hayes, S. C. (2009). Values in acceptance and commitment therapy: A comparison with four other approaches. *Hellenic Journal of Psychology, 6*(3), 244–272.

Part IV
Special Topics

Role of the Chaplaincy

Richard Braswell and Angela Beamer

Chaplains play a vital role in communities and are a valuable asset within first responder agencies. Militaries began utilizing chaplains centuries ago to improve organizational functioning. In recent years, their role has expanded to hospitals, correctional facilities, police departments, and fire departments (Bachrach, 2004). The chaplain's role within these settings can include addressing spiritual needs, well-being, crisis intervention, death notifications, funeral arrangements, community relations, and specific correctional requests (Braswell et al., 2016).

A chaplain is defined as a religious official attached to a branch of the military, an institution, a family, or a court (Merriam-Webster, n.d.). In order to serve as a chaplain, the individual must hold a college degree, preferably in religious studies, and be familiar with various religious sects and traditions to serve individuals of all faiths. Chaplains working with first responders and military populations need to complete a background check and obtain security clearance. Those chaplains who work in military settings should also obtain an ecclesiastical endorsement, critical incident stress management (CISM) certification, incident command system (ICS) certification, and continuing education credits. Chaplaincy requirements will vary among departments and are typically specified in the particular department's policies and procedures.

R. Braswell (✉)
Dallas Baptist University, Religion, Dallas, TX, USA

Plantation Police Department, Plantation, FL, USA

A. Beamer
Nova Southeastern University, College of Psychology, Davie, FL, USA

M. L. Bourke et al. (eds.), *First Responder Mental Health*,
https://doi.org/10.1007/978-3-031-38149-2_17

Historical Impacts

Although chaplains have historically been utilized for spiritual needs, they can address overall well-being including mental, physical, and emotional concerns. The military was the first organization to utilize chaplains to improve the functioning of its members even as far back as the 1200s (Bachrach, 2004). More recently, chaplains have been deployed for disaster relief, crisis intervention and have been embedded into first responder organizations. However, the roles of the chaplain and their place within a departmental team is evolving.

Several major historical events have shaped how chaplains function and how they respond to trauma. Prior to the tragic events of 9/11, chaplains responded to a specific organization (e.g., prison, hospital, military, police, fire) for a particular purpose (e.g., family counseling, officer shooting, death). Post-9/11, the field of chaplaincy expanded to bring various first responder groups together. The chaplain no longer worked as an independent individual with one organization but rather as a part of a team. The chaplain's role primarily as a minister shifted to the role of a caregiver who relied on collaborating with various other professionals, including mental health experts. This integrative approach to crisis impacted many professions relatively quickly due to the urgency and necessity for support following 9/11. Training units began to incorporate a chaplain as part of the team, including peer support and CISM.

Additional tragedies, such as the mass shootings at schools, churches, and nightclubs, brought terror from a large scale to more intimate settings. This created the need for local chaplains to work together with national crisis response teams. The term "chaplain" was no longer just a title or position, but rather a role, that had to adapt flexibly for the kinds of situations chaplains may be called upon to deal with.

The COVID-19 pandemic added another layer of isolation, depression, and anxiety for many individuals and exacerbated preexisting mental health conditions. Chaplains were not able to visit individuals or families in the hospital and had to find new ways to provide support. Complicated grief arose due to a lack of counseling and services, and final wishes were interrupted due to pandemic restrictions. Communities were unable to gather together during times of celebration and loss to garner the support they needed. Chaplains utilized technology in new ways to communicate via phone or video.

The condominium collapse that occurred on June 24, 2021, in Surfside, Florida, also demonstrated a unique crisis response. Crisis teams came from various locations within the state of Florida, other regions of the U.S., and even internationally to assist in the rescue and recovery efforts. This collaboration was evidence that crisis teamwork has not only become a national phenomenon but a global one. Crisis is unique in that it brings individuals together due to death, trauma, and subsequent resilience. Each individual affected by these issues holds personal spiritual and religious beliefs that the chaplain must accommodate differently.

The new emphasis for a chaplain's job must incorporate aspects of teamwork, creativity, technology, adaptability, diversity, inclusiveness, and a willingness to learn. Society is always changing, and the chaplain must find ways to change with it, to continue to foster mental, emotional, physical, and spiritual well-being.

Chaplains in First Responder Populations

A chaplain's role can vary depending on the first responder population and is defined both by what the agency deems necessary, and what the particular situation entails. Chaplains are often integrated into first responder populations due to the stress and trauma that emergency workers are exposed to. The chaplain serves as a resource for the department to call on when dealing with the community, but also to assist the employees themselves. Some specific populations that often include a chaplain are law enforcement, fire service, corrections, and the military.

Law Enforcement

Chaplains who are employed in law enforcement settings serve several purposes that can vary depending on the organization. It is important to ensure officer well-being by providing a safe place where the officer can express how they feel about their personal and professional lives. The chaplain is bound by confidentiality, which allows for trust regarding department grievances. Chaplains form personal connections with members of the department through attendance at roll calls, participating in ride-alongs, and offering to assist with outside events (e.g., weddings and funerals). The head of the law enforcement agency may also call upon the chaplain to assist in crisis situations and death notifications. One of the most relevant roles for a law enforcement chaplain in recent years is fostering the relationship between the law enforcement agency and the community. The community liaison position can be strengthened by attending community outreach events and being a public figure for the department.

Fire Service

Similar to law enforcement chaplains, a chaplain who works in the fire service, makes themselves available around the clock for emergencies and counseling services. Many chaplains refer to their availability for both critical incidents and social celebrations as *ministry of presence* (Yancy et al., 2022). The fire service is unique due to the types of relationships that are formed and the teamwork that is established by living together at the firehouse. Therefore, there may need to be a more collectivistic approach to solving problems and incorporating families into the services that are provided. Attending events, such as a potluck dinner, can be an important opportunity to bond so the chaplain is already familiar with the firefighters when a crisis arises.

Corrections

Inmates have certain religious and spiritual rights that are outlined in the Religious Freedom Restoration Act and can be fulfilled with the assistance of a chaplain (Coleman, 2014). Individuals who are incarcerated often explore spirituality to find a higher purpose and to deal with the psychological demands of being imprisoned. Additionally, some inmates are seeking forgiveness for crimes they have committed. Chaplains can provide spiritual guidance and instill hope for the future (Chui & Cheng, 2014). Another service correctional chaplains offer is ensuring accessibility to religious texts and accommodating dietary restrictions (Warner-Robbins, 2013). Correctional facilities that staff full-time, part-time, or volunteer chaplains may also request that the chaplain manage additional volunteers (Coleman, 2014).

Military

Chaplaincy in the military has been well-vetted in all branches and is an essential position to provide care for those who serve. Many first responders have military experience and hold either active duty or veteran status. Due to the nature of their work in the military (e.g., structure, command, and high risk), many veterans find it easier to adapt to an occupation that is para-militaristic such as law enforcement, corrections, or fire service. Employees who have bridged a career in the military with first response have needs that may be different than their nonmilitary colleagues, including specific trauma, adapting to a civilian lifestyle, lack of structure in nonmilitary settings, ongoing deployment, and identifying a purpose for their new mission as a first responder. The chaplain can be a useful tool for guiding and supporting these transitions.

Roles of the First Responder Chaplain

Chaplains can operate in many capacities depending on the needs of the department and their commitment to serve. Due to the flexibility of the position, they often are not assigned a single role. Therefore, it is essential for the chaplain to define the particular roles they will fill for an agency and the boundaries of where their role ends. Some roles a chaplain in a first responder setting can fulfill are community relations, crisis intervention, department and first responder well-being, line of duty death, suicide, death notifications, and disaster relief.

Community Relations

First responder groups and communities can be plagued by mutual misunderstandings and mistrust. Chaplains can serve as intermediaries to communicate needs and deliver resources. One essential component of chaplaincy involves building relationships with local religious figures, hospital administrators, and community leaders (Adcock et al., 1998). When crises occur, chaplains access this network to provide multifaceted support to victims who may not be emotionally stable enough to know what resources are available or how to mobilize them. This network is established by assisting with weddings, funerals, invocations, volunteering, and disaster relief. A proactive chaplain will seek out events they may attend to build relationships such as at community centers, religious organizations, hospitals, and senior centers. Over time, the chaplain's familiarity as a pillar of the community is reassuring to individuals because they can trust them in times of crisis.

Crisis Intervention

Law enforcement agencies often employ a crisis response team (CRT) and a chaplain should be included as part of this response. The Critical Incident Stress Management (CISM) model also incorporates the use of a chaplain for debriefings. Chaplains have experience counseling individuals during trauma and grief and can assist with defusing emotions and stress management (McDearis, 2009). The crisis intervention skills a chaplain possesses can be beneficial for victims who are in crisis, as well as for first responders dealing with secondary trauma (Koch, 2010). Chaplains can also support families, communities, and administrative personnel through counseling services and referrals to mental health professionals and local clergy (Braswell et al., 2016):

> A motorcycle accident left one boy dead and drew a throng of over 30 people. The crowd included many emotional witnesses, friends, and family members expressing anger, fear, sadness, guilt, and confusion. A chaplain arrived and began using phrases, such as "Please help me" and "Love and care for each other," to manage the group and direct them away from the crash site. The chaplain identified the most rational individuals, used their influence to unite the crowd over their shared loss, and led them in an impromptu prayer service. This calmed them and enabled law enforcement officers to investigate without interference. After the incident, the chaplain notified family members and assisted with funeral arrangements.

Department and First Responder Well-Being

There are a variety of ways for a chaplain to establish rapport with employees including providing counseling, attending roll calls and meetings, facilitating weddings and funerals, and assisting with crisis response. The chaplain can also assist the department as a whole by engaging in community outreach events and acting as a liaison to various businesses, organizations, and places of worship. One way a chaplain can show support for employees is to make hospital visits when the employee or employee's family member is sick or injured. The flexibility of a chaplain's work schedule and the wide variety of their roles can assist in building relationships with individuals who work in the department. Chaplains can foster well-being by providing hope and support. Additionally, a chaplain can provide spiritual guidance to help an individual identify their underlying values and sense of purpose. Aside from individual support, a chaplain can support the department by identifying community needs and keeping apprised of current events:

> Following the motorcycle accident that resulted in the young boy's death, the chaplain felt concerned for the well-being of officers at the scene of the crash. The chaplain identified officers with children around the same age as the boy who died and monitored their reactions over the next month by communicating with the on-scene supervisor and attending roll calls.

Line of Duty Death

One of the most tragic occurrences for a department is a line of duty death. A chaplain may respond with the chief to notify the family of the fallen first responder and provide ongoing support to assist with funeral arrangements. In order to support the family appropriately with their grief, the chaplain needs to identify the family's particular cultural and religious customs. Continued support can be provided by the chaplain on the anniversary of the death to assess the emotional and financial needs of the family. When a department loses one of its own, there are particular traditions that are carried out at the funeral that the family may be unaware of. The chaplain can serve as a liaison between the department and the grieving family during this difficult time:

> A chaplain received a call to respond to the hospital in reference to a deputy who was shot multiple times. The chaplain arrived with the sheriff and command staff and they were advised the deputy's injuries were going to be fatal. They notified the sheriff's department in the county where the wife resided and were escorted to her residence without lights and sirens to avoid disturbing the community or making them aware of their presence. The chaplain knocked on the door at 3:10 am and the wife knew by their presence something terrible had occurred. She was informed by the chaplain, "Your husband has been in an accident and has been shot." The priority was for the wife to respond to the hospital prior to her husband's passing so she could say goodbye. While at the house, the chaplain received a notification the husband had succumbed to his injuries. The interaction shifted and

became a death notification for the wife and her three children who were asleep upstairs. The oldest daughter awoke and came downstairs where she was notified of her father's passing. The chaplain asked who he could call to come sit with them to support them at this difficult time. A deputy from the county where the family resided was at the home for the notification and was a family friend. This deputy stayed to support the family and additional friends and neighbors responded to support the grieving children. Although it was very early in the morning, these friends were asked to respond as soon as possible.

The chaplain called the American Red Cross to notify the adult son (via chain of command) who was serving as an active member of the United States Marine Corps. The son was officially notified, called his mother over the phone, and made arrangements to return home immediately. At this time the second oldest daughter awoke and was notified her father was killed while on duty. The house was full of support from loved ones and friends and the chaplain offered to call a local clergy member, but the family stated they would rather contact them at a later time. The news of the deputy's passing reached the agency where he worked and the larger community. The chaplain responded to assist grieving employees and deputies who were close friends of his. The chaplain's primary role is to maintain peace with the family, ensure they are taken care of, and do not become overwhelmed. The chaplain's role then shifts and they are responsible for helping, comforting, and encouraging the department and the larger community. The hospital employees, sheriff's department employees, and community members had created assembly areas where they brought food to gather together to love and support one another. The chaplain encouraged them to, "Give each other a shoulder to cry on and don't be ashamed or afraid to show your emotion or tears, because today we lost a member of our family." During the planning of the funeral arrangements, the chaplain met the family at the funeral home and was available to assist and care for them while they made decisions for the service based on family wishes and law enforcement traditions. The chaplain helped secure a location large enough for multiple law enforcement agencies and their honor guards to attend. On the day of the service, there were 4,000 individuals in attendance. The chaplain needs to be available and totally committed to ensure the family is ministered to and cared for until the service is completed and long after. The chaplain and the family are still in contact over a decade later. When the chaplain is asked, "Is that what you do?" his response is, "That's who I am."

Suicide

First responders are at greater risk for suicide than the civilian population and one factor is their occupational risk (e.g., exposure to trauma, unpredictability of shiftwork, marital difficulties, and unwillingness to disclose mental health issues) (Tiesman et al., 2021). Although stress from work may contribute to mental health issues and suicidality, most agencies do not currently consider suicide a result of working conditions that qualify the individual for life insurance benefits or line of duty death funeral services. The suicide may even occur while the first responder is on duty, in uniform, at their place of work, and/or include their service weapon.

The families of these first responders may experience grief, confusion, anger, and embarrassment. The chaplain should respond to carry out a next of kin notification and may use the phrase "took their life" to describe the manner in which the death occurred. The chaplain is there as a support to the family and not as a medical professional to answer detailed questions about the means of death. Therefore, it should be cautioned that a chaplain should never indicate the death was a suicide if there is an active investigation that has not yet determined the cause of death. The family may experience anger at their loved one or anger at God when the questions of "how" and "why" arise. If the family asks *why* this occurred the chaplain may choose to respond, "We do not know why" and if they ask *how* the response could be, "It is still under investigation." The chaplain should refer the family to their personal religious leader to assist them with the stages of grief and to answer specific questions about afterlife beliefs. Typically, these deeper questions arise once emotions have settled and as the funeral approaches. The chaplain may also refer the family to counseling with a mental health professional, especially if they were privy to the underlying reasons the suicide occurred or are experiencing survivor's guilt because they feel they should have taken action to protect their loved one sooner. Although the chaplain's primary roles are similar to a line of duty death, there are nuanced differences when dealing with a suicide.

Death Notifications

Line of duty deaths and suicides within a department are unique circumstances that require specific protocols and delicacy in how the situation is handled. Another role the chaplain fills for an agency is assisting with civilian death notifications. The chaplain may accompany first responders when someone in the community dies and the notification must be made. Chaplains provide first responders assistance with delivering the news, navigating the grief process, and providing options for the funeral service. This allows first responders to have additional time to fulfill other duties. If the family does not have a local clergy member whom they trust, the chaplain may even offer to officiate the funeral service. Death notifications are at the heart of the real chaplain ministry – to help the family get in touch with core values.

Disaster Relief

Disasters, such as those caused by weather, terrorism, mass vehicle accidents, train derailments, plane crashes, mass shootings, explosions, and structural collapse, lead to panic, trauma, grief, and suffering. A major component of disaster relief is contacting networks, governmental agencies, and businesses to allocate resources where they are most needed. Chaplains can be placed at reunification or relief centers to provide aid to civilians. Additionally, chaplains should be part of the CISM team to provide defusings and debriefings for employees providing crisis response (e.g., search and rescue pilots and crews who responded to hurricane Ian). Emergency operations procedures should be outlined well in advance of a crisis at the municipal, county, and state levels. Attempting to assign roles and delegate steps to take during an emergency will slow response times and exacerbate trauma due to a lack of resources. A chaplain's role in these disaster relief efforts can be invaluable, and their network of support should be called upon to provide the community with the best possible response:

> A transcontinental plane flight crashed during landing at a layover, killing all but 27 passengers. Three of the 11 crew members survived, but did not serve as crew on a flight after this incident. In the county where the flight originated, the airport contacted the local sheriff's office, and the sheriff made contact with the department chaplain. The chaplain had established a volunteer clergy corps for emergencies such as this, consisting of a Christian minister, a rabbi, an imam, and a Catholic priest. This team assembled at the airport in a large conference room where the families of the loved ones aboard the flight could return to the airport and assemble. Airport security was notified to allow the families access to re-renter the airport and gather in this room. The airport staff provided information as well as food, drinks, and tissues for the families while they received news of their loved ones. Telephones were provided for families to contact loved ones around the country and communicate information regarding their family member who was aboard the flight. The volunteer clergy corps were stationed at various points around the room as a resource for individuals of different faiths to receive information and comfort. These religious leaders also made contact with the families' local clergy, at their request, via phone or extended an invitation for them to respond to the airport directly. This on-site resource was instrumental in helping individuals engage immediately with their faith and receive consolation. There were also translators available representing various languages for families to communicate directly in their native language. The airport provided accommodations at a nearby hotel for families to relocate for dinner and to stay overnight if they did not reside locally. The communication between the airport, sheriff's office, chaplain, and volunteer clergy corps is an example of being situationally aware and ready for disaster relief. A chaplain who is prepared has made these connections with religious leaders in the community and has assembled this team long before an emergency occurs.

Stress and Burnout

As outlined above, the chaplain's roles involve counseling individuals and families, conducting death notifications, and managing critical incident stress and trauma. Trauma can transfer vicariously from an individual in crisis, to a first responder, and then to the chaplain counseling the first responder group. The chaplain's occupation puts them at increased risk of burnout. Maslach and Jackson (1981) describe burnout as chronic psychological strain and emotional exhaustion due to increased interactions with the public and is associated with mental and physical health problems (e.g., insomnia, fatigue, family discord, personal distress). When an individual experiences burnout, it can lead to decreased empathy, or "compassion fatigue." Chaplains should be especially vigilant to watch for signs of burnout since empathy and compassion are core components of a chaplain's work. It should be noted that not every individual experiences burnout as a result of their work due to individual factors such as age, personality, coping skills, and resiliency. Signs of burnout may include psychological reactions (e.g., anger, anxiety, job dissatisfaction), physical reactions (e.g., headaches, gastrointestinal issues, decreased immune response), and behavioral reactions (e.g., accidents, substance use, absenteeism) (Kelty & Gordon, 2015). In first responder communities, there is a tendency to identify as heroes who help others, with a lack of awareness they may need to help themselves. The first responder chaplain is embedded in this culture and should maintain awareness of the vulnerability to also identify with these beliefs.

Recommendations for Effective Chaplaincy

There are several recommendations for an agency to utilize a chaplain effectively. First responder chaplains should be thoroughly vetted (i.e., academics, religious endorsements, security clearances, background checks). The agency's chaplain must be trusted with various types of confidential information that are unique to first responder communities and they must represent the department with integrity. When speaking with individuals in crisis, always ask permission to call local clergy. It is imperative for the chaplain to get involved and network with community and religious leaders to assist with these referrals. Through these personal connections, the chaplain builds, they will have contacts for various types of emergencies and disasters. A chaplain should work with diverse populations so they are able to serve the community's diverse needs. Some agencies task chaplains with coordinating volunteers, and the chaplain should also be willing to offer volunteer clergy support at events (e.g., weddings, funerals). Similar to many other professions, chaplains must continue to seek out additional training and continuing education courses so they are well-informed of changes in the field. Most importantly, the agency chaplain should follow through on all matters they are involved in and never promise something they are unwilling or unable to deliver. Chaplaincy should be something one is *called* to do and never just a job, title, or position. It must be the person behind the uniform who serves with compassion, patience, understanding, and the willingness to sacrifice themselves so other people can be cared for. The chaplain is the right person, at the right place, at the right time.

Limitations

Chaplains' roles are varied and diverse, but there are limitations to their roles. The chaplain must not pressure individuals to adopt specific religious beliefs or endorse a particular religion (D'Angelo, 2010). Accepting all faiths, and those who do not identify as spiritual or religious, is critical for assisting individuals in crisis with identifying appropriate resources. A chaplain who works with a first responder agency must serve all employees of the agency, not just the first responders. Additionally, the chaplain should not interfere with department functioning by conducting investigations or excessively participating in ride-alongs (Braswell et al., 2016). Occasionally, individuals show up on scene at large incidents and identify themselves as clergy for self-serving purposes, such as media attention. It is important for clergy who are affiliated with an agency to carry proper credentials to avoid confusion. It should be conveyed that meeting with a chaplain for any type of service is not mandatory, but rather is an available option that is part of the chaplain's open-door policy. Chaplains should make themselves available 24 hours a day, 7 days a week, because the nature of emergencies dictates they do not occur on a set schedule. Confidentiality must be maintained at all times, even when pressured by agency administration. Having a written policy in place, such as a standard operating procedure, outlining the job functions of an agency chaplain is an asset. It is essential for chaplains to understand their job roles, but it is just as important for them to understand their boundaries while working within the parameters of an agency.

Summary

Chaplains hold varied roles depending on the agency and first responder population with which they are working. The size of the agency and its financial resources often determines the capacity in which a chaplain is called upon. The primary aim of a chaplain should be to encourage, support, and comfort those to whom they are ministering. Due to the power and prestige that can accompany working with first responder agencies, there is a temptation to identify with the perks of the job (e.g., badge, car, media attention). However, there needs to be an emphasis on the heart of what a chaplain does, as opposed to the status of working with these particular groups. The essence of chaplaincy is evolving due to the nature of our ever-changing world. Technological advances and multiple casualty incidents are making it a necessity for a chaplain's role to be flexible and adaptive. Hopefully, future collaborations and training will lead to a greater understanding of new areas chaplains may be utilized and innovative ways to incorporate a chaplain as part of a crisis response team. Additionally, due to chaplains' repeated exposure to grief and trauma, future research could identify the cumulative effect this work has on chaplaincy. This would aid in recognizing common stressors and mental health issues, as well as resiliency factors, to design prevention and intervention programs specifically for chaplains.

References

Adcock, K. F., Baker, D. J., & Padilla, R. (1998). Initiating a chaplaincy program for a hospital police department. *Journal of Healthcare Protection and Management, 14*(2), 113–116.

Bachrach, D. S. (2004). The friars go to war: Mendicant military chaplains, 1216-c. 1300. *The Catholic Historical Review, 90*(4), 617–633. https://doi.org/10.1353/cat.2005.0003

Braswell, R., Steinkopf, B., & Beamer, A. T. (2016, Nov). Law enforcement chaplains: Defining their roles. *FBI Law Enforcement Bulletin*, 11–16.

Chui, W. H., & Cheng, K. K.-Y. (2014). Self-perceived role and function of Christian prison chaplains and Buddhist volunteers in Hong Kong prisons. *International Journal of Offender Therapy and Comparative Criminology, 57*(2), 154–168. https://doi.org/10.1177/0306624X11432128

Coleman, L. L. (2014, March 1). Options for providing mandated religious/spiritual services in a jail. *Corrections Today,* 72–73.

D'Angelo, J. D. (2010). Friedman, Cary A., Spiritual survival for law enforcement: Practical insights practical tools. *Journal of Police and Criminal Psychology, 25*(1), 56–57. https://doi.org/10.1007/s11896-009-9062-y

Kelty, S. F., & Gordon, H. (2015). No burnout at this coal-face: Managing occupational stress in forensic personnel and the implications for forensic and criminal justice agencies. *Psychiatry, Psychology and Law, 22*(2), 273–290.

Koch, B. J. (2010). The psychological impact on police officers of being first responders to completed suicides. *Journal of Police and Criminal Psychology, 25*(2), 90–98. https://doi.org/10.1007/s11896-010-9070-y

Maslach, C., & Jackson, S. E. (1981). The measurement of experienced burnout. *Journal of Organizational Behavior, 2*(2), 99–113.

McDearis, T. R. (2009). Wounded warriors and the Virginia Tech tragedy: A police chaplain's view. *FBI Law Enforcement Bulletin, 78*(1), 13–19.

Merriam-Webster. (n.d.). Chaplain. In *Merrian-Webster.com dictionary*. Retrieved 10 Nov 2022, from https://www.merriam-webster.com/dictionary/chaplain

Tiesman, H. M., Elkins, K. L., Brown, M., Marsh, S., & Carson, L. M. (2021, April 6). *Suicides among first responders: A call to action*. Centers for Disease Control and Prevention. https://blogs.cdc.gov/niosh-science-blog/2021/04/06/suicides-first-responders/#_ednref2

Warner-Robbins, C. (2013). A calling to all jail chaplains. *American Jails, 26*(6), 78–79.

Yancy, A., Molskness, B., & Duncan, J. (2022). *Developing a successful fire chaplain service in your fire department*. International Association of Fire Chiefs Volunteer and Combination Officer Section.

Mental Health of Retired First Responders

Jordana Pepper and Emily M. Cnapich

Retirement, defined as an individual's exit from the workforce signaling a decreased psychological commitment to work (Wang & Shi, 2013), is undoubtedly a complex and often jarring shift in the lives and routines of many. For some, it marks the transition to days of leisure and liberation. In others, the change can lead to a disruption of identity and decline in both physical and psychological health (Clouston & Denier, 2017). Research regarding retirement from the civilian workforce is plentiful, but inconclusive as to whether retirement marks a positive or negative shift; this seems to depend on the presence of certain internal characteristics and external factors. For example, retirement is often conceptualized as a life crisis with numerous studies highlighting mental health problems in retirees of all ages (Gill et al., 2006). Further, type of retirement, namely, forced or early, also has the potential to negatively affect psychological well-being (Börsch-Supan & Schuth, 2014; Dave et al., 2006; Park & Kang, 2016; van der Heide et al., 2013). Personal resilience, social support, community involvement, and financial preparedness, however, are considered protective factors against psychological decline post-retirement across numerous studies. Many highlight that positive adjustment to retirement is contingent on available resources both financially and psychologically (Kubicek et al., 2011). Regardless of the nature of retirement, it is considered a life event requiring coping and adaptation, which could lead to many challenges in which psychological health is compromised (Lindwall et al., 2017).

These findings may be useful when considering first responder groups. However, based on the unique nature of a first responder's job (i.e., increased exposure to

---

J. Pepper (✉)
Federal Bureau of Prisons, Lompoc, CA, USA
e-mail: jpepper@bop.gov

E. M. Cnapich
College of Psychology, Nova Southeastern University, Fort Lauderdale, FL, USA

M. L. Bourke et al. (eds.), *First Responder Mental Health*,
https://doi.org/10.1007/978-3-031-38149-2_18

trauma and intense physical and psychological stress), more research specifically examining this subgroup of retirees is still needed.

Empirical and qualitative research consistently highlight a distinct culture that characterizes public safety personnel, revealing undertones of tight-knit brotherhood and cynicism (Kronenberg et al., 2008). First responder culture regularly leads its members to integrate their personal and professional identities, with professional roles often taking precedence over outside relationships (Kronenberg et al., 2008; Shannon, 2016). For example, firefighters, who comprise a large subset of first responders/emergency personnel, often describe themselves as firefighters first and everything else second (Pepper et al., 2022). In these situations, where work and employment are the primary sources of an individual's self-identity, the act of retirement can bring about profound psychological upset to the retiree (Latif, 2011). As the close bond shared by first responders is figuratively severed by retirement, concerns for the psychological well-being of retirees ensue. Because of the unique characteristics that define these professionals, retirement often poses challenges, as former public safety personnel strive to create new, meaningful, social identities and roles.

There is existing evidence supporting the contributions of identity and self-image to psychological well-being (Lodi-Smith & Roberts, 2010; Sharma & Sharma, 2010). In police officers, the shift to retirement can be difficult due to the loss of their professional identity which is central to their self-concept (Muthondeki et al., 2014). This deviation can be detrimental for a group of individuals who are already deemed at greaert risk for developing a multitude of mental health problems. Similar trends are found in firefighters, who are often the first group of responders on the scene of any emergency. Law enforcement officers, firefighters, and other first responder groups are exposed to numerous traumatic and stressful events over the course of their careers (Karaffa et al., 2015). In fact, their frequent exposure to traumatic events, combined with abnormal and erratic sleep schedules inherent in shift work, pose a significant threat to their mental health throughout their careers and beyond (Stanley et al., 2017). Exposure to traumatic events, in conjunction with other occupational and everyday stressors, leaves first responders at risk of experiencing behavioral and mental health problems such as depression (Henderson et al., 2016; Wang et al., 2010), substance abuse (Menard & Arter, 2014), posttraumatic stress disorder (Henderson et al., 2016; Klimley et al., 2018), and suicide (Violanti, 2010). Nonetheless, first responders as a group tend to exhibit great resilience, and there is evidence this may carry over into retirement (Pole et al., 2006). The majority of research concerning these issues, however, focuses primarily on first responders in active-duty roles. Consequently, there is a need to investigate how retirement may impact these risk factors for psychopathology and suicidality post-retirement.

Retirement and Mental Health

Retirement marks a significant milestone in the lives of many. Because of its prominence, researchers have sought to understand the impact of retirement on both physical and psychological functioning. Many studies have produced inconclusive or contradictory results regarding the association between retirement and psychological well-being. These conflicting findings are rooted in two opposing theories surrounding retirement's impact on identity and psychological functioning: continuity theory (Atchley, 1993) and role theory (Latif, 2011; Miller, 1965). According to Atchley (1993), continuity theory proposes that individuals fulfill many roles throughout their lives and that the "work" role may be the least central to identity and life satisfaction. Thus, retirement is viewed as a positive shift as individuals are able to spend a greater amount of time fulfilling more meaningful life roles, leading to improved psychological well-being (Latif, 2011). By contrast, Miller (1965) contends that according to role theory, employment creates a significant source of meaning and self-efficacy, and greatly contributes to the formation of one's identity. When individuals retire, psychological well-being declines as this important role comes to an end, and other roles (e.g., those tied to family or leisure) cannot provide the same sense of self-efficacy as the work role (Latif, 2011).

Both theoretical frameworks account for much of the discrepancy in the literature examining the impact of retirement on civilians. However, research has made it clear that the careers of those in public safety vastly differ from those in the civilian workforce (Baka, 2015; Graf, 1986; Hartley et al., 2013). For example, the profession of policing is engulfed in a deep-seated culture that promotes loyalty, brotherhood, and family-like ties among its members (Loftus, 2010; Westmarland, 2005). Additionally, police culture perpetuates an "us versus them" mentality that is not often seen in civilian workforce populations, shaping the identities of its members. Because of the unique cultural identity shared by law enforcement personnel, role theory seems to best explain the impact retirement can have on the psychological well-being of police officers. As officers' work roles comes to an end, so does a source of their self-respect and identity, which could potentially lead to significant psychological upset among retirees.

A similar conclusion can be drawn among firefighter groups as well, where brotherhood and social bonding is deeply rooted. In fact, the concept of brotherhood in the fire service is characterized by inherent dedication, love, respect, support for one another, living by a code of unspoken duty, trust, honor, loyalty, and the establishment of close relationships, connections, and bonds (Carey et al., 2011). The experience of belonging to a specific professional group is central to the men and women who live with their fellow firefighters, with all that entails, several days a week (Stanley et al., 2018). When that connection is lost, it could signal a reduction in mental wellness, unstable self-views, and increased depression and anxiety (Smith et al., 1996).

Despite the characteristic and theoretical differences between first responder groups and civilian employees, the literature surrounding general workforce retirement and its implications on mental health and functioning still provides valuable findings. When examining how age at retirement, reason for retirement, and pre-retirement education programs influence mental health outcomes among retirees, it was found that forced retirement led to increased risk for adverse mental health consequences post-retirement (Sharpley & Layton, 1998). Indeed, numerous studies have also reflected the increased risk for adverse mental and physical health outcomes following forced retirement (Dave et al., 2006; Drentea, 2002). Additionally, research suggests that pre-retirement trainings that focus on topics other than financial changes prove beneficial in lowering retirees' risk of developing symptoms of anxiety, depression, or stress after retiring. These findings are crucial to developing workforce retirement procedures and training programs. While they may stem from a civilian sample, it is likely that these results are generalizable to first responder populations as well.

Extant literature provides ample evidence outlining a general decline in physical and mental well-being, notably occurring across a window of 6 years post-retirement (Dave et al., 2006). Retirement may also lead to a decline in cognitive processing abilities, as individuals who retired in a 14-year period had worse overall physical and cognitive health compared to those who remained employed during this time (Clouston & Denier, 2017).

Type of retirement (i.e., early, voluntary, involuntary) can also impact psychological well-being and life satisfaction. Whether retirement is deemed voluntary or involuntary is based on the degree of perceived choice or control employees have over the act of retiring (Szinovacz & Davey, 2005). For example, retirement due to injury or illness is often labeled as "involuntary." In other circumstances, workers who feel "pushed out" or pressured to retire by their employers may also perceive retirement as forced or involuntary (Szinovacz & Davey, 2005). Instances of involuntary retirement are typically viewed as highly stressful, often due to the lack of predictability or control over a major life event and change (van der Heide et al., 2013). Because of the sudden and uncontrollable nature of involuntary retirement, it is not uncommon for these individuals to conceptualize their general health as worse or declining after involuntary retirement occurs (Mosca & Barrett, 2016; van der Heide et al., 2013).

More specifically than general health, those who experience involuntary retirement are at greater risk for developing depressive symptoms when compared to those who retire voluntarily (Park & Kang, 2016). The negative impact of involuntary retirement is of particular relevance to law enforcement and first responder personnel, as the myriad of health problems due to the physical nature of the job places these men and women at greater risk for experiencing this type of retirement. The negative impact of forced retirement on mental health, along with preexisting risks for mental health problems in first responders, should shift the well-being of retirees to the forefront of department mental health initiatives.

Early retirement entices many with various benefits and supportive income while simultaneously removing the constraints of employment, promising more time for leisure and enjoyable activities (Börsch-Supan & Schuth, 2014). Although voluntary in many cases, early retirement may still negatively impact cognitive abilities and psychological well-being. Börsch-Supan and Schuth (2014) hypothesized that declines in cognition and subjective well-being are a result of diminished social networks post-retirement. Results of their study supported this hypothesis, revealing that those who retired early (i.e., before the average retirement age for each country from which data were collected) exhibited more rapid cognitive decline when compared to those who retired at, or after, the average retirement age. Similarly, early retirees also had smaller social networks than those who continued to work. Time elapsed since early retirement had the most significant negative correlation with cognition and social network size and was positively correlated with increases in depressive symptoms. Consistent with other findings, larger social networks appeared to be associated with greater subjective well-being regardless of retirement type.

Despite abundant research highlighting retirement's negative impact on psychological and physical health, numerous studies have drawn opposite conclusions, supporting continuity theory's theoretical underpinning that retirement marks a transition to a more fulfilling era of life (Atchley, 1993; Latif, 2011). With the framework of continuity theory in mind, Drentea (2002) sought to examine retirement's impact on perceived control, subjective distress, symptoms of depression, positive outlook, and anxiety. Overall, retirement was associated with fewer symptoms of depression, anxiety, overall distress, and higher levels of positive outlook. However, retirement appeared to be associated with less sense of control, which the authors attributed to a diminished exposure to situations requiring problem-solving. A systematic review of the literature by van der Heide et al. (2013) drew similar conclusions, reporting that 10 of the 12 studies examining retirement's impact on mental health found it to be beneficial. However, this review revealed several discrepancies and gaps in the literature. Many studies failed to examine the role of employment characteristics and retirement type when examining the impact on psychological well-being, which the authors identify as a causal factor for inconsistent findings among studies of this nature. Whether retirement serves as a positive life shift seems to depend on the circumstances surrounding the transition to retired life, as well as the quality of social networks maintained throughout retirement.

Law Enforcement Retirees

Literature concerning the mental health of law enforcement retirees is scarce and inconclusive. However, anecdotal reports from retired officers often detail the difficulties faced while transitioning from their public safety role. Re-integration into civilian life may pose significant challenges for many law enforcement retirees and is regarded as a highly stressful event (Muthondeki et al., 2014; Shannon, 2016). As previously reported, officers who experience forced retirement endorse more depressive symptoms, which are positively correlated with time since retirement (Tuohy et al., 2005). In addition to increased susceptibility to depression, retirees may also experience interpersonal difficulties. An examination of retired police officers in Kenya revealed that nearly 40% of interviewees experienced loneliness, and approximately 30% reported frustration associated with perceived difficulties integrating into civilian roles (Muthondeki et al., 2014). Additionally, cardiovascular disease was 70% more prevalent among retired officers than their civilian counterparts, likely due to chronic exposure to stress throughout their careers (Ramey et al., 2009).

In a series of structured interviews with retirees from Queensland, Australia, four significant contributors towards subjective well-being in retirement were apparent: social support, positive emotional state, family stability, and financial security. The most prominent coping strategies used by participants included some form of social networking (i.e., volunteering, friendships outside of work, hobbies). Consistent with other findings, officers who experienced mandatory retirement displayed poorer coping skills and appeared to have more difficulty adjusting to retirement than those who retired voluntarily (Carney et al., 2021).

Resilience appears to play a significant role in easing the transition to retirement among police officers. In fact, by employing fewer distancing coping strategies (i.e., suppressing or avoiding emotional discomfort), and being open about their professional lives with friends and family, retirees may be able to exhibit higher levels of resilience post-retirement (Pole et al., 2006). Similarly, building and maintaining positive relationships with friends and family outside of their careers as law enforcement officers also promotes resilience and well-being among retirees (Parnaby & Weston, 2020). Understanding specific predictors of resilience in retirement is crucial, as it appears to be the most powerful predictor of life satisfaction for retired officers (Parnaby & Weston, 2020).

Indeed, retirement from police work can result in great psychological distress, as reflected by cases in which retired officers fall victim to increased substance abuse, residual PTSD, and even suicide. Early pre-retirement intervention programs that emphasize integration with other roles outside of policing to ensure a smoother transition into retired life are crucial. While the adjustment to retirement can be a semi-traumatic experience in itself, adequate preparation and access to mental health resources can protect against the negative outcomes that follow this shift (Violanti, 2007).

Firefighter Retirees

Firefighters are a subset of professional rescue workers who are often exposed to intense physical pain, trauma, and psychological stress from repeated exposure to both human suffering and death (Psarros et al., 2018). Additionally, firefighting has one of the highest injury rates of first responder and rescue personnel and is considered one of the most dangerous jobs in the world (National Institute for Occupational Safety and Health, 2001). While repeated exposure to trauma, injury, and death often predisposes firefighters to numerous mental health problems including PTSD, depression, sleep problems, substance use, and suicidality (Boxer & Wild, 1993;

Heyman et al., 2018; Psarros et al., 2018; Stanley et al., 2018), retirement and a loss of self-concept clarity are additional, less explored, risk factors for the development of psychological problems for firefighters when they leave the workforce.

First responder culture, especially in the fire service, is narrowing in the sense that firefighters typically place their sole reliance for both social and emotional support on other first responders (Sunderland, 2014). Understandably, when the ease of access to these social supports provided by working is lost to retirement, a sense of thwarted belongingness is likely to ensue. In fact, according to Chu et al. (2016), this sense of thwarted belongingness, which is amplified by the loss of an environment that once provided support and stability, likely increases the risk of depression and suicidality in this group of first responders. An abrupt change in social roles may also contribute to a decline in psychological well-being for retired firefighters who typically define themselves by their professional roles. When they are no longer able to view themselves as a "firefighter first," social and family discord can result. In fact, many firefighters see their places of work as a "haven" from stressful home and social environments (S. Pepper, personal communication, March 15, 2020). Limited, or even restricted, access to this haven can amplify family discord and further contribute to a possible decline in the psychological well-being of this group of first responders.

An individual's group affiliations are important in the formation of a person's self-concept (Slotter et al., 2015). Group membership loss, such as the loss suffered through retirement, has the potential to profoundly disrupt the clarity of one's self-concept, which is defined as the extent to which the contents of a person's identity makeup are clearly and confidently defined, internally consistent, and temporally stable (Campbell, 1990). High self-concept clarity is characterized by high self-esteem, improved life satisfaction, and overall contentment (Suszek et al., 2018). However, when self-concept clarity is low, people have the tendency to exhibit increases in both anxiety and depression (Suszek et al., 2018).

In one of the first studies examining the overall psychological functioning of retired firefighters, which included an investigation of the impacts of self-concept clarity on psychological well-being, Pepper et al. (2022) found that out of 300 retirees, retired firefighters were more than twice as likely to suffer from depression. Further, 23.7% of all respondents suffered from a diagnosable substance use disorder, 16.3% experienced elevated levels of anxiety, 11.1% met full criteria for PTSD, and 11.4% endorsed active suicidal ideation, showing their rates of suicidality are slightly higher than the general population for same aged peers, which is between 1.9% and 8.7% (Nock et al., 2008; Pepper et al., 2022). In addition, of the 300 participants in the study, 23.5% had difficulties with life satisfaction, 16.2% endorsed mania or hypomania, 17.1% suffered from impaired social functioning, 21.5% had problems with sexual functioning, and a staggering 37.8% reported significant difficulties with sleep (both falling and staying asleep) (Pepper et al., 2022).

When examining social and personal characteristics contributing to psychological well-being post-retirement, Pepper et al. (2022) found that the older the firefighter, the longer they served on active duty, and the longer they were in their retirement, all correlated with better overall psychological functioning. Additionally, those who were forced into retirement had higher levels of daily physical pain, and those who felt they did not have access to affordable health care all experienced poorer overall psychological functioning. Finally, Pepper et al. (2022) found that the higher the self-concept clarity a firefighter experienced post-retirement, the better their overall psychological functioning. Data also revealed that self-concept clarity significantly moderated the association between overall psychological functioning and feelings of financial stability, type of retirement, and daily levels of pain, such that as self-concept clarity increased in strength, the relationship between overall psychological functioning and the previously mentioned independent variables became weaker and non-significant. Interestingly, self-concept clarity also served as a statistically significant mediator in the relationship between overall psychological functioning, the number of years retired, and daily levels of pain. These findings suggest that retired firefighters with a strong sense of self-concept have a greater ability to more flexibly adjust to changes in social roles and are more protected from poor psychological functioning when faced with life challenges such as loss of a job, physical discomfort, financial instability, and lack of access to affordable healthcare (Pepper et al., 2022).

Summary and Conclusion

Literature concerning retired first responder groups is scarce and limited in scope. However, research relating to active-duty public safety personnel reveals a myriad of mental health problems that are often a result of prolonged exposure to stressful and traumatic situations. Substance abuse, physical health complications, depression, PTSD, and suicide occur at high rates in this population. Several studies have found these concerns continue into retirement (Ramey et al., 2009; Renck et al., 2002; Tuohy et al., 2005). First responders' preexisting risk for these mental health problems can be exacerbated by the difficult transition to retirement, warranting the creation and structure of pre-retirement resources for officers.

The effect of retirement on psychological well-being is unclear. While many studies conclude that retirement can lead to a decline in cognitive functioning and psychological well-being (Clouston & Denier, 2017; Dave et al., 2006), others contend that retirement can lower the risk of experiencing depressive or anxiety symptoms (Drentea, 2002; van der Heide et al., 2013). For law enforcement and firefighter retirees specifically, limited research points to an increase in depressive symptoms (Tuohy et al., 2005), cardiovascular disease (Ramey et al., 2009), and difficulty transitioning to civilian life after retirement (Muthondeki et al., 2014; Violanti, 2007). Regardless of the relationship between retirement and psychological well-being, it is certain that retirement impacts the social identity and roles of these groups as well. During retirement, understanding and conceptualization of the self may become unstable as the roles and expectations change (Sharpley & Layton, 1998). Moreover, loss of identity or group membership during retirement can also lead to a decline in psychological well-being (Praharso et al., 2017; Violanti, 2007).

In summary, the shift to retired life can be a challenge for many individuals, including those in public service. These findings provide essential information that can be integrated into pre-retirement education for both police officers and firefighters. While retirement preparation usually focuses primarily on financial planning, taking steps to promote well-being and resilience following this transition is of equal importance (Sharpley & Layton, 1998). As research notes that fostering current social roles and forming new identities after stressful events is of great importance (Praharso et al., 2017), first responders preparing to retire should be provided with avenues and resources to find meaning through other roles and identities outside the field of public safety. Anecdotally, many retirees have noted that retirement severs the bond between active-duty personnel and those who have retired. Creating avenues (e.g., social media groups, events and activities specifically for retirees) for former first responders to remain connected with each other post-retirement may ease the challenge of this transition.

References

Atchley, R. C. (1993). Continuity theory and the evolution of activity in later life. In J. R. Kelly (Ed.), *Activity and aging: Staying involved in later life* (pp. 5–16). Sage.

Baka, L. (2015). The effects of job demands on mental and physical health in the group of police officers: Testing the mediating role of job burnout. *Studia Psychologica, 57*(4), 285–299.

Börsch-Supan, A., & Schuth, M. (2014). Early retirement, mental health, and social networks. In D. A. Wise (Ed.), *Discoveries in the economics of aging* (pp. 225–250). University of Chicago Press.

Boxer, P. A., & Wild, D. (1993). Psychological distress and alcohol use among firefighters. *Scandinavian Journal of Work and Environmental Health, 19*(2), 121–125. https://doi.org/10.5271/sjweh.1497

Campbell, J. D. (1990). Self-esteem and clarity of the self-concept. *Journal of Personality and Social Psychology, 59*(3), 538–549. https://doi.org/10.1037/0022-3514.59.3.538

Carey, M. G., Al-Zaiti, S. S., Dean, G. E., Sessanna, L., & Finnell, D. S. (2011). Sleep problems, depression, substance use, social bonding, and quality of life in professional firefighters. *Journal of Occupational and Environmental Medicine, 53*(8), 928–933. https://doi.org/10.1097/JOM.0b013e318225898f

Carney, C., Bates, L., & Sargeant, E. (2021). Exploring the impact of retirement on police officers wellbeing. *Police Practice and Research, 22*(1), 257–273.

Chu, C., Buchman-Schmitt, J. M., Hom, M. A., Stanley, I. H., & Joiner, T. E., Jr. (2016). A test of the interpersonal theory of suicide in a large sample of current firefighters. *Psychiatry Research, 240*, 26–33. https://doi.org/10.1016/j.psychres.2016.03.041

Clouston, S. A., & Denier, N. (2017). Mental retirement and health selection: Analyses from the U.S. health and retirement study. *Social Science & Medicine, 178*, 78–86.

Dave, D., Rashad, I., & Spasojevic, J. (2006). *The effects of retirement on physical and mental health outcomes*. (No. w12123). National Bureau of Economic Research.

Drentea, P. (2002). Retirement and mental health. *Journal of Aging and Health, 14*(2), 167–194.

Gill, S. C., Butterworth, P., Rodgers, B., Anstey, K. J., Villamil, E., & Melzer, D. (2006). Mental health and the timing of men's retirement. *Social Psychiatry Psychiatric Epidemiological, 41*, 515–522. https://doi.org/10.1007/s00127-006-0064-0

Graf, F. A. (1986). The relationship between social support and occupational stress among police officers. *Journal of Police Science & Administration, 14*(3), 178–186.

Hartley, T. A., Sarkisian, K., Violanti, J. M., Andrew, M. E., & Burchfiel, C. M. (2013). PTSD symptoms among police officers: Associations with frequency, recency, and types of traumatic events. *International Journal of Emergency Mental Health, 15*(4), 241–253.

Henderson, S. N., Van Hasselt, V. B., LeDuc, T. J., & Couwels, J. (2016). Firefighter suicide: Understanding cultural challenges for mental health professionals. *Journal of Professional Psychology: Research and Practice, 47*(3), 224–230.

Heyman, M., Dill, J., & Douglas, R. (2018). *Mental health and suicide of first responders* [White Paper]. https://rudermanfoundation.org/white_papers/police-officers-and-firefighters-are-more-likely-to-die-by-suicide-than-in-line-of-duty/

Karaffa, K., Openshaw, L., Koch, J., Clark, H., Harr, C., & Stewart, C. (2015). Perceived impact of police work on marital relationships. *The Family Journal, 23*(2), 120–131.

Klimley, K. E., Van Hasselt, V. B., & Stripling, A. M. (2018). Posttraumatic stress disorder in police, firefighters, and emergency dispatchers. *Aggression and Violent Behavior, 43*, 33–44.

Kronenberg, M., Osofsky, H. J., Osofsky, J. D., Many, M., Hardy, M., & Arey, J. (2008). First responder culture: Implications for mental health professionals providing services following a natural disaster. *Psychiatric Annals, 38*(2), 114–118.

Kubicek, B., Korunka, C., Raymo, J. M., & Hoonakker, P. (2011). Psychological well-being in retirement: The effects of personal gendered contextual resources. *The Journal of Occupational Health Psychology, 16*(2), 230–246. https://doi.org/10.1037/a0022334

Latif, E. (2011). The impact of retirement on psychological well-being in Canada. *The Journal of Socio-Economics, 40*(4), 373–380.

Lindwall, M., Berg, A. I., Bjälkebring, P., Buratti, S., Hansson, I., Hassing, L., Henning, G., Kivi, M., König, S., Thorvaldsson, V., & Johansson, B. (2017). Psychological health in the retirement transition: Rationale and first findings in the health, ageing and retirement transitions in Sweden (HEARTS) study. *Frontiers in Psychology, 8*, 1634. https://doi.org/10.3389/fpsyg.2017.01634

Lodi-Smith, J., & Roberts, B. W. (2010). Getting to know me: Social role experiences and age differences in self-concept clarity during adulthood. *Journal of Personality, 78*(5), 1383–1410.

Loftus, B. (2010). Police occupational culture: Classic themes, altered times. *Policing and Society, 20*(1), 1–20.

Ménard, K. S., & Arter, M. L. (2014). Stress, coping, alcohol use, and posttraumatic stress disorder among an international sample of police officers: Does gender matter? *Police Quarterly, 17*(4), 307–327.

Miller, S. J. (1965). The social dilemma of the aging leisure participant. In W. A. Peterson & A. M. Rose (Eds.), *Older people and their social world* (pp. 72–92). F.A. Davis Company.

Mosca, I., & Barrett, A. (2016). The impact of voluntary and involuntary retirement on mental health: Evidence from older Irish adults. *IZA Discussion Papers, 19*, 33–44.

Muthondeki, D., Sirera, M. A., & Mwenje, M. (2014). Psychosocial challenges faced by retired police officers: A case of retired administration police officers in Kenya. *IOSR Journal of Humanities and Social Science, 19*(8), 55–63.

National Institute for Occupational Safety and Health. (2001). *Firefighter injury and fatality data.* http://www.cdc.gov/niosh/ar01contents.html

Nock, M. K., Borges, G., Bromet, E. J., Cha, C. B., Kessler, R. C., & Lee, S. (2008). Suicide and suicidal behavior. *Epidemiologic Reviews, 30*(1), 133–154. https://doi.org/10.1093/epirev/mxn002

Park, H., & Kang, M. Y. (2016). Effects of voluntary/involuntary retirement on their own and spouses' depressive symptoms. *Comprehensive Psychiatry, 66*, 1–8.

Parnaby, P., & Weston, C. (2020). Rethinking role residual: Retired police officers and the inertia of habitus. *Canadian Review of Sociology, 57*(2), 223–242.

Pepper, J. S., Van Hasselt, V. B., Black, R. A., & Schneider, B. A. (2022). Assessment of psychological functioning in retired firefighters. *Psychological Services*. https://doi.org/10.1037/ser0000703

Pole, N., Kulkarni, M., Bernstein, A., & Kaufmann, G. (2006). Resilience in retired police officers. *Traumatology, 12*(3), 207–216.

Praharso, N. F., Tear, M. J., & Cruwys, T. (2017). Stressful life transitions and wellbeing: A comparison of the stress buffering hypothesis and the social identity model of identity change. *Psychiatry Research, 247*, 265–275.

Psarros, C., Theleritis, C., Kokras, N., Lyrakos, D., Koborozos, A., Kakabakou, O., Tzanoulinos, G., Katsiki, P., & Bergiannaki, J. D. (2018). Personality characteristics and individual factors associated with PTSD in firefighters one month after extended wildfires. *Nordic Journal of Psychiatry, 72*(1), 17–23. https://doi.org/10.1080/08039488.2017.1368703

Ramey, S. L., Downing, N. R., & Frankie, W. D. (2009). Milwaukee police department retirees: Cardiovascular disease risk and morbidity among aging law enforcement officers. *AAOHN Journal, 57*(11), 448–453.

Renck, B., Weisaeth, L., & Skarbö, S. (2002). Stress reactions in police officers after a disaster rescue operation. *Nordic Journal of Psychiatry, 56*(1), 7–14.

Shannon, J. (2016). *Retirement for cops, part I: The challenges*. Calibre Press.

Sharma, S., & Sharma, M. (2010). Self, social identity and psychological well-being. *Psychological Studies, 55*(2), 118–136.

Sharpley, C. F., & Layton, R. (1998). Effects of age of retirement, reason for retirement, and pre-retirement training on psychological and physical health during retirement. *Australian Psychologist, 33*(2), 119–124.

Slotter, E. B., Winger, L., & Soto, N. (2015). Loss without each other: The influence of group identity loss on the self-concept. *Journal of Group Dynamics: Theory, Research, and Practice, 19*(1), 15–30. https://doi.org/10.1037/gdn0000020

Smith, M., Wethington, E., & Zhan, G. (1996). Self-concept clarity and preferred coping styles. *The Journal of Personality, 64*(2), 407–434. https://doi.org/10.1111/j.1467-6494.1996.tb00516.x

Stanley, I. H., Boffa, J. W., Hom, M. A., Kimbrel, N. A., & Joiner, T. E. (2017). Differences in psychiatric symptoms and barriers to mental health care between volunteer and career firefighters. *The Journal of Psychiatric Research, 247*, 236–242. https://doi.org/10.1016/j.psychres.2016.11.037

Stanley, I. H., Hom, M. A., Chu, C., Dougherty, S. P., Gallyer, A. J., Spencer-Thomas, S., Shelef, L., Fruchter, E., Comtois, K. A., Gutierrez, P. M., Sachs-Ericsson, N. J., & Joiner, T. E. (2018). Perceptions of belongingness and social support attenuate PTSD symptom severity among firefighters: A multi-study investigation. *Journal of Psychological Services, 16*(4), 543–555. https://doi.org/10.1037/ser0000240

Sunderland, K. J. (2014). *Officer safety after the badge: Preretirement mental health training for law enforcement officers* [Unpublished doctoral dissertation]. Retrieved from: http://search.proquest.com.ezproxylocal.library.nova.edu/docview/1709218635?accountid=6579. Order number: AAI3639556.

Suszek, H., Fronczyk, K., Kopera, M., & Maliszewski, N. (2018). Implicit and explicit self-concept clarity and psychological adjustment. *The Journal of Personality and Individual Differences, 123*, 253–256. https://doi.org/10.1016/j.paid.2017.11.038

Szinovacz, M. E., & Davey, A. (2005). Predictors of perceptions of involuntary retirement. *The Gerontologist, 45*(1), 36–47.

Tuohy, A., Knussen, C., & Wrennall, M. J. (2005). Effects of age on symptoms of anxiety and depression in a sample of retired police officers. *Psychology and Aging, 20*(2), 202–210.

van der Heide, I., van Rijn, R. M., Robroek, S. J., Burdorf, A., & Proper, K. I. (2013). Is retirement good for your health? A systematic review of longitudinal studies. *BMC Public Health, 13*(1), 1–11.

Violanti, J. M. (2007). *Police suicide: Epidemic in blue*. Charles C. Thomas Publisher.

Violanti, J. M. (2010). Suicide or undetermined? A national assessment of police suicide death classification. *International Journal of Emergency Mental Health, 12*(2), 89–94.

Wang, M., & Shi, J. (2013). Psychological research on retirement. *The Annual Review of Psychology, 65*, 209–233. https://doi.org/10.1146/annurev-psych-010213-115131

Wang, Z., Inslicht, S. S., Metzler, T. J., Henn-Haase, C., McCaslin, S. E., Tong, H., Neylan, T. C., & Marmar, C. R. (2010). A prospective study of predictors of depression symptoms in police. *Psychiatry Research, 175*(3), 211–216.

Westmarland, L. (2005). Police ethics and integrity: Breaking the blue code of silence. *Policing and Society, 15*(2), 145–165.

Employee Assistance Programs

Judy Couwels

Definition of Employee Assistance Programs

> The Employee Assistance Professional Association (EAPA) defines an EAP as a worksite-based program designed to assist (1) work organizations in addressing productivity issues and (2) "employee clients" in identifying and resolving personal concerns, including, but not limited to, health, marital, family, financial, alcohol, drug, legal, emotional, stress, or other personal issues that may affect job performance. EAPA was established in 1971 and represents the largest international membership organization for EA professionals. (EAPA, 2022, p. 1)

The definition of an Employee Assistance Program (EAP) varies depending on where (type of industry or agency) the EAP is functioning and what standards are being applied. It is important to have a working definition of an EAP. The definitions of an EAP will vary, depending on the type of EAP (internal vs. external), the nature of the services offered, and how the EAP operates. EAPs, in general, are worksite-based programs designed to help individual employees and the organization. "EAPs are a professional assessment and referral and/or short-term counseling services offered to employees with alcohol, drug, or mental health problems that may affect their jobs" (Masi, 2000). Employees may self-refer to the EAP or be referred by supervisors/managers.

J. Couwels (✉)
Bureau of Human Resources, Broward Sheriff's Office (Ret.), Fort Lauderdale, FL, USA

M. L. Bourke et al. (eds.), *First Responder Mental Health*,
https://doi.org/10.1007/978-3-031-38149-2_19

EAP Core Technology

When discussing the definition of EAPs, it is important to describe the Core Technology. The EAP Core Technology was based on research conducted by Paul Roman and Terry Blum in 1988. Their research was intent on establishing a standardization of what constitutes EAP services and "identify those unique functions of the EAPs that differentiate them from other human resource activities in the workplace" (Roman & Blum, 1988). It is recognized that these eight components are essential to an EAP: (1) consultation with, training of, and assistance to work organization leadership (managers, supervisors, and union officials) seeking to manage troubled employees, enhance the work environment, and improve employee job performance; (2) active promotion of the availability of EA services to employees, their family members, and the work organization; (3) confidential and timely problem identification/assessment services for employee clients with personal concerns that may affect job performance; (4) use of constructive confrontation, motivation, and short-term intervention with employee clients to address problems that affect job performance; (5) referral of employee clients for diagnosis, treatment, and assistance, as well as case monitoring and follow-up services; (6) assisting work organizations in establishing and maintaining effective relations with treatment and other service providers and in managing provider contracts; (7) consultation to work organizations to encourage availability of and employee access to health benefits covering medical and behavioral problems including, but not limited to, alcoholism, drug abuse, and mental and emotional disorders; and (8) the evaluation of the effects of EA services on work organizations and individual job performance.

EAP History in the United States: Mid 1970s

The term "EAP" was coined by the NIAAA (National Institute on Alcohol Abuse and Alcoholism). The acronym grew out of the original name: ALMACA (Association of Labor-Management Administrators and Consultants on Alcoholism), which was the precursor of EAPA. To promote the use of EAPs, the NIAAA funded two occupational program consultants (OPCs) for each state.

These OPCs (known as the "Thundering 100") were charged with helping employers develop EAPs. The original focus of the EAP was largely concerned with addressing alcohol issues with employees. The shift from Occupational Alcohol Programs (OAP) to a more comprehensive EAP led to many changes in the field. The broader based focus on addressing other problems besides alcohol, including depression, mental health, parent/child issues, and family issues. This change in strategy emphasized a more informal one that effectively encouraged worker self-referrals. This period also saw an increased number of referrals to outside agencies and resources. Staff for these programs are largely now mental health professionals with a state license and master's degrees, which replaced the paraprofessionals of the OAPs who were, themselves, often recovering alcoholics.

Labor unions in many industries utilize an employee-based "member assistance program" (MAP) to assist employees with addictions and other personal issues. Often, the MAP will work in conjunction with the organization's EAP to provide assessment, referral, and follow-up services. MAP members are very invested in helping their members get assessment, access treatment, and maintain a supportive recovery network to help them maintain their jobs.

EAP History in the United States: EAPs Today and Future Trends

Modern day EAPs often offer a variety of resources, depending on the type of program model. External EAPs, often funded through the employer's insurance, publish a telephone number via pamphlets, literature mailed to employees' homes, work site posters, and email blasts. Some EAPs provide websites with a great deal of information for their client companies to access. EAPs are also in the forefront in offering telephone, telehealth, and email counseling. Since 9/11, EAPs have been repeatedly called upon to provide responses to traumatic incidents with an in-person response. Due to longer working hours and two-career couples, the workplace has been forced to address issues such as childcare, eldercare, financial stress, legal issues, and other employee needs that formerly would have been provided in the community. The resulting attempt to help employees meet these needs is the "Work/ Life Program."

Structure

Internal Versus External

Not all EAPs are created equal. Frequently, the title EAP can have multiple definitions. Original EAPs were designed as an internal, "in-house" entities. The EAP consisted of company/agency employees with mental health/substance abuse training hired to provide hands on services: assessment and referral, in service training, crisis intervention, management consultation, and overseeing supervisory/command referrals. Advantages of internal EAPs include knowledge of agency culture, familiarity with jargon, and understanding of the intricacies of the politics. Effective internal EAPs offer services consistent with the business model or agency practices, can become familiar with employees, and can be perceived as "part of the first responder community." As department employees, staff are more likely to have a long-term commitment to the agency, ease in obtaining management support, and a greater chance of institutionalizing the program.

Disadvantages of internal programs stem from employees seeing the EAP as a tool of management with concerns about confidentiality, risk of dual relationships, and additional costs or limitations placed on EAP by departmental supervisors.

External EAPs

First responders may be less likely to view outside employees with suspicion, and the program costs may be cheaper. Additionally, the outside employee may have greater autonomy and be less likely to have dual relationships. The downside to an external program could include staff not being familiar with first responder culture/stress, not perceived as institutionalized, and could be vulnerable to budget cuts.

Hybrid EAPs

A hybrid EAP contains the advantages of both internal and external programs. The agency can have a full-time in-house administrator who directs the program and supervises the external, off-site psychologists. Many external providers were compelled to shift treatment services to telehealth during the pandemic. After Covid-19 pandemic, many providers continue to offer therapy services via telehealth. The in-house administrator can conduct assessment and referral for employees with counseling referral options to the agency psychologist and/or mental health providers available through the agency insurance. An internal person can offer behavioral health in-service trainings, new supervisor orientation, and oversight of the peer support program.

The EAP model utilized for a first responder agency should provide EAP staffing to reflect the unique challenges and obstacles for a 24-hour operation. First responders' calls for EAP services are often urgent in nature, especially if precipitated by a crisis. For example, an internal EAP could have an "away" message recording for after hour calls suggesting that the caller should contact the insurance company phone number and in an emergency call 911 or proceed to your local emergency room. This advice would not be received well in a first responder agency with law enforcement, communications, detention, and fire/paramedic services, all of which are 24-hour operations. If your agency is 911, you can't ask employees in crisis to call 911.

Unique Challenges to EAPs and First Responders

There are some unique demands for EAPs in a governmental or municipal setting which retains first responders. First responders' definition includes law enforcement, firefighters, paramedics, and communications operators. First responders' requests for services can involve crisis intervention from an EAP in the form of a critical incident. A critical incident is any event that is outside the realm of ordinary human experience and has the potential to overwhelm one's usual coping skills (Everly & Mitchell, 2000). Critical incidents can involve accidents with children, injury or death of co-workers, or situations with someone they may know. An example of a child-related event would involve a pediatric drowning, which could affect the call taker in 911 who heard the mother's screams for help, the responding law enforcement personnel who pulled the child out of the water and began the CPR, or the firefighter/paramedic who took over CPR and raced the child to the hospital.

Another unique but difficult stressor with first responders is "sanctuary trauma." Both law enforcement and fire service promote the concept of "family" among the troops. Employees are frequently disappointed about their "family" when under an internal affairs investigation or suspension. The employee may have strong feelings about how they were treated. McKay and Gravel (2016) characterize this sentiment as "sanctuary trauma," also known as "betrayal trauma." "This type of trauma occurs when an individual, who thought he or she was safe and supported within the organization in a time of need, discovers that the organization – and their colleagues – are not trustworthy or supporting them at all. They become angry and bitter, and find it difficult to trust anyone, especially those in a position of authority in the organization" (McKay & Gravel, 2016, p. 15).

Culture

There is a distinct sense of a closed group better known as "cop culture." Part of this closed society credo is based on the shared belief that no civilian or outsider could possibly understand what they go through on a day-to-day basis. There is a formal and informal police culture that can exert considerable influence on the individual. Police organizations apply pressure on officers to conform to the behaviors consistent with the "police role." The outcome of this process is a "collective pool of knowledge that determines what is appropriate behavior, directs understanding, and gives guidance on how to resolve problems" (Kampanakis, 2000, p. 129). Informal police culture expects loyalty; an officer never "rats" on another officer, and the code of secrecy remains very influential. Experiences shared by group members result in knowledge on how to act and how to think about work. Cynicism and a cynical notion of reality remains a persistent theme among law enforcement. The socialization process into the police role begins early in the police training. The sense of a superhuman emotional strength (Violanti, 1990) suggests that they can handle anything and never need emotional assistance. Once identified with the police role, they can begin to see and interact with the world exclusively through this lens. This can create a narrow perspective, which limits emotional response options, and in turn affects intimate and family relationships, as well as diminishes any help-seeking behavior.

Marketing

Marketing an EAP program requires ongoing efforts to bring and keep awareness of programs. These efforts can include giveaways: stress balls, key chains, job aids with self-help reminders, and printed materials. Visibility or showing up on work sites increases and maintains awareness. Often employees will remark, "I have been meaning to call you" and by being present, they are able to receive timely information. EAPs need to tailor marketing strategies to the organization and utilize interventions that the leadership recognizes as acceptable services and promotional activities. Monthly newsletters with timely topics, internal "learning management systems" to impart some basic mental health training and supervisory training. Regular sessions of "EAP introduction and overview" keeps up EAP awareness and can be offered to new supervisors, sergeants, and lieutenants, as well as incoming/graduating academy classes for law enforcement, detention, and communications. The EAP needs to be sensitive to how the organization manages its preference for problem-solving in its day-to-day operation and functions. Some organizations use careful succession planning vs. crisis management and these elements can inform planning to maximize the marketing approach within the organization.

Specialized Programs/Interventions

Unions

Police departments, sheriff's offices, and fire rescue departments have long traditions of unions. Over 70% of all rank-and-file officers are covered by some form of collective bargaining agreement today (Levine, 1988). Police are still highly unionized in the United States in the twenty-first century, in contrast to the declining union membership of other professions in both the public and private sectors. High union membership rates among police and other law enforcement officers compel the EAP to develop a working relationship with the associated union.

The International Association of Fire Fighters (IAFF) has more than 316,000 members in its more than 3200 affiliate organizations (International Association of Fire Fighters, 2018). The IAFF is a labor union representing paid full-time firefighters and emergency medical services personnel in the United States and Canada. They provide comprehensive administrative support, discipline, fraternity, and benefits.

EAPs need to develop relationships with Union leadership and representatives. It is important for the union to understand how the EAP works to provide the shared value of employee well-being both physically, psychologically, and emotionally. Effective EAPs work closely with union representatives to coordinate care and provide support and direction for their members in crisis. The EAP can often help facilitate the necessary treatment (mental health and/or substance abuse) for the member to aid them in getting back to work.

Law Enforcement Officers and EAP

Limited research exists on the relationship between EAPs and law enforcement officers. What does exist points to the importance of EAPs marketing their existence and availability. Asen and Colon (1995) surveyed 82 police officers from four municipalities with a common external EAP. Most respondents (70%) had seen the policy, only 22% reported using their EAP, and 15.9% reported usage for a family member. A review of gender differences found a significant difference in willingness to use an EAP, with females more likely than males to report utilization. (This is consistent with women seeking mental health services at a much higher rate than men).

Goldstein (2006) discussed officers' hesitancy regarding accessing available EAP services, noting that police officers often report not being interested or willing to seek help for problems associated with their jobs. Donnelly et al. (2015) found 16% of surveyed police officers and deputy sheriffs used their EAP in spite of 56% reporting knowledge of the EAP's resources. This population was 70% male and 56% white. Their findings indicated that officers who did not know enough about how to access their EAP were in substantially more distress than those who did. This finding points to the importance that lack of knowledge can be a barrier preventing officers in distress from accessing their EAP services.

Stigma reduction for seeking services needs to be a "top-down" effort. Commands should endorse training on issues of mental health and physical health and wellness as part of regular in-service training. Additionally, providing information on how to access and use the EAP should be incorporated in the hiring and "onboarding" process for all employees. Colegrove (2020) cites first responder culture fosters a "stay quiet about emotional or mental distress" (p. 25). Early on the culture implicitly ingrains the first responder "to accept the inevitability of organizational stress and dysfunction, debilitating stress symptoms, emotional upheaval, sleep disruption and disorders, marriage problems and divorce, and substance use and abuse" (Colegrove, 2020, p. 25). The maladaptive coping mechanism often modeled includes drinking, use of prescription drugs, risky behavior, avoidance, and dark humor.

How EAP Works

The EAP functions as a triage of requests for services from first responder employees and family members from phone calls or walk-ins. Often their request for counseling contains a vague description of the problem and unfamiliarity with the most appropriate type of mental health treatment. Their requests can be fine-tuned via questions, familiarity with the work stressors aids, identifying the issues, and giving a better referral recommendation. The term first responder can include law enforcement, firefighter/paramedic, detention deputies, and communications operators. Bearing in mind their unique job functions, it is important to conduct a preliminary needs assessment. Knowledgeable EAP clinicians make it their business to familiarize themselves with the various job demands, personalities, and unique stressors of their specialty. A "culturally competent" EAP knows the jargon, command structure, unwritten rules, and humor of a first responder culture. This kind of knowledge largely comes about through direct interaction in the workplace, such as regular visits to the jail, doing ride-alongs with law enforcement, having coffee in the fire stations, and "plugging in" with communications operators. Besides learning the culture, these interactions initiate the beginning of a relationship, increased awareness of the EAP, and essentially functions as a marketing tool as well.

EAPs need to be familiar with, and make referrals to, therapists who are familiar with first responder culture. There are training programs available now to familiarize therapists with first responders' personalities and needs, which teach them to become "culturally competent."

Communication Operators

Communications operators possess many skills, not the least of which require multitasking and attention to detail. They are essentially "the first" of the first responders taking thousands of 911 calls in a month, hearing people in crisis on the worst day of their lives, along with dispatching calls for service to responding deputies and/or firefighter/paramedics. They often request assistance for themselves following a difficult call such as a child drowning, a high-profile car chase, or at the urging of a supervisor. Referrals include issues arising from stress due to long work hours (12-hour shifts), mandatory overtime resulting in sleep deprivation, and sometimes discipline from frequently calling in sick.

> Susie, while a seasoned call taker/dispatcher, requested assistance with a traumatic call. A woman called 911 from her car stating she had just hit a man who ran in front of her car. Newer car models utilize Bluetooth technology, so the conversation was played on the car stereo speakers. The woman's young child in the car became hysterical crying "Mommy, did you kill the man?" Hearing the child's distress intensified the dispatcher's distress.

Communication operators spend many hours "attached" to a computer, taking hundreds of calls per shift, and hopeful to get a good chair (finding a good chair is of paramount importance). Stress arises from the auditory: screaming voices, crying babies, hysterical parents, and desperate drug addicts. Communication operators create the "picture" of what's happening, which can be worse than the reality. Stress also emanates from the oft-felt sense of helplessness when attempting to get assistance and resources in a crisis. Despite many years of experience, some calls can be emotionally difficult to manage.

> Barb, a mother of two small children, reported a call that kept playing in her head. The caller described her horror in seeing her young child and her mother at the bottom of the pool. Grandmom had tried to save the child, and both drowned as the grandmother could not swim. The dispatcher's reaction, while normal, represented an unpleasant side effect of the job.

Detention Deputies

Detention deputies working in a jail setting perform all their duties without the use of deadly force weapons, rather, requiring good interpersonal communications skills and pepper spray. Detention or correctional officers are charged with the 3 C's: care, control, and custody of inmates. They provide 24-hour supervision, feeding, headcount, medication rounds with nurses, and scheduled recreation and visitation. Everything in the jail runs on a schedule. "It's a stressful job being locked in with people whose primary objective is to get out" (Kirschman et al., 2014, p. 239). Inmates pose a potential threat to detention staff along with supervisory demands, mandatory overtime, staffing shortages, overcrowding, conflicts with co-workers, and the risk of being sued. Detention staff participate in training sessions to gain a working knowledge of high-risk suicide situations, how to respond, and important steps to potentially avert suicide. Detention deputies can be called on to handle suicide attempts in the jail which can be a very stressful situation.

> The "first time" experience with cutting down an inmate or seeing a dead body can present as a critical incident and a unique challenge. Detention staff do not encounter death at anywhere near the rate of law enforcement and fire rescue personnel. Some suicide attempts are experienced as critical incidents and require knowledge of acute stress reactions following these types of events. EAPs can be called upon to conduct debriefings for staff and frequently require follow-up services.

Long-term exposure to inmate populations can place detention personnel at risk for burnout, depression, anxiety, and behavior problems. Becoming overly identified with inmates could produce what Gilmartin (2002) called the "Correctional Officer Stockholm Syndrome." A detention deputy with unresolved personal issues may develop relationships with inmates that can lead to "loyalty slippage." The deputy could be at risk for ethical breaches, such as sex with an inmate, assisting with an escape, or granting special privileges. These behaviors could result in loss of family, job, and facing criminal charges.

Firefighters/Paramedics

Firefighters/paramedics frequently function on a 24-hour work schedule with two days off in between. They live in a fire "house" with meals, grocery shopping, and household responsibilities. They essentially have two families. Family and marital difficulties can arise due to perceptions of allegiance to the "work" family and not the real family. Firefighter families often feel like they "play second fiddle" to the job. Firefighters miss cherished family rituals, such as dinner and bedtime, not to mention birthdays, recitals, holidays, and other important family functions. One spouse has continuous child-care responsibilities and household chores. Spouses can feel "abandoned" at home with the children and unsupported by their fire service partners.

> Sergio recalls the multiple panicked phone calls from his wife during the shift citing problems with the broken down hot water heater, homework crisis, and the adolescent daughter's boyfriend break up. The wife and daughter were crying on the phone requesting him to come home, leave his shift. The wife threatened to call the divorce attorney if he didn't come home, citing he was emotionally unavailable and not part of the family. Several hours later she called him saying, stay at work, don't bother coming home – seems he prefers his work buddies to his family. He is not sure marriage counseling will resolve this dilemma, or if he even wants to work on the marriage.

Exposure to stressors at work can have a "spillover" from the job to home. Firefighters often report responding to calls after midnight resulting in sleep deprivation. After a shift, the firefighter may be unable or unwilling to jump into household chores upon walking in the door. Many first responders coming off shift report the struggle of making the transition from work to home; "shifting gears", as it were. Firefighter families struggle with understanding the "other" (organizational or political) stress. Many hours of any given shift can be occupied by discussions around the kitchen table discussing the rumor mill and attendant "what if's." Effective EAPs need a level of familiarity with the fire service command structure, culture ("let's keep all the dirty laundry in the house"), and the impact of promotions, transfers, and retirements. Firefighters are exposed to numerous critical incidents and chiefs should be sensitive to requesting follow-up debriefings, as warranted.

Law Enforcement

Law enforcement culture dictates that the stoic first responder should always be in control, make good decisions, and know how to handle every crisis. Based on this mentality, any requests for personal mental health assistance would be considered a sign of weakness and possibly imply they are not fit for duty. The stigma associated with seeking mental health would suggest that they are "crazy", and maybe "unstable", or "incompetent." Yet, the trauma from work can cause an emotional and mental "wound", despite the many years of learning how to compartmentalize emotions. Resistance to seeking treatment can result in "stuffing down all the garbage", which does not magically disappear. Rather, if left untreated, the memories, nightmares, and flashbacks can fester and intensify. These can be the makings of Posttraumatic Stress Disorder (PTSD); fortunately, this is treatable.

Untreated PTSD can contribute to suicide risk. According to Violanti et al. (2017), more officers die by suicide every year than are killed in the line of duty. Effective EAPs bear in mind the stigma attached to mental health and utilize a variety of informal and formal methods of providing referrals. Training front-line supervisors to identify high-risk behaviors, patterns of self-destructive behavior, and/or poor attendance, is crucial. Three key risk factors for suicide include access to a firearm, substance abuse, and marital/relationship difficulties. Supervisory referrals can be completed on a voluntary basis, or compelled if warranted.

> Joe found himself drinking his favorite adult beverage most nights after work. As the months passed, he consumed more than he planned and frequently woke up with a hangover. He chalked this up to increased pressures from his ex-wife for child support, his recent pass over party where he was "passed over" for promotion, and the nagging sergeant always on his case about reports. Joe had more than 15 years on the job, lacked any post high school education, and had no interest in changing professions. He felt stuck, miserable, and was unprepared for the cost and humiliation that came from his DUI arrest.

Despite the negative stigma attached to mental health, utilizing the EAP can be a very useful resource for navigating the requirements associated with a DUI charge. Besides the driver's license hearing, the process includes the criminal defense component, and finally the agency administrative investigation (internal affairs).

Resources for First Responders

Peer Support

These programs provide an informal, but effective, mechanism for bridging the fear of being exposed. Providing trained peers to first responders can be instrumental in mitigating the negative consequences of exposure to traumatic events. Peers are trained in identifying risk factors for suicide and can serve as a guiding/supportive hand in seeking professional mental health. Peers can listen, offer support, and reach out to fellow employees involved in personal or professional crises. They can assist following a critical incident with critical incident stress management defusing (shortly after the event) or a formal debriefing conducted with a mental health professional about 3 days after the incident.

Chaplain Services

These offer first responders emotional and spiritual assistance, especially in times of personal loss. Spirituality can offer an enormous foundation of strength, resiliency, perspective, and hope to people in crisis and pain.

Conclusion

While first responders represent a challenging group to engage, productive and well-utilized EAPs can customize their services to address the emotional and psychological issues, which often emerge from the hazardous and adverse work conditions. EAPs need to offer programs and structure delivery services that reflect the diversity of employees' needs, interests, and operational necessities. Effective EAPs can aid in promoting positive organizational change and the improvement of first responders' lives.

References

Asen, J., & Colon, I. (1995). Acceptance and use of police department employee assistance programs. *Employee Assistance Quarterly, 11*(1), 45–54.

Colegrove, K. (2020). *Mindfulness for warriors: Empowering first responders to reduce stress and build resistance*. Mango.

Donnelly, E., Valentine, C., & Oehme, K. (2015). *Law enforcement officers and employee assistance programs*. Florida State University Libraries.

Employee Assistance Professional Association. (2022). *Definition of EAP*. http://www.eapassn.org/public/pages/

Everly, G. S., Jr., & Mitchell, J. T. (2000). The debriefing "controversy" and crisis intervention: A review of lexical and substantive issues. *International Journal of Emergency Mental Health, 2*(4), 211–225.

Gilmartin, K. M. (2002). *Emotional survival for law enforcement*. E-S Press.

Goldstein, D. B. (2006). Employee assistance for law enforcement: A brief review. *Journal of Police and Criminal Psychology, 21*(1), 33–40.

International Association of Fire Fighters. (2018). *A history of firefighter unions*. https://iaff1775.org/our-union/iaff-affiliation/2202-a-history-of-firefighter

Kampanakis, J. (2000). Police organizational culture and policemen's integrity. In M. Pagon (Ed.), *Policing in Central and Eastern Europe: Ethics, integrity and human rights*. College of Police and Securities Studies.

Kirschman, E., Kamena, M., & Fay, J. (2014). *Counseling cops: What clinicians need to know*. Guilford Press.

Levine, M. (1988). Historical overview of police unionization in the United States. *Police Journal, 61*(4), 334–343.

Masi, D. A. (2000). *Evaluating your employee assistance and managed behavioral care program*. Dallen, Inc.

McKay, B., & Gravel, S. (2016). *Walk the talk: First responder peer support*. Syd A. Gravel/Budd Publishing.

Roman, P., & Blum, T. (1988). *Private sector internal EAP profiles*. https://archive.hshsl.umaryland.edu/handle/10713/13275

Violanti, J. (1990). Post trauma vulnerability: A proposed model. In J. T. Reese, J. M. Horn, & C. Dunning (Eds.), *Critical incidents in policing*. U.S. Government Printing Office.

Violanti, J. M., Charles, L. E., McCanlies, E., Hartley, T. A., Baughman, P., Andrew, M. E., Fekedulegn, D., Ma, C. C., Mnatsakanova, A., & Burchfiel, C. M. (2017). Police stressors and health: A state-of-the-art review. *Policing, 40*(4), 642–656. https://doi.org/10.1108/PIJPSM-06-2016-0097

Suicide Prevention and Intervention

Ennio Ammendola, Justin Baker, Edwin Szeto, and David Englert

Suicide is one of the leading causes of death worldwide, with approximately 700,000 people who die from suicide each year. There appears to be an unfortunate upward trend with US suicide rates increasing 30% between 2000 and 2020, from 10.4 per 100,000 in 2000, peaking in 2018 at 14.2, with the most recent rates for 2020 coming down slightly to 13.5 (Garnett et al., 2022). In 2019, suicide was the tenth leading cause of death for all ages, the second for ages 10–34, and the fourth for ages 35–54. Thus, suicide remains a leading public health crisis in the United States, as highlighted in a recent call to action by the Office of the Surgeon General for a National Strategy for Suicide Prevention (Office of Surgeon General, 2021), which encourages suicide prevention efforts to be specifically tailored for disproportionately affected groups.

First responders, including police officers, firefighters, and emergency medical technicians (EMTs), are disproportionately affected by suicide (Peterson et al., 2020; Stanley et al., 2016). Law enforcement officers are 54% more likely to die by suicide than non-law enforcement professionals. Among firefighters, 46% reported experiencing lifetime suicide ideation, and 15.5% have attempted suicide at least once during their careers (Stanley et al., 2015). Wildland firefighters demonstrated an even greater risk of suicide, with 55% of wildland firefighters (compared to 32% of non-wildland firefighters) reporting clinically elevated symptoms of suicide (Stanley et al., 2018). Statistics for police officers and EMTs were similarly elevated, with 25% of female and 23.1% of male officers reporting lifetime suicide ideation and a lifetime suicide ideation prevalence rate of 28% for EMTs (Stanley et al., 2016). These rates are contrasted with those from the general public in the

E. Ammendola (✉) · J. Baker · E. Szeto
The Ohio State University Wexner Medical Center, Columbus, OH, USA
e-mail: ENNIO.AMMENDOLA@osumc.edu

D. Englert
Uniformed Services University of the Health Sciences (USUHS), Navarre, FL, USA

M. L. Bourke et al. (eds.), *First Responder Mental Health*,
https://doi.org/10.1007/978-3-031-38149-2_20

United States, where only 13.5% of the population indicate they have experienced suicidal ideation in their lifetime (Stanley et al., 2016).

A recent review of first responder causes of death revealed that in 2017, more police officers and firefighters died by suicide than in the line of duty (Heyman et al., 2018). Law enforcement officers and firefighters also demonstrated elevated rates of workplace suicide; 5.3 per million police and firefighters took their life at their work site, compared to the national occupational average of 1.5 per million people. In addition, the suicide rate of EMTs in the United States from 2009 to 2015 was 5.3%, compared to 2.2% in the non-EMT population, indicating that EMTs are 1.39 times as likely to die by suicide (Vigil et al., 2019).

One reason first responders demonstrate elevated rates of suicide is the prevalence of men in these professions. Most first responders are White males between the ages of 25 and 54 years. Across first responder occupations, 3 out of 4 EMTs, 7 out of 8 police officers, and 19 out of 20 firefighters identify as male (Schafer et al., 2015). From 2000 to 2020, suicide rates for all civilian US males were three to four times the rate for all females, highlighting a well-documented gender difference, whereby men are more likely to die by suicide and women report higher rates of suicide ideation and attempts (Canetto & Sakinofsky, 1998; Murphy, 1998; Schrijvers et al., 2012).

Men die by suicide at higher rates than women due to their proclivity for using more lethal means, including firearms (Steele et al., 2018). For example, in 2017, half of all suicides were with a firearm, and more than 60% of all firearm-related deaths resulted from suicide (Kochanek et al., 2019). This adds up to men being more than six times as likely as women to die following a self-inflicted gunshot injury versus other means. Police officers, in particular, demonstrated elevated firearm-related death rates, with 91.5% of suicide deaths attributable to a self-inflicted gunshot wound (O'Hara et al., 2013).

Gender differences make determining causal relationships between occupational stressors inherent to first responders and suicide difficult. Recent meta-analyses found suicide rates for law enforcement officers to be no different from non-law enforcement civilians (Loo, 2003; Marzuk et al., 2002). At the same time, other studies have demonstrated elevated rates of suicide among first responders (Violanti et al., 2013). Another confounding variable is that suicide rates for first responders are likely underreported. Organizations like the Firefighter Behavioral Health Alliance, which has an online repository for anonymous reporting of firefighter suicide, estimate that current suicide numbers of firefighters account for only 40% of the actual number of suicides (Heyman et al., 2018). Currently, there exists no comprehensive tracking database for first responder suicides. The National Violent Death Reporting System (NVDRS), a state-level surveillance system, collects data on all types of violent deaths. However, the information gathered lacks critical data elements to fully understand the nature of suicides among first responders.

In 2020, the US House of Representatives and the US Senate approved funding for the Helping Emergency Responders Overcome (HERO) Act. The HERO Act, in part, is intended to develop and maintain a data system called the Public Safety Officer Suicide Reporting System that will collect data on suicide incidence among public safety officers. This data, combined with existing surveillance systems like the NVDRS, will allow for improved collection of necessary data elements specific to first responders to help fill in knowledge gaps of current suicide fatalities. This will hopefully shed additional light on the causes of elevated suicide rates in first responder occupations.

Trauma Exposure, Posttraumatic Stress Disorder, and Occupational Stressors

First responders are exposed to traumatic events more often than their civilian counterparts (Marmar et al., 2006; Norris, 1992). Approximately 80% of first responders report experiencing traumatic events in the line of duty, and 10–15% of first responders indicate they have been diagnosed with posttraumatic stress disorder (PTSD; Klimley et al., 2018). According to the *Diagnostic and Statistical Manual of Mental Disorders* (5th ed.; DSM-5; American Psychiatric Association, 2013), PTSD is defined by four clusters of symptoms in response to a life-threatening or stressful event:

1. Re-experiencing
2. Avoidance
3. Negative alterations in cognitions and mood
4. Alterations in arousal and reactivity

PTSD is a known correlate of death by suicide and distinguishes those with suicidal ideation from those who made a suicide attempt (May & Klonsky, 2016). Elevated symptoms of PTSD also have been linked with an increased risk of alcohol use and suicidal ideation in police officers (Violanti et al., 2004) and a greater risk of reporting lifetime suicidal ideation and prior attempts in firefighters (Boffa et al., 2017).

However, others have demonstrated that factors like administrative inefficiency, poor management, and other workplace-driven stressors may be to blame for elevated rates of suicide in first responders (Chae & Boyle, 2013). For example, in 2012, work-related legal problems accounted for approximately 13% of police suicides, the second-highest reported reason (O'Hara et al., 2013). In the same study, work-related trauma accounted for only 3% of probable reasons for suicide. Other studies have demonstrated similar findings. Barron (2010), for example, found that 31.5% of those who died by suicide had documented work performance issues, and 23% were under investigation preceding their suicide. Thus, clinicians who work with first responders should not assume that the first responder's exposure to trauma is the primary driver of any observed or reported distress. While trauma certainly could be a potential contributing factor, clinicians working with first responders must remain cognizant of the fact that, just as within the civilian population, personal problems are often the primary source of distress.

Suicide Treatment

Suicide Prevention with First Responders

Effective suicide risk reduction requires a multifaceted approach. When done well, suicide prevention recognizes the complex interaction among the first responder's prior mental health history, including any prior suicide attempt(s), mood disorders, and substance abuse; environmental factors, such as access to lethal means and mental health care, interpersonal dynamics with family, friends, and other forms of social support; and other individual factors, including one's ability to regulate emotions and employ problem-solving skills.

The impact of suicide and the costs to individuals, families, and societies are increasingly being recognized, particularly for first responders – our communities' frontline defense. Direct costs are incurred by emergency rooms, first responders, outpatient clinical services, and the family (e.g., funeral expenses). Indirect costs include lost economic outputs, such as premature deaths or injuries, and voluntary activities. The implementation of suicide prevention efforts may help reduce individual, community, and economic losses (Blasco-Fontecilla & De Leon, 2021).

Suicide prevention interventions must be able to target both short- and long-term risk reduction efforts at the individual and community levels. Wilcox and Wyman (2016) emphasize the value of suicide prevention strategies that intervene at the primary, secondary, and tertiary levels. This model is simple in its application and is associated with short- and long-term goals in suicide prevention. *Primary prevention* focuses on reducing the incidence of suicide behaviors by eliminating or decreasing risk factors while optimizing known protective factors. These phase implementations include suicide awareness initiatives, training to improve coping skills, and lethal means restriction (like firearms, which we will analyze in more detail later in this chapter). *Secondary prevention* strategies are aimed at lowering the prevalence of already-existing mental disorders through early detection. Some of these phase implementations are screening techniques and gatekeeper training. Finally, *tertiary prevention* efforts focus on reducing the incidence of relapses through rehabilitation services.

Other prevention programs offer practical suggestions for developing effective strategies to reduce suicide risk (Wasserman, 2019). These include offering mental health services, using psychiatric diagnostic tools earlier in treatment, identifying psychosocial stress factors, conducting regular follow-up appointments, and providing full rehabilitation for those who have made previous suicide attempts. Although many researchers and clinicians continue to focus on cognitive or behavioral solutions for people at risk of suicide, a fundamental social approach also involves providing more practical solutions, such as assisting in social welfare, mental health, indigenous people's health, education, and lethal means restriction. The most crucial aim is to combine cognitive, behavioral, and emotional solutions with solid environmental protective factors.

Evidence-Based Suicide Interventions with First Responders

With suicide rates alarmingly high, it is imperative to implement targeted evidence-based suicide prevention treatments with first responders. Cognitive Behavioral Therapies (CBTs) effectively reduce suicidal thoughts and related behaviors (Fox et al., 2020). Brief Cognitive Behavior Therapy (BCBT) for Suicide Prevention is one CBT modality. BCBT was developed in 2009 as a 12-session therapy protocol to prevent follow-up suicide attempts (Rudd et al., 2015). To remain within the scope and breadth of this chapter, we will highlight a few critical interventions from this treatment modality that can be readily adapted and utilized in therapy cases with first responders. For further training and learning of BCBT, we would direct readers to the *Brief Cognitive Behavioral Therapy for Suicide Prevention* treatment manual by Craig J. Bryan and M. David Rudd.

Telling Their Stories

Good suicide intervention begins with a well-informed clinical assessment of the current suicide risk. Within the framework of BCBT, this is facilitated via the *narrative assessment*. Unlike traditional interviews that utilize lists and structured prompts, the narrative assessment invites the first responder to "tell their story," in their own words, about their most recent suicidal crisis. By initiating the narrative assessment in this way, the therapist can center treatment on the first responder and prioritize their experience. This experience may be a recent attempt, worsening suicidal thoughts during the past week that prompted them to seek professional care or some other related crisis.

After prompting the first responder to tell their story, the therapist engages in active listening and empathic reflection. Listening can be challenging, of course, even for clinicians. Listening is even more challenging when our anxiety and concern for the first responder's wellbeing is heightened, which can often occur when we are sitting with first responders struggling with suicide. As clinicians, we may experience difficulty managing our own reactions to the unconscious biases of first responders as protectors, the individuals who typically are offering help, not receiving it. Maybe our thoughts take us to their easy access to firearms, and we begin to wonder what safety measures need to be put in place. Whatever reactions we may have as providers, the narrative assessment allows for good active listening, increases rapport building with the first responder, and reduces anxiety for both the first responder and the clinician facilitating the assessment.

A study conducted in 2018 found that a narrative approach to suicide risk assessment, compared with a traditional structured interview, led to increased empathy ratings from the patient; higher affective synchrony and emotional co-regulation between the patient and the clinician; and decreased speech complexity (Bryan et al., 2018). In other words, the individual felt more connected to their provider; the provider and the patient were emotionally “in sync” and, in turn, less anxious; and the provider used less jargon, another indicator of increased empathy and connection. In addition, by centering the assessment on the first responder’s experience, the provider can obtain the necessary information to decide on risk while helping the first responder regulate their distress.

Throughout the narrative assessment, interjecting brief comments may assist the first responder to describe their suicidal event. Phrases such as “What happened next?” can help them organize the retelling of their story in chronological order. This allows the clinician to listen and gather information about what transpired. Often the crisis is an overwhelming and confusing time for the first responder and asking them to narrate what happened helps them begin to make sense of their distress. Having space to honestly discuss and explore what is often experienced as a low point in life is validating and starts the healing process. Other helpful prompts include, “What were you feeling during the crises?” “What thoughts did you notice having?” “What physical sensations did you experience throughout the crisis?” “What did you do or try to manage the distress?” These questions help the clinician investigate the contextual variables that contributed to the first responder’s overall distress and led to their suicidal crisis.

Finally, eliciting the first responder’s cooperation is essential. It is more easily obtained if the clinician avoids “why” questions. Regardless of the role the first responder has, they often get “why” questions such as, “Why don’t you shoot them in the leg?” and “Why didn’t you use a tourniquet?” During the narrative assessment, the clinician may be tempted to ask “why” questions; however, in the experience of the authors who have provided therapy to this population, these queries are much more likely to result in defensiveness and frustration.

Developing a Crisis Response Plan

Following the narrative assessment, it is beneficial to develop a crisis response plan (CRP). The CRP is a brief intervention within the BCBT framework that is designed to address the stress reactions associated with specific events immediately. M. David Rudd initially developed the CRP in the mid-1990s as part of his outpatient treatment to work with individuals at risk of suicide. The CRP focuses on all the potential planning and action first responders take to address crises, critical incidents, and unexpected tragic events. The CRP is not focused on a specific event. Rather, it is focused on the general planning and actions that first responders can take when facing actual incidents to restore the biopsychosocial equilibrium and thus minimize the occurrence of potential future crises.

The CRP is crucial because first responders are continuously exposed to challenging events that generate intense emotional and cognitive crises, which could easily lead them to experience significant psychological distress. Our clinical experience has shown us that completing a CRP is critical; without one, first responders under stress may make poor decisions and may unintentionally worsen the ongoing crisis. Paying attention to the CRP means implementing constructive actions that may be the key to the first responders' survival. We want to stress that the CRP is not a substitute for psychotherapy but rather represents an emotional stand-off intervention that first responders can easily access. It is crucial that the CRP includes and integrates current best practices into mental health professionals' delivery of crisis intervention services.

A study in 2017 showed that individuals who received the CRP were 76% less likely to make suicide attempts during the 6-month follow-up period (Bryan et al., 2018). In the same research, the CRP also contributed to a faster reduction in suicidal ideations. An additional study (Rozek et al., 2020) showed that discussing an individual's reason for living in the CRP increases hope, reduces suicidal intent, and decreases the likelihood of psychiatric hospitalization. Additional investigations are underway to further test the CRP and improve its effects.

If we consider the hypothetical case scenario illustrated in Table 1, a clinician works with a first responder to collaboratively create the CRP. The clinician invites the first responder to use an index card in a session to handwrite several sections of the CRP. The CRP is comprised of five key sections: personal warning signs, self-management strategies, reasons for living, social support, and professional crisis support. In our case, the first responder – a New York City police officer serving in Queens – found himself in several hazardous situations related to domestic

Table 1 The five-steps of the crisis response plan (CRP)

CRP key sections	Description	Clinician	First responder
Personal warning signs	Personal indicators of an emerging emotional crisis.	What are some of the symptoms that you feel when you are going through an emotional crisis?	Pacing Feeling irritable Isolation Difficulty sleeping
Self-management strategies	Strategies that can be used to help reduce stress or serve as a distraction.	What are some of the activities you could do by yourself to reduce your stress?	Go for a walk Play with my dog Lift weights
Reasons for living	Things that provide a sense of purpose or meaning in life.	What are your reasons for living?	My wife My kids My parents
Social support	People who provide support or elevate one's mood during crises.	Who are the people in your life that can provide emotional support?	Call my wife Call my mom Call my best friend (name and phone #)
Professional crisis Support	Contact information for health care providers, crisis hotline, and emergency services.	What are some of the professional supports that you can contact when in crisis?	Call my therapist Call 988 Go to the hospital Call 911

violence. He felt emotionally overwhelmed and was unable to manage his stress, which was manifesting as insomnia, impulsiveness, and intermittent suicidal ideations without planning. The officer asked for help from a clinician specializing in BCBT, who invited the officer to complete the CRP during a session.

Means Safety Counseling

Means Safety Counseling Principles

We recommend using a clinical framework of reference when using *means safety counseling*, which is ideal for describing first responders' incremental willingness to change. This framework is best described by the stages of change model that DiClemente and Prochaska developed in the late 1970s. The idea behind the stages of change model is to identify the degree of change the first responder expresses and, in terms of the implementation of the means safety plan, to identify the same therapy goal for the clinicians and the first responder. In terms of the assessment, the first responder will be assessed as being part of one of these stages: *precontemplation* (the first responder has not yet acknowledged a problem behavior needs to be changed); *contemplation* (the first responder recognizes a problem exists but is not yet ready to make a change); *preparation/determination* (the first responder is getting ready to change); *action/willpower* (the first responder implements a changed behavior); and *maintenance* (the first responder maintains the behavior) and, an unofficial sixth stage: *relapse* (the first responder returns to older behaviors and abandons the new changes).

In terms of identifying a collaborative therapy goal for both the clinicians and the first responder, the stages of change incrementally move the first responder closer and closer to the actual behavioral changes because of their mutual understanding of three major points in the therapeutic process: (1) clinicians explain how change occurs, and first responders come to understand this; (2) both the clinician and the first responder consider the pros and cons of change, stressing that the pros of change are valued over the cons; and (3) both the clinician and the first responder have the same commitment to the level of confidence required to execute and maintain a positive change despite the temptation for relapse.

When we implement the means safety counseling, we have noticed that most firearm owners are at the precontemplation stage. No problem has been identified as an area of concern, yet. Under these circumstances, the first responder usually communicates: "I am not necessarily motivated to make a change." We then try to transition the firearm owner to the next contemplation stage by asking, "Now that we've identified an issue worth talking about and we're contemplating change, what can we do to increase your actual motivation?" In our clinical practice, we have noticed that the transition from one stage to another does not happen on a linear trajectory. Instead, it is characterized by several fluctuations of suicide activation that produce behavioral or psychological changes throughout the administration of therapy. Furthermore, the first responder acquires new skills, knowledge, and strategies during the transitions. With each subsequent attempt at making a behavior change, the first responder becomes better equipped to maintain that change over the long term.

After the above considerations, we can state without a doubt that the essential aspect of means safety counseling is the way in which we have conceptualized the variable of the motivation to change. We conceptualize motivation as having two main dimensions: (1) the perceived importance of the change and (2) the perceived confidence with which first responders can make that change. We can assess this during a clinical encounter by asking how important it is for them, on a scale from 0 to 10, to change how they store their firearms.

We believe the means safety counseling model assists first responders in promoting decisional balance, where we help them understand they could weigh the pros and cons of making a change and then compare those with the pros and cons of not making the change. For example, in the specific case of firearms, we explain the benefits and costs of locking up their guns or temporarily removing them from the house, the pros and cons of not doing this, and the advantages and disadvantages of having loaded weapons readily accessible in the household.

To decrease the likelihood that the first responder will grab a gun as an impulsive and volatile act, clinicians should encourage them to create a "waiting period" between their suicidal thinking and their ability to gain access to a firearm. We know suicidal crises are often short-lived and are characterized by ambivalence. Thus, by delaying immediate access to firearms, clinicians create a safer environment where first responders are more willing to use the CRP or other clinical tools to help themselves. In addition, clinicians target the first responders' decisional balance by directly calling attention to both sides of ambivalence with these competing perspectives: I will lock up my guns versus I will not lock up my guns.

Securing firearms reduces the risk factor for injury or death. The best practice for safely storing guns is to store them unloaded and locked, secured in a gun safe or similar device, with the ammunition stored separately in another locked container (Grossman et al., 2005).

Households that locked guns and ammunition separately had a 78% lower risk of self-inflicted gun injuries compared to those that locked neither (Monuteaux et al., 2019). Therefore, we would like to provide the first responder with a clear message: "Delaying your access to guns could save your life!"

Means Safety Counseling Components

Once the clinician has determined if the first responder is at a low, intermediate, or high risk of suicide, a new clinical framework based on therapeutic suicide risk management will determine who will be the most appropriate candidate to receive lethal means safety counseling. Means safety counseling is a process that is discussed collaboratively in the session between the clinician and the first responder.

The clinician first asks the suicidal first responders if they are willing to participate in the therapeutic process to reduce their suicide risk. This process is best delivered through one-on-one interaction. Means safety counseling has two main aims: strictly educating first responders about the hazards of having access to harmful items and limiting their access to and the availability of lethal items. This is a crucial component of suicide risk reduction in clinical practice because it is well established that firearm access increases the risk of suicide. One non-threatening way to address that risk is by promoting safe firearm storage (Britton et al., 2016).

Clinicians could help first responders by working harder to engage them in talking about "gun safety" rather than "gun control." While this may seem a semantic detail, clinicians could uncomplicate this issue to make communication in sessions more productive and lessen resistance.

One of the main advantages of means safety counseling is that it can be used with any demographic group. It is not restricted to those more at risk, such as older adults and men, or groups that unfortunately avoid mental health care altogether because they underreport their thoughts of suicide. We also believe that means safety counseling should be conceptualized within a risk management framework focusing on the risk component of suicide prevention. This is because first responders who complete suicide using firearms are more likely than first responders who use other methods to die in their first suicide attempts.

Our clinical practice has allowed us to notice one of the most critical components of suicide intervention while administering means safety counseling that other clinicians sometimes underestimate. We are referring to a situation where both clinicians and first responders must overcome resistance to any discussions about the Second Amendment to the United States Constitution. The first responders should not perceive being deprived of their firearms forever as being against their constitutional rights. A gentle approach will embrace the part of them that still values self-preservation. Also, this approach considers safety as existing along a spectrum and consequently does not prescribe first responders to do "A," "B," or "C." This is because many aspects related to the risk of suicide result from risk fluctuations between the low and imminent risk of suicide.

Bryan (2021) reported that thoughts about death and suicide vary over time. Kleiman et al. (2017) examined real-time fluctuation in suicidal ideations and their risk factors using an ecological momentary assessment to understand how change processes naturally occur. His results showed that many people exhibited significant shifts in suicidal thinking during time frames as short as a few hours. This outcome has tremendous implications for clinicians who work with first responders and who may attempt to assess suicide risk accurately. It can be implied that instead of asking first responders, "Have you experienced suicidal thoughts for the past week or month?" it would be more clinically sound like asking, "Have you experienced any fluctuations in your suicidal thinking, even if only for a few hours?" The latter approach will allow clinicians better understanding of the various components of the patterns of change related to suicidal thoughts. It is imperative to teach first responders that even small changes in these fluctuation patterns could lead to a big difference in the results and, in a worst-case scenario, to suicide attempt or death.

Another crucial component of the means safety counseling used within the framework of BCBT consists of the practical opportunity for first responders to identify the most critical steps when developing a plan with safety steps. The following process characterizes the means safety counseling: (a) identify the name of the provider to consult; (b) in the case of an emergency, call the suicide hotline at 988; (c) provide the patient's name as well as the support person's name and telephone number if this person needs to be contacted; (d) identify the various aspects of the means safety plan; (e) highlight when the plan ends; and finally, (f) close the document with the patient's signature. One of the most critical components is collaboratively discussing with the first responder when the plan ends. Within a client-centered approach, having a collaborative approach ensures that some of the most crucial factors in therapy are honored, such as honesty, transparency, mutual trust, respect, and decisional empowerment for both the clinician and the first responder. The means safety counseling is crucial because clinicians and first responders engage in a meaningful conversation about promoting change.

This process is completed in a very egalitarian way by putting clinicians and first responders on the same level. We should note that we have used this protocol not only with first responders who have access to firearms but also with first responders who have access to other forms or methods of suicide that could be deemed less lethal than firearms, such as medications or knives.

Understanding from a First Responder Perspective

A supplemental research bulletin (2018) on first responders and their health concerns from the Substance Abuse and Mental Health Services Administration's Disaster Technical Assistance Center reported that approximately 30% of first responders presented symptoms related to depression and PTSD. More alarming, 37% of fire and emergency medical service professionals have contemplated suicide. These numbers reinforce the importance of implementing suicide prevention programs with this population. Designing these programs around a delivery system tailored to their psychological needs would be beneficial. Additionally, the delivery should be relatable to their language to maximize its effectiveness.

Before clinicians attempt to implement a suicide prevention program with first responders, it is strongly advised that they get to know the culture to better address their psychological needs. Otherwise, it could be challenging to work in these communities. Mental health professionals who want to learn about specific first responder culture should be asked to sit in on educational classes; assist and observe confined spaces, tactical or other specialized training; and participate in ride-along. Such activities would allow the clinician to ask the "why" questions to understand their mindset better. In addition, being present and available will help clinicians build relationships and trust within the first responder community as they attempt to deliver the suicide prevention program.

Further, since language is an essential part of first responder culture, we suggest learning the first responder's unique phrasing, acronyms, and numerical codes. This understanding will alleviate a host of misunderstandings and reduce the need to clarify terminology, which often marks an individual as not part of the community. We cannot stress enough the importance of establishing a relationship with the first responder department. This type of professional alignment is the most successful way to overcome the first responder community's resistance to speaking with providers, which often is reflected in the members' belief that someone outside of their community cannot understand them. Understanding the culture includes learning how first responders communicate, and one of their main ways of communicating is using humor. Albert Ellis, the founder of Rational Emotive Behavior Therapy, used humor in therapy for decades as an emotive technique; he felt this allowed individuals to create and hold to their dysfunctional beliefs, emotions, and behaviors in a forceful and powerful way. Ellis would have used humor as a coping mechanism primarily for situations related to PTSD to help first responders learn how to distract themselves from their crises (Dryden & Hill, 1993).

Clinicians need to understand that for many first responders, their humor is often "dark" and could be seen as inappropriate outside their communities. While it is often used as a coping strategy, they usually keep these stories within the circle of first responders and trusted others. Thus, when the first responders feel comfortable enough to share their humor with the clinician, it reflects acceptance. An additional practical component is to use a flexible schedule to deliver a suicide prevention program because first responders have irregular schedules. This means conducting meetings or sessions outside the conventional 9-to-5 workday.

Finally, we would like to anticipate a situation that often happens when working with first responders: "What should I do as a clinician if a first responder decides to come to the office for our session carrying their gun?" First, we would like to stress that this situation is quite different from finding out that a regular client in the office is carrying a gun. For most law enforcement officers, a gun is an extension of their uniform and the role they hold in the community. Also, demanding to come to the office without carrying a gun could prevent the first responder from being able to protect themselves or others if necessary. Also, for some departments, the requirement to carry a firearm when in uniform may be dictated by policy. Therefore, we recommend that clinicians anticipate this scenario and self-assess if they feel comfortable working with first responders who may be armed during the session.

Risk and Protective Factors for Suicide Among First Responders

First responders share many of the same risk factors that members of the general public face. Relationship distress, legal or financial difficulties, social withdrawal or isolation, and substance use are everyday stressors reported by individuals struggling with suicide. Among police officers, personal problems (83%), followed by legal problems (13%), accounted for the top two reasons for suicide (O'Hara, et al., 2013). However, as outlined in a meta-analytic review, Stanley et al. (2016) noted several occupational-related risk factors unique to first responders, which may contribute to increased suicide risk. These include the following: (1) exposure to trauma and other occupational hazards, (2) ready access to firearms and other lethal means, (3) increased capability for suicide, (4) irregular shift schedules, (5) the stigma surrounding help-seeking behaviors, (6) a culture of putting others before self, (7) multiple high-risk duties and frequent career transitions, (8) a lack of mental health access for smaller departments, and (9) current or prior military service. Clinicians working with first responders should balance identifying occupational-related stressors with universally experienced stressors.

Note that first responders have many protective factors that should be included in treatment and recognized as potential avenues for help seeking. They are resilient and tend to have high levels of social support, family connectedness, and friendship networks in the community (Chae & Boyle, 2013). Resilience is essential because it allows first responders to react in the face of unexpected adversities. The most important protective factors for first responders can be organized around social and environmental support in terms of feeling connected to others in the family, community, and work.

Consequently, clinicians must assess protective factors in the treatment of first responders because they could antagonize the risk factors, allowing the first responders to lessen their risk. Clinicians should consider stressing how protective factors can serve as the opposites of risk factors. When they become aware of protective factors, first responders become more willing and able to use them as buffers against potential suicide risk. First responders can learn in treatment that protective factors can be used in a single event or when several events are involved.

How to Make Treatment Culturally Relevant

Our answer to the provocative question: "Can cultural competence in suicide prevention programs be distinguished from competency in general?" is a resounding "yes." For example, several studies found that ethnic minority clients rated their therapists higher in multicultural competency if the therapists scored high on therapeutic alliance and empathy (Fuertes et al., 2022).

Interventions for suicide prevention with first responders must be culturally relevant. Therefore, clinicians should recognize the diversity of first responders from different ethnic backgrounds and consider teaching methods that take their differences into account. One of the consequences of this premise is that clinicians who are willing to get involved in suicide prevention programs need to study cultural diversity to understand the various perspectives within the world of first responders.

When it comes to suicide prevention, clinicians need to become more "internationalized" when thinking about making progress in suicide prevention. Kassin et al. (2016) wrote that we do not have minds without cultural participation. When clinicians work with patients to prevent suicide, it is necessary to become aware of their country of origin, region of the country, ethnicity, religion, gender, and profession. However, the therapist also must assess their degree of *acculturation* into the predominant culture. Adherence to traditional customs, beliefs, and values can vary considerably even between two first responders who are "from" the same ethnic group.

We are also glad APA accreditation requires programs to cover cultural competence, and many states require such training for licensure. Any program in suicide prevention needs to adopt a model of training that strongly focuses on learning how to adapt one's clinical skills to various populations by adhering to the following:

1. **Learning about themselves**: All clinicians need to explore their historical roots, beliefs, and values. A self-assessment exercise is critical because it makes clinicians aware of their session-related experience and helps them to be more aware of their biases as they explore first responders' lives.
2. **Learning about different cultures**: Any clinician who is involved in suicide prevention programs and knows they will provide therapy to people with unfamiliar backgrounds and values should immediately educate themselves through journal articles and books. This is one of the best ways to learn first responders' values and understand their language. In addition, this will allow them to develop a better understanding of how first responders' upbringing shapes their current behaviors.
3. **Interacting with diverse groups**: It is essential for clinicians to interact with others to relate and work with people from unfamiliar cultures. Volunteering in community centers may provide opportunities to fully understand diverse cultural experiences. One could also interact with other family members and involve them in social situations, such as parties, weddings, and cultural events.
4. **Attending diversity-focused conferences**: Another essential way to become culturally competent is to receive formal training on diversity. Conferences and training events allow clinicians to learn about the latest research on the issues being addressed in treatment sessions.
5. **Becoming aware of the work environment**: If the clinician notices that training in any specific area of becoming culturally competent needs to be added to the curriculum, they should advise their supervisor.

In short, if a mental health provider decides to implement suicide prevention intervention but feels unprepared in the five building blocks of cultural competence (open attitude, self-awareness, awareness of others, cultural knowledge, and cultural skills), we strongly recommend they make an effort to increase their cultural competency in any of the identified areas.

Overcoming Roadblocks When Working with First Responders

When working with first responders, it is imperative to understand that one of the primary barriers for them, when they are experiencing difficulty, is that seeking help is perceived as a weakness or, worse, may imply they are unfit for their job. As a result, they may be reluctant to seek mental health treatment since seeking help is often contrary to accepted ethos and social norms (Chae & Boyle, 2013). This reluctance is particularly true among police officers who rarely seek professional care from embedded psychologists or psychiatrists, even when struggling with suicide or PTSD. Although most police officers report having experienced at least one traumatic event, less than half disclosed this to their agency, with most indicating that if they needed professional help, they would seek care elsewhere (Fleischmann et al., 2018). Consequently, they may minimize the symptoms or avoid discussing PTSD by indicating they feel fine and are not experiencing any PTSD symptoms.

There are many contributing factors to why first responders may hesitate to seek care. One consideration is the influence of traditional masculine gender roles. As mentioned, nearly 90% of police officers, 95% of firefighters, and 75% of EMTs and paramedics are male (Schafer et al., 2015). As a result, men are less likely to seek care, instead prioritizing self-reliance due to a fear of being perceived as weak (Sagar-Ouriaghli et al., 2019). Other contributing factors include stigma around receiving mental health care and fear of negative occupational consequences such as removal of firearms, loss of a promotion, or receiving an undesirable duty assignment (Copenhaver & Tewksbury, 2018).

It is recommended that clinicians address these concerns and fears head-on at the outset of treatment when working with first responders. Start with normalizing the first responders' experiences by asking questions such as "How do you feel?" "How do you handle stress?" or "Do you feel that your stress has been building up to the point that you have seen some changes in how your days go on?" Clinicians must reassure first responders that they should feel free to share even the most horrific experiences in the context of the therapeutic relationship. It is important for the patients to understand that the therapy setting is a safe place where difficult issues and psychological experiences can be discussed nonjudgmentally. It would be helpful to avoid extremely reactionary statements such as "I cannot believe what you are telling me right now! That must have been awful for you." One area we would like to highlight for clinicians is to become very aware of facial expressions when working with first responders. It is essential for clinicians not to look shocked or terrified when first responders share their life experiences; such reactions likely will shut down the first responders. On the contrary, providing comments that reinforce their crucial role in helping others is compelling.

Another relevant area of clinical competence is ensuring therapists understand of how personal emotional responses to traumatic experiences can vary based on each individual's level of distress tolerance. Even if only 50–75% of people are exposed to a traumatic event during their lifetime, approximately 7.8–9.8% will develop PTSD or other clinical syndromes (Bleich et al., 1997).

We want to advance the hypothesis that first responders predisposed to significant emotional dysregulation have less psychological ability to tolerate stress (see Trafton & Gifford, 2008). First responders with higher stress tolerance are better equipped to emotionally regulate post-trauma exposure reactions. In our clinical work, we have noticed that first responders with a low level of distress tolerance tend to maintain their maladaptive beliefs, which could easily result in "I cannot stand the pain; I am going to kill myself to stop it." One of the difficulties we encounter in our work with first responders is that emotion regulation responses occur unconsciously and automatically (Gross, 1998), which could justify why so many first responders think they do not have any psychological problems.

Furthermore, it is not unusual in therapy for first responders to say that they feel emotionally numb, which could relate to the development of PTSD and, eventually, suicidal thinking. Consequently, it is imperative to address emotional regulation skills using relaxation, mindfulness, and sleeping hygiene strategies to attenuate symptoms of PTSD that could lead to developing suicidal ideation.

As previously mentioned, another priority is reducing the first responder's resistance to therapy by avoiding the "why" questions because they tend to be followed by simplified answers rather than a descriptive narrative. As a result, first responders can feel pressure to justify their actions or to provide a socially acceptable solution. Instead, clinicians should promote "how" questions to invite first responders to discuss the circumstances under which they made specific decisions. The "how" questions will reduce the language of ambivalence in therapy and amplify the identification of practical decision-making skills.

Finally, based on everything we have written in this chapter, we would emphasize the importance of the following when tailoring suicide prevention interventions to first responders: listen actively, develop a safe environment, reduce first responders' anxiety and stress levels by building resilience, find concrete ways of translating clinical speech into first responders' everyday language, educate how the brain processes traumatic experiences, teach breathing and mindfulness exercises, and use language and practices that are consistent with the person's professional identity and cultural background.

References

American Psychiatric Association. (2013). *Diagnostic and statistical manual of mental disorders* (5th ed.). https://doi.org/10.1176/appi.books.9780890425596

Barron, S. (2010). Police officer suicide within the New South Wales police force from 1999 to 2008. *Police Practice and Research: An International Journal, 11*(4), 371–382.

Blasco-Fontecilla, H., & De Leon, J. (2021). Scales for the evaluation of suicide risk. In D. Wassermann (Ed.), *Oxford textbook of suicidology and suicide prevention* (2nd ed., pp. 369–374). Oxford University Press.

Bleich, A., Koslowsky, M., Dolev, A., & Lerer, B. (1997). Post-traumatic stress disorder and depression: An analysis of comorbidity. *The British Journal of Psychiatry, 170*(5), 479–482.

Boffa, J. W., Stanley, I. H., Hom, M. A., Norr, A. M., Joiner, T. E., & Schmidt, N. B. (2017). PTSD symptoms and suicidal thoughts and behaviors among firefighters. *Journal of Psychiatric Research, 84*, 277–283.

Britton, P. C., Bryan, C. J., & Valenstein, M. (2016). Motivational interviewing for means restriction counseling with first responders at risk for suicide. *Cognitive and Behavioral Practice, 23*(1), 51–61.

Bryan, C. J. (2021). *Rethinking suicide: Why prevention fails, and how we can do better*. Oxford University Press.

Bryan, C. J., Baucom, B. R., Crenshaw, A. O., Imel, Z., Atkins, D. C., Clemans, T. A., Leeson, B., Burch, T. S., Mintz, J., & Rudd, M. D. (2018). Associations of patient-rated emotional bond and vocally encoded emotional arousal among clinicians and acutely suicidal military personnel. *Journal of Consulting and Clinical Psychology, 86*(4), 372–383.

Canetto, S. S., & Sakinofsky, I. (1998). The gender paradox in suicide. *Suicide and Life-threatening Behavior, 28*(1), 1–23.

Chae, M. H., & Boyle, D. J. (2013). Police suicide: Prevalence, risk, and protective factors. *Policing: An International Journal of Police Strategies & Management, 36*(1), 91–118.

Copenhaver, A., & Tewksbury, R. (2018). Predicting state police officer willingness to seek professional help for depression. *Criminology, Criminal Justice, Law & Society, 19*(1), 60–74.

Dryden, W., & Hill, L. K. (Eds.). (1993). *Innovations in rational-emotive therapy*. SAGE Publications.

Fleischmann, M. H., Strode, P., Broussard, B., & Compton, M. T. (2018). Law enforcement officers' perceptions of and responses to traumatic events: A survey of officers completing crisis intervention team training. *Policing and Society, 28*(2), 149–156. https://doi.org/10.1080/10439463.2016.1234469

Fox, K. R., Huang, X., Guzmán, E. M., Funsch, K. M., Cha, C. B., Ribeiro, J. D., & Franklin, J. C. (2020). Interventions for suicide and self-injury: A meta-analysis of randomized controlled trials across nearly 50 years of research. *Psychological Bulletin, 146*(12), 1117.

Fuertes, J. N., Stracuzzi, T. I., Bennett, J., Scheinholtz, J., Mislowack, A., Hersh, M., Garnett, M. F., Curtin, S. C., & Stone, D. M. (2022). *Suicide mortality in the United States, 2000–2020*. NCHS Data Brief, no 433. National Center for Health Statistics. https://doi.org/10.15620/cdc:114217. Retrieved from https://www.cdc.gov/nchs/data/databriefs/db433.pdf

Garnett, M. F., Curtin, S. C., & Stone, D. M. (2022). *Suicide mortality in the United States, 2000–2020*.

Gross, J. J. (1998). Antecedent-and response-focused emotion regulation: Divergent consequences for experience, expression, and physiology. *Journal of Personality and Social Psychology, 74*(1), 224.

Grossman, D. C., Mueller, B. A., Riedy, C., Dowd, M. D., Villaveces, A., Prodzinski, J., & Harruff, R. (2005). Gun storage practices and risk of youth suicide and unintentional firearm injuries. *JAMA, 293*(6), 707–714.

Heyman, M., Dill, J., & Douglas, R. (2018). *The Ruderman white paper on mental health and suicide of first responders* (Vol. 41). Ruderman Family Foundation.

Kassin, S., Fein, S., & Markus, H. R. (2016). *Social psychology*. Cengage Learning.

Kleiman, E. M., Turner, B. J., Fedor, S., Beale, E. E., Huffman, J. C., & Nock, M. K. (2017). Examination of real-time fluctuations in suicidal ideation and its risk factors: Results from two ecological momentary assessment studies. *Journal of Abnormal Psychology, 126*(6), 726.

Klimley, K. E., Van Hasselt, V. B., & Stripling, A. M. (2018). Posttraumatic stress disorder in police, firefighters, and emergency dispatchers. *Aggression and Violent Behavior, 43*, 33–44.

Kochanek, K. D., Murphy, S. L., Xu, J., & Arias, E. (2019). Deaths: Final data for 2017. *National Vital Statistics Report, 68*(9).

Loo, R. (2003). A meta-analysis of police suicide rates: Findings and issues. *Suicide and Life-threatening Behavior, 33*(3), 313–325.

Marmar, C. R., McCaslin, S. E., Metzler, T. J., Best, S., Weiss, D. S., Fagan, J., et al. (2006). Predictors of posttraumatic stress in police and other first responders. *Annals of the New York Academy of Sciences, 1071*(1), 1–18.

Marzuk, P. M., Nock, M. K., Leon, A. C., Portera, L., & Tardiff, K. (2002). Suicide among New York City police officers, 1977–1996. *American Journal of Psychiatry, 159*(12), 2069–2071.

May, A. M., & Klonsky, E. D. (2016). What distinguishes suicide attempters from suicide ideators? A meta-analysis of potential factors. *Clinical Psychology: Science and Practice, 23*(1), 5–20.

Monuteaux, M. C., Azrael, D., & Miller, M. (2019). Association of increased safe household firearm storage with firearm suicide and unintentional death among U.S. youths. *JAMA Pediatrics, 173*(7), 657–662.

Murphy, G. E. (1998). Why women are less likely than men to commit suicide. *Comprehensive Psychiatry, 39*(4), 165–175.

Norris, F. H. (1992). Epidemiology of trauma: Frequency and impact of different potentially traumatic events on different demographic groups. *Journal of Consulting and Clinical Psychology, 60*(3), 409.

O'Hara, A. F., Violanti, J. M., Levenson, R. L., Jr., & Clark, R. G., Sr. (2013). National police suicide estimates: Web surveillance study III. *International Journal of Emergency Mental Health and Human Resilience, 15*, 31.

Peterson, C., Sussell, A., Li, J., Schumacher, P. K., Yeoman, K., & Stone, D. M. (2020). Suicide rates by industry and occupation—National Violent Death Reporting System, 32 states, 2016. *Morbidity and Mortality Weekly Report, 69*(3), 57.

Rozek, D. C., & Bryan, C. J. (2020). Integrating crisis response planning for suicide prevention into trauma-focused treatments: A military case example. *Journal of Clinical Psychology, 76*(5), 852–864.

Rudd, M. D., Bryan, C. J., Wertenberger, E. G., Peterson, A. L., Young-McCaughan, S., Mintz, J., Williams, S. R., Arne, K. A., Breitbach, J., Delano, K., Wilkinson, E., & Bruce, T. O. (2015). Brief cognitive-behavioral therapy effects on post-treatment suicide attempts in a military sample: results of a randomized clinical trial with 2-year follow-up. *American Journal of Psychiatry, 172*(5), 441–449.

Sagar-Ouriaghli, I., Godfrey, E., Bridge, L., Meade, L., & Brown, J. S. L. (2019). Improving mental health service utilization among men: A systematic review and synthesis of behavior change techniques within interventions targeting help-seeking. *American Journal of Men's Health, 13*(3), 1557988319857009. https://doi.org/10.1177/1557988319857009

Schafer, K., Sutter, R., & Gibbons, S. (2015). *Characteristics of individuals and employment among first responders*. U.S. Department of Labor.

Schrijvers, D. L., Bollen, J., & Sabbe, B. G. (2012). The gender paradox in suicidal behavior and its impact on the suicidal process. *Journal of Affective Disorders, 138*(1–2), 19–26.

Stanley, I. H., Hom, M. A., Hagan, C. R., & Joiner, T. E. (2015). Career prevalence and correlates of suicidal thoughts and behaviors among firefighters. *Journal of Affective Disorders, 187*, 163–171.

Stanley, I. H., Hom, M. A., & Joiner, T. E. (2016). A systematic review of suicidal thoughts and behaviors among police officers, firefighters, EMTs, and paramedics. *Clinical Psychology Review, 44*, 25–44. https://doi.org/10.1016/j.cpr.2015.12.002

Stanley, I. H., Hom, M. A., Gai, A. R., & Joiner, T. E. (2018). Wildland firefighters and suicide risk: Examining the role of social disconnectedness. *Psychiatry Research, 266*, 269–274.

Steele, I. H., Thrower, N., Noroian, P., & Saleh, F. M. (2018). Understanding suicide across the lifespan: a United States perspective of suicide risk factors, assessment & management. *Journal of Forensic Sciences, 63*(1), 162–171.

Substance Abuse and Mental Health Service Administrator. (2018). *Disaster technical assistance center supplemental research bulletin first responders: behavioral health concerns, emergency response, and trauma*. SAMHSA.

Trafton, J. A., & Gifford, E. V. (2008). *Biological bases of distress tolerance* (pp. 80–102). Theory, Research, and Clinical Applications.

Vigil, N. H., Grant, A. R., Perez, O., Blust, R. N., Chikani, V., Vadeboncoeur, T. F., et al. (2019). Death by suicide—The EMS profession compared to the general public. *Prehospital Emergency Care, 23*(3), 340–345.

Violanti, J. M. (2004). Predictors of police suicide ideation. *Suicide and Life-threatening Behavior, 34*(3), 277–283.

Violanti, J. M., Robinson, C. F., & Shen, R. (2013). Law enforcement suicide: A national analysis. *International Journal of Emergency Mental Health and Human Resilience, 15*(4), 289–298.

Wasserman, D., & Cyranka, K. (2019). Difficulties in preventing suicidal behaviours in spite of existing evidence-based preventive methods—An overview. *Archives of Psychiatry and Psychotherapy, 1*, 7–12.

Wilcox, H. C., & Wyman, P. A. (2016). Suicide prevention strategies for improving population health. *Child and Adolescent Psychiatric Clinics, 25*(2), 219–233.

Trauma and Posttraumatic Stress Disorder Among First Responders

Maya Zegel, Samuel J. Leonard, Nathaniel A. Healy, and Anka A. Vujanovic

Trauma

First responders represent a unique and understudied population at heightened risk for chronic occupational stress and exposure to potentially traumatic events (PTEs; e.g., attending to fires, medical emergencies, and violent crimes; Bowers et al., 2019; Vujanovic & Tran, 2021). While the majority of first responders are remarkably resilient, weathering extreme stress and potentially traumatic experiences and 'bouncing back' more readily than individuals in the general population (Kilpatrick et al., 2013), chronic exposure to intense occupational demands has the potential to translate to deleterious mental health outcomes, including posttraumatic stress disorder (PTSD). Per the *Diagnostic and Statistical Manual of Mental Disorders, 5th Edition (DSM-5)*, a PTE is defined as "exposure to actual or threatened death, serious injury, or sexual violence," through either direct experience, witnessing the event, learning the event has happened to a close family member or friend (if the event is violent or accidental), or having repeated or extreme exposure to distressing details of a traumatic event (p. 271, American Psychiatric Association, 2013).

The vast majority of first responders, including police and law enforcement officers, firefighters, emergency medical services (EMS) personnel, detention officers, and dispatch operators, experience PTEs (Carleton et al., 2019), yet few large-scale epidemiologic studies are available to provide definitive estimates of PTE exposure

M. Zegel (✉) · S. J. Leonard · N. A. Healy
Department of Psychology, University of Houston, Houston, TX, USA
e-mail: mzegel@uh.edu

A. A. Vujanovic
Department of Psychology, University of Houston, Houston, TX, USA

Department of Psychological & Brain Sciences, Texas A&M University, College Station, USA
e-mail: avujanovic@tamu.edu

M. L. Bourke et al. (eds.), *First Responder Mental Health*,
https://doi.org/10.1007/978-3-031-38149-2_21

and PTSD across first responder populations. A large study ($N = 4441$) in Canada estimated that first responders experience an average of approximately 11 PTE types, with the most distressing events involving sudden, violent, or accidental deaths (Carleton et al., 2019). Furthermore, police (Royal Canadian Mounted Police, $M = 11.64$, SD = 3.04; municipal/provincial police, $M = 11.36$, SD = 3.16), paramedics ($M = 11.59$, SD = 2.86), and dispatchers ($M = 10.96$, SD = 3.56) reported experiencing a significantly greater number of average PTEs compared to correctional workers ($M = 9.88$, SD = 3.88) and firefighters ($M = 10.22$, SD = 2.84; Carleton et al., 2019). Self-reported rates of current (i.e., past month) PTSD varied by occupation with the Royal Canadian Mounted Police ($N = 1069$) and correctional workers ($N = 576$) demonstrating the highest rates of approximately 30%, significantly greater than the 24.5% prevalence reported among paramedics ($N = 609$) in this sample, followed by 19.5% among municipal/provincial police ($N = 1148$) and 18.3% among dispatchers ($N = 201$). All occupations evinced a significantly higher rate compared to firefighters ($N = 682$) in this sample, 13.5% of whom reported experiencing symptoms consistent with a diagnosis of current PTSD (Carleton et al., 2018a, b); however, all aforementioned prevalence rates greatly exceed the 1.4% worldwide prevalence of current PTSD among general population samples (Koenen et al., 2017).

However, it is important to note that first responder roles are not always clearly defined. For example, firefighters and police may perform EMS roles as a part of their job or by nature of the call. Some may work concurrently in multiple roles across different departments (e.g., firefighter and part-time as a dispatcher in another municipality) or may transition to a different first responder role due to injury or retirement (e.g., former firefighter becoming a dispatch operator). Thus, the discrete categorizations of first responder careers may not fully represent the experience of first responders; therefore, it is important for future work to comprehensively evaluate first responders' occupational roles and duties to foster a more granular understanding of associations between role(s) and behavioral health.

Therefore, the aims of the present chapter are three-fold: First, we will summarize, based on the available literature, the prevalence of exposure to PTEs and subclinical and diagnostic PTSD among various subpopulations of first responders, with the caveat that most estimates are not based on representative epidemiological data. For brevity, we focus on North American samples and include samples from other regions if and when there is no other available literature (estimates across nations do not vary widely). Second, we will discuss major risk and vulnerability factors for PTSD and common psychiatric and medical comorbidities of PTSD among first responder populations. Finally, we will enumerate key clinical considerations and future directions necessary to inform evidence-based assessment, intervention, and prevention efforts for PTSD, specifically tailored to the unique needs of first responder populations.

Police Officers

Among police officers in the U.S. and Canada, the prevalence of PTE exposure has been estimated to range from 59% to 82%, with some estimates as high as 100% (Covey et al., 2013; Maguen et al., 2009; Soomro & Yanos, 2018). A prospective study conducted across four U.S. cities found that police officers ($N = 233$) reported experiencing an average of 6 PTEs in the first two years on the job (Yuan et al., 2011), while a study of police officers in the midwestern U.S. ($N = 193$) reported an average of 9 PTEs in which there was a threat to others and 6 PTEs in which there was a threat to themselves (Chopko et al., 2021).

Firefighters

Firefighters (some of whom provide emergency medical services) are estimated to have experienced approximately 8 to 13 PTE types (Langtry et al., 2021; Paulus et al., 2018).

Emergency Medical Service Personnel (EMS)

EMS personnel may include ambulance drivers with basic life support training, emergency medical technicians (EMTs), and paramedics, each with increasing levels of training and job responsibility. It is important to note that some departments require cross-training (e.g., firefighters who are required to pursue paramedic certification and serve in that role for a specified number of years/shifts) and/or riding in units with different capacities (i.e., an ambulance staffed with EMTs will provide basic life support while an ambulance with a paramedic on staff can provide more advanced services). Ambulance workers experience disproportionate rates of PTE exposure as their calls are typically in response to acute medical crises, life-threatening events, serious injuries, or acts of violence. Calls involving pediatric events are consistently reported as the most distressing, as well as mass casualty events, calls regarding sexual violence and rape, and calls where a loved one is experiencing a life-threatening event (Boland et al., 2018; Rybojad et al., 2016). Among EMS workers from the midwestern U.S. ($N = 190$), 68% reported being assaulted by a patient during a shift, and 43% reported being threatened with a gun or other weapon (Boland et al., 2018).

Detention Officers and Dispatch Operators

Broadly, there is a dearth of research examining PTE exposure among detention officers and dispatch operators. One study reported on the prevalence of PTE exposure among correctional and forensic mental health staff in Australia (*N* = 138), with 96% reporting vicarious trauma, or traumatization resulting from repeated exposure to details and materials related to PTEs experienced by others, as a result of their jobs (Newman et al., 2019). Among 9-1-1 telecommunicators in the midwestern U.S. (*N* = 171), participants endorsed experiencing an average of 15 PTE types (Pierce & Lilly, 2012).

Posttraumatic Stress Disorder (PTSD)

A relatively small subset of individuals who experience a PTE may develop PTSD, if they experience symptoms of trauma-related intrusions (e.g., nightmares, intrusive memories), avoidance of internal (e.g., thoughts, memories) and external trauma-related cues, trauma-related negative alterations in cognition and mood (e.g., difficulty feeling positive emotions, feeling inappropriate shame or guilt), and trauma-related alterations in arousal and reactivity (e.g., hypervigilance, startle response, sleep disturbance) for at least one month or more, per the *DSM-5* (American Psychiatric Association, 2013). A systematic review of PTSD among rescue workers (i.e., ambulance personnel, firefighters, police officers exposed to natural disasters, and other rescue teams [e.g., rescue divers, helpers/volunteers, etc.]), estimated the worldwide prevalence of current (i.e., past-month or past-six-month) *DSM-IV* PTSD to be 10% (Berger et al., 2012), significantly greater than the estimated 1.4% worldwide prevalence of past-month *DSM-IV* PTSD among trauma-exposed individuals (Koenen et al., 2017). It is important to note that individuals experiencing PTSD symptoms subthreshold for diagnosis evince relatively equivalent levels of functional impairment as those with diagnostic PTSD (Pietrzak et al., 2011), highlighting the importance of understanding the full spectrum of PTSD symptomatology.

Police

A national study among active-duty U.S. police officers (*N* = 296) demonstrated that approximately 21% self-reported symptoms consistent with PTSD per *DSM-5* criteria (Soomro & Yanos, 2018). Among active-duty Canadian police (*N* = 138), the self-reported prevalence of *DSM-IV* PTSD is estimated to be approximately 32% (Asmundson & Stapleton, 2008). These rates are consistent with other U.S.-based research (Austin-Ketch et al., 2012; Violanti et al., 2006); however, extant literature is mixed on rates of PTSD, in part due to the use of various assessment measures (e.g., clinician-administered and self-report measures), different cutoff scores for probable PTSD based on individual self-report measures, and varying *DSM* criteria over time (e.g., *DSM-IV* vs. *DSM-5*). Thus, rates may signify actual differences in prevalence, or they may be an artifact of assessment type. Future work with representative samples using more consistent measurements is needed for accurate cross-national comparisons.

Notably, rates of trauma and PTSD may be higher for police officers seeking treatment (van der Meer et al., 2017). Further, the duration of PTE exposure may be a factor in the evaluation of PTSD prevalence rates. For example, a large, longitudinal study of 9/11 police responders documented that the prevalence of PTSD doubled between the 2–3 years and the 5–6 years post-9/11 assessment time points (Bowler et al., 2012). A notable body of research has sought to examine mental health outcomes among police who have experienced a specific PTE, such as a natural disaster (Kerswell et al., 2019) or terror attack (Motreff et al., 2020; Whealin et al., 2022). Although difficult to generalize across countries, these studies document psychological distress and PTSD symptoms among police between 4 weeks to 1 year after the specific PTE (Kerswell et al., 2019; Motreff et al., 2020).

Firefighters

A systematic review reported the worldwide prevalence of PTSD among firefighters ranges from 4% to 54%, with an average prevalence of 14.25% and a median prevalence of 10.25% (Wagner et al., 2021). Among a national sample of U.S. firefighters, PTSD prevalence was estimated to be 32% (Boffa et al., 2017), while the national prevalence of PTSD among Canadian firefighters has been estimated to be approximately 17% (Carleton et al., 2018a, b). These rates are consistent with literature among trauma-exposed firefighters who provide both fire suppression and EMS services in the southern U.S. (Paltell et al., 2019; Zegel et al., 2022). The literature is mixed regarding the associations between event type, trauma severity, or number of PTEs and PTSD among firefighters (Heinrichs et al., 2005; Wagner et al., 2021). Overall, studies of higher methodological quality (e.g., recruitment methods, sample size, measurement, and analysis fit; Munn et al., 2014) are associated with higher PTSD prevalence rates (Wagner et al., 2021), underscoring the need for greater rigor and consistency in research methodology across studies (e.g., clinician-administered assessments).

Emergency Medical Service Personnel

A systematic review and meta-analysis of rescue workers worldwide reported that ambulance workers demonstrate PTSD rates greater than those reported by police and firefighters (Berger et al., 2012). Research has documented a PTSD prevalence of approximately 22% among EMTs/paramedics in Canada (Carleton et al., 2018a, b); however, rates have been reported as high as 42% among pre-hospital providers (i.e., paramedics, EMTs, flight nurses, and paramedics) in Texas (*N* = 546; Luftman et al., 2017). It is possible that pre-hospital providers, compared to in-hospital providers (e.g., physicians and nursing staff), are more likely to encounter dangerous and unpredictable situations in a minimally controlled environment as part of their jobs, which may contribute to higher rates of PTSD.

Detention Officers and Dispatch Operators

Reported rates of PTSD among detention officers and dispatch vary widely across studies. Among a study of corrections employees in the northwest U.S., an estimated 19% met *DSM-5* criteria for PTSD (James & Todak, 2018), while among correctional workers in Canada, the prevalence of PTSD was estimated to be approximately 25% (Carleton et al., 2018a, b). Per *DSM-IV* criteria, rates of PTSD have been reported as high as 53% among rural and urban jail correctional officers in the midwestern U.S. (*N* = 320; Jaegers et al., 2019). Similarly, research on PTSD prevalence among emergency dispatch operators is scant. Among emergency dispatch operators in the U.S., studies with sample sizes ranging from 90 to 205 demonstrated rates of PTSD between 13% and 17%, which is consistent with the estimated national prevalence of PTSD of 19% among Canadian dispatchers (Carleton, et al., 2018a, b).

Predictors of PTSD

First responder populations experience unique levels and types of PTEs. Although not all individuals who experience a PTE develop PTSD (Klimley et al., 2018), the cumulative nature of these events, the severity of the traumas endured, and other contextual factors contribute to the likelihood of PTSD outcomes among first responders (Haugen et al., 2012; Kleim & Westphal, 2011). For example, research has sought to examine numerous resilience and vulnerability factors that may mitigate or exacerbate the likelihood that an individual might develop PTSD in the aftermath of PTE exposure (Skogstad et al., 2013). These variables can be broadly divided into two categories: non-occupational and occupational factors (Lewis-Schroeder et al., 2018). Non-occupational factors can be further divided into subcategories of sociodemographic and cognitive-affective factors, as well as pretraumatic, peritraumatic, and posttraumatic factors. Generally, prospective longitudinal studies that follow first responders from academy training through retirement are lacking, and such studies are important to bolster our understanding of the temporal relations between PTE exposure and PTSD symptomatology (and related conditions) through the occupational lifespan.

Sociodemographic Factors

First responders who are younger, single, identify as female, and identify with historically marginalized racial/ethnic populations have a greater risk of developing PTSD (Kleim & Westphal, 2011; Marmar et al., 2006). Younger and non-married first responders are more likely to develop PTSD, potentially due in part to lower levels of emotional and social support when compared to their older, married peers (Kleim & Westphal, 2011; Salleh et al., 2020). Future work might explore the effects of family, including romantic partners and children, on first responders' recovery following PTE.

Gender differences have been documented in the prevalence of PTSD among police officers and EMS personnel, with some studies reporting higher rates among men (Bennett et al., 2005; Kerswell et al., 2019) and others reporting higher rates among women (Darensburg et al., 2006; Rybojad et al., 2016). These documented rates contradict a well-established literature focused on the general population that elucidates higher rates of PTSD among women than men (American Psychiatric Association, 2013). This discrepancy may be due to underreporting among women first responders, perhaps due to significant mental health stigma and gender discrimination in the first responder workforce. Therefore, such stigma may be especially salient among women first responders who may feel greater pressure to "not complain" and prove themselves capable of performing their work duties in a male-dominated field.

Additionally, first responders with lower levels of education and a family history of mental health issues have an elevated risk of developing PTSD (Lewis-Schroeder et al., 2018; Rybojad et al., 2016). Among general populations, a family history of psychopathology increases one's risk of developing PTSD after experiencing a PTE. Poor educational attainment is also associated with an increased risk for PTSD, potentially due to factors related to socioeconomic status, cognitive ability, access to healthcare resources, familial support regarding mental health issues, and/or mental health 'literacy' or awareness (Brewin et al., 2000; Ozer et al., 2003).

Further, disparities in PTSD prevalence have been documented across racial and ethnic groups of first responders. For example, among police officers who responded to the World Trade Center following the 9/11 terror attacks, white police officers experienced a significantly lower rate of PTSD (8.7%) compared to Latino/police officers (10.4%) and Black police officers (9.8%; Whealin et al., 2022). One study among Hispanic male firefighters (N = 551) reported a PTSD prevalence rate of approximately 11% and emphasized the need to examine differences in PTSD prevalence across racial and ethnic groups within first responder subpopulations (Arbona et al., 2017). Future research is needed to explore the intersection of cultural (e.g., Verbeek & van der Velden, 2016) and gender differences related to the manifestation/reported rate of PTSD among first responders, as well as the role of discrimination (e.g., sexism, racism) and related stress in the etiology and maintenance of symptoms.

Cognitive-Affective Factors

Various cognitive-affective factors have been identified as etiological or maintenance processes relevant to PTSD among first responders. These factors include but are not limited to distress tolerance (i.e., a diminished capacity to withstand distressing emotions; Leyro et al., 2010), mindfulness (i.e., purposeful awareness of and focus on the current moment and the non-judgmental acceptance of unfavorable affective states; Baer et al., 2006), anxiety sensitivity (i.e., increased fear of anxiety-related sensations and cognitions; Reiss et al., 1986), resilience (i.e., the capability to adapt in the face of adversity, trauma, or significant threat; Horn et al., 2016), and emotion regulation difficulties (i.e., problems with modulating emotional reactions when faced with psychological stressors; Gratz & Roemer, 2004). Studies have documented significant relations between these factors and PTSD symptom severity (e.g., Grupe et al., 2021; Lebeaut et al., 2021; Zegel et al., 2019), but most of this work has been cross-sectional and focused on police or firefighter/EMS populations. Heightened PTSD symptomatology is associated with a lower ability to tolerate negative emotion states (i.e., distress tolerance; Vujanovic & Zegel, 2020) and a lower ability to be nonjudgmentally aware of the present moment (i.e., mindfulness; Banks et al., 2015) and vice versa. Further, heightened PTSD symptomatology is associated with greater emotion regulation difficulties and heightened fear of anxiety-related sensations (i.e., anxiety sensitivity; Vujanovic et al., 2018). High levels of resilience are protective against the development of PTSD in firefighters as well (Lee et al., 2014). The moderating (i.e., exacerbating) and mediating (i.e., explanatory) effects of each of these cognitive-affective factors have been documented between PTSD and highly prevalent correlates, including alcohol use and suicide risk (e.g., Boffa et al., 2018; Lebeaut et al., 2021). Longitudinal studies and ecological momentary assessment methodologies may be particularly useful in helping to elucidate the interplay of these factors over time and in the context of the workplace versus home environments.

Pre-, Peri-, and Post-Traumatic Factors

In terms of pre-traumatic events, historical backgrounds of childhood adversity and abuse, as well as previous history of psychiatric impairment and substance use issues are associated with the risk of developing PTSD in first responders (Lewis-Schroeder et al., 2018). Experiences during a PTE that predict PTSD in these populations include the individual and social context of the event, personal interpretation of trauma severity (i.e., whether the individual believes the event qualifies as being traumatic; Ricciardelli et al., 2020), dissociation during the event, sustaining an injury during the event, and perceiving the trauma as life-threatening (Kleim & Westphal, 2011; Lewis-Schroeder et al., 2018). Following the PTE, low perceived social support, limited access to mental health treatment, and the experience of various post-trauma stressors (e.g., medical illnesses, interpersonal conflicts) are all correlated with the risk of developing PTSD in first responders (Kleim & Westphal, 2011; Lewis-Schroeder et al., 2018).

Occupational Factors

Certain occupational factors specific to first responder populations have been identified as related to PTSD, including lower levels of job training, lower service rank, limited workplace social support (Lewis-Schroeder et al., 2018; Marmar et al., 2006) as well as work versus contract status (e.g., self-employed paramedics or volunteer firefighters; Rybojad et al., 2016). First responders are typically given specialized training that prepares them for the job and provides skills training to cope with regular exposure to physical and psychological stressors (Klimley et al., 2018). Research has shown that when first responders receive minimal or inadequate training, they are at a higher risk of developing mental health issues, including PTSD (Klimley et al., 2018). Lower-ranking first responders are more likely to experience a PTE and develop PTSD symptoms, potentially because they are more likely to engage in more direct emergency work compared to higher-ranking peers (Salleh et al., 2020). The importance of camaraderie and social support in the workplace (e.g., colleagues, peer support programs) and at home (e.g., romantic/marital partners, family members) are also protective factors against the development of PTSD, particularly among firefighters (Lewis-Schroeder et al., 2018). Shift work and the impact on sleep are associated with increased stress and difficulty managing emotions, potentially hindering first responders' ability to process their experience of PTEs (Feldman et al., 2021). Poor sleep and the impact on emotion regulation may also interfere with first responders' social support, by straining their relationships with spouses/romantic partners, for example (Casas & Benuto, 2022; Palmer & Alfano, 2017).

In terms of work/contract status, self-employed paramedics and volunteer firefighters are more likely to develop PTSD when compared to professional full-time employed first responders. This risk might result from limited job resources (e.g., salary, equipment), training, and/or accessibility of mental health treatment (Klimley et al., 2018; Rybojad et al., 2016). Additionally, hazardous occupational exposures (e.g., exposure to fire, smoke, and carcinogens) increase PTSD risk in part due to alterations in physiological stress responses and decreases in overall physical health (Lewis-Schroeder et al., 2018). Finally, numerous occupational stressors contribute to PTSD risk among first responder populations. These occupational stressors can include conflict with co-workers and supervisors, demanding shift schedules, chronic sleep disturbance, as well as both discrimination and stigmatization based on an individual's gender identity, sexual orientation, or race/ethnicity (Kleim & Westphal, 2011; Lewis-Schroeder et al., 2018). Wagner et al. (2020) found that the clearest predictive associations for the development of PTSD symptoms following a PTE among EMS workers were exposure-related and organizational factors, whereas individual-difference factors had weaker associations with the development of PTSD symptoms.

Psychiatric and Medical Comorbidities

Approximately 80% of individuals with PTSD meet the criteria for another mental disorder (American Psychiatric Association, 2013), and first responders are no exception (Bowler et al., 2016). The first responder literature does not distinguish pre-morbid (i.e., pre-PTE) diagnoses versus symptoms and psychiatric diagnoses that evolve following PTE. Most available research is cross-sectional and does not query the timing of PTE and/or the onset of symptoms of PTSD or other conditions. For example, first responders may enter the occupation with clinical symptomatology and/or a history of exposure to PTE, and this may place them on paths of risk or resilience given the often chronic stress and PTE exposure in first responder occupations. Clinically, it is important to consider whether first responder prevention or intervention approaches might differ for those who experienced PTE (e.g., childhood abuse, interpersonal violence) or behavioral health symptoms (e.g., PTSD, sleep disturbance, anxiety, alcohol use disorder) prior to their first responder roles, compared to those who encounter PTE or develop behavioral health symptoms for the first time in the workplace.

Emotional Symptoms and Disorders

Emotional disorders, such as depression and anxiety, co-occur with PTSD at high rates. It is estimated that among individuals with PTSD, the rate of depression ranges from 21% to 94% and the prevalence of anxiety ranges from 39% to 97% (Spinhoven et al., 2014). For example, among police officers (N = 243) who responded to the 9/11 terrorist attacks, approximately 25% demonstrated comorbid

PTSD and depression, while nearly 50% demonstrated comorbid PTSD, depression, and anxiety (Bowler et al., 2016).

Substance Use

Substance use disorders, including alcohol use disorder, have been identified as one of the most common comorbidities with PTSD, particularly among men (American Psychiatric Association, 2013). Among first responders, much of the literature has focused on the comorbidity of PTSD and alcohol use (e.g., Smith et al., 2020), likely due to the greater acceptance of alcohol use in first responder culture compared to other substance use, as well as likely underreporting of other substance use due to concerns about work-related consequences of such disclosure. For example, it has been estimated that 50% of firefighters report engaging in excessive alcohol use (Haddock et al., 2015) and 58% report binge drinking (Carey et al., 2011), which is further substantiated by estimates that approximately 47% of firefighters meet criteria for a lifetime alcohol use disorder (North et al., 2002). In a study of French police officers hospitalized for alcohol-related concerns ($N = 133$), approximately 38% reported symptoms consistent with PTSD (Brunault et al., 2019). A high rate of alcohol use was documented among volunteer EMS workers in the northeast U.S., as approximately 50% reported drinking alcohol as a coping strategy (Essex & Scott, 2008).

Extant research among first responders suggests that elevated alcohol consumption may be associated with drinking to cope with work-related (e.g., injury) and PTSD symptomatology (Haddock et al., 2017; Zegel et al., 2019), which is consistent with the self-medication hypothesis (Khantzian, 1997). This is noteworthy, as research has demonstrated that probable co-occurring PTSD and alcohol use disorder among firefighters/EMS evinces greater clinical and functional outcome-related difficulties (e.g., depression, suicide-related thoughts, and behaviors) compared to either disorder alone (Zegel et al., 2022).

Suicide Risk

There has been a growing body of literature regarding the increased risk for suicide among first responder populations. Stanley et al. (2015) estimated that among a sample of career and volunteer firefighters, 46.8% thought about suicide, 19.2% made a suicide plan, and 15.5% made a suicide attempt; notably higher than the estimated rates of 5.6–14.3%, 3.9%, and 1.9–8.7% rates, respectively, among the general U.S. population (Nock et al., 2008). Studies have indicated associations between PTSD and heightened suicide risk, including among police, firefighters, paramedics/EMTs, and corrections officers (Healy & Vujanovic, 2021; Stanley et al., 2016; Violanti et al., 2013). Furthermore, research has provided evidence to suggest that a lifetime diagnosis of PTSD differentiates those who make suicide attempts from those experiencing suicidal thoughts (Nock et al., 2009).

Pain

A large study of public safety personnel in Canada (*N* = 5093) documented elevated rates of PTSD among first responders with chronic pain compared to those without chronic pain, and these findings were consistent across occupational groups (i.e., police, firefighters, paramedic/EMTs, correctional workers), except for dispatchers who reported similar rates of PTSD regardless of chronic pain status (Carleton, et al., 2018a, b). The majority of extant literature regarding pain among first responders has focused on firefighters. Firefighters have reported elevated rates of acute and chronic pain when compared to the general population (Bos et al., 2004; Kim et al., 2007) as well as, elevated rates of a work-related injury, chronic musculoskeletal disorder (e.g., low back pain) (Carleton, et al., 2018a, b; Katsavouni & Bebetsos, 2016; Lebeaut et al., 2022). Research has suggested that shared vulnerability factors along with an increased rate of experiencing trauma exposure events may account for these elevated rates of pain (Rogers et al., 2019). This heightened risk has been suggested to result from the exposure to many highly stressful, dangerous, and potentially traumatic events, as well as various occupation-related duties, including the utilization and movement of onerous work-related equipment (e.g., portable oxygen tanks and fire-retardant gear) and the 'polarizing' transition between physically demanding (e.g., fighting fires) and low-level (e.g., time off between calls) activities (Kim et al., 2019; Rogers et al., 2019).

Cardiovascular Risk

Extant literature has cited findings that PTSD has been found to predict future increased cardiovascular risk (Boscarino, 2008; Burg et al., 2017; Kubzansky et al., 2007). Much of the literature exploring cardiovascular risks among first responders has focused on police and firefighters. A prominent study of police officers conducted by Violanti et al. (2006) indicated that the risk for cardiovascular harm was elevated among officers with PTSD and found an association between PTSD and a collection of cardiovascular disease-related risk factors (e.g., blood pressure, triglycerides, HDL cholesterol), and police officers with severe PTSD symptoms were approximately three times more likely to have the collection of cardiovascular risk factors. Studies have shown that cardiovascular symptoms were common among firefighters following a PTE, with additional supporting evidence to suggest that these symptoms were greater among those with PTSD compared to those without PTSD (Milligan-Saville et al., 2017; Ranney et al., 2020). A separate study identified that 42% of all firefighter duty-related fatalities have been attributed to cardiac issues within the previous 10 years (Smith et al., 2019). Taken together, these findings underscore the need for continued research into associations between cardiovascular health and PTSD among other first responder populations.

Examining First Responder Culture

While considering the numerous factors and mechanisms that may contribute to the development and expression of the various psychopathological symptoms and/or comorbidities previously described in this chapter, we must contextualize these insights with respect to the culture that subsumes this uniquely vulnerable subpopulation. Investigations into these cultural elements reveal that only about 8% of career and volunteer firefighters identify as female (Evarts & Stein, 2020), facilitating a generally cisgender male organizational culture often characterized by "traditionally masculine" qualities, which include but are not limited to heroism, physical strength, rationality, hardiness, "toughness," focus, and self-reliance established upon a foundational sense of teamwork and camaraderie (Evarts & Stein, 2020; O'Neill & Rothbard, 2017; Vujanovic & Tran, 2021). Although some characteristics may be protective against negative mental health outcomes (e.g., camaraderie engendering greater social support), many of these traits fuel reputational concerns of being embarrassed or the fear of being perceived as "unfit for duty" if the first responder were to have an emotional reaction or struggle with their mental health (Hom et al., 2016; Kim et al., 2018; Vujanovic & Tran, 2021). Prior work has posited how this culture may serve a key role in the development and maintenance of mental health stigma, which may discourage the seeking of mental health or other medical care-related services (Vujanovic & Tran, 2021). Thus, first responders are likely to have lower emotional expressiveness which may be associated with generally decreased emotional awareness. First responders may also be less inclined to label a PTE as "traumatic", given the frequency with which they encounter these events in their line of work. For a first responder who is hesitant to label an event as traumatic but is experiencing mental health sequelae from the PTE, clinicians may consider using behavioral anchors (i.e., changes in PTSD symptomatology) pre- and post-PTE to emphasize the impact of the event and facilitate initiation of treatment services.

Clinical Considerations

First responder culture may promote the expectation or idealization of resilience when enduring experiences of extreme psychological distress. Further, first responders may differ from other populations due to their perceptions of inadequate workplace social support (Lewis-Schroeder et al., 2018), stressors related to interpersonal conflict (e.g., discrimination, harassment, and criticism), poor resourcing (e.g., inadequate income and/or access to mental health services), and fewer opportunities for consultation, communication, and confidentiality (Collins & Gibbs, 2003; Maguen et al., 2009; Thompson et al., 2006). Limited workplace support may affect first responders' desire or accessibility to engage in mental health treatment services. Furthermore, shift work, concerns of stigma, and negative changes to job-related duties and pay may contribute to workplace stress (Haugen et al., 2012). In addition to the challenges with seeking departmental social support, first responders might face difficulties receiving social support from external sources (e.g., family, friends, and relationship partners). Reasons for these additional difficulties with external sources of support include: (1) incongruent job-related scheduling and demands (e.g., challenges in coordinating and balancing childcare due to shift work), (2) differential coping, communication, and problem-solving skills and strategies, (3) a lack of job-related shared experiences, and (4) concerns regarding mental health stigma.

Moreover, it is important to consider the nuances both between and within first responder occupational subgroups. For example, each of the previously referenced subgroups (e.g., police officers, firefighters, dispatch operators) has received various forms of training that enable the development and implementation of distinct skills and strategies in response to an emergency. Generally, first responder trainings may have a deleterious impact on the development and utilization of self-coping strategies *if implemented rigidly across contexts*, due to reinforced encouragement of persevering through highly distressing situations. It is worth noting that some of these subgroups may share more similar characteristics or training (e.g., firefighters and police officers) when compared to others (e.g., correctional officers and dispatch operators). In some cases, dispatch operators may have previously served as police or firefighters while some might be civilians, underscoring further the complex task of differentiating occupational groups. The job- and pay-related structures among first responder departments also differentiate them from other careers. Specifically, first responders provide their services via a career, volunteer, or combination (i.e., career and volunteer) capacity, each with varying levels of financial and contractual obligations. Career first responders may work as either part-time or full-time employees. First responders employed in a career or combination capacity may be provided with increased access to additional benefits, including health insurance and corresponding resources for seeking psychological services or support, as compared to volunteers. Emerging research suggests that volunteer firefighters, as compared to career firefighters, report more severe mental health symptoms, for example (Johnson et al., 2020; Stanley et al., 2017). Future research is needed to explore these population-specific characteristics and, as the similarities and discrepancies both between and within first responder occupational subgroups may be relevant when contextualizing the etiological or maintenance mechanisms associated with psychological outcomes, including PTSD, and culturally tailored best-practice treatment approaches.

Future Directions

First responders are invaluable to our society, and yet the impact of their stressful occupational demands on mental health and well-being has been historically understudied, including the potential impact of chronic exposure to PTEs and the experience of PTSD symptomatology. First responder culture is unique and requires a deeper understanding by mental health professionals. Extant research has documented significant rates of PTSD and co-occurring psychiatric and medical comorbidities. Many first responders continue to report mental health stigma and hesitation to seek out mental health services. Furthermore, pragmatic barriers such as shift work, overnight shifts, long commutes, and financial concerns may prevent many first responders from accessing mental health services.

While there are numerous evidence-based treatment options for the most common psychological symptoms reported by first responders (e.g., PTSD, alcohol use disorder), relatively few randomized clinical trials have been conducted to evaluate such interventions among first responders, specifically (e.g., Alghamdi et al., 2015; Skeffington et al., 2016; Trombka et al., 2021). Programs, such as Stress First Aid, have been developed for firefighters and emergency medical services personnel (Watson et al., 2012) to quickly assess and respond to acute stress reactions in oneself or others. Many departments use critical incidents stress management and peer support to address stress in the immediate aftermath of potentially traumatic events, although efficacy in reducing or preventing mental health concerns has not been unequivocally established (e.g., Johnson et al., 2020). Cognitive processing therapy (CPT) or prolonged exposure therapy for PTSD may be indicated (Watkins et al., 2018). CPT may be more applicable for firefighters who either cannot recall an event due to a traumatic brain injury or who may not report a single index traumatic event but rather a chronic series of exposures to work-related traumas (Asmundson et al., 2019; Powers et al., 2010).

Transdiagnostic treatment approaches may be relevant if first responders are presenting with PTSD and emotional disorders, such as depression and anxiety (e.g., Barlow et al., 2017). Mindfulness-based interventions may be useful for concurrent management of stress and pain. First responders with comorbid PTSD and substance or alcohol use problems may benefit from integrated PTSD/SUD treatments, such as Concurrent Treatment of PTSD/SUD with Prolonged Exposure (e.g., Ruglass et al., 2017). Psychopharmacological intervention may also be indicated in some circumstances and may require care coordination with primary care physicians or psychiatrists (Fraess-Phillips et al., 2017).

Notably, first responders may face significant pragmatic and psychological barriers to treatment access, initiation, and maintenance that should be addressed to enhance engagement and decrease attrition rates (Johnson et al., 2020). To address pragmatic barriers, providers might consider teletherapy options (e.g., video, telephone), after-hours or weekend care, structured peer support, and family involvement (e.g., couples therapy). Transparent communication about fees, health insurance coverage for mental health services, and scheduling are important from the outset, especially for first responders with PTSD symptomatology who may experience altered beliefs about trust (e.g., "No one can be trusted"), safety (e.g., "The world is not a safe place"), power and control ("If I disclose my trauma, I will lose control of my emotions"), esteem (e.g., "I am damaged"), and intimacy ("I cannot get close to people because if they knew what I am really like, they won't want anything to do with me"; Resick et al., 2016). First responders may be more likely to cancel at the last minute due to work-related duties and crises, and a clear framework for cancellations and tardiness is important. Relatedly, clarifying limits to confidentiality early and often is important so that first responders understand the parameters and legal standards in place to protect their personal health information, reaffirming their sense of perceived control and contextual safety and predictability. This careful orientation to confidentiality and its limits is intended to avoid unexpected circumstances in which the first responder might feel shamed or surprised when the clinician must initiate crisis management protocols (e.g., police wellness checks and psychiatric inpatient care) to reduce safety risks. Such transparency is especially important for first responders with PTSD who might experience such uncontrollable or surprising circumstances as trauma-related triggers or cues.

Finally, first responders with PTSD might find it difficult to relate to mental health professionals. In some instances, connecting first responders to peer support programs may be effective as a first step toward help-seeking and mental health treatment for PTSD. One-on-one meetings or workshops, led by firefighter peers, for example, have demonstrated promise, and peer support can offer an effective collaborative partnership with mental health professionals (Bowers et al., 2019). The development of self-help resources and self-assessment tools, online or via apps, may also enhance the dissemination of evidence-based information, assessment, and treatment of trauma and PTSD to first responders. Continuing education on mental health-related topics, offered through first responder departments, can further target stigma and bridge the gap between first responders and effective mental health services (Isaac & Buchanan, 2021). As part of this effort, increasing engagement in conversations, from the command staff and through the ranks, about mental health can be effective in promoting awareness and improving service initiation, engagement, and maintenance.

References

Alghamdi, M., Hunt, N., & Thomas, S. (2015). The effectiveness of Narrative Exposure Therapy with traumatised firefighters in Saudi Arabia: A randomized controlled study. *Behaviour Research and Therapy, 66*, 64–71. https://doi.org/10.1016/j.brat.2015.01.008

American Psychiatric Association. (2013). *Diagnostic and statistical manual of mental disorders: DSM-5* (5th ed.). American Psychiatric Association.

Arbona, C., Pao, C., Long, A., & Olvera, N. (2017). Perceived stress in Black and Latino male firefighters: Associations with risk and protective factors. *Ethnicity and Disease, 27*(4), 421–428. https://doi.org/10.18865/ed.27.4.421

Asmundson, G. J., & Stapleton, J. A. (2008). Associations between dimensions of anxiety sensitivity and PTSD symptom clusters in active-duty police officers. *Cognitive Behaviour Therapy, 37*(2), 66–75. https://doi.org/10.1080/16506070801969005

Asmundson, G. J., Thorisdottir, A. S., Roden-Foreman, J. W., Baird, S. O., Witcraft, S. M., Stein, A. T., et al. (2019). A meta-analytic review of cognitive processing therapy for adults with posttraumatic stress disorder. *Cognitive Behaviour Therapy, 48*(1), 1–14.

Austin-Ketch, T. L., Violanti, J., Fekedulegn, D., Andrew, M. E., Burchfield, C. M., & Hartley, T. A. (2012). Addictions and the criminal justice system, what happens on the other side? Post-traumatic stress symptoms and cortisol measures in a police cohort. *Journal of Addictions Nursing, 23*(1), 22–29. https://doi.org/10.3109/10884602.2011.645255

Baer, R. A., Smith, G. T., Hopkins, J., Krietemeyer, J., & Toney, L. (2006). Using self-report assessment methods to explore facets of mindfulness. *Assessment, 13*, 27–45.

Banks, K., Newman, E., & Saleem, J. (2015). An overview of the research on mindfulness-based interventions for treating symptoms of posttraumatic stress disorder: A systematic review. *Journal of Clinical Psychology, 71*(10), 935–963.

Barlow, D. H., Farchione, T. J., Bullis, J. R., Gallagher, M. W., Murray-Latin, H., Sauer-Zavala, S., et al. (2017). The unified protocol for transdiagnostic treatment of emotional disorders compared with diagnosis-specific protocols for anxiety disorders: A randomized clinical trial. *JAMA Psychiatry, 74*(9), 875–884.

Bennett, P., Williams, Y., Page, N., Hood, K., Woollard, M., & Vetter, N. (2005). Associations between organizational and incident factors and emotional distress in emergency ambulance personnel. *British Journal of Clinical Psychology, 44*(2), 215–226.

Berger, W., Coutinho, E. S., Figueira, I., Marques-Portella, C., Luz, M. P., Neylan, T. C., et al. (2012). Rescuers at risk: A systematic review and meta-regression analysis of the worldwide current prevalence and correlates of PTSD in rescue workers. *Social Psychiatry and Psychiatric Epidemiology, 47*(6), 1001–1011. https://doi.org/10.1007/s00127-011-0408-2

Boffa, J. W., Stanley, I. H., Hom, M. A., Norr, A. M., Joiner, T. E., & Schmidt, N. B. (2017). PTSD symptoms and suicidal thoughts and behaviors among firefighters. *Journal of Psychiatric Research, 84*, 277–283. https://doi.org/10.1016/j.jpsychires.2016.10.014

Boffa, J. W., Stanley, I. H., Smith, L. J., Mathes, B. M., Tran, J. K., Buser, S. J., et al. (2018). Posttraumatic stress disorder symptoms and suicide risk in male firefighters: The mediating role of anxiety sensitivity. *Journal of Nervous and Mental Disease, 206*(3), 179–186. https://doi.org/10.1097/NMD.0000000000000779

Boland, L. L., Kinzy, T. G., Myers, R. N., Fernstrom, K. M., Kamrud, J. W., Mink, P. J., & Stevens, A. C. (2018). Burnout and exposure to critical incidents in a cohort of emergency medical services workers from Minnesota. *Western Journal of Emergency Medicine, 19*(6), 987–995. https://doi.org/10.5811/westjem.8.39034

Bos, J., Mol, E., Visser, B., & Frings-Dresen, M. (2004). Risk of health complaints and disabilities among Dutch firefighters. *International Archives of Occupational and Environmental Health, 77*(6), 373–382.

Boscarino, J. A. (2008). A prospective study of PTSD and early-age heart disease mortality among Vietnam veterans: Implications for surveillance and prevention. *Psychosomatic Medicine, 70*(6), 668.

Bowers, C. A., Beidel, D. C., & Marks, M. R. (2019). *Mental health intervention and treatment of first responders and emergency workers*. IGI Global.

Bowler, R. M., Harris, M., Li, J., Gocheva, V., Stellman, S. D., Wilson, K., et al. (2012). Longitudinal mental health impact among police responders to the 9/11 terrorist attack. *American Journal of Industrial Medicine, 55*(4), 297–312.

Bowler, R. M., Kornblith, E. S., Li, J., Adams, S. W., Gocheva, V. V., Schwarzer, R., & Cone, J. E. (2016). Police officers who responded to 9/11: Comorbidity of PTSD, depression, and anxiety 10–11 years later. *American Journal of Industrial Medicine, 59*(6), 425–436.

Brewin, C. R., Andrews, B., & Valentine, J. D. (2000). Meta-analysis of risk factors for posttraumatic stress disorder in trauma-exposed adults. *Journal of Consulting and Clinical Psychology, 68*(5), 748.

Brunault, P., Lebigre, K., Idbrik, F., Mauge, D., Adam, P., El Ayoubi, H., et al. (2019). Posttraumatic stress disorder is a risk factor for multiple addictions in police officers hospitalized for alcohol. *European Addiction Research, 25*(4), 198–206. https://doi.org/10.1159/000499936

Burg, M. M., Brandt, C., Buta, E., Schwartz, J., Bathulapalli, H., Dziura, J., et al. (2017). Risk for incident hypertension associated with PTSD in military veterans, and the effect of PTSD treatment. *Psychosomatic Medicine, 79*(2), 181.

Carey, M. G., Al-Zaiti, S. S., Dean, G. E., Sessanna, L., & Finnell, D. S. (2011). Sleep problems, depression, substance use, social bonding, and quality of life in professional firefighters. *Journal of Occupational and Environmental Medicine, 53*(8), 928–933. https://doi.org/10.1097/JOM.0b013e318225898f

Carleton, R. N., Afifi, T., Taillieu, T., Turner, S., El-Gabalawy, R., Sareen, J., & Asmundson, G. (2018a). Anxiety-related psychopathology and chronic pain comorbidity among public safety personnel. *Journal of Anxiety Disorders, 55*, 48–55.

Carleton, R. N., Afifi, T. O., Turner, S., Taillieu, T., Duranceau, S., LeBouthillier, D. M., et al. (2018b). Mental disorder symptoms among public safety personnel in Canada. *Canadian Journal of Psychiatry. Revue Canadienne de Psychiatrie, 63*(1), 54–64. https://doi.org/10.1177/0706743717723825

Carleton, R. N., Afifi, T. O., Taillieu, T., Turner, S., Krakauer, R., Anderson, G. S., et al. (2019). Exposures to potentially traumatic events among public safety personnel in Canada. *Canadian Journal of Behavioural Science / Revue canadienne des sciences du comportement, 51*(1), 37–52. https://doi.org/10.1037/cbs0000115

Casas, J. B., & Benuto, L. T. (2022). Work-related traumatic stress spillover in first responder families: A systematic review of the literature. *Psychological Trauma: Theory, Research, Practice and Policy, 14*(2), 209–217. https://doi.org/10.1037/tra0001086

Chopko, B. A., Palmieri, P. A., & Adams, R. E. (2021). Trauma-related sleep problems and associated health outcomes in police officers: A path analysis. *Journal of Interpersonal Violence, 36*(5–6), NP2725-NP2748. https://doi.org/10.1177/0886260518767912

Collins, P., & Gibbs, A. (2003). Stress in police officers: A study of the origins, prevalence and severity of stress-related symptoms within a county police force. *Occupational Medicine, 53*(4), 256–264.

Covey, T. J., Shucard, J. L., Violanti, J. M., Lee, J., & Shucard, D. W. (2013). The effects of exposure to traumatic stressors on inhibitory control in police officers: A dense electrode array study using a Go/NoGo continuous performance task. *International Journal of Psychophysiology, 87*(3), 363–375. https://doi.org/10.1016/j.ijpsycho.2013.03.009

Darensburg, T., Andrew, M. E., Hartley, T. A., Burchfiel, C. M., Fekedulegn, D., & Violanti, J. M. (2006). Gender and age differences in posttraumatic stress disorder and depression among Buffalo police officers. *Traumatology, 12*(3), 220–228.

Essex, B., & Scott, L. B. (2008). Chronic stress and associated coping strategies among volunteer EMS personnel. *Prehospital Emergency Care, 12*(1), 69–75.

Evarts, B., & Stein, G. P. (2020). *US fire department profile 2018*. National Fire Protection Association Quincy.

Feldman, T. R., Carlson, C. L., Rice, L. K., Kruse, M. I., Beevers, C. G., Telch, M. J., & Josephs, R. A. (2021). Factors predicting the development of psychopathology among first responders: A prospective, longitudinal study. *Psychological Trauma: Theory, Research, Practice and Policy, 13*(1), 75–83. https://doi.org/10.1037/tra0000957

Fraess-Phillips, A., Wagner, S., & Harris, R. L. (2017). Firefighters and traumatic stress: A review. *International Journal of Emergency Services, 6*(1), 67–80. https://doi.org/10.1108/ijes-10-2016-0020

Gratz, K. L., & Roemer, L. (2004). Multidimensional assessment of emotion regulation and dysregulation: Development, factor structure, and initial validation of the difficulties in emotion regulation scale. *Journal of Psychopathology and Behavioral Assessment, 26*(1), 41–54.

Grupe, D. W., McGehee, C., Smith, C., Francis, A. D., Mumford, J. A., & Davidson, R. J. (2021). Mindfulness training reduces PTSD symptoms and improves stress-related health outcomes in police officers. *Journal of Police & Criminal Psychology, 36*(1), 72–85. https://doi.org/10.1007/s11896-019-09351-4

Haddock, C. K., Day, R. S., Poston, W. S., Jahnke, S. A., & Jitnarin, N. (2015). Alcohol use and caloric intake from alcohol in a national cohort of U.S. career firefighters. *Journal of Studies on Alcohol and Drugs, 76*(3), 360–366.

Haddock, C. K., Poston, W. S. C., Jahnke, S. A., & Jitnarin, N. (2017). Alcohol use and problem drinking among women firefighters. *Women's Health Issues, 27*(6), 632–638. https://doi.org/10.1016/j.whi.2017.07.003

Haugen, P. T., Evces, M., & Weiss, D. S. (2012). Treating posttraumatic stress disorder in first responders: A systematic review. *Clinical Psychology Review, 32*(5), 370–380.

Healy, N. A., & Vujanovic, A. A. (2021). PTSD symptoms and suicide risk among firefighters: The moderating role of sleep disturbance. *Psychological Trauma: Theory, Research, Practice, and Policy, 13*, 749.

Heinrichs, M., Wagner, D., Schoch, W., Soravia, L. M., Hellhammer, D. H., & Ehlert, U. (2005). Predicting posttraumatic stress symptoms from pretraumatic risk factors: A 2-year prospective follow-up study in firefighters. *American Journal of Psychiatry, 162*(12), 2276–2286.

Hom, M. A., Stanley, I. H., Ringer, F. B., & Joiner, T. E. (2016). Mental health service use among firefighters with suicidal thoughts and behaviors. *Psychiatric Services, 67*(6), 688–691.

Horn, S. R., Charney, D. S., & Feder, A. (2016). Understanding resilience: New approaches for preventing and treating PTSD. *Experimental Neurology, 284*(Pt B), 119–132. https://doi.org/10.1016/j.expneurol.2016.07.002

Isaac, G. M., & Buchanan, M. J. (2021). Extinguishing stigma among firefighters: An examination of stress, social support, and help-seeking attitudes. *Psychology (Savannah, Ga.), 12*(03), 349–373. https://doi.org/10.4236/psych.2021.123023

Jaegers, L. A., Matthieu, M. M., Vaughn, M. G., Werth, P., Katz, I. M., & Ahmad, S. O. (2019). Posttraumatic stress disorder and job burnout among jail officers. *Journal of Occupational and Environmental Medicine, 61*(6), 505–510. https://doi.org/10.1097/JOM.0000000000001600

James, L., & Todak, N. (2018). Prison employment and post-traumatic stress disorder: Risk and protective factors. *American Journal of Industrial Medicine.* https://doi.org/10.1002/ajim.22869

Johnson, C. C., Vega, L., Kohalmi, A. L., Roth, J. C., Howell, B. R., & Van Hasselt, V. B. (2020). Enhancing mental health treatment for the firefighter population: Understanding fire culture, treatment barriers, practice implications, and research directions. *Professional Psychology: Research and Practice, 51*(3), 304–311. https://doi.org/10.1037/pro0000266

Katsavouni, F., & Bebetsos, E. (2016). The relationship between burnout, PTSD symptoms and injuries among ambulance personnel. *Sport Science, 9*(1), 7–13.

Kerswell, N. L., Strodl, E., Johnson, L., & Konstantinou, E. (2019). Mental health outcomes following a large-scale potentially traumatic event involving police officers and civilian staff of the Queensland police service. *Journal of Police and Criminal Psychology, 35*(1), 64–74. https://doi.org/10.1007/s11896-018-9310-0

Khantzian, E. J. (1997). The self-medication hypothesis of substance use disorders: A reconsideration and recent applications. *Harvard Review of Psychiatry, 4*(5), 231–244. https://doi.org/10.3109/10673229709030550

Kilpatrick, D. G., Resnick, H. S., Milanak, M. E., Miller, M. W., Keyes, K. M., & Friedman, M. J. (2013). National estimates of exposure to traumatic events and PTSD prevalence using DSM-IV and DSM-5 criteria. *Journal of Traumatic Stress, 26*(5), 537–547. https://doi.org/10.1002/jts.21848

Kim, J. M., Suh, B. S., Jung, K. Y., Kim, D. I., Kim, W. S., Cho, H. S., et al. (2007). The study for musculoskeletal symptoms and job stress in firemen. *Journal of Korean Society of Occupational and Environmental Hygiene, 17*(2), 111–119.

Kim, J. E., Dager, S. R., Jeong, H. S., Ma, J., Park, S., Kim, J., et al. (2018). Firefighters, posttraumatic stress disorder, and barriers to treatment: Results from a nationwide total population survey. *PLoS One, 13*(1), e0190630. https://doi.org/10.1371/journal.pone.0190630

Kim, M.-J., Jeong, Y., Choi, Y.-S., Seo, A.-R., Ha, Y., Seo, M., & Park, K.-S. (2019). The association of the exposure to work-related traumatic events and work limitations among firefighters: A cross-sectional study. *International Journal of Environmental Research and Public Health, 16*(5), 756.

Kleim, B., & Westphal, M. (2011). Mental health in first responders: A review and recommendation for prevention and intervention strategies. *Traumatology, 17*(4), 17–24.

Klimley, K. E., Van Hasselt, V. B., & Stripling, A. M. (2018). Posttraumatic stress disorder in police, firefighters, and emergency dispatchers. *Aggression and Violent Behavior, 43*, 33–44. https://doi.org/10.1016/j.avb.2018.08.005

Koenen, K. C., Ratanatharathorn, A., Ng, L., McLaughlin, K. A., Bromet, E. J., Stein, D. J., et al. (2017). Posttraumatic stress disorder in the World Mental Health Surveys. *Psychological Medicine, 47*(13), 2260–2274. https://doi.org/10.1017/S0033291717000708

Kubzansky, L. D., Koenen, K. C., Spiro, A., Vokonas, P. S., & Sparrow, D. (2007). Prospective study of posttraumatic stress disorder symptoms and coronary heart disease in the Normative Aging Study. *Archives of General Psychiatry, 64*(1), 109–116.

Langtry, J., Owczarek, M., McAteer, D., Taggart, L., Gleeson, C., Walshe, C., & Shevlin, M. (2021). Predictors of PTSD and CPTSD in UK firefighters. *European Journal of Psychotraumatology, 12*(1), 1849524. https://doi.org/10.1080/20008198.2020.1849524

Lebeaut, A., Zegel, M., Leonard, S. J., Bartlett, B. A., & Vujanovic, A. A. (2021). Examining transdiagnostic factors among firefighters in relation to trauma exposure, probable PTSD, and probable alcohol use disorder. *Journal of Dual Diagnosis, 17*(1), 52–63. https://doi.org/10.1080/15504263.2020.1854411

Lebeaut, A., Zegel, M., Healy, N. A., Rogers, A. H., Buser, S. J., & Vujanovic, A. A. (2022). PTSD symptom severity, pain intensity, and pain-related disability among trauma-exposed firefighters: The moderating role of mindfulness. *Mindfulness, 13*(3), 786–798.

Lee, J.-S., Ahn, Y.-S., Jeong, K.-S., Chae, J.-H., & Choi, K.-S. (2014). Resilience buffers the impact of traumatic events on the development of PTSD symptoms in firefighters. *Journal of Affective Disorders, 162*, 128–133.

Lewis-Schroeder, N. F., Kieran, K., Murphy, B. L., Wolff, J. D., Robinson, M. A., & Kaufman, M. L. (2018). Conceptualization, assessment, and treatment of traumatic stress in first responders: A review of critical issues. *Harvard Review of Psychiatry, 26*(4), 216.

Leyro, T. M., Zvolensky, M. J., & Bernstein, A. (2010). Distress tolerance and psychopathological symptoms and disorders: A review of the empirical literature among adults. *Psychological Bulletin, 136*(4), 576–600. https://doi.org/10.1037/a0019712

Luftman, K., Aydelotte, J., Rix, K., Ali, S., Houck, K., Coopwood, T. B., et al. (2017). PTSD in those who care for the injured. *Injury, 48*(2), 293–296. https://doi.org/10.1016/j.injury.2016.11.001

Maguen, S., Metzler, T. J., McCaslin, S. E., Inslicht, S. S., Henn-Haase, C., Neylan, T. C., & Marmar, C. R. (2009). Routine work environment stress and PTSD symptoms in police officers. *Journal of Nervous and Mental Disease, 197*(10), 754–760. https://doi.org/10.1097/NMD.0b013e3181b975f8

Marmar, C. R., McCaslin, S. E., Metzler, T. J., Best, S., Weiss, D. S., Fagan, J., et al. (2006). Predictors of posttraumatic stress in police and other first responders. *Annals of the New York Academy of Sciences, 1071*(1), 1–18.

Milligan-Saville, J. S., Paterson, H. M., Harkness, E. L., Marsh, A. M., Dobson, M., Kemp, R. I., et al. (2017). The amplification of common somatic symptoms by posttraumatic stress disorder in firefighters. *Journal of Traumatic Stress, 30*(2), 142–148.

Motreff, Y., Baubet, T., Pirard, P., Rabet, G., Petitclerc, M., Stene, L. E., et al. (2020). Factors associated with PTSD and partial PTSD among first responders following the Paris terror attacks in November 2015. *Journal of Psychiatric Research, 121*, 143–150. https://doi.org/10.1016/j.jpsychires.2019.11.018

Munn, Z., Moola, S., Riitano, D., & Lisy, K. (2014). The development of a critical appraisal tool for use in systematic reviews addressing questions of prevalence. *International Journal of Health Policy and Management, 3*(3), 123.

Newman, C., Eason, M., & Kinghorn, G. (2019). Incidence of vicarious trauma in correctional health and forensic mental health staff in New South Wales, Australia. *Journal of Forensic Nursing, 15*(3), 183–192. https://doi.org/10.1097/JFN.0000000000000245

Nock, M. K., Borges, G., Bromet, E. J., Cha, C. B., Kessler, R. C., & Lee, S. (2008). Suicide and suicidal behavior. *Epidemiologic Reviews, 30*, 133–154. https://doi.org/10.1093/epirev/mxn002

Nock, M. K., Prinstein, M. J., & Sterba, S. K. (2009). Revealing the form and function of self-injurious thoughts and behaviors: A real-time ecological assessment study among adolescents and young adults. *Journal of Abnormal Psychology, 118*(4), 816–827.

North, C. S., Tivis, L., McMillen, J. C., Pfefferbaum, B., Spitznagel, E. L., Cox, J., et al. (2002). Psychiatric disorders in rescue workers after the Oklahoma City bombing. *American Journal of Psychiatry, 159*(5), 857–859.

O'Neill, O. A., & Rothbard, N. P. (2017). Is love all you need? The effects of emotional culture, suppression, and work–family conflict on firefighter risk-taking and health. *Academy of Management Journal, 60*(1), 78–108.

Ozer, E. J., Best, S. R., Lipsey, T. L., & Weiss, D. S. (2003). Predictors of posttraumatic stress disorder and symptoms in adults: A meta-analysis. *Psychological Bulletin, 129*(1), 52.

Palmer, C. A., & Alfano, C. A. (2017). Sleep and emotion regulation: An organizing, integrative review. *Sleep Medicine Reviews, 31*, 6–16. https://doi.org/10.1016/j.smrv.2015.12.006

Paltell, K. C., Bing-Canar, H., Ranney, R. M., Tran, J. K., Berenz, E. C., & Vujanovic, A. A. (2019). Anxiety sensitivity moderates the effect of posttraumatic stress disorder symptoms on emotion dysregulation among trauma-exposed firefighters. *Journal of Psychopathology and Behavioral Assessment, 41*(3), 524–535. https://doi.org/10.1007/s10862-019-09731-4

Paulus, D. J., Gallagher, M. W., Bartlett, B. A., Tran, J., & Vujanovic, A. A. (2018). The unique and interactive effects of anxiety sensitivity and emotion dysregulation in relation to posttraumatic stress, depressive, and anxiety symptoms among trauma-exposed firefighters. *Comprehensive Psychiatry, 84*, 54–61. https://doi.org/10.1016/j.comppsych.2018.03.012

Pierce, H., & Lilly, M. M. (2012). Duty-related trauma exposure in 911 telecommunicators: Considering the risk for posttraumatic stress. *Journal of Traumatic Stress, 25*(2), 211–215. https://doi.org/10.1002/jts.21687

Pietrzak, R. H., Goldstein, R. B., Southwick, S. M., & Grant, B. F. (2011). Prevalence and Axis I comorbidity of full and partial posttraumatic stress disorder in the United States: Results from Wave 2 of the National Epidemiologic Survey on alcohol and related conditions. *Journal of Anxiety Disorders, 25*(3), 456–465. https://doi.org/10.1016/j.janxdis.2010.11.010

Powers, M. B., Halpern, J. M., Ferenschak, M. P., Gillihan, S. J., & Foa, E. B. (2010). A meta-analytic review of prolonged exposure for posttraumatic stress disorder. *Clinical Psychology Review, 30*(6), 635–641.

Ranney, R. M., Bing-Canar, H., Paltell, K. C., Tran, J. K., Berenz, E. C., & Vujanovic, A. A. (2020). Cardiovascular risk as a moderator of associations among anxiety sensitivity, distress tolerance, PTSD and depression symptoms among trauma-exposed firefighters. *Journal of Psychosomatic Research, 139*, 110269.

Reiss, S., Peterson, R. A., Gursky, D. M., & McNally, R. J. (1986). Anxiety sensitivity, anxiety frequency and the prediction of fearfulness. *Behaviour Research and Therapy, 24*(1), 1–8.

Resick, P. A., Monson, C. M., & Chard, K. M. (2016). *Cognitive processing therapy for PTSD: A comprehensive manual*. Guilford Publications.

Ricciardelli, R., Czarnuch, S., Afifi, T. O., Taillieu, T., & Carleton, R. N. (2020). Public Safety Personnel's interpretations of potentially traumatic events. *Occupational Medicine (Oxford, England), 70*(3), 155–161. https://doi.org/10.1093/occmed/kqaa007

Rogers, A. H., Shepherd, J. M., Orr, M. F., Bakhshaie, J., McHugh, R. K., & Zvolensky, M. J. (2019). Exploring anxiety sensitivity in the relationship between pain intensity and opioid misuse among opioid-using adults with chronic pain. *Journal of Psychiatric Research, 111*, 154–159. https://doi.org/10.1016/j.jpsychires.2019.02.004

Ruglass, L. M., Lopez-Castro, T., Papini, S., Killeen, T., Back, S. E., & Hien, D. A. (2017). Concurrent treatment with prolonged exposure for co-occurring full or subthreshold posttraumatic stress disorder and substance use disorders: A randomized clinical trial. *Psychotherapy and Psychosomatics, 86*(3), 150–161.

Rybojad, B., Aftyka, A., Baran, M., & Rzonca, P. (2016). Risk factors for posttraumatic stress disorder in polish paramedics: A pilot study. *Journal of Emergency Medicine, 50*(2), 270–276. https://doi.org/10.1016/j.jemermed.2015.06.030

Salleh, M. N. B. M., Ismail, H. B., & Yusoff, H. B. M. (2020). Prevalence and predictors for PTSD among firefighters. A systematic review. *International Journal of Public Health Research, 10*, 1183–1194.

Skeffington, P. M., Rees, C. S., Mazzucchelli, T. G., & Kane, R. T. (2016). The primary prevention of PTSD in firefighters: Preliminary results of an RCT with 12-month follow-up. *PLoS One, 11*(7), e0155873. https://doi.org/10.1371/journal.pone.0155873

Skogstad, M., Skorstad, M., Lie, A., Conradi, H. S., Heir, T., & Weisaeth, L. (2013). Work-related post-traumatic stress disorder. *Occupational Medicine (Oxford, England), 63*(3), 175–182. https://doi.org/10.1093/occmed/kqt003

Smith, D. L., Haller, J. M., Korre, M., Sampani, K., Porto, L. G. G., Fehling, P. C., et al. (2019). The relation of emergency duties to cardiac death among US firefighters. *The American Journal of Cardiology, 123*(5), 736–741.

Smith, L. J., Zegel, M., Bartlett, B. A., Lebeaut, A., & Vujanovic, A. A. (2020). Posttraumatic stress and alcohol use among first responders. In *Mental health intervention and treatment of first responders and emergency workers* (pp. 32–48). Medical Information Science Reference/ IGI Global.

Soomro, S., & Yanos, P. T. (2018). Predictors of mental health stigma among police officers: The role of trauma and PTSD. *Journal of Police and Criminal Psychology, 34*(2), 175–183. https://doi.org/10.1007/s11896-018-9285-x

Spinhoven, P., Penninx, B. W., van Hemert, A. M., de Rooij, M., & Elzinga, B. M. (2014). Comorbidity of PTSD in anxiety and depressive disorders: Prevalence and shared risk factors. *Child Abuse and Neglect, 38*(8), 1320–1330. https://doi.org/10.1016/j.chiabu.2014.01.017

Stanley, I. H., Hom, M. A., Hagan, C. R., & Joiner, T. E. (2015). Career prevalence and correlates of suicidal thoughts and behaviors among firefighters. *Journal of Affective Disorders, 187*, 163–171. https://doi.org/10.1016/j.jad.2015.08.007

Stanley, I. H., Hom, M. A., & Joiner, T. E. (2016). A systematic review of suicidal thoughts and behaviors among police officers, firefighters, EMTs, and paramedics. *Clinical Psychology Review, 44*, 25–44. https://doi.org/10.1016/j.cpr.2015.12.002

Stanley, I. H., Boffa, J. W., Hom, M. A., Kimbrel, N. A., & Joiner, T. E. (2017). Differences in psychiatric symptoms and barriers to mental health care between volunteer and career firefighters. *Psychiatry Research, 247*, 236–242. https://doi.org/10.1016/j.psychres.2016.11.037

Thompson, B. M., Kirk, A., & Brown, D. (2006). Sources of stress in policewomen: A three-factor model. *International Journal of Stress Management, 13*(3), 309.

Trombka, M., Demarzo, M., Campos, D., Antonio, S. B., Cicuto, K., Walcher, A. L., et al. (2021). Mindfulness training improves quality of life and reduces depression and anxiety symptoms among police officers: Results from the POLICE study—A multicenter randomized controlled trial. *Frontiers in Psychiatry, 12*, 112.

van der Meer, C. A., Bakker, A., Smit, A. S., van Buschbach, S., den Dekker, M., Westerveld, G. J., et al. (2017). Gender and age differences in trauma and PTSD among Dutch treatment-seeking police officers. *Journal of Nervous and Mental Disease, 205*(2), 87–92. https://doi.org/10.1097/NMD.0000000000000562

Verbeek, I. C., & van der Velden, P. G. (2016). Police studies on PTSD in Spanish-speaking nations: A systematic review. *Traumatology, 22*(4), 233–241. https://doi.org/10.1037/trm0000084

Violanti, J. M., Fekedulegn, D., Hartley, T. A., Andrew, M. E., Charles, L. E., Mnatsakanova, A., & Burchfiel, C. M. (2006). Police trauma and cardiovascular disease: Association between PTSD symptoms and metabolic syndrome. *International Journal of Emergency Mental Health, 8*, 227.

Violanti, J. M., Robinson, C. F., & Shen, R. (2013). Law enforcement suicide: A national analysis. *International Journal of Emergency Mental Health and Human Resilience, 15*(4), 289–298.

Vujanovic, A. A., & Tran, J. K. (2021). Providing psychological services to firefighters. *Journal of Health Service Psychology, 47*, 137–148. https://doi.org/10.1007/s42843-021-00041-6

Vujanovic, A. A., & Zegel, M. (2020). Distress tolerance and posttraumatic stress. In M. T. Tull & N. A. Kimbrel (Eds.), *Emotion in posttraumatic stress disorder: Etiology, assessment, neurobiology, and treatment* (pp. 343–376). Guilford Press.

Vujanovic, A. A., Farris, S., Bartlett, B., Lyons, R., Haller, M., Colvonen, P., & Norman, S. (2018). Anxiety sensitivity in the association between posttraumatic stress and substance use disorders: A systematic review. *Clinical Psychology Review, 62*, 37–55.

Wagner, S. L., White, N., Regehr, C., White, M., Alden, L. E., Buys, N., et al. (2020). Ambulance personnel: Systematic review of mental health symptoms. *Traumatology, 26*(4), 370–387. https://doi.org/10.1037/trm0000251

Wagner, S. L., White, N., Buys, N., Carey, M. G., Corneil, W., Fyfe, T., et al. (2021). Systematic review of mental health symptoms in firefighters exposed to routine duty-related critical incidents. *Traumatology, 27*(3), 285–302. https://doi.org/10.1037/trm0000275

Watkins, L. E., Sprang, K. R., & Rothbaum, B. O. (2018). Treating PTSD: A review of evidence-based psychotherapy interventions. *Frontiers in Behavioral Neuroscience, 12*, 258. https://doi.org/10.3389/fnbeh.2018.00258

Watson, P., Gist, R., Taylor, V., Nash, W. P., Westphal, R. J., & Litz, B. (2012). *Stress First Aid (SFA) student manual for firefighters and emergency medical services personnel.*

Whealin, J. M., Ciro, D., Dasaro, C. R., Udasin, I. G., Crane, M., Moline, J. M., et al. (2022). Race/ethnic differences in prevalence and correlates of posttraumatic stress disorder in World Trade Center responders: Results from a population-based, health monitoring cohort. *Psychological Trauma: Theory, Research, Practice and Policy, 14*(2), 199–208. https://doi.org/10.1037/tra0001081

Yuan, C., Wang, Z., Inslicht, S. S., McCaslin, S. E., Metzler, T. J., Henn-Haase, C., et al. (2011). Protective factors for posttraumatic stress disorder symptoms in a prospective study of police officers. *Psychiatry Research, 188*(1), 45–50. https://doi.org/10.1016/j.psychres.2010.10.034

Zegel, M., Tran, J. K., & Vujanovic, A. A. (2019). Posttraumatic stress, alcohol use, and alcohol use motives among firefighters: The role of distress tolerance. *Psychiatry Research, 282*, 112633.

Zegel, M., Lebeaut, A., Healy, N., Tran, J. K., & Vujanovic, A. A. (2022). Mental health correlates of probable posttraumatic stress disorder, probable alcohol use disorder, and their co-occurrence among firefighters. *Behavior Modification, 46*(2), 395–421.

Part V
Advocacy

First Responder Families: Identifying Stressors and Building Support

Lisa Berg Garmezy

A gloomy superstition among first responders holds that divorce rates "can be as high as seventy percent," as a 2021 *FBI Bulletin* warned (Haddock et al., 2016; Wetherington, 2021). The available data point to a different conclusion. The divorce rate was 16.4% in the general population in the 2000 census, versus 14.1% for firefighters, 15.0% for police, and 23.9% for dispatchers. Haddock et al. (2016), in a sample of 1456 firefighters, found the prevalence of divorce for men in the sample was 11.8%, slightly higher than the rate of 9.4% in the general population. Among the 49 women, the divorce rate was much higher than in the general population, with a rate of 32.1% compared to 10.1%. Responder populations, because of steady incomes, pre-employment screening, and pre-employment psychological examinations (for police officers and a minority of other responders) may show a "healthy worker" effect that elevates the likelihood of marital stability. Undeniably, however, their choice of career alters their relationships and their families.

Clinical writings and personal experience are integrated here with the scant available research literature, which is limited by a focus on white male responders with female spouses who are not first responders themselves. Women make up 4% of career firefighters, 11% of volunteer firefighters, less than 13% of police officers and detectives, and 21% of paramedics and EMTs (Fahy et al., 2022; Rineer et al., 2022). Female responders, responders belonging to communities of color, and LGBTQ+ responders and their spouses were often absent from past research and are still under-represented in analyses. Researchers typically obtained responders' spouses' input only when responders informed them of the projects, introducing additional bias to relevant literature. Findings may have been subject to confirmation bias. Civilian police and fire paraprofessionals were studied infrequently. Although many of these employees encounter the job-related stressors and potentially traumatic events (PTEs) discussed here, they typically hold lower

L. B. Garmezy (✉)
Independent Practice, Houston, TX, USA

M. L. Bourke et al. (eds.), *First Responder Mental Health*,
https://doi.org/10.1007/978-3-031-38149-2_22

organizational status, are less prepared for PTEs, and feel less supported by the public, other responders, and their own departments.

The term "responder" is used in this chapter to refer to police, fire, and emergency medical personnel and a minority of civilian employees in these agencies who work under risky or emergency circumstances, including dispatchers, crime scene analysts, and others. Although responders are often discussed collectively, some caution must be used in generalizing from one profession to another. Space does not permit discussion of important differences, for example, that firefighters tend to be a younger, less educated population than police officers. The narrower term "police" is preferred here to "law enforcement officer" (LEO) but the latter term is reproduced where it appeared in the literature. For brevity and clarity, the terms "spouse" and "marriage" are used exclusively, although the material also pertains to unmarried partners in other relationships. Significant acute stressors are referred to by the purposefully broad term "potentially traumatic experiences," capturing the devastating scenes that endanger responders' lives and expose them to injury, death, and tragedy.

This chapter explains the consequences for the responder family of common job stressors, the "wear and tear" of day-in, day-out exposure to PTEs, and the maladaptive coping strategies traditionally sanctioned by responder culture. The discussion of distinctive stressors and the dysfunctional patterns that evolve around them is followed by suggestions that may mitigate their impact. Responder marriages can be rocked by PTEs that bring physical, spiritual, emotional, and behavioral changes, including anger, apathy, burnout, detachment, exhaustion, questioning of faith, questioning of self-worth, self-blame, social withdrawal, secondary trauma, and other symptoms and problems (Landers et al., 2020; Van Hasselt et al., 2022; Violanti, 2021). Admittedly, not all responder careers are debilitating or traumatic. PTEs do not necessarily impact family life more severely than living with danger or stressors such as shift work. Generally, chronic stress can impact the family as severely as acute life events (Compas et al., 2019).

The reader should note that the dyadic dysfunction described here is common in responders presenting for therapy, not responders in general. The responder culture, discussed as problematic below, must also be applauded for valuing and promoting honesty, loyalty, duty, leadership, teamwork, and civic responsibility.

Understanding a Culture

In healthy responder marriages, support and respect are mutual. Without losing their identities, spouses respect the responder's work, and the spouse's labor, paid or unpaid, is valued in return. Career-related stressors are accepted as the price of financial security and personal fulfillment and, in many cases, the cost of service to others. In fact, cognitive dissonance theory predicts that the more the career negatively impacts family members, the more they will value it, in order to rationalize the responder's continued involvement. This is especially true for the half of firefighters who are unpaid volunteers, who accept the risks and unpredictable call-ups without the justification of a paycheck.

Spouses are expected to toughen and "marry the profession" by bonding with other responders and their spouses (Campbell et al., 2022; Landers et al., 2020). They often develop civic-mindedness and pride in the employing agency (Porter & Henriksen, 2016). They need to trust that its protocols and equipment will ensure the responder's safety. They may acquire a sense of responsibility for the responder's physical and psychological safety. Failure to embrace responder culture can be isolating since new responders frequently break ties with former associates in light of scheduling conflicts, disapproval of "outsider" behavior, and the belief that others cannot understand what they face.

Civilian family members are usually shielded from the work's graphic aspects. When the home is treated as a sanctuary, responders protect themselves (e.g., from retraumatization), as well as their spouses. Typically, both parties protect each other by concealing fears about the responder's safety (Campbell et al., 2022; Sharp et al., 2022). Responder wives fear physical injuries more than psychological ones; for responders, the reverse appears to be true (Campbell et al., 2022).

Colleagues become a second family, buffering the impact of stress and trauma (Bohl-Penrod & Clark, 2017). The close ties and camaraderie may elicit jealousy or disapproval from spouses. Traditionally, these male-dominated professions have been influenced by a "fraternity culture" that condones coping with stress in unhealthy ways, notably drinking and casual sexual encounters (S. J. Buser, personal communication, Jan. 25, 2019). This may be more pronounced in environments where men are present in higher numbers.

To the extent responders risk their lives for the common good, they are legitimate heroes. Still, strict allegiance to the ideal of the responder as a glorified hero, as seen in some families, complicates personal and family adjustment, since three detrimental beliefs can follow. First, if a responder is a more special or important person than the spouse, it follows that his or her needs take precedence over those of the spouse, who assume a subordinate position. Chronic neglect of spouses' needs is likely to play a role in their high rates of pathology, reviewed in a later section. Second, the relevant cultural narrative dangerously dictates that heroes must bear the weight of burdens silently and alone, pretending to be invulnerable (Allison et al., 2019). Third, the hero myth can create unattainable expectations of the responder, for example, that the knight in shining armor will unfailingly face adversity wisely and bravely, protecting the family against all evils. This belief can amplify disappointments, leaving the responder devastated by perceived failure.

A subset of unhappy responder relationships seems to exist in part because both parties embrace hero mythology. In these partnerships, a reciprocal attraction grows when a responder who is a would-be rescuer, usually male, supports and solves problems for a needy civilian encountered on duty (Garmezy, 2020; Violanti & Samuels, 2007). The dependence of the rescued person is gratifying to the would-be hero and may bolster shaky self-confidence or promise relationship stability (Lamia & Krieger, 2009). Needy citizens of both genders embrace responders as symbols of safety and stability, as advised in the bumper sticker, "Feel safe -- sleep with a cop." The presumption of unequal competence in these relationships can be mutually satisfactory at first and will remain so for some couples. The unilateral growth of either partner, however, disrupts the relationship. If partners do not move together beyond the established pattern, the rescued partner may be frustrated either by unsuccessful attempts to gain autonomy or by unwanted pressure to do so. The responder in the hero's role may be distressed by a dysfunctional spouse's pathology, may try to preserve the relationship by discouraging the spouse's growth, or, in the wake of greater spousal independence, may seek a new partner who provides needed validation.

Much like the hero myth, the traditionally masculine role encompasses strength, courage, and concealing vulnerability (Di Bianca & Mahalik, 2022). Responder cultures have traditionally expected conformity to the masculine role, although this pressure may be waning as departments diversify. Hegemonic masculinity has been associated with hyper-independence, emotional suppression, a need to deny pain, avoidance of help-seeking, a greater risk of perpetrating violence, and the acceptance of risky behavior such as excessive drinking (Di Bianca & Mahalik, 2022; Pappas, 2019). Embracing traditional male role norms may come at a price. Jakubowski and Sitko-Dominik (2021) found that firefighters experiencing probable posttraumatic stress disorder (PTSD) endorsed these norms (e.g., toughness) more than their peers.

Work Stressors and the Family

In addition to cultural considerations, practical job necessities stress responder families. Typically, firefighters work multiday rotating shifts, such as 24 hours on duty, followed by 48 hours off duty. At the extreme, 43.4% of 1841 wildland firefighter spouses said they felt they functioned without their spouses for seven months or more per year. Almost half, 49.3%, said they had considered separation because of the demands of the career (Grassroots Wildland Firefighters, 2021). Absences, particularly lengthy absences, may necessitate a period of adjustment when responders return home. Spouses who have developed new competencies -- for example, in budgeting -- may be reluctant to surrender their authority. Resentment and exhaustion on both sides can mar reunions.

Shiftwork, rotating shifts, unorthodox schedules, and missed holidays and special occasions can wreak havoc on personal lives. Responders may be unavailable during family members' illnesses and deaths and must tend to others when disaster strikes. Nightshift workers and employees with rotating shifts or erratic callouts face higher expenses and more limited options for childcare. Further, mistrust of others may complicate the process of choosing childcare providers (Agocs et al., 2015). Responder wives give up career plans because arranging childcare proves too difficult, or their careers cannot "compete" with the responders' (Campbell et al., 2022; Regehr et al., 2005). Schedules put satisfying sexual relationships at risk: Spouses eventually lose patience with being awakened in the middle of the night.

Sexual desire may increase with elation at surviving a dangerous encounter and diminish after disturbing encounters such as working sex crime cases.

Time together is reduced because responders, particularly in single-earner families, often work overtime or second jobs to supplement income. Couples may not agree that the extra income justifies the absences. A lifestyle dependent on supplemental income means financial hardship if injury or other events interrupt it. Excessive spending may be rationalized as compensation for the responder's long hours, generating more bills, more absences, and more family tension. Among firefighter fathers, satisfaction with children's behavior decreased with additional hours worked (Shreffler et al., 2011).

One bright spot is that responder parents sometimes can be more available to school-aged children than employees with more traditional schedules, with fathers taking a more hands-on role (Shows & Gerstel, 2009). Couples with shifts that do not overlap can facilitate more paternal involvement (Brayfield, 1995, as cited in Shreffler et al., 2011). Unfortunately, dual-responder couples on separate shifts share few waking hours.

Responders and family members alike may feel stressed by depleted public trust and collective anger, made plain by citizens brandishing cell phone cameras. When community and responder cultures clash, as has happened after the fatal shootings of unarmed Black men and the banning of LGBTQ+ responders from Pride parades, divided loyalties may cause stress. Spouses and children can be battered by identity conflicts, hostility, and bullying related to the responder's profession (Sharp et al., 2022).

Responders who are female, people of color, or who belong to the LGBTQ+ community or other marginalized communities often face the additional challenges of exclusion, harassment, and discrimination (Holmes, 2021). Holmes (2021) interviewed 10 LEOs and 2 non-LEO partners in six lesbian couples. They described unequal treatment felt by the families; for example, a supervisor acknowledged heterosexual officers' wives at a promotional ceremony but announced a lesbian wife as a "friend."

Although research has not established that extramarital affairs are more frequent in responders than in the general population, they seem endemic among often-absent responders, presenting a temporary antidote to blunted emotions. First responders are, after all, risk-takers. Boredom is rampant. Each shift is likely to bring encounters with admiring citizens and colleagues who share and understand experiences in a way that civilian spouses do not. Concealing harsher aspects of one's working life also may contribute to infidelity. The gap between what happens and what is reported to family members -- for example, telling a child, "Mommy fell," when an on-duty injury required stitches (Agocs et al., 2015) -- might begin a pattern of deception. Betrayal has special significance in this population since others' unreliability can be disastrous.

Most first responders face multiple dangers on a daily, or nightly, basis. Fertility, pregnancy, and breastfeeding bring special risks. Responders may conceal pregnancies to evade department policies experienced as restrictive or disruptive, or welcome light-duty status. Pregnant responders worry about exposure to violence, contagion, street drugs, and the known and unknown risks of chemical exposure. Exposed to heat and toxins, firefighters of both sexes have higher rates of infertility than the general population (Hollerbach, 2020; Women in Fire, n.d.). Poorly fitting protective gear used by women firefighters in some departments increases exposure to harmful airborne particulates, a particular concern during pregnancy. Female firefighters experienced more than double the number of miscarriages seen in a comparable sample of nurses, and more premature births (Jung et al., 2021). Causes could include stress and physical strain in addition to heat and toxins. Breastfeeding firefighters are currently advised to discard breast milk for 72 hours after fighting a structural fire (Hollerbach, 2020). And appropriate efforts are not always made to accommodate the needs of breastfeeding responders. For example, in 2019 a Tucson paramedic was awarded $3.8 million after her request for an appropriate place to express breast milk was met with discrimination and retaliation (Schmidt, 2019). A U.S. Department of Justice conference on women in policing concluded that eliminating rotating shifts, granting parental leave, and making accommodations for postnatal nursing, among other recommendations, were likely to help hire, support, and retain female officers, a needed applicant pool (National Institute of Justice, 2019).

Police officers have higher rates of cardiovascular disorders, metabolic syndrome, and other health problems than the general population (Violanti, 2021). Firefighters die more often from cancer and cardiac disorders, and experience higher rates of psychiatric illness, compared to the general population (Henderson et al., 2016; Van Hasselt et al., 2022). Shift work, particularly rotational shift work, has been linked to increased sleep disturbance, cardiovascular risk, risk of metabolic disorders, cancer risk, and other negative health outcomes, as well as decreased alertness (Violanti, 2021). The impaired emotion modulation, judgment, concentration, and impulse control associated with sleep disturbance in firefighters could jeopardize any romantic or parental relationship (Healy & Vujanovic, 2021).

Responder families live with caregiver stress, loss, and the frightening specters of injury, disability, and early death. Colleagues' tragedies resonate through these tight-knit communities. The link between cancer in firefighters and occupational exposure to toxins in smoke, protective gear, and firefighting materials is sufficiently strong that many states presume certain cancers to have been acquired in the line of duty and award benefits accordingly. Actor Steve Buscemi (2021, p. 21), when raising awareness of health problems in 9/11 responders, claimed to represent "every former firefighter who cannot laugh without coughing, and every family member who pretends not to notice." Line-of-duty deaths are feared. Tragically, death by suicide is more common than other acute line-of-duty deaths for both police and firefighters and is increasingly understood as an occupational hazard (Henderson et al., 2016; Violanti, 2021). Suicide risk may be increased by a host of factors including moral injury, desensitization to the fear of death, or the perception that the act -- like other responder behavior -- is a eusocial sacrifice made for the good of others, in this case, the family (Bryant, 2021; Henderson et al., 2016; Ringer et al., 2021).

Of course, the effect of the responder's work on the family is not unidirectional. Family responsibilities may curtail career advancement. Unsupportive family relationships increase the perceived negative impact of stress (Neff & Karney, 2009). Family stress can spill over into work performance (Casas & Benuto, 2022), potentially endangering responder functioning. This threat gives rise to self-censoring by family members, who may blame themselves for diluting the responder's concentration after adverse events. And, as a responder might say, for most, family makes it all worthwhile, bolstering the responder's resilience.

Bringing the Job Home

Behaviors that are favorable to performing the responder role can be detrimental to performing the roles of partner and parent. For Kirschman et al. (2014), the "police officer's paradox" is that skills that are desirable or essential on the job, in their assessment, hypervigilance, emotional control, and cynicism, are potentially damaging to relationships. Hypervigilance and emotional suppression appear to be common among responders, whereas cynicism may have disproportionate significance for police (since firefighters and EMTs are lied to less often). Police recruits show a small, significant increase in cynicism after entry into the profession (Gerber & Ward, 2011). The level of cynicism in active officers is not high (Gerber & Ward, 2011), although cynicism may be more prevalent among officers seeking treatment, as noted by previous clinicians (Kirschman et al., 2014).

The responder's vigilance is often so ingrained that it is never fully turned off. For example, he or she is likely to automatically note the location of emergency exits in a restaurant. The high level of physiological arousal required for sustained attention and readiness on duty lingers after a shift, particularly after a difficult shift. Feeling "keyed up," "on edge," irritable, or impatient can interfere with intimacy or prompt self-medication.

Responders habitually suppress or disregard emotions on the job to prevent losing their equilibrium and adhere to community norms (Bryant, 2021). Persistent efforts to avoid engaging with negative emotions may work too well. At home, this may result in a lack of self-awareness, a devastating inability to register or respond to a spouse or child's emotional state, a restricted range of affect, difficulty modulating emotional expression, and/or the absence of symptoms of suicidality (Violanti & Samuels, 2007). Responders may become detached and appear numb to spouses' daily problems, which can seem trivial when compared to citizens' suffering or tasks such as retrieving burned bodies. Skilled problem-solving by a responder with no apparent affect is likely to be interpreted by spouses as rejection or indifference. Less often, hyperawareness of negative emotion may be observed.

Beyond the Kirschman et al. (2014) list, the need for rapid decision-making on duty can lead to a habit of dichotomous black-and-white thinking without shades of grey, for example, people are good or bad, or things are useful or not. In relationships, this cognitive distortion discards important information and is not conducive to nuanced discussions or compromise (Dattilio, 2010). Catastrophizing minor misconduct such as a teen's single use of marijuana can result.

Perhaps more than the other attributes listed, the first responder's practice of quickly taking control is essential at work but damaging to the family. Responders' exposure to random horrific events may cause them to crave control at home, to balance the helplessness experienced at work, and prevent adverse outcomes in their own families. Some controlling behavior may be habitual. Family members may be addressed in the same authoritative, directive manner used with citizens on duty (Kirschman, 2004). Responder marriages are disrupted by "bringing the job home" and continuing to "give tickets." Firefighters may find fault with family members who fail to maintain firehouse standards of order and cleanliness. Some responders bring home serious coercive or intimidating behaviors such as barking orders, name-calling, and the invasion of personal space. These "authoritarian spillover" behaviors, useful for establishing a potentially life-saving command presence on duty, can upset, anger, and frighten civilian spouses and children (Stinson & Liederbach, 2013). Responders are desensitized to aggression and trained to take orders without question; family members are not.

The desire for and reliance on control, combined with vigilance and an awareness of danger, may lead to the overprotection of spouses or children and/or adopting an authoritarian parenting style. Family members' subsequent subtle or overt resistance can contribute to relationship breakdown. Research has not found authoritarianism associated with rigidity or intolerance in police officers but has found an "authority orientation" – a higher-than-usual acceptance of yielding decision-making power to those who are knowledgeable and experienced (Gerber & Ward, 2011). Officers may similarly expect family members to yield to them. Responders may limit family members' activities because danger is perceived. They may use job skills to surveil children or spouses, for example, tracking their computer usage or vehicle movements. These behaviors become more probable when responders cast as heroic rescuers believe they are mandated to direct and repair family life. Clearly, verbal and psychological aggression, surveillance, stalking, and control maneuvers such as isolating the spouse from former friends who are deemed unsuitable can develop into or constitute abuse.

Alcohol, violence, trauma, and other problems (e.g., gambling and corruption) affect responder families like other families. These escalated concerns are correlated with negative, hostile, or disrupted parenting and can fuel a marital conflict that indirectly compromises children's adjustment. They can occur in the absence of specific trauma, but in responder populations higher trauma exposure is correlated with greater responder distress (Bartlett et al., 2018; Merlino, 2011). The problems named often co-occur. The physiological reactivity, irritability, anger, and deficits in interpersonal problem-solving of PTSD make it an established risk factor for relationship dysfunction and intimate partner violence (IPV; Taft et al., 2011). Stress, PTEs, and PTSD all increase the likelihood of alcohol abuse or dependence (Smith et al., 2019), which in turn increases the likelihood of IPV (McCrady & Epstein, 2015).

Approximately 20% of firefighters and paramedics will develop PTSD at some point during their careers (International Association of Fire Fighters [IAFF] Center of Excellence Staff, 2019). PTSD is estimated to develop in 7–19% of police officers (Violanti, 2021), 13.3–15.6% of dispatchers (Steinkopf et al., 2018), and as high as 35% of EMTs (Russ, 2022). PTSD, which may develop more often in individuals with insecure attachments to others, typically lessens the individual's ability to engage with others and can quintuple divorce rates (Bryant, 2021; Godfrey et al., 2022). In veterans, severe PTSD has been linked to wives' reports of IPV, relationship dissatisfaction, stress, sadness, isolation, and anger (Mansfield et al., 2014). In active and former military personnel, parenting with PTSD has been associated with emotional numbing, lower engagement with children, and increased use of physical aggression (Creech & Misca, 2017; Taft et al., 2011). First responder families may be similarly impacted.

Subsyndromal PTSD, or what might be called "walking PTSD," also causes family discord and distress. Bryant (2021) found 7–16% of first responders show subsyndromal PTSD, which he noted can cause as much dysfunction as the full disorder. Violanti (2021) estimated that a much higher 34% of LEOs show subsyndromal symptoms. The job spillover behaviors identified earlier overlap with diagnostic criteria for PTSD, often signaling the presence of subsyndromal PTSD. That is, a responder with subsyndromal PTSD may exhibit hypervigilance (with or without re-experiencing symptoms), which can manifest as overprotectiveness, as well as negative changes in cognition or mood. The DSM-V's negative cognitions or mood criterion can be met by emotional numbness, feelings of detachment from others, and cynicism. "The world is completely dangerous," an outlook a responder might hold, is provided as an example of negative cognitions in the manual (American Psychiatric Association, 2013, p. 272). The avoidance of trauma cues is seen less often. When trauma is job-related, avoidance proves difficult.

Regardless of a responder's trauma history, alcohol use that may be culturally sanctioned blurs negative emotions and memories, eases access to constricted emotions, and disinhibits behavior, often facilitating communication and assertiveness in relationships (McCrady & Epstein, 2015). Alcohol's usefulness in smoothing interpersonal interactions, including sexual expression, may decrease one or both partners' interest in reducing its use. Approximately 47% of firefighters report an alcohol use disorder in their lifetimes (Smith et al., 2020). Miller and Galvin (2016) determined that 33.4% of police and firefighter survey respondents engaged in binge drinking (i.e., consumed five or more drinks in a session) in the previous month. Spouses of people with alcohol use disorders are at elevated risk of mood disorders, somatic concerns, abuse, and low marital satisfaction (Rodriguez et al., 2013). Alcohol use problems and relationship problems reoccur and increase in a feedback loop, with drinkers underestimating the harm done to marital adjustment (Rodriguez et al., 2013). Injuries, chronic pain, and access elevate responders' risk of abusing opioids and other substances as well, although random testing may suppress usage.

Approximately 24% of American women and 14% of American men are victims of IPV, which increases in the presence of poor emotional regulation, high physiological reactivity, and high exposure to violence, as well as the demand-withdrawal cycles and chronic stress seen in many responder marriages (Rowe & Jouriles, 2019). The hegemonic masculine role's demand for toughness, desensitization to aggression (Di Bianca & Mahalik, 2022), and/or a power imbalance associated with the hero myth may present additional risk factors. Only in police officers has the subject been studied extensively (Pasca & Wagner, 2021; Sharp et al., 2022).

Stinson and Liederbach's (2013) analysis suggested that among police, "authoritarian spillover" behaviors increase with higher exposure to violence, which in turn increases the risk of IPV. The exposure may foster a desire for control and obedience, a habit of intimidation, and desensitization, perhaps appearing as early as the training academy (Meffert et al., 2014). Authoritarian spillover may be less common among officers who are women or people of color, perhaps resulting in lower rates of officer-perpetrated family violence (Anderson & Lo, 2011). A 2016 review of seven studies estimated family violence was perpetrated by 21.2% of police officers, including against their children (Mennicke & Ropes, 2016). A later literature review found rates of officer-perpetrated family violence varied from 4.8% to 28%, concluding that its prevalence might not exceed rates in the general population (Russell & Pappas, 2018). Sharp et al.'s (2022) review of 10 U.S. police studies found a frightening 8.1–8.9% of respondents self-reported violence against children. It supported a link between exposure to violence and perpetration.

The possibility of job loss discourages responder and spouse from entering treatment: Legislation enacted in 1994 and 1996 prohibited the owning of firearms by anyone convicted of a qualifying family violence offense. Threats, fear of retaliation, fear of being outed if in closeted same-sex relationships, and the anticipation of unfair treatment by the responder's cohort in the justice system also silence victims. Economic necessity can motivate silence; so can love or the wish to avoid single parenthood. Either party may be reluctant to "dishonor" the profession. The author's clients have expressed that reporting IPV seems too vindictive, given the severity of the consequences.

Parkinson and Zara (2013) interviewed Australian firefighters and civilians, among them firefighter spouses, who were impacted by a weeks-long bushfire. The authors concluded that IPV rose in part because firefighters could not "live up to society's demands of their masculinity" (Parkinson & Zara, 2013, p. 30). They added, "Community members, police, case managers, trauma psychologists and family violence workers empathized with traumatized and suffering men—men who may have been heroes in the fires—and encouraged women to wait it out" (Parkinson & Zara, 2013, p. 28). Police departments, in the past, concealed IPV under the guise of "handling it informally," allowing offenders to plead guilty to lesser assault charges (Russell & Pappas, 2018).

Coping, Spousal Trauma, and a Crisis

More positively, the undeniable power of a partner's love, empathy, and care to buffer the stress of the first responder career has long been recognized (Landers et al., 2020; Regehr et al., 2002). Casas and Benuto's (2022) meta-analysis of 16 studies found the varied responder groups turned primarily to friends, family, and coworkers for support. Formal peer support programs earned mixed reviews (the meta-analysis included Landers et al., 2020; Meffert et al., 2014; Porter & Henriksen, 2016; and Regehr et al., 2005, discussed separately in this chapter). Regehr et al. (2002) found 79.1% of a sample of paramedics regarded their significant others as supportive or very supportive; only a third said the same about other family members. Rennebohm et al. (2021) found positive relationship quality seemed to mitigate posttraumatic stress in firefighters: Venting and denial-based coping, initially considered maladaptive emotional coping, had an unexpected buffering effect. Police officers gave positive ratings to post-critical incident interventions after they found sharing their stories with spouses, as recommended, was beneficial (Violanti, 2014). A spouse may prompt a responder to find meaning in a PTE or affirm the responder's primary identity or personal efficacy (Chen et al., 2022).

Spousal support is not always available, even to those who are partnered, nor is it necessarily sought or preferred (Morman et al., 2020). Moral injury in responders is linked to low perceived social support, perhaps because those injured, beset by shame, conceal their involvement and distance themselves from support providers (Bryant, 2021). Supervisor support may create an environment conducive to processing PTEs healthily and therefore be more beneficial (Setti et al., 2016). Firefighters who live and work together 24 hours per day place high value on the informal collegial support they obtain (Johnson et al., 2020) although rural firefighters, wildfire firefighters, and volunteers who disperse after a call-up may have little or no access to it. When peers are absent, when perceived peer support is limited to recommending stoicism, when support vacillates after highly distressing or controversial events, or when support feels less available (e.g., to women [Arble & Arnetz, 2017]), the importance of spousal support may grow.

Spouses seem to know without being told when the responder has experienced a particularly difficult shift and is disturbed by it; that is, it is tacitly communicated to them (Regehr et al., 2005). Following responders' exposure to PTEs or a community trauma such as line-of-duty death, they provide instrumental support, such as taking on more parenting and household chores, to allow the responder time to recuperate (Campbell et al., 2022; Landers et al., 2020). Sharp et al. (2022) concluded after reviewing 43 papers that spouses avoided conflict and subdued their own needs to balance the emotionality or challenges of the responder. This "placed a huge emotional burden upon them causing withdrawal and negative well-being outcomes" (Sharp et al., 2022, p. 9). Casas and Benuto (2022) similarly found spouses took on more household responsibility after responders' trauma exposure, to support recovery and avoid or reduce "emotional volatility." Doing so frequently "led spouses to feel isolated, lonely, and as if their needs were unimportant or illegitimate" (Casas & Benuto, 2022, p. 215).

The actions of a police wife after her husband was injured in the January 6, 2021 assault on the U.S. Capitol are illustrative. She tried to "spare her husband exposure to stress, spare them all his reactions to that stress . . . so she stayed up late, folding every piece of laundry, writing more lists for the coming week, making sure that her son's baseball uniform was where it needed to be so there would be no last-minute panic, no hassle, no outbursts" (Dominus & Broadwater, 2022, p. 44). Apprehension about emotional volatility is implied.

Some accommodation is positive and routine, such as subduing a busy household to benefit a nightshift worker trying to sleep. Flexibility and adaptability are characteristics of healthy families. Compas et al. (2019) describe dyadic coping, whereby stress in one partner triggers coping responses in the other, with the shared goal of relationship stability. Problems arise when responder spouses continually overaccommodate because of the level or chronicity of their partners' stress, and if or when the hero myth relegates them to a subordinate position that requires ignoring their own needs. E. Kirschman (personal communication, April 14, 2022; see frsn.org) believes the largely female partners of responders she sees at residential retreats have habitually met responders' needs at the expense of their own, often resulting in anger and loss of identity.

Dyadic interactions may diminish the flow of spousal support just when it is most needed. Campbell et al. (2022) found a mutual lack of emotional response in couples after PTEs, resulting in a tension-inducing "withdraw-withdraw pattern." Spouses may experience a range of negative emotions they are unwilling to share, including fear and grief for lost ideals. They may show reciprocal negativity in response to bad moods, sleep deprivation accompanied by weak emotional control, and other symptoms that responders can show after stress and trauma. A police wife described her husband after a fatality response, as "horrible…just rude and mean and short-tempered and just completely crabby" (Landers et al., 2020, p. 313).

After a PTE, responders may choose to withdraw. A responder shaken by a PTE such as an on-the-job injury may feel unable to empathize with a spouse who is also responding to the event. PTSD or the feeling that one's presence is burdensome or toxic to family members can motivate withdrawal. Responders may wish to avoid judgment, hide occupational dangers, bury perceived inadequacies, or simply rest. Spouses oppose withdrawal out of concern for their partners and children and because of their own practical and emotional support needs. The pairing of persistent efforts by responders to create emotional distance with spousal insistence on interaction can fuel harmful demand-withdrawal cycles.

The negative interactions described can foster social disconnectedness, which has been linked to poorer emotional regulation and a higher level of PTSD symptoms in firefighters (Leonard & Vujanovic, 2022). That is, disconnection can lead to dysregulation ("crabbiness") and relationship dysfunction, which can lead to further disconnection in a destructive cycle.

In short, living with responders does not leave spouses unscathed. Friese (2020) found 70% of LEO wives reported significant stress related to their husbands' profession, noting that the LEOs' selection of healthy or unhealthy coping styles could add to spousal stress. A study by Landers et al. (2020) of eight LEO couples identified hypervigilant behavior, nausea, intrusive thoughts, anxiety, and worry in the spouses. Other law enforcement spouses provided needed support.

Secondary trauma resulting from empathic responses to the responders' trauma leads to symptoms like those seen in primary traumatic stress, including sleep disturbance, confusion, mood changes, and fear (Casas & Benuto, 2022; Landers et al., 2020). In one case, a military wife developed hypervigilance as she monitored her environment for triggers for her husband's panic attacks (Strzalkowski, 2018). In their meta-analysis, Casas and Benuto (2022) concluded that secondary traumatic stress and psychopathology were "common" in responder spouses, who endured the repetitive and cumulative effects of their partners' trauma exposure and subsequent emotional and behavioral changes. A study of firefighters' wives found 21% had secondary trauma and an additional 4% manifested other disorders (Gawrych, 2011). Alrutz et al. (2020) identified apparent secondary trauma in 20% of responder spouses; more than half felt unsupported in their roles. Hero mythology, to the extent that it discourages self-care among spouses, may contribute to these statistics. The harm done to spouses by responders' career-related stress and pathology and the family dysfunction that ensues constitute an unacknowledged crisis.

Building Stronger Families

This chapter turns now to strategies that may mitigate or prevent the damage done by some of the stressors discussed when used with evidence-based treatments as needed. Helping responders to identify, own, and accept their needs, emotions, and limitations creates a truer self-image for the responder, a path to richer emotional experience, and in turn a stronger foundation for relationships. The contribution of the hero myth to negative patterns such as overaccommodation or overprotection must be explored without denigrating the genuine sacrifices made by responders. A core irrational belief that may be the target of intervention is, "I can prevent all harm to my family" (Bryant, 2021). Among the author's cases, an officer who learned of his child's molestation by a neighbor, and another who terminated a parent's life support, each experienced devastating self-blame when they could not safeguard all family members in all circumstances.

Therapeutic work should gauge whether the negative interactions described here are disrupting a relationship or a family's well-being, assessing the reciprocal flow of support between responder and spouse. Equitable consideration of both partners' needs will be beneficial to couples, and equitable provision of support will foster relationship closeness. When spouses are in treatment, any conflicting emotions they have about compromises made to sustain the responder's career must be untangled. They may hold the irrational belief that "My well-being is less important than the responder's."

Clients easily grasp that job spillover behaviors such as commanding vocal tones create strain at home. They can be coached to implement positive spillover, potentially transferring emotional control and communication skills from the workplace to the home. A critically important teachable skill for this population is emotional self-regulation through relaxation, deep breathing, attention and cognition management, anger management training (anger being a culturally permissible emotion), or other approaches. Mobile apps developed for veterans are helpful, portable, and reputable. Symptoms such as heightened arousal and diminished emotional responsiveness can often be modified with treatments designed for PTSD.

Initial clinical assessment should include exploration of aggression, for example, questions about having to restrain the partner "for her own good," or about times the responder felt out of control. The storage and display of weapons are important; aggressive responders may toy with weapons, perhaps threatening self-harm, to intimidate or manipulate partners. Safety planning may be complicated by the presence of weapons and responders' access to shelter information. The possibility of bidirectional IPV should be considered, particularly in two-responder couples.

Couples need to collaboratively determine whether and how negative aspects of the responder's job will be discussed at home, setting aside mythology about invulnerability and recognizing the damage caused by silence. Regehr et al. (2005) found that their sample of fourteen firefighter wives said their husbands "never" talked about PTEs; one learned at a party that her husband had fallen through a roof. Bryant (2021, p. 62) quotes a paramedic who asks, "What does she want me to do? Tell her about the decapitated babies I find in cars on the freeway?" The paramedic's wife wants him to share emotions, not gory specifics. Responders feel misunderstood but hesitate to open up in a way that might ease understanding. A default recommendation for uncertain couples is that they "share the headlines" of shifts, omitting details, to foster honesty and acceptance and help the spouse recognize when the responder's stress management capacity has been breached. One police wife said her husband told her, "It was just not a good day," which led her to conclude, "I just kind of know the fact that something happened and I don't want to know anyway" (Landers et al., 2020, p. 313). This couple's shorthand is more conducive to intimacy than false cheer.

Reframing techniques promote adopting a novel perspective to attain therapeutic goals (Dattilio, 2010). The following reframes have proved valuable to responders and spouses, at least in defusing initial blame or tension (reiterating some recommendations outlined in Garmezy, 2020). First, clients can shift to viewing the responder's overprotectiveness as fear for a beloved family as much as a need to control and understand that fear as entirely consistent with the responder's experience of the world as a dangerous place. The couple can accept without judgment that they have different lived experiences resulting in different world views. Some excessive vigilance can be treated as an inescapable, well-intended side effect of the career, not criticism of family members' judgment. Clients then can review any "safety behaviors," for example, following a teen's vehicle.

Time spent with others can be recognized as a conduit to life-saving social support rather than a frivolous or questionable activity, particularly when peer support is scarce. Social support for spouses is also essential to their mental health. Positive experiences with community members, such as a faith community, are a lifeline in crises and offset cynicism. Outside networks also buffer the losses associated with retirement.

The impact of the job on the responder can be reframed: Some withdrawal on the part of the responder can be viewed as decompression or self-care, rather than selfishness or disregard. While the clinician remains alert for excessive withdrawal, “excused absences” from family life can be beneficial. A standard recommendation is building reentry time into the responder’s schedule, for example, a minimum of 30 minutes after returning home to separate from work physically and psychologically before the demands of family life begin.

Berne’s (1985) Parent-Adult-Child transactional analysis offers clients another fresh perspective. In Berne’s framework, one spouse (the responder) may function as a nurturing, authoritative, and at times authoritarian Parent, for example, framing a budget, while the other spouse is a naive, playful, and at times irresponsible Child. More Child-like behavior begets more Parent-like behavior, and vice versa. The P-A-C formulation reminds clients that to heal a marriage, begin with oneself, that is, shift into dependable Adult mode. The challenges of actual parenting are addressed next.

Children and teens may share the ability of spouses to sense when a PTE has occurred without being told, noticing unusual parental behavior or alterations in routines that indicate accommodation. High-profile events should be discussed with children; if parents do not, others will. Media coverage of events should be viewed jointly by children and parents and in limited quantities. After PTEs, parents can explicitly teach coping strategies and values, for example, “Let’s pray about it and then go to the park” (Compas et al., 2019). Children should not be allowed to feel overly responsible for ensuring a responder is rested or calm, or (in most circumstances) assume caretaking roles.

Responders appear more likely than other professionals to adopt authoritarian parenting styles. They may expect the immediate obedience they require on scenes, with a display of the respect for authority and hierarchical organization they were taught. These expectations can exacerbate typical parent-child power struggles. Moreover, vigilant, hypervigilant, or frightened responders may be loath to grant developing children and teens the increased independence they seek, leading to resentment, resistance, and the risk of lowered self-efficacy or social competence in their offspring. These possible outcomes and the futility of teaching obedience without decision-making skills can be explored with the client. Communication may be enhanced by acknowledging to the family that career experiences have bred atypical caution. Bryant (2021) recommends behavioral experiments allowing children progressively more freedom.

Responder parents may consider themselves responsible for instilling a high level of discipline in children or stepchildren. Responders’ partners may have wished, consciously or not, for a hero to maintain order in either a biological family or a stepfamily. Healthy stepfamily formation may be impeded when a responder stepparent, perhaps responding to spousal cues, attempts to exercise authority too rigidly or too quickly. In both types of families, problems develop when expectations are not met or rules are inconsistently enforced. The spouse may become the more acquiescent, flexible parent, compensating for what is perceived as the harshness of the responder. The responder, in turn, may consider the spouse naïve or feel undermined. In other cases, a frequently absent responder is reluctant to set limits. Partners can be coached on consistency tempered by flexibility, best practices for stepparenting, and the utility of phrasing ("we decided…") that highlights shared authority, despite a co-parent's absence.

Worried children and teens need accurate age-appropriate information about their parents' professions. The functioning of protective equipment can be explained to emphasize how responders are safeguarded. Similarly, responders should point out that they are protected by their teams within their own agencies and the added support, such as medical care, of other professionals on scenes. Visits to the workplace and descriptions of innocuous calls or activities help to counteract sensational media imagery.

When responders' children experience anxiety, depression, or other problems, these conditions are seldom solely related to parents' absences or occupations, but the possibility of an association should be considered. Modeling in the home may be unhelpful, and if so, parents will need to be educated about the issue and supported in dealing with their own concerns or trauma. Secondary trauma may be present in children and teens following exposure to disturbing content in the home, in the media, or – rarely – from accompanying a parent when the responder acts spontaneously in a critical incident off-duty. Children whose caretakers participated in the manhunt following the Boston Marathon attack showed elevated rates of hyperactivity/ inattention and emotional problems and experienced rates of PTSD that were 5.7 times higher than those of children whose caretakers were not involved (Comer et al., 2014). Of course, inattention and restlessness, seen with anxiety, also can be indicative of Attention-Deficit/Hyperactivity Disorder (ADHD) and other disorders. The prevalence of ADHD and academic problems may be higher than that seen in the general population, as responders' children have parents who chose professions that de-emphasized deskwork and extensive academics (and may have had learning difficulties, themselves).

Specialized support programs are available to survivors after line-of-duty deaths; for example, the children's programming and retreats sponsored by Concerns of Police Survivors and the National Fallen Firefighters Foundation. Facilitating widow-to-widow connections has a documented positive effect (Sharp et al., 2022). With the passing of time, bereaved families may remain a cared-for part of the responder community or come to feel they are unsettling reminders of worst-case scenarios.

To offer effective treatment to responder families at any stage of life, clinicians must examine their own positive and negative biases about first responders. They must learn from clients the meanings of independence, power, and gender roles in different cultures and identity groups, professional and nonprofessional while pursuing further understanding through other avenues. They can neither disparage clients' understanding of masculinity nor presume that all responders embrace a hegemonic masculinity ideal. Clinicians may find responders are overcontrolling in sessions, or that they are concerned the civilian clinician has sided with the civilian spouse against the responder. Limits to confidentiality must be made clear to clients and agencies and preserved carefully to maintain trust. Therapists who are integrated into responder communities and who earn their living via that community's patronage must at times disturb the system by reporting abuse, initiating involuntary hospitalizations, or making other unwelcome-to-departments but ethically required decisions, including nondisclosure of the serious misconduct that angry spouses can divulge.

Improving the resilience of responder families requires changing occupational cultures and organizations, not just employees and their families (Steinkopf et al., 2018). More organizational support for pregnancy, postnatal care, and parenting, such as stabilizing shifts where possible, will benefit all responders (National Institute of Justice, 2019). Limiting overtime remains a controversial policy (International Association of Chiefs of Police [IACP], 2021). Websites, orientation programs, training courses, and other communication vehicles can offer preventive educational interventions and resources to reduce the impact of the career on families. Leadership can combat the threats of suicide, PTSD, substance abuse, and IPV with training at the pre-service and in-service levels, and the implementation of model policies and programs, for example, *Preventing Officer-Involved Domestic Violence* (2020). Departments can promote the use of formal peer support programs, chaplaincy programs, and mental health services with professionals who have developed satisfactory cultural competence.

Department-sponsored programs foster vital connections among family members that potentiate social support, including open houses, fundraisers, recreational events, ceremonies, CPR classes, financial literacy training, spouse support groups, and relationship or parenting skills classes open to responders, recent retirees, couples, and unaccompanied spouses. "Family" should be left to the responder to define, with welcomes extended to unmarried partners and multigenerational family members. Direct outreach, such as through social media, prevents unsupportive responders from serving as gatekeepers. Significant others educated on topics such as PTSD can become de facto screeners, perhaps prompting responders to find needed help (IACP, 2021).

National organizations have published helpful guides to building responder family resilience, and many of them are useful across professional boundaries. For example, a guide for EMT families produced in conjunction with the National Child Traumatic Stress Network offers excellent recommendations on communicating with children, and the International Association of Chiefs of Police published an online guide to starting family support groups in 2019. In 2021, an online guide to "family-friendly" policies followed, recommending supporting postnatal care and sharing information about mental health resources at frequent family programs, among other innovations (IACP, 2021).

Responder careers cannot be rid of their inherent stress and danger. Those who serve can be strengthened by social connections and strong relationships, both of which clearly promote individual health (Schetter, 2017). This review reminds us that responders' well-being will be enhanced by helping them to fulfill their hopes for their families. Those who wish to aid the responder community should adopt the goal of increasing support for spouses, to improve coping, prevent pathology, limit the debilitating effects of secondary trauma, and enable them to support responders and other family members more fully. The critical role loved ones play in responder health cannot be ignored, particularly while the responder professions lack reliable methods of preventing PTEs from negatively impacting personnel. As the occupational hazards discussed in this chapter imperil family bonds, responders and their loved ones swim against the current to maintain remarkably robust marriages and families. The mental health professionals who are privileged to know them are obliged to assist in their efforts.

References

Agocs, T., Langan, D., & Sanders, C. B. (2015). Police mothers at home: Police work and danger-protection parenting practices. *Gender & Society, 29*(2), 265–289. https://doi.org/10.1177%2F0891243214551157

Alrutz, A. S., Buetow, S., Cameron, L. D., & Huggard, P. K. (2020). What happens at work comes home. *Healthcare, 8*(3), 350. https://doi.org/10.3390/healthcare8030350

Allison, S. T., Goetals, G. R., Marrinan, A. R., Parker, O. M., Spyrow, S. P., & Stein, M. (2019). The metamorphosis of the hero: Principles, processes, and purpose. *Frontiers in Psychology, 10*. https://doi.org/10.3389//fpsyg.2019.00606

American Psychiatric Association. (2013). *Diagnostic and statistical manual of mental disorders* (5th ed.). https://doi.org/10.1176/appi.books.9780890425596

Anderson, A. S., & Lo, C. C. (2011). Intimate partner violence within law enforcement families. *Journal of Interpersonal Violence, 26*(6), 1176–1193. https://doi.org/10.1177/0886260510368156

Arble, E., & Arnetz, B. B. (2017). A model of first responder coping: An approach/avoidance bifurcation. *Stress and Health, 33*, 223–232. https://doi.org/10.1002/smi.2692

Bartlett, B. A., Jardin, C., Martin, C., Tran, J. K., Buser, S., Anestis, M. D., & Vujanovic, A. A. (2018). Posttraumatic stress and suicidality among firefighters: The moderating role of distress tolerance. *Cognitive Therapy and Research, 42*(4), 483–496. https://doi.org/10.1007/s10608-018-9892-y

Berne, E. (1985). *Games people play: The basic handbook of transactional analysis*. Ballantine Books.

Bohl-Penrod, N. K., & Clark, D. W. (2017). Peer support in public safety organizations. In C. L. Mitchell & E. H. Dorian (Eds.), *Police psychology and its growing impact on modern law enforcement* (pp. 237–251). IGI Global.

Brayfield, A. (1995). Juggling jobs and kids: The impact of employment schedules on fathers' caring for children. *Journal of Marriage and Family, 57*(2), 321–332. https://doi.org/10.2307/353686

Bryant, R. A. (2021). *Treating PTSD in first responders*. American Psychological Association.

Buscemi, S. (with Vick, K.) (2021, September 20). The Ground Zero death toll is still climbing. *Time*, 21.

Campbell, A. R., Landers, A. L., & Jackson, J. B. (2022). I have to hold it together: Trauma in law enforcement couples. *Family Relations*, 1–26. https://doi.org/10.1111/fare.12661

Casas, J. B., & Benuto, L. T. (2022). Work-related traumatic stress spillover in first responder families: A systematic review of the literature. *Psychological Trauma: Theory, Research, Practice, and Policy, 14*(2), 209–217. https://psycnet.apa.org/doi/10.1037/tra0001086

Chen, J., Li, W., An, Y., Zhang, Y., Du, J., & Xu, W. (2022). Perceived social support mediates the relationships of dispositional mindfulness to job burnout and posttraumatic stress disorder among Chinese firefighters. *Psychological Trauma: Theory, Research, Practice, and Policy, 14*(7), 1117–1123. https://psycnet.apa.org/doi/10.1037/tra0000534

Comer, J. S., Kerns, C. E., Elkins, R. M., Edson, A. L., Chou, T., Dantowitz, A., Miguel, E., Brown, B., Coxe, S., & Green, J. G. (2014). Adjustment among children with relatives who participated in the manhunt following the Boston marathon attack. *Depression and Anxiety, 31*(7), 542–550. https://doi.org/10.1002/da.22281

Compas, B. E., Murphy, L. K., Yarboi, J., Gruhn, M. A., & Watson, K. H. (2019). Stress and coping in families. In B. H. Fiese, M. Celano, K. Deater-Deckard, E. N. Jouriles, & M. A. Whisman (Eds.), *APA handbook of contemporary family psychology: Vol. 1. Foundations, methods, and contemporary issues across the lifespan* (pp. 37–55). American Psychological Association.

Creech, S. K., & Misca, G. (2017). Parenting with PTSD: A review of research on the influence of PTSD on parent-child functioning in military and veteran families. *Frontiers in Psychology, 8*. https://doi.org/10.3389/fpsyg.2017.01101

Dattilio, F. M. (2010). *Cognitive-behavioral therapy with couples and families: A comprehensive guide for clinicians*. Guilford Press.

Di Bianca, M., & Mahalik, J. R. (2022). A relational-cultural framework for promoting healthy masculinities. *American Psychologist, 77*(3), 321–332. https://doi.org/10.1037/amp0000929

Dominus, S., & Broadwater, L. (2022). The Capitol Police and the scars of Jan. 6. *The New York Times Magazine, 26–33*, 44–47.

Fahy, R., Evarts, B., & Stein, G. P. (2022, September). *U.S. Fire Department Profile 2020*. National Fire Protection Association, www.nfpa.org

Friese, K. M. (2020). Cuffed together: A study on how law enforcement work impacts the officer's spouse. *International Journal of Police Science and Management, 22*(4), 407–418.

Garmezy, L. B. (2020). Swimming upstream: The first responder's marriage. In C. A. Bowers, D. C. Beidel, & M. R. Marks (Eds.), *Mental health intervention and treatment of first responders and emergency workers* (pp. 16–31). IGI Global.

Gawrych, A. L. (2011). *PTSD in firefighters and secondary trauma in their wives*. [Abstract]. Hofstra University. Dissertation Abstracts International: Section B: The Sciences and Engineering, *71*(10-B), 6438. http://search.proquest.com.ezproxy.lib.uh.edu/dissertations-theses/ptsd-firefighters-secondary-trauma-their-wives/docview/756455723/se-2?accountid=7107

Gerber, G. L., & Ward, K. C. (2011). Police personality: Theoretical issues and research. In J. Kitaeff (Ed.), *Handbook of police psychology* (pp. 421–436). Routledge.

Godfrey, D. A., Zegel, M., Babcock, J. C., & Vujanovic, A. A. (2022). Posttraumatic Stress Disorder and relationship satisfaction among firefighters: The role of emotion regulation difficulties. *Jouranal of Aggression, Maltreatment and Trauma, 31*(3), 356–369. https://doi.org/10.1080/10926771.2022.2043973

Grassroots Wildland Firefighters. (2021). *Wildland firefighter partner/spouse perspective survey data summary*. http://www.grassrootswildlandfirefighters.com

Haddock, C. K., Jahnke, S. A., Carlos Poston, W. S., Jitnarin, N., & Day, R. S. (2016). Marriage and divorce among firefighters in the United States. *Journal of Family Issues, 37*(16), 2294–2308. https://doi.org/10.1177/0192513X15583070

Healy, N. A., & Vujanovic, A. A. (2021). PTSD symptoms and suicide risk among firefighters: The moderating role of sleep disturbance. *Psychological Trauma: Theory, Research, Practice, and Policy, 13*(7), 749–758. https://psycnet.apa.org/doi/10.1037/tra0001059

Henderson, S. N., Van Hasselt, V. B., LeDuc, T. J., & Couwels, J. (2016). Firefighter suicide: Understanding cultural challenges for mental health professionals. *Professional Psychology: Research and Practice, 47*(3), 224–230. https://doi.org/10.1037/pro0000072

Hollerbach, B. S. (2020). Occupational risk factors and the mental health of women firefighters. In C. A. Bowers, D. C. Beidel, & M. R. Marks (Eds.), *Mental health intervention and treatment of first responders and emergency workers* (pp. 86–102). IGI Global.

Holmes, K. L. (2021). *Where my girls at? A phenomenological study of the lived experiences of lesbian law enforcement couples* [Unpublished doctoral dissertation]. Sam Houston State University. ProQuest Dissertations and Theses Global. http://search.proquest.com.ezproxy.lib.uh.edu/dissertations-theses/where-my-girls-at-phenomenological-study-lived/docview/2572566976/se-2?accountid=7107

IAFF Center of Excellence Staff. (2019, March 20). *Trauma, firefighting, and PTSD*. IAFF Center of Excellence for Behavioral Health Treatment and Recovery. https://www.iaffrecoverycenter.com/blog/trauma-firefighting-and-ptsd/

International Association of Chiefs of Police. (2021). *Family matters: Executive guide for developing family-friendly policies, procedures, and culture*. IACP Office of Community Oriented Policing Services.

Jakubowski, T. D., & Sitko-Dominik, M. M. (2021). The impact of the traditional male role norms on the posttraumatic stress disorder among Polish male firefighters. *PLoS One, 16*(10). https://doi.org/10.1371/journal.pone.0259025

Johnson, C. C., Vega, L., Kohalmi, A. L., Roth, J. C., Howell, B. R., & Van Hasselt, V. B. (2020). Enhancing mental health treatment for the firefighter population: Understanding fire culture, treatment barriers, practice implications, and research directions. *Professional Psychology: Research and Practice, 51*(3), 304–311. https://psycnet.apa.org/doi/10.1037/pro0000266

Jung, A. M., Jahnke, S. A., Dennis, L. K., Bell, M. L., Burgess, J. L., Jitnarin, N., Kaipust, C. M., & Farland, L. V. (2021). Occupational factors and miscarriages in the US fire service: A cross-sectional analysis of women firefighters. *Environmental Health, 20*(1), Article 116. https://doi.org/10.1186/s12940-021-00800-4

Kirschman, E. (2004). *I love a fire fighter: What the family needs to know*. Guilford Press.

Kirschman, E., Kamena, M., & Fay, J. (2014). *Counseling cops: What clinicians need to know*. Guilford Press.

Lamia, M. C., & Krieger, M. J. (2009). *The white knight syndrome: Rescuing yourself from your need to rescue others*. New Harbinger Publications.

Landers, A. L., Dimitropoulos, G., Mendenhall, T. J., Kennedy, A., & Zemanek, L. (2020). Backing the blue: Trauma in law enforcement spouses and couples. *Family Relations, 69*(2), 308–319. https://doi.org/10.1111/fare.12393

Leonard, S., & Vujanovic, A. A. (2022). Thwarted belongingness and PTSD symptom severity among firefighters: The role of emotion regulation difficulties. *Behavior Modification, 46*(2), 352–373. https://doi.org/10.1177/01454455211002105

Mansfield, A. J., Schaper, K. M., Yanagida, A. M., & Rosen, C. S. (2014). One day at a time: The experiences of partners of veterans with posttraumatic stress disorder. *Professional Psychology: Research and Practice, 45*(6), 488–495. https://psycnet.apa.org/doi/10.1037/a0038422

McCrady, B. S., & Epstein, E. E. (2015). Couple therapy and alcohol problems. In A. S. Gurman, J. L. Lebow, & D. K. Snyder (Eds.), *Clinical handbook of couple therapy* (5th ed., pp. 555–584). Guilford.

Meffert, S. M., Henn-Haase, C., Metzler, T. J., Qian, M., Best, S., Hirschfeld, A., McCaslin, S., Inslicht, S., Neylan, T. C., & Marmar, C. R. (2014). Prospective study of police officer spouse/partners: A new pathway to secondary trauma and relationship violence? *PLoS One, 9*(7), 1–8. https://doi.org/10.1371/journal.pone.0100663

Mennicke, A. M., & Ropes, K. (2016). Estimating the rate of domestic violence perpetrated by law enforcement officers: A review of methods and estimates. *Aggression and Violent Behavior, 31*, 157–164. https://doi.org/10.1016/j.avb.2016.09.003

Merlino, J. P. (2011). Rescuing ourselves: Self-care in the disaster response community. In F. J. Stoddard Jr., A. Pandya, & C. L. Katz (Eds.), *Disaster psychiatry: Readiness, evaluation, and treatment* (pp. 35–48). American Psychiatric Publishing.

Miller, T. R., & Galvin, D. M. (2016). Assessing and responding to substance misuse in law enforcement. *Southern Illinois University Law Journal, 40*, 475–499.

Morman, M. T., Schrodt, P., & Adamson, A. (2020). Firefighters' job stress and the (un)intended consequences of relational quality with spouses and firefighter friends. *Journal of Social and Personal Relationships, 37*(4), 1092–1113. https://doi.org/10.1177/0265407519886355

National Institute of Justice. (2019). *Women in policing: Breaking barriers and blazing a path.* U.S. Department of Justice Office of Justice Programs. https://www.ojp.gov

Neff, L. A., & Karney, B. R. (2009). Stress and reactivity to daily relationship experiences: How stress hinders adaptive processes in marriage. *Journal of Personality and Social Psychology, 97*(3), 435–450. https://psycnet.apa.org/doi/10.1037/a0015663

Pappas, S. (2019). APA issues first-ever guidelines for practice with men and boys. *Monitor on Psychology, 50*, 34–39.

Parkinson, D., & Zara, C. (2013). The hidden disaster: Domestic violence in the aftermath of natural disaster. *Australian Journal of Emergency Management, 28*(2), 28–35. search.informit.org/doi/10.3316/informit.364519372739042

Pasca, R., & Wagner, S. L. (2021). Firefighters and spouses: Hostility, satisfaction, and conflict. *Journal of Family Issues, 0*, 1–19. https://doi.org/10.1177/0192513X211055116

Porter, K. L., & Henriksen, R. C. (2016). The phenomenological experience of first responder spouses. *The Family Journal, 24*(1), 44–51. https://doi.org/10.1177/1066480715615651

Preventing officer-involved domestic violence. (2020). *Community Policing Dispatch, 13*(10) https://cops.usdoj.gov/recentreleases

Regehr, C., Goldberg, G., & Hughes, J. (2002). Exposure to human tragedy, empathy, and trauma in ambulance paramedics. *American Journal of Orthopsychiatry, 72*(4), 505–513. https://doi.org/10.1037/0002-9432.72.4.505

Regehr, C., Dimitropoulos, G., Bright, E., George, S., & Henderson, J. (2005). Behind the brotherhood: Rewards and challenges for wives of firefighters. *Family Relations, 54*(3), 423–435. http://doi.org/b6h9cc

Rennebohm, S. B., Dolezal, M. L., Bentley, J. A., Edwards-Stewart, A., Thoburn, J. W., & Holguin, J. (2021). The moderating effect of coping behaviors on posttraumatic stress and first responder romantic relationships. *Couple and Family Psychology: Research and Practice,* no pagination specified. https://doi.org/10.1037/cfp0000165

Rineer, J., Taniguchi, T., Duhart Clarke, S. E., Hoogesteyn, K., & Craven, K. (2022). Ten steps for recruiting more women police. *Police Chief, 89*(12), 30–35.

Ringer, F. B., Rogers, M. L., Podlogar, M. C., Chu, C., Gai, A. R., & Joiner, T. E. (2021). To support and defend: A eusociality-based account of suicide in U.S. military service members and first responders. *Clinical Psychology: Science and Practice, 28*(4), 380–390. https://psycnet.apa.org/doi/10.1037/cps0000033

Rodriguez, L. M., Overup, C. S., & Neighbors, C. (2013). Perceptions of partner's problematic alcohol use affect relationship outcomes beyond partner self-reported drinking: Alcohol use in committed romantic relationships. *Psychology of Addictive Behaviors, 27*(3), 627–638. https://psycnet.apa.org/doi/10.1037/a0031737

Rowe, L. S., & Jouriles, E. N. (2019). Intimate partner violence and the family. In B. H. Fiese, M. Celano, K. Deater-Deckard, E. N. Jouriles, & M. A. Whisman (Eds.), *APA handbook of contemporary family psychology: Vol. 1. Foundations, methods, and contemporary issues across the lifespan* (pp. 399–416). American Psychological Association.

Russ, T. (2022). Post-traumatic stress disorder comparison between fire and EMS personnel. *Journal of Emergency Medical Services*. https://www.jems.com

Russell, B. L., & Pappas, N. (2018). Officer involved domestic violence: A future of uniform response and transparency. *International Journal of Police Science & Management, 20*(2), 134–142. https://doi.org/10.1177/1461355718774579

Schetter, C. D. (2017). Moving research on health and close relationships forward—A challenge and an obligation: Introduction to the special issue. *American Psychologist, 72*(6), 511–516. https://doi.org/10.1037/amp0000158

Schmidt, C. (2019, April 23). City of Tucson ordered to pay $3.8M to paramedic deprived of adequate lactation space. *Arizona Daily Star*. https://www.tucson.com

Setti, I., Lourel, M., & Argentero, P. (2016). The role of affective commitment and perceived social support in protecting emergency workers against burnout and vicarious traumatization. *Traumatology, 22*(4), 261. https://psycnet.apa.org/doi/10.1037/trm0000072

Sharp, M.-L., Solomon, N., Harrison, V., Gribble, R., Cramm, H., Pike, G., & Fear, N. T. (2022). The mental health and wellbeing of spouses, partners and children of emergency responders: A systematic review. *PLoS One, 17*(6). https://doi.org/10.1371/journal.pone.0269659

Shows, C., & Gerstel, N. (2009). Fathering, class and gender: A comparison of physicians and emergency medical technicians. *Gender and Society, 23*(2), 161–187. https://doi.org/10.1177/0891243209333872

Shreffler, K. M., Meadows, M. P., & Davis, K. D. (2011). Firefighting and fathering: Work-family conflict, parenting stress, and satisfaction with parenting and child behavior. *Fathering, 9*(2), 169–188.

Smith, L. J., Paulus, D. J., Gallagher, M. W., Norman, S. B., Tran, J. K., & Vujanovic, A. A. (2019). Perceived stress and probable alcohol misuse in firefighters: The role of posttraumatic stress. *International Journal of Stress Management, 26*(4), 367–377. https://doi.org/10.1037/str0000118

Smith, L. J., Zegel, M., Bartlett, B. A., Lebeaut, A., & Vujanovic, A. A. (2020). Postraumatic stress and alcohol use among first responders. In C. A. Bowers, D. C. Beidel, & M. R. Marks (Eds.), *Mental health intervention and treatment of first responders and emergency workers* (pp. 32–48). IGI Global.

Steinkopf, B., Reddin, R. A., Black, R. A., Van Hasselt, V. B., & Couwels, J. (2018). Assessment of stress and resiliency in emergency dispatchers. *Journal of Police and Criminal Psychology, 33*(4), 398–411. https://doi.org/10.1007/s11896-018-9255-3

Stinson, P. M., & Liederbach, J. (2013). *Fox in the henhouse: A study of police officers arrested for crimes associated with domestic or family violence.* Bowling Green State University Criminal Justice Faculty Publications. https://scholarworks.bgsu.edu/crim_just_pub/6

Strzalkowski, B. (2018, June 19). His war, her PTSD: Caregivers admit to experiencing secondary PTSD symptoms. *Military Families Magazine*. https://www.militaryfamilies.com

Taft, C. T., Watkins, L. E., Stafford, J., Street, A. E., & Monson, C. M. (2011). Posttraumatic stress disorder and intimate relationship problems: A meta-analysis. *Journal of Consulting and Clinical Psychology, 79*(1), 22–33. https://psycnet.apa.org/doi/10.1037/a0022196

Van Hasselt, V. B., Bourke, M. L., & Schuhmann, B. B. (2022). Firefighter stress and mental health: Introduction to the special issue. *Behavior Modification, 46*(2), 259–266. https://doi.org/10.1177/01454455211064955

Violanti, J. M. (2014). *Dying for the job: Police work exposure and health*. Charles C. Thomas.

Violanti, J. M. (2021). *Occupation under siege: Resolving mental health crises in police work.* Charles C. Thomas.

Violanti, J. M., & Samuels, S. (2007). *Under the blue shadow: Clinical and behavioral perspectives on police suicide*. Charles C. Thomas.

Wetherington, J. (2021, Feb 11). Officer wellness spotlight: The law enforcement family. *FBI Law Enforcement Bulletin*. https://www.leb.fbi.gov

Women in Fire. (n.d.). *Reproductive health and the fire service*. https://womeninfire.org. WIFReproHealth-Infographic_poster_Citations_QR-Code_FINAL.pdf.

Role of the Law Enforcement Administrator

Larry L. Massey Jr.

The research underscores the complexity of suicide as a problem impervious to easily understood solutions. Consequently, intervention strategies must include initiatives ranging from mitigating circumstances contributing to an event to addressing underlying causes at the individual level (Hawton & Pirkis, 2017). Statistics consistently show that more first responders commit suicide each year than die in the line of duty (Tiesman et al., 2021). Further, studies reveal that they have higher rates of severe anxiety, depression, and posttraumatic stress disorder (PTSD) than the general population. Yet, there has been little formal recognition nor a determination of the most appropriate approach to solving this problem. The critical question is, what role do agency administrators play in crisis intervention strategies?

This chapter aims to offer a personal perspective that augments the empirical research cited extensively throughout this book, with more than three decades of practical field experience working in municipal, tribal, and academic public safety settings. However, unlike researchers relying on outside sources or materials to study phenomena, the perspective offered here draws upon the experience of managing death scenes and delivering notifications to closest living relatives. Unfortunately, many other sheriffs, police chiefs, and fire chiefs can share similar stories that mark a major change in their lives and that of others.

Without a doubt, the job will continuously touch off memories of past traumatic events among first responders while causing them to simultaneously live new ones. Although there are many developmental sequences in the exposure to trauma, residency requirements for new hires and decisions by some retirees to settle in the jurisdiction where they perform services may increase the risk of emotional aftershocks because of the lingering memories triggered by their surroundings. Often

L. L. Massey Jr. (✉)
Abraham S. Fischler College of Education, School of Criminal Justice, Nova Southeastern University, Fort Lauderdale, FL, USA
e-mail: lm2315@nova.edu

M. L. Bourke et al. (eds.), *First Responder Mental Health*,
https://doi.org/10.1007/978-3-031-38149-2_23

overlooked, however, is how agency leadership and customs contribute to employee mental health, which is a difficult conversation. Nevertheless, discussing the role of the administrator in mental health may lead to a better evaluation of the adequacy of efforts applied historically to employee resilience. In practical terms, leaders must be capable of drawing lines of distinction between individual behavior and the agency's contribution to poor mental health.

Levels of tolerance to emotional strain and patterns of conduct change over the course of an individual's career. The core position taken here is that the influence of crisis intervention strategies might obstruct pathways underlying suicide. The challenge administrators face is recognizing mental health issues when exposure to trauma manifests differently in every person or at various stages of their career. Hence, this chapter focuses on the role that agency administrators play within the mental health framework of two intervention strategies: organizational culture and crisis response teams. It ends with a few words of advice for clinicians.

At one level, organizational culture influences thinking and shapes the behavior of others (Schein, 2010). On another, the early identification of troubled individuals enables crisis response (or intervention) teams to take precautionary steps that lessen the potential of harm or acts of violence from occurring. At the same time, partnerships with mental health experts are gaining greater acceptance beyond training police officers to make de-escalating decisions in the field when encountering a person experiencing a mental health crisis. Contemporary administrators are bringing clinicians into the broader conversation by asking them to educate all first responder groups and help them understand the consequences of exposure to acute and chronic trauma. Clinicians are also having a profound effect on removing the stigmatizing label that otherwise causes some first responders to avoid seeking professional help.

Culture

Defining culture will, hopefully, remove some ambiguity associated with its general meaning. Organizational culture typically originates from an agency's policies, procedures, and more importantly, practices (Schein, 2010). These are all aspects of the things a department values most. For the same reason, these standards create a work environment that employees come to view as normal. Our definition of culture embodies articulated beliefs, shared ideologies, and underlying assumptions on how to carry out the work. In powerful ways, culture influences patterns of behavior in the workplace, not all of which are easily perceptible or desirable (Schein, 2010).

Some scholars who study culture, like Edgar Schein (2010), propose that customs are a distinctly *organizational* phenomenon, not an *occupational* one. The rationale is that each agency has its own leadership, administrative structure, labor relations, history, traditions, hiring requirements, and tolerance of misconduct. Further, although line-level personnel develop subcultures, they typically have little control over how the larger agency operates, which often contributes to their occupational stress. For instance, in addition to external factors, applying agency policies, assigning shift work, maintaining staffing levels, administering the promotional process, and handing out discipline all take a toll on the mental well-being of first responders. Administrators who pay attention to fairness in applying agency rules, discipline, and promotions might be able to reduce incidents of self-harm.

The attitudes and behaviors prevalent in the cultures of police and fire departments are often intolerant and resistant to change. Tradition is important and carries a special intensity, particularly when socializing new hires into the organization. It is unrealistic to assume that all departments have a healthy culture or one strongly supportive of crisis intervention techniques. Attitudes vary among administrators across jurisdictions leading to dramatic differences in the workplace, not to mention conflict in deciding on intervention strategies to address mental health issues. The character and emotional development of first responders is shaped by independent forces, with agency leadership being one.

Understanding the Leadership Stool

Readers may benefit from a basic understanding of the general structure utilized by many agencies in law enforcement and the fire service. First, they are established and strictly governed by law. Next, they customarily function as paramilitary organizations regulated by comprehensive policies, procedures, behavior standards, and conduct rules. Occasionally, accrediting agencies oversee voluntary compliance with leading industry standards or best practices, but not all agencies seek certification by external regulators.

Moreover, many states have enacted strict procedural due process laws to protect first responders from false allegations or overzealous administrators. These laws grant property rights in continued employment to first responders while mandating the legal steps necessary before administrators can take disciplinary action against them. This constitutes a very complex area of the law, but one worth mentioning here because some first responders feel that receiving mental health counseling is akin to administering punishment.

Like the military, departments traditionally adopt a rigid, hierarchical chain of command using ranks to distribute power and responsibilities. Senior leaders are supposed to share knowledge, offer guidance, and provide support, but that depends on the willingness of the individual occupying the position. Some administrators are reluctant to relinquish control or delegate authority. Worse, they insist on clinging to old ways. Fortunately, most administrators excel at cultivating the next generation of transformational leaders who demonstrate a genuine concern for the professional growth and emotional needs of employees.

Ultimately, the overall mission of agency leadership among first responders is to inspire a diverse group of individuals to work hard together to improve the quality of life for everyone in their community. Regrettably, recognizing employees as equally deserving community members sometimes gets lost in translation. At issue is the enduring tension between operational styles centered on getting the job done and the psychological protection of individual employees.

Although sheriffs are elected officials, agency directors, police chiefs, and fire chiefs are politically appointed. Junior leaders are promoted because they possess the requisite formal education, operational experience, and career development necessary to manage an agency. Over the last few years, highly vocal special interest groups have manipulated public sentiment toward first responders, mainly the police. To restore legitimacy, police leaders are looking at trust as a means of improving community interactions. However, problems can arise when administrators focus more on building trust with the community than developing honest relationships within the workforce.

As history demonstrates, it is not uncommon for line-level workers to complain that agency leadership no longer understands them because of the abstract distinction of being too far removed from the streets. Agency critics quickly point out that fieldwork involves tremendous uncertainty, not the predictability or stability administrators enjoy in the office environment. Accordingly, with an air of mistrust, some first responders insulate themselves from outside influences to cope with a world they feel most people could not possibly understand. If there is a disconnect between the traditional notion of labor and management, it is generally found here. The degree of discontent within a department might sway the willingness of its employees to seek mental health services out of fear that doing so could impact perceptions of their fitness for duty. Consequently, they rank their emotional health of secondary importance to the faulty opinions of others.

Next, imagine the image of an agency head sitting on a three-legged stool. Each leg represents an often-competing interest. One group consists of local politicians. The next are agency employees or the unions representing them. The last are members of the community, including activists and crusaders. On some issues, all the groups align to fully support the leader. On other matters, the interests, and values among the various groups conflict. When this happens, each group fights for dominance. If the agency head cannot simultaneously support the principles of all groups, they find themselves in peril.

The agency head can lose the support of any one leg at a time and survive. However, their leadership collapses at the loss of two. The agency head should expect a very public yet unceremonious firing if this situation occurs. Professional survival, therefore, demands the ability to manage competing interests effectively. With this understanding, a crisis among first responders generally comes about in one of two ways: a single, emotionally significant event that attracts a lot of publicity (acute) or the more subdued, cumulative effect of repetitive exposure to adverse circumstances (chronic).

One of the most punishing aspects of the job occurs whenever an administrator is forced to stand before the media, community, department, and politicians to justify the agency's actions. Managing unanticipated, chaotic, and rapidly changing events that garner a lot of attention strains agency leadership, which could also intensify negativity for first responders. The actions of street-level personnel and supervisors are often harshly called into question when things go wrong. Complaints, usually premature to any official investigation, rapidly accumulate. These circumstances create the type of setting that could lead to a temporary mental health crisis for first responders.

Two notable examples are the mass school shootings in Parkland, Florida, and Uvalde, Texas. Here, an elected sheriff and an appointed police chief both faced heavy criticism from political leaders for their agency's reputedly failed response. The ensuing media attention invited the condemnation of the community, thus resulting in their removal from office. Simultaneously, first responders continued to face an avalanche of disparaging appraisals of their performance. With agency leadership in disarray, they had no one publicly supporting them.

To prevent the stool's legs from being kicked out beneath them, administrators focus on areas exerting the most pressure, sometimes at the expense of ignoring others. Also, compared to the more subdued cumulative effect of repetitive exposure to adverse circumstances, high-profile events will likely mushroom throughout a toxic social media cloud. Anonymous posters abuse first responders by directing hateful, dangerous comments toward them. Even worse, they publish the responder's home address or threaten their family, encouraging others to join the pursuit. This variation of cyber-stalking can catapult first responders to an even darker place psychologically. Conscientious leaders should never allow the mental health of first responders to lose supremacy to all the noise.

Early Lessons

Leaders have all gone through essentially the same training as other members of the organization. Yet, the actual exercise of leadership varies tremendously within departments and across agencies. So does the operational tempo, which describes the speed, intensity, and volume of events unfolding, forcing some departments to adopt a strictly reactive response. Leadership within the first responder profession often involves confusion, incomplete or inaccurate information, and fragmented communication through a hierarchal chain of command. Moreover, leaders are stretched to their limits while under tremendous political pressure to accomplish a great deal with a retrenchment in resources. This reality helps to explain why no administrator has the capacity or knowledge of everything happening across a variety of settings to make a meaningful difference in mental health. Coordinated leadership must play a vital role in reshaping public safety and reforming troublesome institutional practices.

The lesson here is not to assign or deflect blame from the mental health crisis, but rather to learn from glaring omissions of the past. Administrators have come to recognize that exposure to traumatic events carries emotional aftershocks. Clinical psychologists often discuss the symbolism of the "invisible backpack" in shining a light on the signs of someone in danger of harming themselves. The backpack is a metaphor for the pathway to PTSD awareness, suicide prevention, and intervention in behavioral problems. The expression ostensibly refers to all the stress, fears, anxiety, loss, and emotional pain a first responder carries from the impact of occupational trauma. The degree of struggle the individual experiences not only hinges on the size and weight of the backpack but what is stored inside. Early leadership lessons from in-service training or career development courses, even having a mental health component, only offered superficial guidance. Administrators should work to make the invisible backpack lighter, not heavier. Once again, the problem is defining what this undertaking actually looks like.

A Fundamental Truth

It is worth remembering that in their daily life, first responders witness the disturbing impact of childhood trauma. They see the victimization of vulnerable populations. They can share stories of homicide, suicide, traffic fatality, accidental death, and animal abuse that crush the human spirit. They can also give eyewitness accounts describing injuries so severe that no person should survive, yet somehow did, thanks in part to the intense conviction of police officers, firefighters, correctional officers, emergency medical technicians (EMTs), and dispatchers. As a special occupational group, their jobs are a true test of determination. Even when scared, they venture beyond relative safety to confront death. Consequently, their psyches are forged through hypervigilance associated with the uncertainty of dangerous, distressing, hands-on experiences. Unfortunately, one of the most important job-related truths is that up until the last decade or so, interest in mental health among first responders was unintentionally a missing component in the concerted leadership of administrators. They remained oblivious, but not indifferent, to the mental health crisis now coming into focus among first responders in the United States. In fairness, these promising leaders were not born with the knowledge of today. However, understanding that meaningful change begins with dissatisfaction over traditional, dubious outlooks and accepting the need for expert help is what separates contemporary administrators from their counterparts of the past.

A Misguided Belief

It is clearly established that first responders are not immune from what happens in the community. Often overlooked, however, is how agency leadership and customs contribute to employee mental health. If suppressed, internal conflict can be destructive and result in the loss of life. To illustrate this point, a "dirty little secret" is often defined as facts known to small groups of people, but not widely shared with others. The rationale for the secrecy is that public disclosure would, by some means, disgrace the reputation of the organization or its leadership. Suicide, for example, was not part of the broader conversation among many police chiefs, fire chiefs, or sheriffs for decades. Administrators ignored the internal and external environmental outlook of how the job affected people. Partly acknowledging the department's piece in the overall narrative of mental health could reflect poorly on agency leadership. Accordingly, administrators frequently adopted the individualistic perspective that suicide was isolated to weak individuals who slipped through the screening process. Under this rationale, an individual's personality places the blame for, or the opposition to PTSD, anxiety, depression, or suicide ideation squarely at the feet of the first responder.

Consequently, some administrators use subjective assessments to categorize these individuals as ill-suited for the job. They label them differently from other first responders. Doubts about whether these individuals can modify their persona to conform with agency expectations mean sometimes treating them as less deserving, thus placing them at an increased risk of decline in their mental state by failing to direct intervention efforts. This outlook could explain why some departments have higher rates of suicide. The clinician must understand that they might be treating an individual exposed to a traumatic event or accumulation of adverse circumstances compounded by the influence of a harmful organizational culture that leaves them feeling alienated.

For example, first responders killed in the line of duty receive a dignified burial service with full ceremonial honors. Throngs of mourners attend, usually under a heavy media presence, to express their deepest gratitude to those who faithfully served. Also, their families are entitled to lucrative survivor benefits. Conversely, first responders who die by suicide receive unceremonious, private funerals usually paid for by family members. Unfortunately, until recently, the profession regarded these individuals as an inferior subscript to those possessing greater resiliency.

Narrowly restricting the characterization of first responders as falling into one of two groups, either "able to cut it" or not, fails to acknowledge a continuum susceptible to intervention. The challenge for supervisors lies in deciding how to intervene and precisely when. The predicament arises because events with adjacent aspects, not perceptibly dissimilar from each other, can have distinctly divergent outcomes. You might even say contradictory extremes. Anytime an administrator or supervisor treats a situation as if it is nothing more than a repeat of something they have handled many times before, they risk unintended consequences that can be devastating.

A Case Study: Missed Opportunities?

While some worrisome behavior reveals itself slowly and incrementally, others are impulsive. The following case study involves police officers, firefighters, EMTs, dispatchers, and crime scene technicians. It provides unexpected insights into the role agency culture, reinforced by administrators, plays in possibly obstructing early intervention during a mental health crisis. Moreover, this case challenges or complicates existing assumptions that a first responder's troubling behavior results entirely from willful misconduct rather than the department conceivably contributing to circumstances leading up to the event.

A police officer assigned to the midnight shift calls out sick. She offers no explanation to her supervisor, and respecting her privacy, he does not ask for one. By all accounts, she is a very good officer. She has no history of poor performance or abuse of the department's sick leave policy. Disturbingly, that same night she stands in the darkness in front of her boyfriend's townhome, screaming obscenities. It is a sweltering, humid night in August. Most people are seeking relief from the heat by closing all windows and relying on central air conditioning to bring them comfort. Still, they can hear the officer yelling angrily.

In what neighbors describe as a state of rage, the officer paces back and forth across the parking lot, becoming increasingly demonstrative over her boyfriend's apparent refusal to allow her inside. She repeatedly shouts, "you killed my baby!", which remains an unsubstantiated declaration alluding to feeling pressured by her boyfriend to terminate a pregnancy under the future promise of marriage, only to be shunned by him immediately afterward.

The police officer and her boyfriend are employed by the same municipality, but he works for the fire department. Fearing that she faces disciplinary action by her employer if someone calls the police over the disturbance she is causing, he takes it upon himself to call the cell phone of a friend who works as a supervisor for the police department. This decision bypasses phone lines in the dispatch center that record every incoming and outgoing call. Otherwise, details of the incident would move out of the shadows and into the bright light of very broad public disclosure laws that anyone can access. The boyfriend's choice also allows him an opportunity to speak privately with a supervisor in the expectation that he will use his influence to discretely remedy the situation.

Because he was off-duty at the time, the friend immediately notified an on-duty police supervisor, alerting him to the situation and asking him to respond to the boyfriend's address. When he gets there, the on-duty supervisor approaches the officer. Without attempting to determine why she is so upset, he orders her to leave. He either ignores or fails to recognize that she is in the throes of a full-blown mental health crisis. Instead, he approaches the situation from a procedural standpoint, treating it like a routine domestic dispute call. However, compared to citizens requiring the assistance of the police, he seems excessively annoyed over having to deal with the questionable behavior of an off-duty officer, one apparently feigning illness, no less. Perhaps the heat is a factor.

He insists that she get into her car at once and go home. She appears defeated, if not disheartened, by his lack of empathy. The officer does not argue with the supervisor nor offer any resistance to his demands. Moreover, the tension between the two individuals suggests the lack of trust one needs before confiding in personal matters. Successful early intervention depends on establishing trust among first responders, perhaps more than anything else, and this is a posited belief worth remembering.

The officer walks away, gets into her vehicle, and drives off. The supervisor follows closely in his patrol car to ensure that she goes home. He watches her drive into the parking lot of the apartment complex where she lives, only about one-half mile from her boyfriend's home. The supervisor sees her pull into a parking space. Satisfied, he drives past her vehicle and leaves. Again, he does not attempt to speak with the officer to see if he can be of any emotional support.

In handling domestic disputes, the police routinely try to separate parties for the night as a cooling-off period to lessen the likelihood of violence. Procedurally, the supervisor accomplishes this objective. However, in the process, he disregards the deteriorating psychological state of the officer.

Now all alone, the police officer enters her apartment. She retrieves her service weapon, a semi-automatic handgun containing a fully loaded high-capacity magazine. Without hesitation, she returns to her vehicle and drives straight to her boyfriend's house. Only minutes have passed since she left. Now armed, she walks around the side of his townhome to a sliding glass door. Finding it locked and unable to see inside, she blindly fires an intense, rapid volley of bullets through the door, shattering the glass, which otherwise remains intact. Then, she crashes through the opening, propelling the broken glass forward where it scatters across the interior floor. Inside, she finds her stunned boyfriend standing just outside his kitchen. Without saying a word, she shoots him to death. Afterward, she continues her uncontrollable fit of rage, destroying items in the home and overturning furniture. Ultimately, she places her service weapon against her head and pulls the trigger. The officer completes suicide, dying only a few feet from the body of her murdered boyfriend. The violence is unrestrained, and the evidence of such is overwhelming, even for seasoned detectives and crime scene investigators. On some level, they experience their own occupational trauma that night.

A good friend visiting the boyfriend's home when the events unfolded is fortunate to survive the encounter. He provides eyewitness testimony to investigators during the ensuing administrative and criminal investigations. When the shooting began, he was seated on a couch adjacent to the glass sliding door. The initial volley of gunshots passed a couple of feet above his right shoulder just before the officer violently bursts into the room. She looks directly at him while extending her handgun, shouting, "where is he!" referring to her boyfriend. Before the frightened witness could even compose an answer, she noticed her boyfriend standing near the kitchen. She turns and shoots him numerous times. Her actions are excessive and indicative of uncontrollable emotions.

During the gunfire, the witness exploits the disorienting chaos and jumps to his feet, fleeing the home through the shattered opening. He reports that the officer gave chase with the intent to kill him as well, but he loses her in the darkness by jumping over a wooden shadow box fence, running through a neighboring backyard, and hiding underneath a row of dense shrubbery. Unable to find him, the panicked officer returns to the boyfriend's home, stands near his body, and completes suicide.

The Aftermath

When he feels sheltered enough, the witness calls 911 via his cell phone. He identifies the killer as an off-duty police officer and pleads with dispatchers for help. Although not discussed here, the witness experiences severe emotional trauma and subsequently struggles psychologically for years. Also, the first police officers responding to the scene were unaware that the offending officer had killed herself. While trying to rescue the witness, locate the officer, and render her harmless, they had to mentally prepare themselves to kill a coworker, if necessary, which is not something they ever trained for, nor ever had to carefully consider. The supervisor who confronted the officer prior to her suicide was the first person on the scene following the shooting. He did his best to perform emergency medical procedures to save both lives while awaiting the arrival of paramedics, but neither person survived. Over the course of the following year, he gradually pulled away from people, lost weight, and ultimately decided to separate from service. Thus, his law enforcement career came to an end.

Courses of Action

First responders are often under tremendous pressure to make split-second decisions. Even if time does permit, it is fleeting, not allowing the benefit of considerable deliberation. Besides, they feel that unless you stand shoulder-to-shoulder with them in the trenches, you cannot possibly understand their painful experiences. Consequently, agency culture and customs can unintentionally obstruct intervention strategies designed to improve mental health. This case study serves as a clear illustration.

To explain further, perhaps more so in policing, first responders pattern themselves after unwritten codes of conduct. Generally understood and informally accepted, these codes find their origins in needing trust or feeling misunderstood by outsiders. For example, there exists a belief that individuals should support one another, regardless of the violation of policy, unless a person's behavior is so outrageous that saving them from administrative harm is futile. Do not misinterpret this assertion as support for unethical or illegal conduct. Nothing could be farther from the truth. The desire here is to allow good people who perform admirably under very demanding conditions to make good-faith mistakes while shielding them from having supervisors unnecessarily place bad things in their personnel files. Therefore, with an eye toward steering clear of discipline rather than a concern for mental health, some employees will not report a coworker's minor misconduct to a supervisor. At the same time, supervisors have different levels of tolerance for minor misconduct. Some elect to address poor performance informally. The types of behavior can include abusing sick leave, neglecting one's appearance, pulling away from people, drinking too much off-duty, and exhibiting mood swings. All of which could signal a decline in mental health. Occasionally, the disciplinary process is a necessary precursor to managing a critical period in mental health.

This case study shows examples of culture unintentionally obstructing mental health in favor of eluding discipline. Recall that the boyfriend circumvented routine procedures for calling the police for assistance because he did not want the police officer getting into trouble for her behavior. Simultaneously, the on-duty supervisor ignored the officer's violation of agency standards of conduct governing off-duty behavior and the possibility that she may have feigned illness to avoid reporting for her assigned shift. At the very least, both circumstances warranted a conversation that never took place. In addition, the state where this murder-suicide occurred has a mental health law known as the Baker Act. This law grants law enforcement officers the authority to take a person into protective custody for a mental health evaluation if the individual exhibits signs that they might be a danger to themselves or others. Using this law for a first responder in a severe crisis could be lifesaving, but also career-ending, which some individuals perceive as discipline. Therefore, it seems rarely used.

In transforming agency culture, administrators are responsible for developing in-service training programs to educate employees and help them understand the consequences of repeated exposure to trauma. They must prepare supervisors to confront the dilemmas inherent in their work so they are not immune from the signs of declining mental health. Otherwise, employees could have a distorted view that discourages them from seeking help because they conflate intervention with discipline.

Until this tragedy, the chief did not fully grasp the conceivability of the work setting contributing to poor mental health. This suicide caused an incremental shift from the former individualistic perspective dominating professional outlooks on suicide toward the environmental perspective. This case also marks the first widespread use of crisis response teams within all the city's public safety sectors. Sadly, the teams never reached the two people who would have benefited the most.

Crisis Response Teams

When this murder-suicide occurred, crisis response teams (CRTs) were just gaining traction. Training at the time focused more on taking armed, barricaded subjects into custody and peacefully ending hostage situations as opposed to helping employees in crisis. Thanks to the dedication and talent of a licensed clinical psychologist providing in-house CRT training to the department, that same night, teams deployed across the city and around the clock to provide urgent mental health counseling to employees.

This event signaled a considerable shift in the evolution of CRT. Not only were teams responding to mental illness calls and decriminalizing the conduct of citizens in crisis, but they also activated along with SWAT for barricaded subjects. Perhaps more importantly, they expanded their role internally to ensure a quick response in providing psychological first aid to employees, thus preventing an emotional descent.

Years later, in Parkland, Florida, a police officer entered a high school in response to a mass shooting in search of the killer, whose whereabouts were unknown at the time. His primary mission was to quickly move through the building's classrooms to locate the killer and render him harmless or risk even more death (17 students and teachers killed, another 17 critically injured). In speaking with the officer the following morning, he sadly said, "I don't get paid enough to step over the bodies of dead and dying children!" The exigency of having to ignore the pleas of children with gunshot wounds begging for help was antithetical to his values, leading to conflicting feelings of regret. Mainly because, at that moment, the children could not possibly understand the importance of his mission to save lives. He worried that for the rest of their lives, the children would remember feeling abandoned or neglected by him when they needed a rescuer.

What a powerful indicator of the trauma the officer experienced, not to mention the inner turmoil and guilt he was feeling. In all the subsequent unrelenting media coverage and harsh criticism of the primary agency's response, administrators prioritized assembling crisis response teams. They did not forget the emotional needs of this officer and the other first responders.

The primary role of administrators in the development of crisis response teams is to embrace the experts and seasoned employees, providing them with the unbridled discretion to identify the right people for the team. Rank has no place here, only skills. Collaboration should gain supremacy over any need to control. While a competent administrator may be called upon to serve as an incident commander, the crisis team leader establishes roles and responsibilities. If necessary, administrators should help the team navigate the political environment to receive the required funding, equipment, and training.

Case Study Two: A Partial Win?

The mother of two teenage children develops a friendly relationship with an employee at her local grocery store. Unknown to her at the time is that the man wants a romantic relationship. More frightening is that he is developing an unhealthy enthusiasm toward her. He subsequently begins to stalk her.

One afternoon he makes an unannounced visit to her home. Both children and the mother's boyfriend are present. Her son answers the door. Without an invitation to come inside, the man enters the house and begins searching for the mother. Sensing danger, the mother immediately grabs her car keys and tells the man that she wants to speak with him privately outside. Her children and boyfriend appear confused. This request is a ruse to get the man out of the home and away from her children. Once outside, the mother jumps into her car and drives off, hoping to lure the man further away. Her plan works. He enters his vehicle and gives chase. The mother's boyfriend also jumps into his car to follow the pair, but it fails to start, leaving him helpless.

The mother immediately calls 911, screaming for help and asking for directions to the police department, which is located only a few blocks away. The dispatcher tells the mother to calm down so she can help, then switches to speaking Spanish, the mother's first language. Unable to gather essential information in time, the dispatcher never puts the emergency call out over the police radio. No one knows that the mother is inbound with a stalker in pursuit.

With no assistance from the dispatcher, the mother finds her way to the police department. She pulls up to a locked gate preventing access into a parking lot reserved for police department personnel only. The stalker is pulling in right behind her. Finding herself boxed in, she leaps from the parked car to run just as the suspect intentionally rams her vehicle from behind. The impact propels her vehicle forward, causing the open driver's side door to spring backward, violently close, and knock her to the ground. This move allows the stalker enough time to exit his vehicle and advance on the mother. Just as she scrambles to her feet, the stalker shoots her for the first time, striking her in the back. Although badly wounded, the mother stays on her feet and runs toward the front door of the police department.

The main entrance of the police department is shaped in a semi-circle constructed of impact-resistant hurricane glass. This design allows for excellent visibility from the lobby to the outside. Fortuitously, a female police officer has stopped by the station on a meal break when she witnesses a man with a gun pursuing a woman. Her observations are all the information she has at that instant. The officer is then captured on surveillance cameras inside the building, running parallel to the man on the outside, with only the high-impact glass separating the two. The panicking mother, with the stalker close behind, runs past the front doors of the police department just as the police officer exits. Observing the man possessing a firearm, the officer draws her service weapon while she is still running and immediately launches a short burst of gunfire at the stalker. To put the high degree of difficulty for the shot into perspective the officer was trying to acquire a moving target in very close proximity to an innocent person that she must not hit, while all three were at a full run.

All the officer's bullets miss their intended target. Almost simultaneously, the man overtakes the mother and shoots her to death. Looking at the officer, he then turns the gun on himself, completing suicide. Everything instantly fell quiet. In disbelief, the police officer found herself alone, staring down at the bodies of the deceased. A total of 94 seconds elapsed from the moment the mother connected with the dispatcher until she was dead…94 seconds!

The recording of the mother's 911 call was released to the media through a public records request, and it garnered international attention for several reasons. First, listeners grew incensed by the tone the dispatcher took while speaking with the mother in trying to take control of the call so that she could quickly obtain essential information. People were also upset with the dispatcher for not alerting police officers to the danger the mother was facing.

Next, the police officer faced condemnation because her bullets missed the stalker, thus failing to save the mother's life. None of her fiercest critics ever considered how badly she was beating up on herself. Ironically, had the officers' rounds found their mark, people would be praising her courage and awarding her a medal. Although the outcome was not the one desired, the police officer demonstrated professionalism and courage in the face of extreme danger.

Both the dispatcher and the police officer experienced severe emotional trauma from this single, acute event that attracted considerable attention. Moreover, they received death threats over their reputedly failed response. Afterward, they shared that the incident kept replaying, looping over and over in their minds. Once again, crisis response team members were called in to assist.

In the end, the dispatcher separated from service. The police officer became more withdrawn. A couple of years later, the police officer violated the public's trust by breaking the law. Arrested, prosecuted, convicted, and sentenced, she lost her career. Questions swirled over whether psychological trauma contributed to her moral collapse.

Although suicide prevention remains the ultimate goal in crisis intervention, these case studies illustrate that even though someone survives trauma they emerge forever transformed. They no longer engage the world in the same way but rather live in a memory.

Advice for Clinicians

A department's organizational culture is an important consideration for clinicians, either training crisis response teams or treating personnel. Be mindful, however, that in addition to saving lives, agencies are concerned with reputation management. An administrator is likely to assess whether the clinician is devoted to promoting positive mental health or loyal to supporting the principles of either side in a conflict. Therefore, the practitioner must maintain neutrality in any disagreement where the lines of distinction blur between individual behavior and the contribution the agency makes to poor mental health. It is logical to presume that clinicians functioning with independence are more likely to earn the requisite unwavering trust of administrators and line-level personnel. That is to say that they do not involve themselves in office politics. Central to developing trust, beyond demonstrating neutrality, is convincing first responders that the clinician has an acute understanding of their painful experiences. Otherwise, for example, why would a physicist discuss String Theory with someone who cannot possibly understand the dynamics?

Historically, administrators have been slow to work in conjunction with mental health professionals to accumulate the occupational and scientific knowledge necessary for crisis intervention, which has far-reaching consequences. First, research is not widely shared outside of academia resulting in limited public awareness by leaders. PTSD, alcohol/drug abuse, and suicide are complex problems resulting from multiple factors across a variety of settings. Moreover, there is a convoluted interplay between individual traits, occupational stressors, and organizational influences. Administrators, therefore, find themselves unable to disentangle the relevance of each. They grapple with finding cures.

Next, there remain occupational outlooks supporting opposition to mandating mental health counseling, mainly through labor unions, because of the apprehensions associated with accessing care. A prevailing misguided belief is that acknowledging the need for care is to risk one's continued fitness for duty. The horrors witnessed by first responders are occupational hazards, not psychological defects. Thankfully, this antiquated outlook is changing through trust, which is coming about by transforming agency culture. Finally, the most destructive consequence of failing to clearly trace the connection between mental health and being a better first responder is suicide.

Summary

The goal of leaders within the first responder profession is to become acutely aware of their responsibilities and devote the agency to psychological well-being. More importantly, it involves connecting individuals who may be incapable of recognizing for themselves that they need care with someone who can provide it. In short, the role of administrators demands a quick response in providing psychological first aid to prevent an emotional descent. These leaders must prioritize the critical issues surrounding mental health while facilitating posttraumatic, transformative growth that might save a life. To accomplish this goal, administrators must re-imagine organizational culture in favor of endorsing and encouraging programs where individuals receive care from someone who understands their experiences.

References

Hawton, K., & Pirkis, J. (2017). Suicide is a complex problem that requires a range of prevention initiatives and methods of evaluation. *British Journal of Psychiatry, 210*(6), 381–383. https://doi.org/10.1192/bjp.bp.116.197459

Schein, E. H. (2010). *Organizational culture and leadership* (4th ed.). Jossey-Bass.

Tiesman, H., Elkins, K. L., Brown, M., Marsh, S., & Carson, L. M. (2021). *Suicide among first responders: A call to action!* Centers for Disease Control and Prevention. https://blogs.cdc.gov/niosh-science-blog/2021/04/06/suicides-first-responders/

Mental Health of Women First Responders: Clinical Considerations

Shelby J. McGrew, Carrington Slaughter, Jana K. Tran, Sam J. Buser, and Anka A. Vujanovic

Women first responders are an understudied population as they comprise a relative gender minority across various first responder roles. The vast majority of first responders, including police, law enforcement, firefighters, paramedics, and emergency medical technicians (EMTs) identify as cis-gender men and the profession has been predominantly characterized by traditionally masculine gender norms (Jones et al., 2020; Pasciak & Kelley, 2013). Recent data from The National Fire and Protection Association (2019) suggests that of the 1,085,800 career and volunteer firefighters in the United States, 88,000 (8%) identified as women. Further, the U.S. Department of Justice (2017) indicates that 12.5% of full-time police officers identified as women. With regard to emergency medical technicians (EMTs), the proportion of women earning EMT certification grew from 28% in 2008 to 35% in 2017 (Crowe et al., 2020).

Despite these data, there is limited empirical research explicitly focusing on women first responders. We acknowledge that gender identity is nonbinary and fluid and that first responders are comprised of individuals who may or may not identify with their assigned sex at birth. We intentionally focus this chapter on women while underscoring the importance of expanding our definitions of gender in first responder

S. J. McGrew (✉) · A. A. Vujanovic
University of Houston, Houston, TX, USA

Texas A&M University, College Station, TX, USA
e-mail: smcgrew@tamu.edu; avujanovic@tamu.edu

C. Slaughter
University of Houston, Houston, TX, USA

J. K. Tran
National Aeronautics and Space Administration, Houston, TX, USA

S. J. Buser
Houston Fire Department (Retired), Houston, TX, USA

M. L. Bourke et al. (eds.), *First Responder Mental Health*,
https://doi.org/10.1007/978-3-031-38149-2_24

communities to envelop the more inclusive spectrum (e.g., transgender, nonbinary, agender, gender-expansive). Presently, our understanding of the needs of first responders who identify with more minoritized gender identities is empirically not well-established and may not be clinically assessed or acknowledged in workplaces, highlighting an important gap in our knowledge and practice.

Mental Health

The mental health of women first responders is an important and growing public health issue. There is a dearth of epidemiological research available to characterize the mental health of women first responders using generalizable, nationally representative samples. We review available literature with the caveat that prevalence rates of mental health conditions vary based on study methodologies and sample sizes. In the mental health realm, the most attention has been devoted to outcomes associated with occupational stress and exposure to potentially traumatic events, which are chronic for many first responder populations.

Occupational Stress and Exposure to Potentially Traumatic Events

Patterns of occupational stress may differ between men and women first responders. Generally, first responders' work-related stressors may involve a range of potentially traumatic events as well as chronic job stressors, such as shift work, sleep disturbance, and unpredictability (Bergen-Cico et al., 2015; Regambal et al., 2015). Indeed, Hartley et al. (2013) found that 27% of women police officers in their sample reported experiencing a potentially traumatic event in the last month. Exposure to potentially traumatic events (e.g., violent crimes, medical injuries, suicide attempts, child abuse) predicts burnout among men and women police officers (McCarty & Garland, 2007). Firefighters and EMTs also may encounter potentially traumatic events as part of their jobs (e.g., line of duty deaths, medical injuries, fire suppression), and women firefighters may provide more distanced and abstracted accounts when discussing critical work events compared to men who provide more "macabre" accounts (Jacobsson et al., 2015, p. 102). Notably, there are a number of issues women first responders may encounter that could uniquely contribute to this stress, including gender discrimination and sexual harassment, which are commonly reported by women first responders (Jahnke et al., 2019). Research on these topics will be discussed in detail later in this chapter.

Posttraumatic Stress Disorder (PTSD)

Compared to men firefighters, women may be at increased risk for PTSD, with approximately 20% of women firefighters reporting elevated PTSD symptoms (Noor et al., 2019). Research focusing on PTSD among women police officers varies; some studies suggest women and men police officers report similar rates of PTSD (Ballenger et al., 2011; Pole et al., 2001), while others suggest women police officers evince higher rates (Bowler et al., 2012). Women civilians may report higher rates of PTSD compared to women police officers (Lilly et al., 2009). This may be due to under-reporting among law enforcement personnel potentially due to the nature of police culture and/or police training (Burke et al., 2006) which might translate to blunted emotional reactions to life-threatening duty-related experiences (Violanti et al., 2017). Notably, empirical research focusing on women emergency medical service (EMS) workers is particularly limited. Extant work among samples from Switzerland and South Africa suggests women EMS workers, compared to men, may be at a greater risk for PTSD (Soravia et al., 2021; Ntatamala & Adams, 2022).

Suicide Ideation and Behavior

Deaths by suicide among first responders, primarily law enforcement officers and firefighters, have risen to levels higher than the general population and may outpace the prevalence of line-of-duty deaths (Heyman et al., 2018). Thus, it is important to advance epidemiological work focused on suicide among women first responders. Available research indicates suicidal ideation may occur at increased rates among women first responders (Stanley et al., 2017a, b). Specifically, women firefighters and police officers may be at an increased risk for suicidal ideation compared to their men counterparts (Noor et al., 2019; Violanti et al., 2009). For example, women firefighters demonstrate high pre-career and career rates of suicidal ideation (28.4%; 37.7%), plans (10.2%; 10.9%), and attempts (11.2%; 9.3%) (Stanley et al., 2017a, b). Among police from a midsized, urban police department, the lifetime prevalence of suicidal thoughts was 25% for women and 23.1% for men (Violanti et al., 2009). It has been suggested that women officers may be more likely to die by suicide than women in the general population (Violanti & Steege, 2020). Work focusing on women EMTs in the U.S. is particularly understudied, but Sterud et al. (2008) estimated that among a sample of Norwegian ambulance workers, 32.4% of women reported the lifetime prevalence of feeling life was not worth living.

Depression

Women police officers often report higher levels of depressive symptoms compared to their men counterparts (Darensburg et al., 2006). Data collected from police officers (21% women) in Oregon and southwest Washington suggest women reported greater levels of burnout (i.e., physical, emotional, and/or mental exhaustion) than men. Women officers with high levels of burnout reported greater depression symptoms (Elliot et al., 2015). Further, Jahnke et al. (2012) found that depression among women firefighters (n = 38) was more prevalent than among community women (22% vs. 10.1%). Findings on EMTs are mixed, with some work suggesting similar rates of depression among men and women (Bennett et al., 2004) and other work positing lower levels among women (Bentley et al., 2013).

Anxiety

Women police officers may be more vulnerable to anxiety and stress-related pathology compared to men officers (Acquadro Maran et al., 2015; Husain, 2014). Research among a primarily women-identifying sample of police officers has demonstrated that anxiety-related pathology is an important factor involved in PTSD symptomatology (e.g., Asmundson & Stapleton, 2008). Stanley et al. (2017a, b) found anxiety pathology is a predictor of PTSD symptomatology and suicide risk among women firefighters. Regarding EMS personnel, women report similar levels of anxiety as men (Bennett et al., 2004), but empirical work is limited. Taken together, there is a very small body of research examining anxiety among women who serve as first responders.

Alcohol Use

In the police and fire services, alcohol is a socially accepted method of building camaraderie and coping with stress, trauma, and sleep disturbance (FEMA, 2019). Research among women police officers has found that they report drinking at similar rates as their men counterparts, but significantly more than women in the civilian population (Ballenger et al., 2011). Younger women officers may be at an elevated risk for hazardous drinking, characterized by a pattern of alcohol consumption that may exacerbate the risk for adverse health events, compared to older women officers (Violanti et al., 2011). A 3-year longitudinal investigation of firefighters revealed that although men reported higher rates of binge drinking (i.e., greater than four drinks for women and five for men in a 2-hour period) initially, binge drinking among women increased over time such that a greater percentage of women (compared to men) firefighters met criteria for problem drinking by the first year (Gulliver et al., 2019). In a sample of Norwegian ambulance personnel, Sterud and colleagues (2007) found that 16.8% of men and 7.4% of women reported hazardous drinking. Results demonstrated that men and women ambulance personnel may drink to cope with negative emotions at similar rates.

Unique Occupational Stressors

The occupational demands of first responders are not unique to women, as they do the same jobs and are exposed to the same stressors as their male counterparts (FEMA, 2019). For example, providing public safety requires 24-hour coverage, so all first responders experience the mental and physical burden of shift work and the resulting sleep deprivation. However, women first responders also face the challenge of navigating a potentially hostile working environment, as the police and fire service are male-dominated and have a hyper-masculine culture that promotes negative attitudes toward women (FEMA, 2019). Gender-based discrimination and harassment are unique and salient job stressors that are encountered by women first responders (FEMA, 2019).

Gender Discrimination

Women first responders are at an elevated risk for gender-based discrimination in their work environment. Somvadee and Morash (2008) found that an alarming number of women police officers experience gender harassment, with 69.2% reporting being treated differently than men officers and over half (53.8%) experiencing perceived condescension due to their gender. Women police officers are routinely viewed as being less competent than men police officers, leading to women feeling the need to prove themselves on the job (Angehrn et al., 2022). Additionally, women police officers must deal with the gendered assignment of duties; for example, women may be excluded from frontline calls, which require physical strength, yet are selected for sexual assault cases, which require listening skills (Angehrn et al., 2022). Research has demonstrated that among a sample of primarily women EMS providers (96%), 83% reported some form of discrimination or harassment and 33% endorsed receiving unequal recognition because of gender (Staats et al., 2021). According to the National Report Card on Women in Firefighting (Hulett et al., 2008), 84.7% of women firefighters reported being treated differently because of their gender, and 50.8% reported incidences of shunning and isolation. Among a large sample of women firefighters, over 40% reported feeling the need to work twice as hard as others to get equal treatment as men firefighters and being watched more closely while performing job-related duties due to their gender (Jahnke et al., 2019). Indeed, there is a "glass ceiling" for women in the fire department, with

36.5% reporting gender barriers related to promotion and advancement (Hulett et al., 2008).

Fire stations were traditionally built for only men and few have been updated to accommodate a diversifying workforce. Thus, women might have to share bathrooms, showers, and sleeping quarters with their men counterparts (Hulett et al., 2008). Approximately 46.2% of women firefighters reported problems related to lacking privacy while changing, showering, and using the restroom while on shift (Hulett et al., 2008). Many fire departments have failed to renovate or even make minor changes, such as adding privacy curtains, thereby sending women the message that they are not full-time, permanent members of the department and their needs and preferences are not important (Hulett et al., 2008).

Additionally, 80% of women firefighters endorsed problems related to ill-fitting gear, (FEMA, 2019; Hulett et al., 2008). Some captains and chair officers may buy gear designed for men and expect women to "adapt," while others may "miss" the opportunity to enhance inclusivity in the fire service by ensuring that all equipment is appropriately fitted and available for firefighters of all genders and sizes. It is imperative that personal protective gear properly fits to minimize the risk of injury (McQuerry et al., 2019). Traditional firefighter gear was designed for a man's body; and it has been suggested that simply resizing gear to be shorter or smaller is an ineffective solution as it does not accommodate the differing proportions of women's silhouettes (McQuerry et al., 2019). Ill-fitting gear creates gaps that increase the risk of thermal and chemical exposure, as well as bulkiness that causes decreased mobility and physical discomfort, particularly in the chest and hip regions (McQuerry et al., 2019).

Harassment

Among women police officers, researchers have found that more than half (58.2%) endorse being a victim of sexual harassment, which may be broadly defined as unwelcome sexual advances, requests for sexual favors, and verbal or physical conduct of a sexual nature (Somvadee & Morash, 2008). Approximately 51% indicated being harassed by men officers with sexist remarks, and 36.7% reported being a victim of unwelcome touching (Somvadee & Morash, 2008). Among a large sample of EMS providers in South Korea, women endorsed significantly greater rates of sexual harassment (28.1%) compared to their men counterparts (5.6%; Yoo et al., 2019).

With regard to women firefighters, Jahnke et al. (2019) found that, among a sample of 1773 firefighters, more than a third reported being verbally harassed while at work. In the same sample, nearly 40% reported being sexually harassed, 12.9% reported being harassed via written means, 16% reported hazing, and 5.1% reported being assaulted while working as a firefighter due to their gender. Historically, fire departments operated with an all-male staff, resulting in a "fraternity-like" atmosphere in which sexual conversations and pornography were commonplace at fire stations (Hulett et al., 2008). Although many fire departments have shifted to a more professional atmosphere, undertones of the original culture persist (Hulett et al., 2008). For example, firefighters often engage in hazing and practical jokes, which are traditionally intended to build rapport among crews (Hulett et al., 2008). However, pranks against women often involve sexist content and might be perceived or intended as a form of intimidation intended to drive them out of the fire service (Hulett et al., 2008). These include pornography and sexually-related messages left in lockers, as well as life-threatening pranks at fires, such as cutting off the water supply (Hulett et al., 2008). Women firefighters also report a general expectation to date or have sex with their fellow firefighters in order to remain crew members (Hulett et al., 2008). Women first responders may experience difficulties establishing professional reputations, and rumors of sexual affairs lead to being further ostracized (Angehrn et al., 2022). As a result, women first responders may file lawsuits or become involved in litigation about sexual harassment in the workplace; such lawsuits can have significant detrimental effects on women's mental health and professional development potentially resulting in disempowerment due to the typically slow and expensive legal processes involved in such legal proceedings.

Barriers to Reporting Discrimination and Harassment

Women first responders often choose not to file an official complaint because the process can be overwhelming or distressing; being asked to repeatedly recount the experience might be psychologically traumatizing (Angehrn et al., 2022). Other women may opt not to report due to fear of losing their job, being further ostracized (e.g., labeled as a "troublemaker"), being retaliated against (e.g., forced to transfer), and/or not being believed (Angehrn et al., 2022; FEMA, 2019; Hulett et al., 2008). Police and fire departments' internal procedures should be regularly reviewed to ensure that policies and procedures are in place for addressing complaints and that any complaints brought forward are not overlooked or dismissed without due diligence (FEMA, 2019). Surveys of women firefighters have found that approximately 65% of women firefighters reported that their department has no procedures that they were aware of for addressing such complaints, and 23.4% endorsed that their supervisors failed to act when gender-related problems were reported to them (Hulett et al., 2008). Women first responders tend to handle situations of discrimination or harassment independently or with the support of mentors, unless the problem is severe, in which they may be more likely to trust outside agencies (e.g., Equal Employment Opportunity Commission, EEOC) than their own department (Hulett et al., 2008).

Other Occupational Demands: Pregnancy and Motherhood

Women first responders experience additional job stressors that are unique to their gender. For example, the work environment can potentially be harmful to women who become pregnant while working as emergency responders. Firefighters, for example, are exposed to fires, toxins, and high temperatures; shift work and physical strain also contribute to reproductive risk (Jahnke et al., 2018). Approximately 27% of firefighter pregnancies result in miscarriage, which is two times higher than the general population (Jahnke et al., 2018). There is a lack of work focusing on the potential reasons for this elevated risk. However, working night shifts and heavy lifting, as well as exposure to environmental toxins in the occupational environment, are characteristic of many first responder roles and have been related to increased risk of miscarriage (Feodor Nilsson et al., 2014; Wong et al., 2009). Moreover, policies related to pregnancy are often poor or may be completely lacking. In a national sample of firefighters, nearly a quarter reported that their department had no policies related to pregnancy or maternity leave (Jahnke et al., 2018). Thus, fire departments should evaluate and develop policies regarding pregnancy that are evidence-based and grounded in best practice guidelines.

Similarly, it is estimated that 20% of police departments do not have policies for maternity leave (Rabe-Hemp & Humiston, 2015). The most common accommodation for pregnant first responders is to remove them from active duty and assign them to desk work, sometimes without their request (Langan et al., 2019). Women should be empowered to request health-related accommodations for pregnancy, as with any health condition, with guidance from their medical providers. First responder departments should move away from imposing general "blanket" policies on women due to health conditions such as pregnancy. Empowering women to take responsibility for their health and bodies with appropriate authorization from their medical providers would provide a more first responder-centric approach.

Notably, removing pregnant women from active duty renders crews/units "short a body," thereby framing pregnancy as a liability to others and fostering feelings of guilt and shame (Angehrn et al., 2022; Langan et al., 2019). In addition, such policies might communicate a message that pregnant women are no longer able to perform their job (Langan et al., 2019). Although some women first responders do not contest light duty, many women resist, because this type of work is typically denigrated in first responder culture (Langan et al., 2019). As such, women first responders are likely to delay disclosing their pregnancies to their departments, meaning they are actively running calls during their first or second trimester of pregnancy (Jahnke et al., 2018; Langan et al., 2019). Shifting the responsibility to pregnant women and their healthcare providers might provide a solution to some of these issues, but larger-scale policy reform might be warranted to provide more detailed guidance that balances health and safety standards with individual health decision-making and autonomy.

The stigma and challenges women first responders face extend beyond pregnancy into motherhood and are similar to those encountered by other mothers who work outside the home, (Dequilla, 2018). For nursing mothers, for example, department policies regarding pumping breaks and private accommodations (e.g., lactation rooms) are severely lacking (Dequilla, 2018). First responder departments should evaluate their policies and designate spaces for lactation rooms, if possible. First responder mothers in a male-dominated organizational culture may also feel uncomfortable storing pumped milk alongside other's personal items in the community refrigerator (Dequilla, 2018). Personal mini-refrigerators might be available for this purpose. Furthermore, it is difficult for women first responders to pump on a regular schedule, as emergency calls occur unexpectedly and can last for hours at a time (Dequilla, 2018). If possible, women first responders who are nursing in the acute months following delivery may request temporary duty changes or shift schedule changes if recommended by their medical providers; such medical guidance might be shared with leadership to inform policy more broadly. Additionally, women firefighters are concerned that the chemicals in the fire environment may be transferred to the infant during breastfeeding (Solle et al., 2021). Since some of these issues are specific to the fire service profession, women first responders are encouraged to discuss safety issues with healthcare providers (e.g., exposure to chemicals while breastfeeding, and irregular pumping schedules).

Securing childcare is also a unique challenge due to shift work. Firefighters, for example, work 24-, 48-, or even 72-hour shifts, which renders reliable childcare arrangements to be exceedingly difficult to arrange, particularly if the first responders are single parents or married to another firefighter (Dequilla, 2018). Being away from family for long periods of time is an additional stressor (Dequilla, 2018). Moreover, women first responders may not get adequate sleep while on duty, and upon returning home after a shift, they must stay awake to care for their children or attend social activities, as women – even those who work outside the home – tend to be primary caregivers (Watkins et al., 2021). Chronic sleep deprivation, coupled with managing work-related trauma, may lead to difficulty being present and providing the full level of care first responder mothers want to give their children (Dequilla, 2018). Spouses and partners of first responders often encourage them to nap or have personal time after a shift, as it is preferred that they be more present with the family (Watkins et al., 2021).

Clinical Considerations

Although women first responders are at increased risk for behavioral health problems, there are multiple barriers to seeking treatment. First and foremost, first responder culture values strength and self-reliance, thereby creating a stigma related to disclosing psychological distress and seeking mental health services (Jetelina et al., 2020; Vujanovic & Tran, 2021). First responders tend to refrain from sharing personal problems even with their peers, as it is often viewed as a vulnerability (Jones et al., 2018). Given the dangerous nature of their job, such disclosures at work may lead peers to question their personal safety (Jones et al., 2018).

Additionally, fear of career repercussions may impact disclosure, as having a mental health diagnosis could lead to being considered unfit for duty (Jetelina et al., 2020). Another barrier to treatment is access to care. Many first responder departments, particularly smaller departments in rural settings, do not offer mental health services (Gulliver et al., 2019). Even if there are mental health professionals on staff, first responders may be distrusting of psychological services, and there are significant concerns about a potential breach of confidentiality within the department (Jetelina et al., 2020). As such, first responders may be more likely to seek private professional services outside of the department (Gulliver et al., 2019). Issues with access to mental health care are therefore not unique to women first responders but are shared across most first responders nationally.

Alongside the aforementioned sense of mistrust, women first responders may doubt that mental health professionals understand their line of work (Jetelina et al., 2020; Jones et al., 2018). Among a large sample of professional firefighters, "clinicians who understand firefighter work culture" was rated as the most important component of an effective behavioral health program (Gulliver et al., 2019). As such, it is critical for clinicians working with this unique population to be competent regarding fire culture (Jones et al., 2018; Vujanovic & Tran, 2021). Interventions not only need to be tailored to meet the needs of first responders (e.g., trauma-informed therapy), but they also must address the nuances of women's experiences in their profession (Jones et al., 2018). For example, clinicians must assess all sources of trauma and stress (e,g., work-related critical incidents, sexual trauma, and history of interpersonal violence). Clinicians also need to be prepared to work with victims of sexual harassment exhibiting symptoms of PTSD. Although it has been argued that sexual harassment does not constitute an index trauma, Avina and O'Donohue (2002) contend that many forms of sexual harassment meet the diagnostic criteria for PTSD. Additionally, clinicians should validate that women first responders may not feel comfortable confronting their harasser(s) or notifying their supervisor(s) (FEMA, 2019). For those who choose to file a formal complaint, clinicians should carefully document this complaint and be prepared to interact with the EEOC and attorneys (FEMA, 2019).

Lack of mental health care may also be attributed to women first responders' difficulties in identifying when they are experiencing a mental health problem (Jetelina et al., 2020). First responders may not know the signs and symptoms of psychological disorders or how to identify when help is necessary (Jones et al., 2018). Such knowledge deficits can be addressed with tailored education programs (Jones et al., 2018). Mental health professionals may deem it necessary for these mental health education programs to be delivered by a mental health expert (Jones et al., 2018). However, first responders may prefer that they be led by an "insider," such as a peer or retiree (Jones et al., 2018).

Indeed, first responder departments have taken the initiative in creating peer support programs, which engage a mental health professional to provide ongoing training and oversee the services provided (FEMA, 2019; Milliard, 2020). Peers are trained to recognize signs of mental health problems and provide an empathic “listening ear,” as they are able to relate to their colleagues’ experiences in the line of duty (Jones et al., 2018; Milliard, 2020). One of the primary goals of peer support programs is to identify individuals who are in psychological distress or crisis and connect them with professional help (Milliard, 2020). Mental health professionals who oversee peer responder teams need to ensure that members are trained on the unique factors facing women first responders (FEMA, 2019). Members should be chosen with careso women feel comfortable approaching them for support, so women are represented in peer support programs (FEMA, 2019). Finally, peers need to ensure conversations are free from judgment and that private information is not shared; otherwise, their services may not be readily used by women first responders, particularly those dealing with gender-related discrimination and harassment, due to apprehensions about confidentiality (Jones et al., 2018; Milliard, 2020).

Future Directions

Despite the growing number of women first responders, small sample sizes often lead to their elimination from research studies (FEMA, 2019). As such, information regarding mental health problems and occupational stressors unique to this population is generally lacking. Furthermore, it is imperative to include issues of intersectionality in first responder work (e.g., women first responders who identify as racial or ethnic minorities) to begin to understand the unique needs of these individuals and to bolster diversity, equity, and inclusion initiatives in first responder organizations, broadly. Thus, future research must increase the representation of diverse women in the study of first responders.

Research should focus on the development of interventions focused on addressing the presenting concerns specific to women first responders. Specifically, treatments tailored for trauma-related symptoms, broadly, as well as PTSD, depression, alcohol use, and sleep disturbance may be helpful. Women first responders also need psychological support in balancing their careers and family and in dealing with gender-based discrimination and sexual harassment (Angehrn et al., 2022). Research on the impact of sexism in the workplace is severely lacking, although some studies suggest negative outcomes on women first responders’ mental health, job satisfaction, and job retention (FEMA, 2019; Hom et al., 2017). To bolster the effectiveness of interventions, these issues should be directly addressed. Moreover, first responder departments should create initiatives to increase women’s physical and mental well-being by fostering cultural and organizational changes to eliminate sexism from the top down (Angehrn et al., 2022).

References

Acquadro Maran, D., Varetto, A., Zedda, M., & Leraci, V. (2015). Occupational stress, anxiety and coping strategies in police officers. *Occupational Medicine, 65*(6), 466–473.

Angehrn, A., Vig, K. D., Mason, J. E., Stelnicki, A. M., Shields, R. E., Asmundson, G. J., & Carleton, R. N. (2022). Sex differences in mental disorder symptoms among Canadian police officers: The mediating role of social support, stress, and sleep quality. *Cognitive Behaviour Therapy, 51*(1), 3–20.

Asmundson, G. J., & Stapleton, J. A. (2008). Associations between dimensions of anxiety sensitivity and PTSD symptom clusters in active-duty police officers. *Cognitive Behaviour Therapy, 37*(2), 66–75.

Avina, C., & O'Donohue, W. (2002). Sexual harassment and PTSD: Is sexual harassment diagnosable trauma? *Journal of Traumatic Stress, 15*(1), 69–75.

Ballenger, J. F., Best, S. R., Metzler, T. J., Wasserman, D. A., Mohr, D. C., Liberman, A., et al. (2011). Patterns and predictors of alcohol use in male and female urban police officers. *The American Journal on Addictions, 20*(1), 21–29.

Bennett, P., Williams, Y., Page, N., Hood, K., & Woollard, M. (2004). Levels of mental health problems among UK emergency ambulance workers. *Emergency Medicine Journal, 21*(2), 235–236.

Bentley, M. A., Crawford, J. M., Wilkins, J. R., Fernandez, A. R., & Studnek, J. R. (2013). An assessment of depression, anxiety, and stress among nationally certified EMS professionals. *Prehospital Emergency Care, 17*(3), 330–338.

Bergen-Cico, D., Lane, S., Thompson, M., Wozny, S., Zajdel, M., Barduhn, M., & Noce, J. (2015). The impact of post-traumatic stress on first responders: Analysis of cortisol, anxiety, depression, sleep impairment and pain. *International Paramedic Practice, 5*(3), 78–87.

Bowler, R. M., Harris, M., Li, J., Gocheva, V., Stellman, S. D., Wilson, K., et al. (2012). Longitudinal mental health impact among police responders to the 9/11 terrorist attack. *American Journal of Industrial Medicine, 55*(4), 297–312.

Burke, R. J., Richardsen, A. M., & Martinussen, M. (2006). Gender differences in policing: Reasons for optimism? *Policing: An International Journal of Police Strategies & Management, 29*(3), 513–523.

Crowe, R. P., Krebs, W., Cash, R. E., Rivard, M. K., Lincoln, E. W., & Panchal, A. R. (2020). Females and minority racial/ethnic groups remain underrepresented in emergency medical services: A ten-year assessment, 2008–2017. *Prehospital Emergency Care, 24*(2), 180–187.

Darensburg, T., Andrew, M. E., Hartley, T. A., Burchfiel, C. M., Fekedulegn, D., & Violanti, J. M. (2006). Gender and age differences in posttraumatic stress disorder and depression among Buffalo police officers. *Traumatology, 12*(3), 220–228.

Dequilla, L. Y. (2018). *Firefighter mothers and social support: Fighting the fires around work-life balance* [Theses and Dissertations]. 943. https://digitalcommons.pepperdine.edu/etd/943

Elliot, D., Garg, B., Kuehl, K., DeFrancesco, C., & Sleigh, A. (2015). Why are women law enforcement officers more burned-out and what might help them? *Occupational Medicine & Health Affairs, 3*(3), 204.

Federal Bureau of Investigation (2017). *Table 74: Full-time Law Enforcement Employees*. https://ucr.fbi.gov/crimein-the-u.s/2017/crime-in-the-u.s.-2017/tables/table-74

Federal Emergency Management Agency. (2019). *Emerging health and safety issues among women in the fire service*. Retrieved from https://www.usfa.fema.gov/downloads/pdf/publications/emerging_health_safety_issues_women_fire_service.pdf

Feodor Nilsson, S., Andersen, P. K., Strandberg-Larsen, K., & Nybo Andersen, A. M. (2014). Risk factors for miscarriage from a prevention perspective: A nationwide follow-up study. *BJOG: An International Journal of Obstetrics & Gynaecology, 121*(11), 1375–1385.

Gulliver, S. B., Zimering, R. T., Dobani, F., Pennington, M. L., Morissette, S. B., Kamholz, B. W., et al. (2019). Alcohol use and mental health symptoms in female firefighter recruits. *Occupational Medicine, 69*(8–9), 625–631.

Hartley, T. A., Sarkisian, K., Violanti, J. M., Andrew, M. E., & Burchfiel, C. M. (2013). PTSD symptoms among police officers: Associations with frequency, recency, and types of traumatic events. *International Journal of Emergency Mental Health, 15*(4), 241.

Heyman, M., Dill, J., & Douglas, R. (2018). *The Ruderman white paper on mental health and suicide of first responders* (Vol. 41). Ruderman Family Foundation.

Hom, M. A., Stanley, I. H., Spencer-Thomas, S., & Joiner, T. E. (2017). Women firefighters and workplace harassment: Associated suicidality and mental health sequelae. *The Journal of Nervous and Mental Disease, 205*(12), 910–917.

Hulett, D. M., Bendick, M., Thomas, S. Y., & Moccio, F. (2008). *A national report card on women in firefighting*. International Association of Women in Fire & Emergency Services.

Husain, W. (2014). The levels of depression, anxiety and stress in police officers. *Academic Research International, 5*(4), 458–465.

Jacobsson, A., Backteman-Erlanson, S., Brulin, C., & Hörnsten, Å. (2015). Experiences of critical incidents among female and male firefighters. *International Emergency Nursing, 23*(2), 100–104.

Jahnke, S. A., Poston, W. S., Haddock, C. K., Jitnarin, N., Hyder, M. L., & Horvath, C. (2012). The health of women in the U.S. fire service. *BMC Women's Health, 12*(1), 1–12.

Jahnke, S. A., Poston, W. S., Jitnarin, N., & Haddock, C. K. (2018). Maternal and child health among female firefighters in the U.S. *Maternal and Child Health Journal, 22*(6), 922–931.

Jahnke, S. A., Haddock, C. K., Jitnarin, N., Kaipust, C. M., Hollerbach, B. S., & Poston, W. S. (2019). The prevalence and health impacts of frequent work discrimination and harassment among women firefighters in the U.S. fire service. *BioMed Research International, 2019*, 6740207. https://doi.org/10.1155/2019/6740207

Jetelina, K. K., Molsberry, R. J., Gonzalez, J. R., Beauchamp, A. M., & Hall, T. (2020). Prevalence of mental illness and mental health care use among police officers. *JAMA Network Open, 3*(10), e2019658.

Jones, S., Nagel, C., McSweeney, J., & Curran, G. (2018). Prevalence and correlates of psychiatric symptoms among first responders in a Southern State. *Archives of Psychiatric Nursing, 32*(6), 828–835.

Jones, S., Agud, K., & McSweeney, J. (2020). Barriers and facilitators to seeking mental health care among first responders: "Removing the darkness". *Journal of the American Psychiatric Nurses Association, 26*(1), 43–54.

Langan, D., Sanders, C. B., & Gouweloos, J. (2019). Policing women's bodies: Pregnancy, embodiment, and gender relations in Canadian police work. *Feminist Criminology, 14*(4), 466–487.

Lilly, M. M., Pole, N., Best, S. R., Metzler, T., & Marmar, C. R. (2009). Gender and PTSD: What can we learn from female police officers? *Journal of Anxiety Disorders, 23*(6), 767–774.

McCarty, W. P., & Garland, B. E. (2007). Occupational stress and burnout between male and female police officers: Are there any gender differences? *Policing: An International Journal of Police Strategies & Management, 30*(4), 6722–6691.

McQuerry, M., Kwon, C., & Johnson, H. (2019). A critical review of female firefighter protective clothing and equipment workplace challenges. *Research Journal of Textile and Apparel, 23*(2), 94–110.

Milliard, B. (2020). Utilization and impact of peer-support programs on police officers' mental health. *Frontiers in Psychology, 11*, 1686.

National Fire Protection Association. (2019). *U.S. fire department profile 2019*. https://www.nfpa.org/-/media/Files/News-and-Research/Fire-statistics-and-reports/Emergency-responders/osfd-profile.pdf

Noor, N., Pao, C., Dragomir-Davis, M., Tran, J., & Arbona, C. (2019). PTSD symptoms and suicidal ideation in U.S. female firefighters. *Occupational Medicine, 69*(8–9), 577–585.

Ntatamala, I., & Adams, S. (2022). The correlates of post-traumatic stress disorder in ambulance personnel and barriers faced in accessing care for work-related stress. *International Journal of Environmental Research and Public Health, 19*(4), 2046.

Pasciak, A. R., & Kelley, T. M. (2013). Conformity to traditional gender norms by male police officers exposed to trauma: Implications for critical incident stress debriefing. *Applied Psychology in Criminal Justice, 9*(2), 137–156.

Pole, N., Best, S. R., Weiss, D. S., Metzler, T., Liberman, A. M., Fagan, J., & Marmar, C. R. (2001). Effects of gender and ethnicity on duty-related posttraumatic stress symptoms among urban police officers. *The Journal of Nervous and Mental Disease, 189*(7), 442–448.

Rabe-Hemp, C. E., & Humiston, G. S. (2015). A survey of maternity policies and pregnancy accommodations in American police departments. *Police Practice and Research, 16*(3), 239–253.

Regambal, M. J., Alden, L. E., Wagner, S. L., Harder, H. G., Koch, W. J., Fung, K., & Parsons, C. (2015). Characteristics of the traumatic stressors experienced by rural first responders. *Journal of Anxiety Disorders, 34*, 86–93.

Solle, N. S., Santiago, K. M., Louzado Feliciano, P., Calkins, M. M., Fent, K., Jahnke, S., et al. (2021). Perceptions of work-related health and cancer rtisks among women firefighters: A qualitative study. *Journal of Occupational and Environmental Medicine, 63*(12), e846–e852.

Somvadee, C., & Morash, M. (2008). Dynamics of sexual harassment for policewomen working alongside men. *Policing: An International Journal of Police Strategies & Management, 31*(3), 465–498.

Soravia, L. M., Schwab, S., Walther, S., & Müller, T. (2021). Rescuers at risk: Posttraumatic stress symptoms among police officers, fire fighters, ambulance personnel, and emergency and psychiatric nurses. *Frontiers in Psychiatry, 11*, 602064.

Staats, K., Counts, C. R., Dyer, K. S., Stemerman, R., Braithwaite, S., Luke, A., & Mercer, M. P. (2021). Characteristics and experiences of women physicians and professionals in NAEMSP. *Prehospital Emergency Care, 26*(5), 689–699.

Stanley, I. H., Hom, M. A., Spencer-Thomas, S., & Joiner, T. E. (2017a). Examining anxiety sensitivity as a mediator of the association between PTSD symptoms and suicide risk among women firefighters. *Journal of Anxiety Disorders, 50*, 94–102.

Stanley, I. H., Hom, M. A., Spencer-Thomas, S., & Joiner, T. E. (2017b). Suicidal thoughts and behaviors among women firefighters: An examination of associated features and comparison of pre-career and career prevalence rates. *Journal of Affective Disorders, 221*, 107–114.

Sterud, T., Hem, E., Lau, B. R., & Ekeberg, Ø. (2008). Suicidal ideation and suicide attempts in a nationwide sample of operational Norwegian ambulance personnel. *Journal of Occupational Health, 50*(5), 406–414.

Violanti, J. M., & Steege, A. (2020). Law enforcement worker suicide: An updated national assessment. *Policing: An International Journal of Police Strategies & Management, 44*(1), 18–31.

Violanti, J. M., Fekedulegn, D., Charles, L. E., Andrew, M. E., Hartley, T. A., Mnatsakanova, A., & Burchfiel, C. M. (2009). Suicide in police work: Exploring potential contributing influences. *American Journal of Criminal Justice, 34*(1), 41–53.

Violanti, J. M., Slaven, J. E., Charles, L. E., Burchfiel, C. M., Andrew, M. E., & Homish, G. G. (2011). Police and alcohol use: A descriptive analysis and associations with stress outcomes. *American Journal of Criminal Justice, 36*(4), 344–356.

Violanti, J. M., Charles, L. E., McCanlies, E., Hartley, T. A., Baughman, P., Andrew, M. E., et al. (2017). Police stressors and health: A state-of-the-art review. *Policing: An International Journal of Police Strategies & Management, 40*(4), 642–656.

Vujanovic, A. A., & Tran, J. K. (2021). Providing psychological services to firefighters. *Journal of Health Service Psychology, 47*, 137–148. https://doi.org/10.1007/s42843-021-00041-6

Watkins, S. L., Shannon, M. A., Hurtado, D. A., Shea, S. A., & Bowles, N. P. (2021). Interactions between home, work, and sleep among firefighters. *American Journal of Industrial Medicine, 64*(2), 137–148.

Wong, E. Y., Ray, R. M., Gao, D. L., Wernli, K. J., Li, W., Fitzgibbons, E. D., et al. (2009). Dust and chemical exposures, and miscarriage risk among women textile workers in Shanghai, China. *Occupational and Environmental Medicine, 66*(3), 161–168.

Yoo, J., Kim, J. H., Yoon, J., & Kim, S. S. (2019). Sexual harassment and its relationship with depressive symptoms: A nationwide study of Korean EMS providers. *American Journal of Industrial Medicine, 62*(1), 74–79.

First Responders of Color: A Qualitative Approach to Understanding Mental Health

Leah J. Belsches and Garry W. Blackmon

Background

This chapter is informed by the authors' collective experience in providing mental health and counseling services to members of a large urban, fire department located in the southern United States. The department is one of the nation's largest with almost 100 stations and around 4000 firefighters. The department provides services to one of the most culturally and ethnically diverse cities of the country. It is considered a "combined services" department, meaning that its members provide both fire suppression and EMS services. The qualitative data that informed this chapter came from interviews of firefighters of color who are or were members of the department. In addition, a lesser number of police and corrections officers of color were interviewed.

Because the data and findings are based largely on experiences with firefighters within one department, we recognize that they do not necessarily generalize to other departments or other first responder groups such as police or corrections personnel. We also acknowledge that this history of inequality based on the region may be related to how first responders of color in this department have responded to our inquiries. However, we suspect that many of the observations about the experience of first responders of color in the sampled department may apply to other groups of first responders of color. The shared commonalities among these groups may relate to conditions in our country as a whole (e.g., a history of systemic racism).

Many individuals who shared with us felt their stories had previously fallen on deaf ears. They felt unheard and unseen. We believe it is important for others to hear

L. J. Belsches (✉)
Houston Fire Department, Houston, TX, USA

G. W. Blackmon
Houston Fire Department (Retired), Houston, TX, USA

M. L. Bourke et al. (eds.), *First Responder Mental Health*,
https://doi.org/10.1007/978-3-031-38149-2_25

their stories, their perspectives, and the obstacles they encounter while serving as a first responder of color. We hope this chapter inspires mental health professionals to continue to acknowledge the system and be advocates for change.

History of Firefighters of Color

Historically, fire departments serve all individuals; however, not all individuals were allowed to serve within fire departments. First responders[1] of color[2] are a newer addition to the history of the fire service. For example, it was not until 1955 that African Americans were allowed to become firefighters in our department; even then, this only happened after the city annexed a primarily black neighborhood (Graves, 2005). The first African American graduates of the fire academy in our department, nine in number, began their careers at what had been a volunteer fire station (Evans & Whitehead, n.d.). Similar to sitting in the back of the bus, these African American firefighters were only allowed to ride on the outside and back of the apparatus, fulfilling the role known as "pipemen" (Graves, 2005). Racial barriers were in place that kept the fire service segregated. It was not until 1964 when President Lyndon B. Johnson signed the Civil Rights Act that the segregation established by Jim Crow laws ended, both in the country at large, and in our department in particular. Prior to 1964, White chauffeurs (drivers) and captains at the station had separate quarters. Black firefighters were not allowed to fill in for these positions in the absence of White chauffeurs and captains. Instead, a White firefighter from another fire station would be temporarily brought in (Graves, 2005). Although ending the ideology of "separate but equal" created space for racial integration, it did not create a shift in the American culture. An ongoing battle until as late as the 1970s, African American firefighters still were profiled and policed. For example, before they were allowed to apply, some Black applicants were asked to submit a letter from the police department affirming they did not have a criminal record.

The national fire service historically has been predominantly staffed by White males. However, there is also a rich history of African Americans, although working separately from Whites, engaging in fire services dating back to 1802. The first Black volunteer fire unit was known as the Good Will Engine Company and was founded in Philadelphia, Pennsylvania (Winkle, 2021). African American fire fighting began out of a desire to help as well as a necessity. Initially, Philadelphians of color could only rely on White firefighters to help maintain their property and homes. This was a gamble as some of these White firefighters were tied to white gangs, mobs, and riot groups that participated in destroying African American places of business (Winkle, 2021). For the next couple hundred years, African

[1] "First responder" refers to both firefighters and EMTs throughout this chapter.

[2] "First responders of color" refers to African American and Hispanic first responders.

American firefighters were often met with extreme opposition, racism, and disdain even when protecting their own property.

Today, fire departments include members of all ethnic and racial groups. However, according to the United States Bureau of Labor Statistics (2022), 84.3% of firefighters identify as White males. This is a larger than expected representation since only 58% of Americans are White. Only 11% of firefighters identify as being of Hispanic/Latinx origin although the percentage of Hispanics in the nation is around 20%. Similarly, about 12% of Americans are Black, but less than 9% of firefighters are Black. Furthermore, while around 6% of Americans are of Asian background, only 2.6% of firefighters identify as Asian American. In short, people of color from all ethnic groups are underrepresented in the fire service, with similar data reflected in law enforcement.

Representation

Do children of color imagine themselves as firefighters? First responders of color often said they did not consider their profession until they saw someone that looked like them doing the job. Such "making the career opportunity visible" is a missing key to recruitment. It is important to note that first responders of color are often recruited through word of mouth or from a mentorship relationship with other minorities (Graves, 2005). Seeing first responders of color on the news, observing them working as Chiefs and officers, having them participate in neighborhood events, attending fire safety days at schools, and showing up at recruiting events for the fire service all are ideal ways to increase exposure of the career to children and people of color. Interestingly, police officers who were interviewed with this question seemed to feel their presence in their career field was more visible and known.

The entrance of first responders of color into the fire service, and more specifically into life at the station, has often been met with a combination of support and mentorship, as well as covert – and at times overt – racism. According to Elias (2015), overt racism is "characterized by blatant use of negative and/or intentionally harmful attitudes/ideas/symbols and actions directed at a specific racial group or groups labelled non-white." African American first responders reported more overt, blatant racism compared to Hispanic respondents. Both African American and Hispanic first responders shared experiencing a greater number of experiences involving covert racism – a subtler form of racism that is often unspoken and more difficult to recognize. Of note, some Hispanic first responders denied experiencing racism at all. This seems aligned with recent research on the experience of racism in the United States during the pandemic (Su et al., 2022).

What amounts to racist behavior has evolved over the years, often becoming more subtle. For some people, racism is only embodied in obvious discrimination such as the image of a "Whites only" water fountain. By arguing that these "rules" no longer apply, some might assume that old-fashioned racism is over. However, racism still exists today (Elias, 2015; Su et al., 2022); it can simply look different, and be less apparent, than during the Jim Crow era (Eschmann, 2019; Milner et al., 2020).

Collective Themes

Several common themes emerged during the collection of data. Understanding these themes is key to working with first responders of color and designing resources to support them.

Stereotypes

The American Psychological Association (n.d.-b) defines stereotype as, "a set of cognitive generalizations about the qualities and characteristics of the members of a group or social category." The APA goes on to state, "Stereotypes, like schemas, simplify and expedite perceptions and judgments, but they are often exaggerated, negative rather than positive, and resistant to revision even when perceivers encounter individuals with qualities that are not congruent with the stereotype."

Numerous stereotypes are encountered within departments; although many are specific to African Americans, some are experienced by members of other races, including Hispanics and Asians. Firefighters of color said they had been described as inferior; they were told they were untrustworthy, lazy, uneducated, and physically strong but never smart enough. They had been accused of being unable to do their job well because of their ethnicity; not doing their part to help around the station, unable to perform their jobs correctly, or giving an emotional rather than a professional response during an emergency situation. Their communities and values had been denigrated; their ethnic group did not take care of their children, and they were unable to afford nice things (e.g., a home or car). Sometimes, their experiences echoed prejudices of an earlier era – being afraid of White men, sexually desirous of White women, and overly superstitious (e.g., being afraid of ghosts and therefore avoiding entering a home with a dead body). Even worse, they had heard that they were inferior to White men, would not make good officers, and were unworthy to be members of the department.

Most first responders of color reported encountering multiple stereotypes on a long-term basis throughout their career. The stress of managing ongoing degradation can lead to psychological distress, depressive symptoms, anxiety, and low morale within the department (Kwate & Goodman, 2015; Pieterse et al., 2012; Pitcan et al., 2018). In addition to creating an "us" and "them" division, a greater issue emerged involving concern for when personal beliefs and opinions influenced professional judgments. Essentially, these stereotypes can take on a life of their own, leading to lower rates of promotion and increased disciplinary acts. A first responder of color shared what he heard when he asked a White captain why he believed his White counterpart would make a better captain. He was told, "Well he's a great guy." While this is an anecdotal example, we heard several other accounts when personal opinions and stereotypes influenced professional decisions.

Microaggressions

The American Psychological Association (n.d.-a) defines microaggressions (first introduced by psychiatrist Chester M. Pierce in 1974) as "brief and commonplace verbal, behavioral, or situational indignities that communicate hostile, derogatory, or negative slights or insults, especially toward members of minority or oppressed groups." The APA states, "Microaggression may be intentional (e.g., calling a transgender person a "she-male") or implicit (e.g., implying that the colleague may have obtained a job through affirmative action)."

Three subtypes of microaggression were identified by psychologist Derald Wing Sue: "*microassaults*, which are purposefully discriminatory actions (e.g., uttering a racial slur); *microinsults*, which are subtle snubs that devalue a person's identity; and *microinvalidations*, which are unintentional exclusions or negations of an individual's thoughts, feelings, or experiences" (Sue et al., 2007). Sue et al. described the effects of experiencing microaggression as feelings of "abnormality, inferiority, invisibleness, powerlessness, or untrustworthiness."

First responders reported implicit microassaults, microinsults, and microinvalidations as part of their experience throughout their career. Statements such as, "I'm glad you showed up on your debit day (rather than calling in sick)," and "You don't seem like a good fit here (because of your ethnicity)," were experienced microaggressions, often in response to first responders of color combating stereotypes. Microinsults included, "You speak well (for someone of your ethnicity)," and "I don't know why anyone would want to live in (ethnic neighborhood) – they should just drop a bomb on it." Examples of microinvalidations were as follows: "You finished paramedic school?" "Why is he driving someone else's new car?" "How did you afford that?" "Why are (ethnic foods) in our fridge?" There were also microassaults such as "You all have two Black Chiefs – stop fighting for more."

Overt/Covert Racism

While overt racism is still present in many parts of our society, the experience of covert racism was more prevalent for first responders of color. Perhaps overt racism is less common in first responder departments now because of years of fighting for equality within these professions. In addition, the importance of diversity has become more recognized among politicians and the command staff/people of power in these departments. Nevertheless, overt racism has not completely disappeared. Our interviewees reported examples of overt racism such as being called the

"N-word," having racial slurs written on the white boards in stations, finding nooses hanging in lockers, and Ku Klux Klan paraphernalia being worn around the station. Covert racism examples included being singled out for disciplinary practices, assumptions that high value items (e.g., cars) did not belong to the member, and racial profiling such as accusations of stealing items from the station. These experiences of overt and covert racism occurred in addition to the microaggressions and stereotypes previously discussed.

Another form of covert racism was evidenced in the treatment and care of minority patients in the community. Research indicates health care professionals, including doctors and nurses, prefer treating White individuals more than other patients (Jones, 2022). Our respondents reported that some White first responders were aggressive, short, dismissive, and demeaning toward minority patients. Sometimes, officers and supervisors were challenged by other first responders on their orders regarding direct care to elderly or minority patients. Such actions quickly led to dissension among the crews. Our interviewees commonly shared that they joined the fire service with a strong desire to help others, especially members of their community. Feelings about how members of one's community are being treated are closely related to community ties and connections, which are often strong within minority communities. If underlying racist beliefs are affecting the actions of first responders, we cannot expect citizens to receive the appropriate care, the crew to be able to do their jobs safely and successfully, or for the community to support the first responders.

Station Life

Stations have reputations based on the word-of-mouth reports of crews and their histories (e.g., how often they respond to fires, major events they have experienced). First responders of color may seek out safer places to work. In this context, "safe" is used to describe a place of mental and emotional security rather than physical safety. Due to long shifts that are often more than 24 hours, desiring a level of comfort and comradery is expected. Through their stories, it was clear that first responders of color sought out stations with supportive crews to avoid the mental exhaustion of covert racism, while reportedly, some White first responders avoided crews that were primarily African American or minority because of stereotypes.

Some stations remain unofficially segregated, while others are the epitome of a melting pot. Certain stations reflect the ethnic backgrounds of the neighborhoods they serve, and their crews are primarily of the same ethnic makeup. At other stations, the first responders are from a mixture of backgrounds. Several first responders of color recalled feeling unwelcome or uncomfortable at certain stations, primarily when they were requested to fill in, or substitute for a member, at that station. A repetitive theme described by our respondents was being turned away from a newly assigned station by a captain or chief when they realized the assignee was African American. In a similar vein, interviewees described being placed in less desirable roles because of their ethnicity or color. Some even recalled being denied various positions at stations and experiencing increased hazing if they were members of minority groups. Informal segregation even occurred at stations with mixed crews. Crew members might avoid preparing meals with or for the first responder of color. Similarly, some respondents reported being excluded from meal purchases, or were not offered a seat at the table. White members reportedly might bring their own tables or sit on the apparatus to eat when they worked at majority black stations. The segregation, or rather voluntary separation, is not an openly addressed topic according to respondents. It is covert and subtle, but present on occasion. "You can tell when people don't want you around," stated a respondent.

The officers assigned to a station are also responsible for maintaining discipline at the station. Disparate treatment of African American and Hispanic firefighters was reported by some respondents. It was felt that officers holding racial biases often found reason to reprimand or prevent firefighters of color from moving beyond the probation stage. A first responder of color discussed how a previous captain implied that because he did not spend enough time with the crew in the common room at the station, he was not an "ideal fit" for the station. Not sharing a meal with other crew members was seen as more significant than his work ethic or test scores. While complaints can be filed about discriminatory experiences, many first responders of color felt they could not complain because the officers who would consider such complaints were perceived to hold racist views and beliefs, themselves. Indeed, at times, the superior officer was the one viewed as being the offender. Research suggests that subordinates may be less likely to report racist or sexist remarks and behavior due to the power differential between themselves and their superiors (Ashburn-Nardo et al., 2014). Thus, while crew members may not complain to their chain of command about perceptions of racism this should not imply they have no such complaints or concerns. Ideally, one would expect those in leadership to follow through on complaints accordingly, regardless of race. However, many of our respondents felt the continuing presence of "the good ol' boys club," leaving them with the frustration and anger of unfair treatment and little recourse. Notably not every first responder of color has this experience. Given the climate of the country, some of our interviewees felt that they have a "50/50 chance" of being assigned to a racist mentor or captain. For the stations that create a safe, multicultural environment, first responders of color reported increased crew cohesiveness and higher job satisfaction. "I couldn't wait to get there; it was like a family."

Promotions

Promotions are highly regarded as they come with a new title, new duties, and a new level of respect. First responders spend extensive hours studying for exams to one day excel in their career. Over the last several decades, there have been numerous lawsuits filed against cities for use of racially biased tests (Moran, 2011).

More recently, testing related to hiring and promotions has come under fire, including those involved in the hiring and promotion of first responders. While this is a hot-button topic for some with political ties, it boils down to science. On numerous occasions, industrial/organizational psychologists have provided strong evidence that racially biased testing not only exists, but has a significant adverse impact. Adverse impact occurs when a selection procedure results in inequitable hiring, promotion, or membership opportunities for members of a race, color, religion, sex, national origin group, or other protected class (Zedeck, 2011). These high-stakes tests have a tremendous impact on professional opportunities, and in turn, economic outcomes. For example, personnel selection instruments such as the Wonderlic Personnel Test (Wonderlic, 2007) have determined access to occupational opportunities for millions of job applicants since their inception (Hicks et al., 2015).

Several lawsuits have proven successful in expanding testing practices to be culturally conscious through the use of assessment centers and skills-based testing. Assessing job knowledge and situational judgment has proven to be a more accurate measure of performance rather than test-taking skills. Fire departments are moving to this format for choosing officers of all ranks for a simple reason: It works! The assessment center mimics a day in the life of the job at hand. The examinee is thrust into the deep end of the pool to either sink or swim. He or she cannot fake it, pay lip service, or pretend. Either they possess the skills, or they do not (Kastros, 2018). Unlike written tests, the assessment process takes practice and training to develop the requisite knowledge, skills, and abilities.

The first responders of color interviewed presented with similar reviews of the assessment process previously used in the department, where only a written exam was used to identify those ready for promotion. One respondent shared, "Some people were promoted without having actually ever fought a fire, but they are now over a fire station. This puts people's lives at risk." While some aligned with the mindset of "let the best man win," others highlighted hidden issues within the written testing process. The main complaint was the allegation that White first responders had access to test questions, both in the academy and prior to promotional exams. Access to test questions was reportedly passed down from "father, brothers, and White test composers." While this accusation may be disputed by fire service administrators, it was a common belief of nearly every participant who was queried about the promotional process.

In some departments, lists are created of people who score the highest on the promotional exams. Some firefighters of color found this process flawed, noting that nepotism took place, names of African Americans were passed over, and there was a reluctance to promote multiple African Americans simultaneously. One recalled, "When two African American firefighters scored number one and number two on the promotional exam, it was assumed they cheated." He said an investigation would take place, and the test results could be held up for months. Many believed the administration did not want to diversify those in leadership roles, but rather desired for first responders of color to "die on the list," meaning the test results would expire without a selection, necessitating retesting to begin the process all over again. After numerous lawsuits and requested changes, skills-based assessment was added to various departments with the goal to "add a component to the promotional exam, not to take anything away."

Mental Health Responses to Stereotypes and Racism

The weight of managing the feeling of exclusion because of one's ethnicity can feel heavy. However, a common theme that emerged as a response to managing the emotional and mental challenges associated with racism was *positivity*. A direct opposite entity of the hate and exclusion brought forth via racist or discriminatory acts, positivity proved to be a powerful reckoning force, primarily for African American first responders. A first responder stated, "For so many years, you've had to look at it in this (positive) lens to process and stay focused." Pitcan et al. (2018) indicated African American men may "censor their self-presentation to conform to White masculine norms for self-preservation and protection." Maintaining a positive disposition and mindset proved helpful for many to "get through the job." While positivity can help maintain day-to-day operations, it is not always a realistic perspective of difficult situations. Ignoring without acknowledging the harsh reality of hearing racial slurs, and even seeing them written in the station houses, can lead to maladaptive coping strategies, such as alcohol use (Zegel et al., 2019).

Isolation was another common response to the racially uncomfortable workspaces. Many suggested they sat alone, ate by themselves, and avoided unnecessary interaction with members. They were there to do their jobs, and that was it. Similar to continuous positivity, isolation can appear ideal in the short term, but it is also a maladaptive coping strategy. Many were willing to take this risk because it often meant safety from derogatory remarks, from stereotypes, and from potentially losing one's job.

Working harder was also a common response to racism on the job. Familial values are instilled in children of color for this very moment in life. Many minority parents plant the seeds of "you have to work twice as hard," in their children. This principle is based on the understanding that because of the color of your skin, you cannot just be good, you have to be great – only then will you have a seat at the table or gain "their" respect, also known as John Henryism (Neighbors et al., 2007). Being the first one in and the last one out or letting one's work speak for themselves was a common coping strategy used to trump negativity and discrimination. But at the end of the day, working twice as hard is exhausting and can lead to burnout. It can also lead to additional feelings of exclusion when hard work is not rewarded equally.

What Do You Do with the Uncomfortable Memories?

The psychological toll of witnessing and experiencing discrimination is often left out of the conversation when first responders of color seek mental health care. People of color experience racism so often that it is frequently labeled as a regular part of life. That does not mean people of color have stopped fighting for equality; rather, it means some people of color have stopped battling their emotional reaction to overt and covert racism. When this happens, the discriminatory experiences are no longer labeled as "traumas." Rather, the experiences are seen as part of the fabric of life, something people of color are forced to manage because they have families to raise, jobs to maintain, and other issues to address. The danger of this kind of minimization is desensitization. People of color can become used to taking the high road, to watching inflictors experience minimal consequences, as they get up each morning to go to work in an unemotional state. Racial discrimination is traumatic, and it is okay to encourage people of color to label it as such (Williams et al., 2021).

People of color may feel there is something weakening about labeling negative racial experiences as "traumas." Some may feel it allows the inflictors to get the reaction they were hoping for. In a sense, this can be a goal of racism – to disarm, dehumanize, and psychologically affect victims. Yet we would argue that discouraging people from speaking about injustice, asking for redress, or seeking treatment for trauma are greater risks.

Seeking Treatment

The stigma against seeking treatment is especially tough for first responders, a largely male population. Our respondents reported that seeing the "shrink" could lead to isolation and labels of "being crazy." Mental health treatment was described as taboo and embarrassing, a secret to be kept. Ideals of self-reliance, remaining unemotional, and not needing help have been described as part of the underpinnings of "toxic masculinity" (Elordi, 2022), and they contribute to the unwillingness of many men to seek mental health care or counseling. These ideas originate long before young men enter their professions. From childhood, stereotypical definitions of masculinity may be passed down creating unrealistic expectations and forming barriers to mental health. There may be additional issues facing young men of color.

Many young men of color are discouraged from showing emotion as a method of providing safety from bullies, racism, and even relationships. Seeds may be planted equating emotion with weakness. With repeated exposure to painful and traumatic events as part of their work as first responders, the risk of mental health challenges can increase. Furthermore, when these first responders of color experience the adverse effects of racism at work, their risk for depression, anxiety, and additional trauma-related symptoms grows (Greer & Cavalhieri, 2019; Pieterse et al., 2012). Williams et al. (2021) stated that these experiences can result in the "cognitive, behavioral, and affective presentations of PTSD in people of color." Higher PTSD symptoms have also been found to be associated with current suicidal intent (Stanley et al., 2019).

There are various perspectives about mental health resources among first responders of color. One common perception offered by our interviewees is that showing emotion while on the job, or after an incident, was unnecessary. While the term "unnecessary" denies natural emotions that may arise and may be related to stereotyped notions of masculinity, there is some truth to the following statement shared by a first responder of color, "You don't have time to dwell on things. You have to be ready for the next one." This is both a sign of possible toxic masculinity and an administrative issue, where the need for appropriate, and sometimes extended, breaks between calls could create the time and space for first responders to process painful or traumatic scenes. Understandably, though, emergencies wait for no one, and staffing issues can arise when first responders are allowed such time.

An additional perspective on the current state of mental health resources for first responders of color was that they simply do not exist. There is truth to this perspective, as well. While police departments have a history of mental health professionals participating in the department, fire departments, and correctional facilities have lagged in this area. There are only a few fire departments that employ full-time staff psychologists to serve their members (other departments may employ part-time mental health professionals or may contract with local professionals for these services). Not surprisingly, rural and smaller first responder departments have even fewer resources than urban and larger ones. Furthermore, many of the mental health professionals who are supposed to provide these services are unfamiliar with the culture and experiences of the first responder world. Correctional facilities often have psychologists or other mental health professionals available to the inmate population, but they are not always available for staff. Correctional officers experience traumatic events that are unreported in the news due to maintaining the confidentiality of inmates or juveniles. They have a significantly dangerous job and are also at an elevated risk for mental health conditions, such as PTSD, depression, and anxiety (Fusco et al., 2021).

The mental health resources that do exist are not enough. Our interviewees were skeptical of the helpfulness of post-incident debriefings. In some cases, these debriefings were focused on operational effectiveness and did not address the emotional aftermath of the events. First responders in these debriefings are not always honest about the emotional or mental toll they are experiencing. In other cases, the first responders participated in crisis debriefings after difficult incidents (e.g., pediatric deaths). These crisis debriefings are usually led by peers trained to assist in addressing the emotional aspects of such events. Sometimes, they are guided or accompanied by mental health professionals. While these debriefings are intended as psychological first aid, rather than long-term care, for many first responders, this is all the care they may receive even after severely traumatic events (e.g., school shootings) due to stigma and a lack of access to mental health professionals. First responders of color who were interviewed shared that these critical incident responses, which were defined as processing through their feelings in the moment, did not feel "enough". These first responders of color with histories of repeated trauma compounded with experiences of racial discrimination may need a more intensive and extensive approach.

Employee Assistance Programs are a needed and helpful resource provided to first responders by many municipalities; however, the services they provide are typically limited to a relatively few free sessions. If the first responders want to continue in treatment, they may be required to pay out of pocket, although possibly at a reduced rate, or find an outside provider. Seeking an outside provider can be huge barrier to first responders. Their schedules do not comport with those of providers and the community providers may be unfamiliar with the culture and demands of first responders. For larger departments, multiple mental health professionals are required to offer the needed and appropriate amount of care.

Cultural Mistrust

A specific challenge for first responders of color is cultural mistrust. Benkert et al. (2006) discuss the treatment disparities between African American populations and non-African American populations, including the fact that African Americans have developed a mistrust of many aspects of society, including mental health treatment, in response to a history of discriminatory treatment. Sampling from a low-income, African American population, the authors concluded that perceptions of racism and mistrust of European Americans, also known as cultural mistrust, have a significant negative effect on the trust and satisfaction with care provided. Specifically, perceived racism had a significant indirect effect on satisfaction with care. This was mediated by cultural mistrust (Benkert et al., 2006). Whaley (2001) provides a possible solution by suggesting that CBT may be extremely helpful when treating a client dealing with cultural mistrust. However, therapists should keep in mind that cultural mistrust has been shown to affect processes and outcomes of mental health treatment including levels of disclosure and early termination with non-African American therapists (Benkert et al., 2006).

Not only is there a lack of data on people of color's response to behavioral treatments in comparison with White individuals, there is even more limited research on first responders of color and their response to treatment. There are also discrepancies that exist in the quality of therapeutic services delivered to White individuals and people of color. People of color are more likely to drop out of treatment and are less likely to receive appropriate treatment when they do participate in therapeutic services (Horrell, 2008; United States Department of Health and Human Services, 2001).

Cultural mistrust must also be taken into consideration when treating people of color, especially if using a behavioral treatment that has not been adapted to their unique characteristics. Whaley (2001) recommends first acknowledging the possibility that cultural mistrust is a valid process of coping with racism and discrimination. As therapists, we should respect our clients' complaints about racism and their life experiences in addition to being open to learning from them in a non-judgmental way. This includes learning about their level of cultural mistrust and how they view their behavioral treatment.

If psychotherapy is to become truly beneficial and culturally responsive, we must develop interventions to include the clients' background, ethnically idiosyncratic features, and in this case, occupation (Hwang, 2009). If treatments become more culturally conscious, mental health professionals must as well.

But working as a mental health professional with first responders requires an additional step, because first responders are a culture unto themselves. Indeed, it actually includes different subcultures (e.g., police, fire, EMS, emergency communications operators, corrections). First responders of color are a subgroup within the overall first responder culture requiring additional understanding for successful treatment. For example, Arbona et al. (2017) discussed that although African American and Latino firefighters report similar levels of stress, there were different predictors of stress for each group. For Latino firefighters, having a lower firefighter rank and working a second job were associated with higher levels of stress; for African American firefighters, having a lower level of education and serving as a caregiver for sick family members were associated with higher levels of perceived stress. Despite different predictors, both Latino and African American firefighters reported utilizing alcohol as a coping mechanism. Thirty percent of Latino firefighters and 24% of Black firefighters reported alcohol abuse (Arbona et al., 2017).

It is highly recommended that mental health providers working with first responders become versed in the lives and experiences of these community servants – understanding the challenges they embrace and the physical and mental toll on their bodies. Mental health providers should spend time at the stations or facilities to gain a better perception of what their lives are like. When working with first responders of color, the mental health professional should introduce topics such as possible discrimination or experiences of covert racism, rather than waiting for the first responder to volunteer such information. Ultimately, recognizing how the trauma experienced on the job can compound with intergenerational experiences of racial injustice is essential. This is especially true given our country's recent record of repeated, unjust killings of men of color, sometimes by first responders. Providing trauma-informed care is key. Training for mental health professionals seeking to work with first responders should include Trauma Focused Cognitive Behavioral Therapy (TF-CBT) and Cognitive Processing Therapy (CPT) as a minimum standard.

Having a diverse staff is not only important within the first responder culture, but also for mental health professionals. Creating a multicultural staff that represents race, gender, and additional diversifying factors increase the chances of first responders of color seeking treatment from someone whom they see as more like them.

Unions

Unions have traditionally been viewed as an organization or organized group of workers coming together to have a stronger voice to maintain and improve working conditions. First responders of color had diverse opinions on the unions that are supposed to represent their interests. Some viewed the union as a source of support, a bargaining chip, and an organization worth joining. Others viewed the union as "smoke and mirrors." First responders of color felt the organization's union avoided involving themselves in racial issues within the department or race-based court cases for fear of being perceived as Pro-Hispanic, Pro-Black, etc. Many felt that they were unable to benefit from their paid dues while others felt that their dues were actually used against them. For example, several first responders of color voiced that union representatives would avoid showing up to various meetings in which they were to represent the member. Some noted that union lawyers had shared that they avoided taking on cases "they knew they would lose." Other first responders of color shared experiences where they felt union funding was used to fight against addressing various racial discriminatory practice cases, especially regarding promotion. Many felt there were prior verbal agreements between those in departmental leadership roles and their friends who were union representatives. This made some members question if they would have a fair shot at justice. One member shared his thoughts on the matter: "If something happens at the station, and I bring a grievance up the chain of command against my captain, but the captain is friends with everyone at the union. So, I get the union to try to represent me against management? But that's their buddy. I'm paying them to work against me."

Future Directions

The majority of first responders of color who were interviewed felt that the atmosphere of the department has progressed in a positive direction. Others believed it was simply different – not necessarily better – compared to several decades ago. Most thought there are now better anti-discriminatory practices in place, more accurate promotional exams, increases in the numbers of people of color being promoted, and a more helpful union administration. One expressed, "We still have to work on inclusion, but upward mobility is improving." Others felt that the progress made was simply not enough. They noted that covert racism is still taking place on the job, that the department and its command staff are still not representative of the populations in most major cities, and that the country itself needs to make more efforts toward preventing and managing racism. So where do we go from here? What are the biggest needs of first responders of color?

Consistency

First responders of color are usually proud to represent their department. Many expressed a tireless commitment to their jobs as they experienced a sense of family and brotherhood and intend to or did, make a career of it. They need a safe and non-toxic work environment. The internal culture that allowed for covert and even overt racism to fester over time needs to be addressed on a continuous basis. The progress that the fire service has already made should be seen as a steppingstone to greater inclusivity. Discipline must be implemented consistently, fairly, and justly. Reporting racially based infractions should be a separate process within departments, not necessarily involving the chain of command. There is a need for a safe space for discussing race-based topics and situations. There is a desire for all rules, guidelines, and regulations to apply to all members. This principle is generally held by most departments, their chiefs, and their command staffs. However, the behavior and decisions that take place at the small unit level in individual stations, out of sight of higher leadership, are where unfair and discriminatory practices are more likely to reside. The power differential between crews and officers can leave crew members with decreased feelings of personal responsibility for intervening when there are problems of discrimination. This can lead to difficulties in deciding how to intervene and weighing the pros and cons of involving themselves in matters of discrimination or prejudice (Ashburn-Nardo et al., 2014).

First responders of color should not only know but also have proof that there is a no tolerance policy for discrimination based on ethnicity. This must include no tolerance for retaliation for complaints about such discrimination. When discipline of these offenders is lenient, minimal, or not implemented, there is a shift in control and decision-making away from command officers to lower ranking, local officers. Transferring members who hold racist, misogynistic, sexist, ableist, or elitist views to another station does not truly solve the problem. These views are deeply rooted in values and beliefs. Education and training are a healthy start for these individuals, but at some point, a decision needs to be made if they belong in the fire or police department. After an investigation, avoiding appropriate consequences to these individuals creates more division in the department and the community.

First responders of color simply want to be seen, heard, and treated like a human being when they come to work. They desire guidelines and policies that are promptly and consistently followed to ensure a healthy working environment. It is important for checks and balances to be created to maintain integrity. Most departments already have something resembling this in place, but is it enforced? Who is monitoring behavior at the stations? For many first responders, there are still stations and captains that are notoriously racist. There needs to be a system put in place to address this. First responders of color recognize that fire and police departments cannot control every citizen in their departments, but they can control who is employed by them.

Resources and Training

Access to trained, culturally sensitive mental health providers and services remain a need for all first responders, regardless of race or gender. Ideally, free, confidential, trauma-informed mental health providers should be available and a part of necessary staff for first responder departments. Psychologists and counselors of diverse backgrounds should be recruited to create a diverse mental health staff, trained in not only responding to trauma, but also to the kinds of trauma specifically experienced by first responders. These services should also be made available to dispatchers, as their trauma often goes unrecognized.

Maintaining accurate promotional assessments, involving both written and hands-on applications, will continue to leave the door open to fair and accurate promotions of a diverse staff. While implicit bias does exist, there is little evidence that implicit bias training produces long-term change or can change a workplace culture (Dobbin & Kalev, 2018; Forscher et al., 2019). There is research suggesting that basic diversity training can produce anger and frustration among White participants, rather than promoting a deepened understanding of inclusivity. Instead, diversity policies must be researched, developed, and implanted within the department to change the internal culture (Dover et al., 2016). Employees should be encouraged to participate in mental health–related programs to understand their own mental health better and supported when they seek available treatment.

As we end this chapter, you may find yourself asking, "Why is the issue always about race?" Racial identity does not go away or come off as easily as one's shirt. It is always present, undergirding our reactions to others, sometimes even outside our awareness. Our country has a long history of inequity, which we are still trying to remedy. That inequity may be reflected in the composition of first responder departments, in the internal processes of those departments, and in the interactions of first responders with the public. If you are uncomfortable with managing these issues or find yourself preferring to be colorblind to race, we urge you to spend additional time understanding the source of your discomfort. Discomfort is not always bad – it can also be a sign of growth. You are encouraged to acknowledge the power you have on employees, friends, and the world to address injustice. Ask yourself, have you contributed to this discussion in a meaningful way? It is never too late to make improvements.

References

American Psychological Association. (n.d.-a). Microaggression. In *APA dictionary of psychology*. Retrieved August 11, 2022 from https://dictionary.apa.org/microaggression

American Psychological Association. (n.d.-b). Stereotype. In *APA dictionary of psychology*. Retrieved August 11, 2022 from https://dictionary.apa.org/stereotype

Arbona, C., Pao, C., Long, A., & Olvera, N. (2017). Perceived stress in Black and Latino male firefighters: Associations with risk and protective factors. *Ethnicity & Disease, 27*(4), 421. https://doi.org/10.18865/ed.27.4.421

Ashburn-Nardo, L., Blanchar, J. C., Petersson, J., Morris, K. A., & Goodwin, S. A. (2014). Do you say something when it's your boss? The role of perpetrator power in prejudice confrontation. *Journal of Social Issues, 70*(4), 615–636. https://doi-org.latech.idm.oclc.org/10.1111/josi.12082

Benkert, R., Peters, R. M., Clark, R., & Keves-Foster, K. (2006). Effects of perceived racism, cultural mistrust and trust in providers on satisfaction with care. *Journal of the National Medical Association, 98*(9), 1532–1540.

Dobbin, F., & Kalev, A. (2018). Why doesn't diversity training work? The challenge for industry and academia. *Anthropology Now, 10*(2), 48–55. https://doi.org/10.1080/19428200.2018.1493182

Dover, T. L., Major, B., & Kaiser, C. R. (2016, January 4). Diversity policies rarely make companies fairer, and they feel threatening to white men. *Harvard Business Review*. https://hbr.org/2016/01/diversity-policies-dont-help-women-or-minorities-and-they-make-white-men-feel-threatened

Elias, S. (2015). Racism, overt. In J. Stone, R. M. Dennis, P. S. Rizova, A. D. Smith, & X. Hou (Eds.), *The Wiley Blackwell Encyclopedia of race, ethnicity, and nationalism* (1st ed.). Wiley. https://doi.org/10.1002/9781118663202.wberen398

Elordi, J. (2022, September 21). *'Toxic masculinity': What does it mean, where did it come from – and is the term useful or harmful?* The Conversation. https://theconversation.com/toxic-masculinity-what-does-it-mean-where-did-it-come-from-and-is-the-term-useful-or-harmful-189298

Eschmann, R. (2019). Unmasking racism: Students of color and expressions of racism in online spaces. *Social Problems*. https://doi.org/10.1093/socpro/spz026

Evans, J., & Whitehead, A. (n.d.). *About the Houston fire department -- HFD history*. City of Houston. https://houstontx.gov/fire/about/history.html

Forscher, P. S., Lai, C. K., Axt, J. R., Ebersole, C. R., Herman, M., Devine, P. G., & Nosek, B. A. (2019). A meta-analysis of procedures to change implicit measures. *Journal of Personality and Social Psychology, 117*(3), 522–559.

Fusco, N., Ricciardelli, R., Jamshidi, L., Carleton, R. N., Barnim, N., Hilton, Z., & Groll, D. (2021). When our work hits home: Trauma and mental disorders in correctional officers and other correctional workers. *Frontiers in Psychiatry, 11*, 493391.

Graves, R. (2005, February 26). First black HFD firefighters reflect on integration. *Houston Chronicle*. https://www.chron.com/news/houston-texas/article/First-black-HFD-firefighters-reflect-on-1490585.php

Greer, T. M., & Cavalhieri, K. E. (2019). The role of coping strategies in understanding the effects of institutional racism on mental health outcomes for African American men. *Journal of Black Psychology, 45*(5), 405–433. https://doi-org.latech.idm.oclc.org/. https://doi.org/10.1177/0095798419868105

Hicks, K. L., Harrison, T. L., & Engle, R. W. (2015). Wonderlic, working memory capacity, and fluid intelligence. *Intelligence, 50*, 186–195.

Horrell, S. C. V. (2008). Effectiveness of cognitive-behavioral therapy with adult ethnic minority clients: A review. *Professional Psychology: Research and Practice, 39*(2), 160–168. https://doi.org/10.1037/0735-7028.39.2.160

Hwang, W. C. (2009). The formative method for adapting psychotherapy (FMAP): A community-based developmental approach to culturally adapting therapy. *Professional Psychology: Research and Practice, 40*(4), 369–377. https://doi.org/10.1037/a0016240

Jones, D. D. (2022). Examining the unconscious racial biases and attitudes of physicians, nurses, and the public: Implications for future health care education and practice. *Health Equity, 6*(1), 375–381. https://doi.org/10.1089/heq.2021.0141

Kastros, A. (2018). Assessment center. *Firefighter Nation*. https://www.firefighternation.com/firerescue/assessment-centers/#gref

Kwate, N. O., & Goodman, M. S. (2015). Cross-sectional and longitudinal effects of racism on mental health among residents of Black neighborhoods in New York City. *American Journal of Public Health, 105*(4), 711–718. https://doi-org.latech.idm.oclc.org/. https://doi.org/10.2105/AJPH.2014.302243

Milner, A., Franz, B., & Henry Braddock, J. (2020). We need to talk about racism—In all of its forms—To understand COVID-19 disparities. *Health Equity, 4*(1), 397–402. https://doi.org/10.1089/heq.2020.0069

Moran, C. (2011, March 22). HFD exam lawsuit settled for 7 black firefighters. *Houston Chronicle*. https://www.chron.com/news/houston-texas/article/HFD-exam-lawsuit-settled-for-7-black-firefighters-1687065.php

Neighbors, H., Njai, R., & Jackson, J. (2007). Race, ethnicity, John Henryism, and depressive symptoms: The National Survey of American Life adult reinterview. *Research in Human Development, 4*(1/2), 71–87. https://doi.org/10.1080/15427600701481004

Pieterse, A. L., Todd, N. R., Neville, H. A., & Carter, R. T. (2012). Perceived racism and mental health among Black American adults: A meta-analytic review. *Journal of Counseling Psychology, 59*(1), 1–9. https://doi.org/10.1037/a0026208

Pitcan, M., Park-Taylor, J., & Hayslett, J. (2018). Black men and racial microaggressions at work. *The Career Development Quarterly, 66*(4), 300–314. https://doi.org/10.1002/cdq.12152

Stanley, I. H., Boffa, J. W., Tran, J. K., Schmidt, N. B., Joiner, T. E., & Vujanovic, A. A. (2019). Posttraumatic stress disorder symptoms and mindfulness facets in relation to suicide risk among firefighters. *Journal of Clinical Psychology, 75*(4), 696–709. https://doi.org/10.1002/jclp.22748

Su, D., Alshehri, K., Ern, J., Chen, B., Chen, L., Chen, Z., Han, X., King, K. M., Li, H., Li, J., Li, Y., Michaud, T., Shi, L., Ramos, A. K., Wen, M., & Zhang, D. (2022). Racism experience among American adults during COVID-19: A mixed-methods study. *Health Equity, 6*(1), 554–563. https://doi.org/10.1089/heq.2022.0070

Sue, D. W., Capodilupo, C. M., Torino, G. C., Bucceri, J. M., Holder, A. M. B., Nadal, K. L., & Esquilin, M. (2007). Racial microaggressions in everyday life: Implications for clinical practice. *American Psychologist, 62*(4), 271–286. https://doi.org/10.1037/0003-066x.62.4.271

United States Bureau of Labor Statistics. (2022, August 13). *Employed persons by detailed occupation, sex, race, and Hispanic or Latino ethnicity.* Labor Force Statistics from the Current Population Survey. https://www.bls.gov/cps/cpsaat11.htm.

United States Department of Health and Human Services. (2001). *Mental health: Culture, race, and ethnicity. A supplement to mental health: A report of the surgeon general*. US Department of Health and Human Services. https://www.ncbi.nlm.nih.gov/books/NBK44243/

Whaley, A. L. (2001). Cultural mistrust: An important psychological construct for diagnosis and treatment of African Americans. *Professional Psychology: Research and Practice, 32*(6), 555–562. https://doi.org/10.1037/0735-7028.32.6.555

Williams, M. T., Osman, M., Gran-Ruaz, S., & Lopez, J. (2021). Intersection of racism and PTSD: Assessment and treatment of racism-related stress and trauma. *Current Treatment Options in Psychiatry, 8*, 167–185. https://doi.org/10.1007/s40501-021-00250-2

Winkle, T. (2021, October 4). *Two objects bring the history of African American firefighting to light* [Blog post]. O Say Can You See? Stories from the Museum. https://americanhistory.si.edu/blog/african-american-firefighting

Wonderlic, E. F. (2007). Wonderlic personnel test-revised: Manual. Los Angeles, CA: Western Psychological Services.

Zedeck, S. (2011). Adverse impact: History and evolution. In J. L. Outtz (Ed.), *Adverse impact: Implications for organizational staffing and high stakes selection* (pp. 3–28). Routledge.

Zegel, M., Tran, J., & Vujanovic, A. (2019). Posttraumatic stress, alcohol use, and alcohol use motives among firefighters: The role of distress tolerance. *Psychiatry Research, 282*, 112633. https://doi.org/10.1016/j.psychres.2019.112633

Veterans as First Responders

Sam J. Buser

Introduction

Lewis and Pathak (2014) found that veterans are more likely to work for state and local governments than nonveterans, and many of them are employed as first responders. According to the Marshall Project (Weichselbaum et al., 2017), a non-profit news organization focused on the criminal justice system, one in five police officers is a veteran. A 2015 US Department of Labor report (Schafer et al., 2015) stated that 10% of our Emergency Medicine Technicians (EMTs), 19% of our fire-fighters and 25% of our police officers are veterans. The percentages of first responders who are veterans are especially high in those areas that offer hiring preferences for veterans.

In considering the ideas in this chapter, the author's background should be considered. While many first responders were in the military prior to becoming a first responder, this is not true for MHPs. Only a few MHPs have themselves served within the military, police, corrections, EMS, or fire service. For most MHPs, the first responder and the military worlds are foreign. The chapter's author is somewhat of an exception in that he has served within the army, commanded a military police detachment, worked as a psychologist for the VA Medical System, and was the staff psychologist for one of the largest fire departments in the country. These experiences have shaped his perspective, and, in turn, the views that are presented in this chapter.

S. J. Buser (✉)
Houston Fire Department (Retired), Houston, TX, USA
e-mail: sam@drsambuser.com

M. L. Bourke et al. (eds.), *First Responder Mental Health*,
https://doi.org/10.1007/978-3-031-38149-2_26

Similarity of Cultures

Former military members sometimes struggle readapting to a civilian world and its very different standards and expectations. This may be especially true for those veterans who have experienced the hardships and dangers of combat. However, there is significant overlap between military culture and the world of first responders. For veterans, joining the paramilitary world of the first responder may bridge the gap between the military and civilian experience.

A Sense of Duty Being in the military, serving one's country and community, is often associated with a sense of duty. Patriotism is not dead or an antiquated concept for these Americans. One Air Force Commander (Archer, 2009) described duty in this way *"What duty really equates to is a moral force that binds you to accomplishing your assigned responsibilities without regard to your own preferences, your own desires, or your own well-being. Duty in the armed forces means not balancing personal obligations, career aspirations, or monetary enhancements with duty, but putting the service duty first."* The desire to continue in a role of duty is very important for many veterans. Such values may have drawn them into the military in the first place, and after discharge, they may seek a new role to continue addressing those ideals. As in the military, the sense of duty to protect one's community is a shared value among most first responders.

Mission Accomplishment Related to a sense of duty is the importance of mission accomplishment. Among both first responders and the military, mission accomplishment is one's paramount duty. It is valued over all other things, including personal safety. Sergeant Major of the Marine Corps, Troy E. Black (Escott, 2019) recently described it this way: *"Mission First, Marines Always…No matter what it is we are tasked to do as Marines, that's what we're required to do, accomplish the mission. It's always mission first, taking care of your Marines and accomplishing that mission, it is what we do each and every day."* In virtually all organizations, leaders are advised to put the mission first (Katpitulik & MacDonald, 2019) (e.g., to improve productivity, increase sales and profits, produce more), but this idea carries a different and more serious meaning within the military and among first responders. Police, fire, corrections, and EMS, like military members, are expected to do their job regardless of weather, despite personal hardship – even putting their lives on the line to accomplish their mission.

Strong Role Identity *"Once a Marine, Always a Marine!" "Hire a vet."* Being in the military tends to create a sense of identity that does not expire upon discharge. Service members tend to identify as a veteran, even if it has been decades since they last donned their uniform. They usually take pride in the military units in which they served and the activities in which they were engaged (e.g., Vietnam veteran bumper stickers, shirts emblazoned with the name of the ship on which they last served). Former servicemembers proudly stand to be recognized at sporting events, attend reunions of their old units, and wear baseball caps identifying their service.

Similarly, first responders often talk about their work as not a job, but a calling. Most feel a strong identity with that role manifested in multiple ways. Frequently, they mainly socialize with other first responders. Go into the home of a first responder, and you are likely to see memorabilia, antiques, and tchotchke associated with their career (e.g., many firefighters keep and restore old fire engines which they proudly drive in community parades and the like). First responders frequently volunteer for additional career connected activities (e.g., Honor Guard, sports teams representing their department, fundraising charities for sick or injured members, supporting the 100 Club for fallen first responders). After retirement, first responders tend to continue their affiliation with other first responders through groups of retired members or even by just dropping by their old departments or stations.

Civilians are often viewed skeptically by military members. Soldiers, sailors, marines, airmen usually live and work in separate facilities, away from civilians. There is no mistaking whether you are at a military installation or "off-post." Indeed, former service members can be closed off even to other veterans who served in a different capacity (e.g., you didn't serve in combat, you were not deployed, you weren't being targeted, you weren't a Marine).

As with military members, first responders frequently lack trust in outsiders (i.e., those who have not served). Police and other first responders usually distinguish themselves from others who are not in their ranks. While not necessarily unfriendly to non-first responders, they tend to be cautious when meeting them. A frequent complaint of first responders is being asked to describe a gory scene or to give their account of a sensational public event (e.g., crime, fire, death). First responder groups (e.g., dispatch vs. line; police vs. fire) are even competitive with each other, seeing the other groups as having it different (and typically better) than they themselves.

Camaraderie Many veterans cite the camaraderie, a sense of cohesion with their fellow service members, as one of the best parts of their service career. Of course, not all units have the same sense of cohesion, and, just as in other walks of life, some people may have trouble fitting in with their unit or comrades. Yet, veterans, especially those who serve in combat together, often speak of their sense of connection. You see this evidenced in the reunions of former service members who served in the same unit or location, and even with the overall identity of being a veteran. Recognizing the importance of interpersonal connections in the military, the US Army even instituted a "battle buddy" program (US Training and Document Command, 2019) in an attempt to ensure that every newly enlisted soldier would have a "best friend" serving in their unit. Furthermore, research (Nevarez et al., 2017) has suggested that good peer relationships during deployments can reduce the incidence of posttraumatic stress disorder (PTSD) among soldiers who are deployed. As noted by Tom Wolfe (2012) in his book about transitioning from the military to the civilian world, "*There is nothing in the civilian workforce that can approximate the bonding that occurs in the wardroom, ready room, or foxhole. Military personnel in those environments put up with much hardship – long hours, stressful working conditions, danger to personal safety, separation from loved ones, and more. … Other than perhaps the professions of law enforcement, firefighting, and emergency* *medicine (notice the common denominator), it would be difficult to find a civilian occupation that approximates the conditions of the foxhole."*

First responders often talk about the importance of connections with others in their department or crew. Firefighters, for example, who must spend 24 hours or more together living and working in close quarters, may transfer stations to be with a "tight crew." Fellow first responders are frequently referred to as "brother" or "sister," and units are often described as a "family."

Adrenaline/Excitement/Danger Another common element in military life is to experience the adrenaline rush and excitement from exposure to danger. Whether those emotional extremes come from being on a carrier deck, jumping out of an airplane, or facing hostile fire, military members frequently experience heightened reactions. In listening to veterans you will frequently hear them recall such terrifying, and, sometimes, thrilling moments. A return to the civilian world with offices, meetings, and "deadlines" may seem far too boring and mundane. These veterans may seek the less predictable and more dangerous world of the first responder where they can again experience the exhilaration of pushing themselves to physical and psychological limits. I recall one of my own military buddies who after leaving the military found it impossible to feel happy in the corporate world. He then found a way to return to service, not in the military, but for a federal intelligence agency doing a dangerous job.

Self-Sufficiency The Rand Corporation (2018) noted that there is a tension between the desire for military members to solve their own problems and their willingness to seek help. The report commented that military members do not always recognize their need for help until their problems are severe. Within the first responder world, there is a similar desire to take care of one's own problems without having to involve others. The unofficial mantra of the Marines "*Improvise, Adapt, and Overcome*," made famous by Clint Eastwood in the movie *Heartbreak Ridge* (Eastwood, 1986), suggests that regardless of the situation, one should use their own resources to address a problem. As with most such exhortations, it is true to a point. It is certainly good to be resilient, to use ingenuity, and to not give up, but there are also times when it is wise to solicit advice, guidance, instruction, and counsel. No man, woman, soldier, or first responder is an island. Indeed, both the military and first responders work in teams to accomplish their mission. This quality of self-sufficiency can, at times, pose problems for first responders and military members as we shall discuss further later in this chapter.

Physical Fitness Both the military and the first responder world place an emphasis on physical fitness. Not everyone can perform the physical tasks required of these jobs. Applicants must pass physical fitness tests to qualify for membership. Strength, endurance, agility, and aerobic conditioning are needed to complete the missions of the military and of first responders. In both cultures, members must continue to demonstrate their ability to physically perform their duties throughout their careers. A loss of those abilities can mean termination. The facilities of both the military and first responders always include fitness equipment, and many service members and first responders compete in races, martial arts, and bodybuilding during their time off. For service members leaving the military, the expectations among first responders of physicality and staying in shape feel familiar, comfortable, and important.

Self-Discipline Inductees to the military, as well as trainees at a first responder training academy, get intensive education in self-discipline. New members of both the first responder and the military world are expected to comply with strict rules for demeanor and behavior. They must meet exacting standards for cleanliness, personal appearance, and punctuality. Violations of those standards can result in discipline by superiors and a loss of social status in the organization. Veterans are familiar with these expectations from their military experience and generally have little trouble continuing to meet them as first responders.

Rituals The rituals common among first responder groups are similar to those in the military: respect for the flag, elaborate funerals, awards for valor. Indeed, many first responder rituals were adapted from military predecessors. These rituals are symbolically important to both first responders and service members. Even in civilian life, many veterans continue to engage in some of those rituals (e.g., flying a flag at their home). For the veteran, the first responder world with its shared traditions and ceremonies is a place of familiarity and comfort.

Clothing and Language The clothing and language unique to a culture denote membership. Group identity is conveyed through style of dress and how one communicates. While the language and dress of the military and first responders are not identical, they are similar. Their language is replete with specialized terms, acronyms, and expressions, some of which are shared by both groups. Their uniforms share commonalities, and there are specific rules about how and when they are to be worn. The variety of civilian dress is replaced by the predictability and standards of uniform dress codes. For the veteran, wearing the uniform of the first responder can be familiar and comforting, identifying them as a member of that unique "tribe." Those who do not dress, talk, or act similarly are denoted as outsiders, and, as such, are viewed as less trusted.

Scarcity of Resources Scarcity of resources, learning how to do more with less, and the importance of flexibility and improvisation in dynamic situations are ubiquitous within both the military and the first responder culture. Dependent on tax dollars and the beneficence of politicians, both groups usually feel underfunded and under-resourced. As one joke heard both among first responders and service members goes: *"We've been doing so much, for so long, with so little, that now we can do everything, with nothing, forever."* Equipped with various protocols to deal with common problems and never enough resouces, they repeatedly train to achieve success. Yet, they frequently face unpredictable circumstances – whether the fog of war, inclement weather, chaotic situations, or the actions of hostiles and criminals. Veterans and first responders have to cope with novel or unforeseen problems, adopt new solutions on the fly, and overcome unique challenges. The ingenuity and can-do-it attitude of the military are also much appreciated within the first responder community.

What Veterans Bring to the Table

Veterans may exhibit personal qualities or experiences that make them interested in subsequently pursuing a career as a first responder. French (2018) cites four things that make veterans good police officers (or for that matter, other kinds of first responders):

1. They are team players. They are accustomed to working together to achieve difficult, sometimes dangerous goals. Veterans are used to depending on each other, rather than being lone wolves.
2. They communicate concisely, confidently, and effectively. The military emphasizes the importance of direct, clear communications. To the civilian, military communication is full of jargon and acronyms. It lacks much expressive language and is much more instrumental in character. While this style is a liability in emotional relationships, it is advantageous in critical, life-and-death situations where time and decisiveness are paramount. Veterans are accustomed to this communication style.
3. They are practiced in being both leaders and subordinates. From early in their service, military members are placed in leadership positions. Simultaneously, they have had to respond to leaders above them and to direct their own subordinates. They understand the chain-of-command concept and the importance of both giving and following orders.
4. They have had to practice stress management, often under extreme circumstances. Stressors, both physical and mental, are common in military service and are often much more severe than those experienced in the civilian world. The stressors of military life are more like those that face first responders than to the stressors of other occupational groups. The stressors for both military and first responders are not arbitrary deadlines or quotas, but life-threatening events.

Others have pointed out that some of the skills learned in the military have application for first responders (Milzarski, 2020). For example, both military and first responders have at least a modicum of medical training. Additionally, comfort and proficiency in using firearms is common for military members and extremely helpful for potential police officers. Some military members are specialists occupying remarkably similar roles to those of civilian first responders. For example, all branches of the military utilize highly trained personnel to provide emergency medicine services, particularly to deal with traumatic injuries. Likewise, some military personnel serve as military and security police or work in military correctional facilities. Military firefighters serve in every branch of the service, and those skills are readily applicable to firefighting in the civilian world.

Challenges for First Responders Who Are Veterans

Most veterans who become first responders are valued for their discipline and the skills they bring to the job. However, some veterans do bring problems with them from their military experience to the squad car, prison, ambulance, or fire truck.

Traumatic Exposure An important risk factor for developing mental disorders or substance abuse is the amount of one's exposure to traumatic events (Davis et al., 2022). Unfortunately, experiencing critical incidents, *"an event which has the potential to overwhelm one's usual coping mechanisms resulting in psychological distress and an impairment of normal adaptive functioning"* (Mitchell & Everly, 1996), is common both for those who serve in the military and among first responders. For veteran/first responders there is an additive effect of potentially traumatic exposure from military experience plus the traumatic exposure from being a first responder.

Mental Disorders While most veterans do not develop mental disorders, there is an increased incidence of a variety of mental disorders among those with prior military service (Seal et al., 2009) in comparison to a civilian cohort. First responders with prior military experience are significantly more likely to develop psychiatric disorders including PTSD, depression, anxiety, stress, panic disorders and suicidal ideation (Groll et al., 2020) than those first responders who are not veterans. In short, being a veteran or a first responder puts you at risk for a psychiatric disorder. If you are both a former service member and a first responder, Groll et al. (2020) found that you were 1.5 times more likely to develop a mental disorder.

PTSD It is well established that veterans, especially those with combat experience, abuse from childhood, or sexual trauma, are at significant elevated risk for posttraumatic stress symptoms and a PTSD diagnosis. There is some indication that veterans who served in wars of different eras may experience varying levels of PTSD (e.g., Kulka et al., 1988; Marmar et al., 2015; Richardson et al., 2010); however, these findings are confounded with other variables such as the age of the veteran, differential mortality rates, length of time since they had served, and differing definitions and instruments used to measure PTSD symptoms (Schnurr, n.d.).

When combat veterans experience further traumatic incidents, the risk of posttraumatic stress symptoms emerging, or reemerging, is elevated (Sachs-Ericsson et al., 2016). Prior exposure to trauma may alter one's sensitivity of the stress-response systems (McLaughlin et al., 2010), making the person more apt to develop PTSD symptoms after encountering additional traumatic situations. Considerable research has been done to examine this altered sensitivity of the stress response system usually referred to as "kindling or sensitization" (e.g., Petr, 2016).

For veterans who become first responders, they are highly likely to engage in or witness further traumatic events. Although in some ways these veterans, based on their previous experience in crisis situations, may be better prepared than others to act or react in the crisis moment, they are also probably more vulnerable to subsequent suffering from experiencing additional trauma.

Substance Abuse Veterans have been found to be at increased risk of developing substance use disorders (Larson et al., 2012; Seal et al., 2011). Likewise, first responders are at heightened risk for developing substance use disorders (SAMHSA, 2018). Both within the military and among first responders, applicants and current members are often required to take random drug tests (typically urinalysis). If an applicant to the military or to a first responder department fails the drug test, they are usually not hired. For current members, those who are found to be abusing substances (other than alcohol), often face dismissal. Despite these prohibitions, substance abuse, especially of alcohol, is a common problem among both military and first responder populations.

Typically, departments do not screen for alcohol use during random drug tests. Although first responders are much more likely to abuse alcohol than other substances, overuse of alcohol is not detected. This also means that veterans with alcohol problems may be admitted as rookie first responders.

Alcohol use, while not officially condoned, is commonplace among first responders and is considered culturally acceptable (Ballenger et al., 2011; Haddock et al., 2022), so long as you are not using while on duty or getting into trouble because of it (e.g., DWI). There is considerable variation in how departments handle alcohol-related problems. Commonly, alcohol overuse is discovered as the result of the member getting into trouble with the law (e.g., DWI). In some departments, being arrested for a driving while intoxicated (DWI) or public intoxication (PI) is automatic grounds for dismissal, while other departments prefer to use demotion, temporary suspension, loss of privileges, or financial penalties to dissuade members from overuse of alcohol. The allowances made for alcohol use and even overuse in the first responder world make it more likely for the veteran with an alcohol problem to continue heavier alcohol use, not surprisingly leading to high incidences of misuse and even dependence.

Physical Health Effects While there has been considerable research documenting the negative effects of combat on mental health, its effects on physical health have been less well studied (Schnittker, 2018). When veterans have sustained service-related disabilities (e.g., traumatic brain injuries and back injuries), those effects are often self-evident and documented. Some of those injuries would prevent the veteran from even qualifying later for first responder jobs. However, Schnittker found that combat experience, especially being exposed to the dead and wounded, is associated with poor physical health outcomes as well, even among those who are not themselves physically wounded. He suggests that the relationship between combat and poor physical health outcomes is related to social and behavioral processes. For example, combat-exposed veterans are more likely to smoke, less likely to be married, and report being less prepared for transitioning back to the civilian world. Similarly, Taylor et al. (2016) found an association between military experience and physical health. Those veterans exposed to hazardous or traumatic experiences reported negative health effects. Thus, first responders who are veterans may be more prone to long-term physical health issues as well as mental disorders.

Anger and Aggression Anger, hostility, and aggression are associated with combat-related PTSD among veterans (Jakupcak et al., 2007). Furthermore, especially among men, depression may be masked by increased anger and irritability (Cochran & Rabinowitz, 1999). Problems in modulating anger or aggression can prove to be a major problem for those veterans wishing to serve as first responders. Gonzalez et al. (2019) found that police officers who had served in the military were more likely to be involved in shootings than non-veteran police officers. Furthermore, those officers who had been deployed to combat zones were almost three times more likely to be involved in such shootings than officers who were not veterans. While not exclusive to veterans who are first responders, there is also research that demonstrates a higher incidence of violent or aggressive behavior among veterans with PTSD, especially if complicated by alcohol misuse (Elbogen et al., 2014).

Suicide First responders are more likely to die by suicide than as the result of a line-of-duty incident (Ruderman Foundation, 2022, June). We also know that suicide among veterans is unfortunately too common (Suitt III, 2021). Research on first responder suicides has not really addressed the potentiating effects of being a member of both high-risk groups, but it seems likely that first responders who are veterans might be especially at elevated risk for contemplating suicide. Other variables common to veterans such as PTSD, combat experience, substance abuse history, and unaddressed mental health problems have been examined as factors in increasing suicidal behavior among veterans. Of these, the presence of mental health issues, including PTSD, seems to have been the variable most consistently found to elevate the risk of suicidal thoughts and actions among veterans (LeardMann et al., 2013). Weichselbaum et al. (2017) reported that veterans who serve as police officers were more likely to engage in self-destructive behavior including suicide than non-veterans.

Combat Experience Most veterans have not had actual combat experience, even when they served during a time of armed conflict. Fewer still have been directly in the line of fire. Combat experience, though, has been repeatedly shown to have particularly deleterious long-term effects on both the mental and physical well-being of the individuals who performed this role (Nasveld et al., 2012). Studies of veteran adjustment, though, often conflate deployment to a war zone (e.g., Quatar) with actual combat experience. Even those who serve in combat vary in terms of the risk they experienced, their exposure to bodies and wounded, casualties in their unit, whether they were themselves wounded, and the amount of emotional support they received after action. To understand these veterans, it is important to ask about their individual experiences while in the military. The MHP who has not served in the military may not fully appreciate the events that some veterans have faced and may underestimate the potential negative effects of their service. For example, one such veteran reported that he had served as a cook while deployed to a combat zone. Such a role, at first glance, would not seem to be particularly dangerous. Further questioning revealed that one of his responsibilities was to drive a supply truck along a road that was well known to be booby trapped with IEDs by the enemy.

Warriors to Guardians Military members are trained to be warriors, to defeat the enemy. Violence is justified, even necessary, to complete this task. The first responder, though, is committed to "protect and serve" as the common slogan on law enforcement vehicles suggests. Police have been called upon to reexamine their role considering several, well-publicized incidents involving deaths of civilians at the hands of the police. Concerns have also been expressed about the militarization of law enforcement through the acquisition of military style vehicles and weapons (Delehanty et al., 2017). *"Law enforcement should embrace a guardian – rather than a warrior – mindset to build trust and legitimacy both within agencies and with the public,"* according to a report on the twenty-first-century policing (President's Task Force, 2015).

The "warrior" mentality in law enforcement seems to be a response to threats to police safety. From this perspective, any encounter with the public may be dangerous, and one must always be prepared to fight. However, others have argued that such a stance increases the risk of avoidable violence directed by police at civilians (van Brocklin, 2019). For the veteran trained to be a warrior, the guardian role may require an adjustment in expectations, attitudes, and behavior (Kindy, 2015).

Paramilitary At times being a veteran in a first responder organization can be frustrating because it is "not military enough". This might be particularly true for those veterans who have served for a number of years in the military and had become more accustomed to those cultural expectations. For them, a lack of adherence to military standards (e.g., of punctuality or accountability) can be very frustrating and disappointing. This is sometimes seen in complaints from veterans about what would have happened in their old military unit if a similar thing would have happened. This can give rise to a higher level of aggression or violence than is expected in an organization that interacts more with civilians than the "enemy".

Ongoing Service Commitments

Among the first responders in many departments are part-time service members: National Guard and Reservists. These veterans may continue to be called up for training, deployments overseas, or domestic duties such as training assignments, responses to natural disasters, or border duties. While these first responders are with their military units, their first responder jobs are typically protected, awaiting their return. While they may be gone for a relatively short time, a few weeks or months, they can be gone for a year or more. In some cases, they may have been deployed to a combat zone and have seen significant fighting during their deployment. When they return, especially if they have been gone for an extended period, these reservists/guard members usually go through some sort of reorientation process. Part of this process is administrative (e.g., human resources, benefits, and the like). They also may be required to retrain to ensure that they can still perform their duties (e.g., weapons requalification, demonstrating medical skills proficiency, practicing fire rescue skills). It is prudent for the MHP working with the department to be part of the reorientation process when these reservists/guard members return to their first responder jobs. In this way, the MHP can determine what the service member experienced (e.g., combat) while on military duty. Typically, these veterans are anxious to get back to their normal duties and view these various reorientation activities as a waste of time, but for the MHP meeting with these returnees, this can be an important moment for clinical assessment and for establishing a connection with the veteran that may facilitate helping in the future.

Providing Help to Veteran/First Responders

Stigma About Seeking Help Traditionally, service members do not want to acknowledge having a psychological problem (Kaplan, 2019). To do so can result in the loss of your security clearance, your specific job, a promotion, or even your career. After a military deployment, those admitting to emotional distress from their experience may be delayed in returning home, separated from their unit, or not allowed to reenlist. Furthermore, military culture discourages showing any form of weakness, even to close friends or buddies. The denial of psychological distress is a career survival tool in the military.

For similar reasons, first responders hold a strong prohibition against admitting psychological problems. According to a survey by the University of Phoenix (2019), 57% of first responders felt that there would be negative repercussions for seeking counseling. Of those, almost half expected that they would receive different treatment from their supervisors and 35% believed they would be viewed as weak by their colleagues or peers. These first responders feared being given a different job assignment and being passed over for promotion. To admit to psychological distress runs against the stereotypical profile of the stoic hero who fights fires or nabs criminals. When the first responder is a veteran as well, they have been steeped with a double dose of "don't show any weakness."

Mental health professionals are familiar with the general stigma that many people hold about not wanting to see a "shrink". Many, if not most, clients are hesitant to begin counseling or to seek therapy for fear of how they might be perceived by others or themselves. The reluctance in seeking psychological care among first responders and veterans is far greater, though, than most MHPs have previously encountered. This stigma is one of the primary obstacles to delivering psychological care to a group that is very vulnerable to mental health problems.

Confidentiality Challenges From their first graduate classes, MHPs are taught to maintain the confidentiality of their clients. While this is important in any clinical setting, it has even greater significance when working with veterans and first responders. If the MHP is working for the same organization (e.g., department) that employs the first responder, that veteran/first responder is likely to be skeptical of assurances that their private conversations with the MHP are secure. Their experience has taught them that is not necessarily true. They may expect the MHP's loyalty to lie with the organization, not the individual. A substantial number of these first responders will never believe that their information will be kept in confidence. If, on the other hand, the MHP is working outside that system (e.g., private practice or separate agency), the MHP may be relatively unfamiliar with the culture, life, and work of the first responder. This, too, is a barrier for the first responder seeking care. Either way, the MHP has an extra burden in earning the trust of the first responder. In my personal experience, MHPs tend to overestimate their understanding of the first responder and underestimate their stigma against seeking help. Many MHPs seem to feel that their natural empathy will make up for a lack of familiarity with first responder culture.

VA Medical System The VA, the nation's largest health care system (US Dept. of Veteran Affairs, n.d.), can be a valuable referral source for the MHP working with first responder veterans. VA psychiatrists may be able to provide medications for those first responder veterans who are struggling with depression and anxiety, and the VA has first-rate programs for treating PTSD. When necessary, the VA also offers inpatient psychiatric care. For those first responder veterans who are struggling with substance abuse, there are alcohol and drug treatment programs available, often on both an inpatient and outpatient basis.

While the Veterans Administration (VA) maintains the biggest medical and psychiatric system to aid veterans, it is not always favorably viewed by them. Qualifying for services from the VA can be an arcane and daunting process, and not every first responder veteran is eligible for services. Furthermore, veterans sometimes see the VA as an extension of the military or the federal government that they may blame for creating the conditions from which they suffer. The negative reputation of the VA among so many vets is not entirely justified, but, as with the stigma about seeking help, it is part of the fabric with which the MHP working with first responder veterans must consider.

The VA system also evaluates potential disability cases of veterans, assigning a percentage of disability related to military service. It is not unusual for veterans who work as first responders to apply for a partial disability based on physical or mental injuries that occurred while on military duty (e.g., PTSD, exposure to toxic chemicals). The MHP working with first responder veterans may be called upon to assist them in applying for a VA disability. This may include production of records or providing letters of support substantiating their claim. A VA-rated disability, though, does not necessarily mean that the veteran is unable to perform a job as a first responder.

Engaging Families of Veterans and First Responders A recent qualitative study (Lawn et al., 2022) examined the experiences of family members of veterans and first responders in supporting their loved ones to get mental health care. The study found that the family played a vital role in getting the veteran or first responder to seek help, but these families felt largely ignored by the military or emergency services organizations that employed their loved ones. The authors suggest that efforts to encourage first responders and veterans to seek help might be more successful if directed at the family level. Six key themes were identified in this phenomenological study of veteran and first responder families:

1. *The job is different from others.*

   Families are required to provide a level of emotional support different from other occupations because of the life-threatening nature of the role.

2. *Making a change first involved recognizing that something was wrong.*

   Loved ones were able to identify changes in their veteran and first responder family members more easily than could professionals or peers. Family members recognized that the behavior of their veteran or first responder had become out of the ordinary for them.

3. *The tipping point – Deciding that something needed to be done*

   Making the decision to utilize professional help was typically not quick or linear. Often the decision was made only after some sort of crisis (e.g., family violence, separation from the kids).

4. *Barriers to help-seeking – A lack of trust in the help-seeking process*

   Once the veteran or first responder agrees to seek help, a sense of urgency is needed before the moment passes. Seeking help from the organization was complicated by a lack of confidence in the competence of available help providers, fears that the first responder might be seen as "weak," and concerns about the potential impacts on the career of the first responder or veteran.

5. *Family support is critical.*

   Decisions about the type of support and how to access help were complex. Families often did not reach out to the support services that might be available to them. The families also felt distrusting of the organization to respond appropriately. Furthermore, the families tended to blame the organization for being complicit in the development of their family member's problems.

6. *What families need from organizations*

   Families wanted first responder and veteran organizations to include families as part of the support team for veterans and first responders. They wanted their organizations to acknowledge and address workplace-related trauma. They also wanted mental health education to be embedded within the organization both for first responders and for family members throughout the career cycle.

Veterans and first responders vary as to whether they share their work experiences with family members (most typically the spouse or romantic partner). Many do not, feeling the need to protect their loved ones from the potentially secondary traumatizing effects of describing what they have seen or done. Those who do share more with their families tend to have spouses or partners who are themselves first responders, seeing them as peers who will understand what it was like. In either case, family members are likely to be the first ones that notice mental health changes (Lawn et al., 2022).

Family members are also the ones most often encouraging the first responder to seek help. Of course, if the family members themselves fear that the first responder will face negative consequences because of help-seeking, those hopes for help may be stymied (Beks, 2016). Likewise, if families feel that the organization is to blame for the problems of the first responder, they are unlikely to reach out for help within the organization. Furthermore, if family members are unaware of helping resources, they, of course, will not try to access them. Because of official communication channels, it is much easier to communicate about helping resources to the first responders than to their families. This points to the importance of MHPs establishing communication channels not only to the first responders but also to their families. The MHP needs to let the families know about available help, about warning signs of problems, and about how to access care. This may be especially important in the case of families with a first responder who is also a veteran.

Tips for the MHP Working with Veteran/First Responders

The following ideas are offered to mental health professionals working with first responders who are also veterans of military service.

Pre-employment Psychological Screenings Advocate for pre-employment psychological screenings for applicants to first responder departments. Veterans should not be discriminated against in the hiring process, but potential problems stemming from prior military service should not be ignored either. Unfortunately, there is a lack of uniformity in pre-employment screening processes for those seeking to become first responders. Police departments are likely to use a screening process, but there is much variability in the application process to become firefighters or EMS. Given the risks of substance abuse, PTSD, anger, and suicide inherent in being a first responder, these should be emphasized in pre-employment background evaluations and psychological pre-employment screenings. Much more research is needed on how to assess positive qualities needed to be a successful first responder as well as how to detect disqualifying criteria.

On-boarding Create an on-boarding process for new recruits who are veterans and for those who are returning from active military duty (e.g., in the reserves or Guard). There should be at least one individual meeting with these veterans as they enter/return to the department. This can be built into the administrative processes in the department for new or returning employees. In the military, when a member and/or their family changes duty stations, it is customary for them to be helped in that transition by an assigned "sponsor". The sponsor acquaints the service member and their family with what is available in the community to help them with their transition. This can include information about housing, schools, medical facilities, recreational activities, etc. The on-boarding process with the MHP working with first responders should seek to establish a similar tone—one of welcoming and assistance during transition. During the on-boarding, the MHP can describe potential helping resources available to the veteran (MHP, EAP, chaplain, veterans' programs). The veteran may also be told about services and programs in the department that are likely to be helpful or of interest to veterans (e.g., the Honor Guard, chaplain). While such information might be included on websites or through pamphlets, a personal approach acknowledging the member's veteran status is likely to be more effective. It is important for this meeting to not be a "mental health screening" but a genuine effort to welcome and assist the veteran. The meeting between the veteran and the MHP should have a feel of sponsorship and welcoming rather than one of "evaluation." The meeting also provides an opportunity for the MHP to establish an initial connection between the veteran and the MHP in case services are needed. The MHP should be aware that veterans who are also first responders are at significantly elevated risk of developing psychiatric problems and substance abuse. Thus, it is important for the MHP to establish that they can be a potential source of help for the veteran/first responder should the need arise.

Veterans Service Officer Consider asking Command to create a Veterans' Service Officer (VSO) within your department. The ideal person for this role is a veteran who already is known and respected in the department. (In most departments, this would be an additional duty, rather than a primary role.) Former military members usually continue to identify with their experience within the service and are often eager to assist fellow veterans. The VSO should serve as an advisor to Command Staff and officers in matters concerning veterans. For example, the VSO might suggest ways to honor veterans on Veterans Day, Marine Corps Birthday, etc. (e.g., feature a member of the department who is a veteran in department websites, describing their military service). The VSO might also informally meet with veterans in the department who are experiencing difficulties and assist them in connecting with appropriate resources either in the department or in the community. The VSO should be involved in the on-boarding process described previously, meeting with new recruits who are veterans as well as with returning active-duty members. First responder departments should not only "hire vets" but also "support vets".

Supporting Veterans in the Department Look at establishing a communication link with veterans in the department using media such as a Facebook Group, a webpage, or e-mail blasts. Find ways to remind your first responder/veterans that you are available to them and that you are sensitive to their needs. Be a visible and outspoken proponent of the needs of veterans within your department.

As the MHP for the department, you will not be able to directly meet all the needs of veterans/first responders. Establish liaisons with VA hospitals, clinics, or programs in your area. Become familiar with how to refer veterans to the VA for additional services. The MHP does not have to become expert on the complexities of qualifying for VA services, but the MHP should be familiar with how to guide the veteran in finding out about qualifying for services. Since not all veterans qualify for VA services, it is vital for the MHP to also know about additional helpful programs and assets for veterans, especially for those that do not qualify for VA services. Such groups include *Wounded Warriors*, *Disabled American Veterans,* and *Combined Arms.*

Service-Connected Disability Become familiar with how disability pensions for military service-connected injuries are handled in your department. In some jurisdictions, PTSD symptoms among first responders are automatically presumed to be connected with their service as first responders. When the first responder is also a veteran, especially one with combat experience, this well-intentioned idea can pose issues for the department and for their retirement plans. Is the pension/retirement fund responsible for providing compensation in this case? Is there any pre-employment screening to determine if applicants have preexisting history or conditions that might lead to a diagnosis of PTSD?

Access to Mental Health Services Try to address the cultural stigma within the department about seeking mental health services. Use focus groups and the like to identify specific reasons for members not seeking help. Tailor messaging/advertising to address the specific feedback given by members about their reluctance to seek help. Seek to address common myths and misbeliefs about seeking help for mental health concerns. Command staff and well-regarded members of the department might be asked to serve as role models, speaking publicly about their support and utilization of mental health services.

Make it easy for first responders to access the MHP. Reduce barriers to access by allowing for direct e-mail and/or phone calls to the MHP rather than employing administrative go-betweens (e.g., receptionists). Remove administrative and bureaucratic barriers (e.g., calling a general number; going through the chain of command; having to submit a request for service) that discourage first responder/veterans and family members from seeking mental health services. Publicize direct communication links (e.g., cell phone numbers; e-mail addresses; Facebook pages) available to first responder/veterans and their family members to utilize in contacting the MHP.

Family Emphasis Find ways to connect with the families of the first responders. Given that veterans and first responders are usually reluctant to seek help for themselves, creating easy access to the MHP for family members increases the likelihood that help can be provided in a timely way. As found in recent research by Lawn et al. (2022), family members are often unaware of the support services available to them. Yet, the family members are the first ones to recognize potential mental health problems. Rather than being seen as ancillary to the veteran/first responder, the family needs to be viewed as a central element in the support systems available to them. In some departments, there are organized or informal networks of spouses that can be conduits for the MHP to communicate with those families.

Offer relationship and family services to the members of your department. The most common reason that first responders and veterans seek mental health assistance is because of relationship problems (e.g., divorce, potential break-up). Even then, that request for services is often only coming at the insistence of their romantic partner. Elements common in the first responder role and the veteran role (e.g., traumatic experiences, shift schedules, missing family events) put additional strains on their family relationships – sometimes erupting into infidelity, severe marital conflicts, and even family violence.

Consider how to assist veteran/first responder families with special needs. First responder families must, of course, deal with the same childhood and family issues of other families (e.g., adolescent behavior problems, developmental delays, chronic childhood illnesses, aging parents). The first responder may be less able to provide care for infants or the sick because of their schedules or duties. It may be more common in these families for them to adopt a more traditional gender role split of responsibilities (e.g., the woman not working outside the home, men providing respite care of children rather than taking on greater parenting responsibilities). Meeting every potential need of first responder/veteran families (e.g., play therapy for young children, adolescent treatment) is likely beyond the scope of the MHP's mission. To help address the MHP's limitations, it is important to identify referral resources in the community that can be of assistance.

Anger Management Anger issues are a common presenting problem among first responders and veterans being referred for treatment. Several factors contribute to this. First, the great majority of first responders and veterans are male, and men more commonly have had trouble managing emotions. Many men have been taught that anger is the one emotion that they can safely express, and some seemingly channel all other emotions into expressions of anger. It is well known that men are more likely than women to get into trouble for inappropriately expressing anger. Secondly, veterans, especially those with combat history or PTSD, often have problems in managing anger (Jakupcak et al., 2007). Anger problems among first responders often present as difficulties in getting along with their peers at the station or as part of a pattern of relationship conflict or domestic violence within the home.

Community resources offering anger management programs may be ill suited to meet the needs of first responders. Weekly appointments for group sessions/classes or individual meetings may be impractical for them. The costs of such treatment, even if available, may be prohibitive, and first responders lack trust in programs that are designed for the general population. Develop anger management programs adapted to the needs of the first responders you serve. Modify proven anger management techniques using language and examples consistent with the culture of the first responders. Offer such programs at times/places that are convenient for first responders rather than expecting them to adapt to the schedule of the MHP.

Emphasis on Alcohol Abuse Treatment Expect that alcohol abuse will be one of the mental health problems that you will most encounter as an MHP working with first responder/veterans. Develop alcohol psychoeducation programs that are integrated into required training modules. Become familiar with the substance abuse treatment programs that exist in your area and establish good working relationships with them for referral purposes. Using evidence-based research lobby command staff for policies that encourage treatment rather than discipline. Those who self-identify with alcohol problems seeking help should be treated differently than those who are detected through infractions of rules or laws. Understand that the science you present on this will be competing with long-standing traditions of cultural acceptance of heavy alcohol use among first responders. There are also strong political forces at work that may hamper your ability to address alcohol abuse as a mental health issue.

It is essential to work with the representatives of labor (e.g., union) to develop a compassionate approach that supports those members with alcohol problems. At the same time, management (i.e., command and politicians) will be concerned about liability, precedence, and public perception of how your department handles substance abusers within its ranks. Your efforts to address alcohol problems in the department must consider the sometimes competing needs of these three disparate groups: labor, management, and the individual who needs help.

Suicide Prevention In light of the high suicide rates among both veterans and first responders, develop an ongoing suicide prevention program for your department. Suicide prevention needs to be viewed as a continuous effort rather than relegated to postvention following a completed suicide among your members. Consider creating a suicide prevention committee or task force that meets periodically to review suicide prevention efforts. The committee might include members of the command staff, the Veterans Service Officer, union representatives, and even family members who have lost first responders to suicide. Connect with larger suicide prevention efforts in the community and nation (e.g., holding events during Mental Health Month and National Suicide Prevention Week). Incorporate veterans in peer support efforts (e.g., CISM) in order to respond to potential suicidal crises among your members who are veterans.

Referrals to Other Providers If you are successful in establishing yourself as a helpful resource for the first responder/veterans in your department, there will be more needs for service than you can meet. Furthermore, regardless of your efforts some members of your department will prefer to go outside the department for mental health care. Identify outside providers and agencies in the community who are well suited to help first responders and veterans. Many community resources, even those serving veterans, are unfamiliar with the culture and needs of first responders. Educate referral sources about the first responder world. Offer free trainings and consultation to enhance their abilities to help first responders. Maintain a list of those who have attended your trainings that includes areas of specialization (e.g., children, women's issues). When providers attend trainings about mental health issues of first responders, you might ask that they offer discounted fees for those first responders who seek services from them.

Summary

For many veterans, becoming a first responder is a logical choice after leaving the military. While the two cultures are not identical, they have many similarities, making for an easier transition from the military world to the civilian one. However, many of the psychological issues faced by military members (e.g., alcohol abuse, PTSD) are also similar to those encountered by first responders. The MHP working within a first responder organization should make special efforts to reach out to military veterans in the organization as they are at increased risk for both physical and psychological issues because of their military service. Furthermore, they have likely been affected by the stigma against seeking help that is prominent in the military. At the same time, though, these veterans have been well prepared by their military service to work as first responders. The veteran/first responder is potentially among the most valuable resources of the department.

References

Archer, S. K. (2009, August 19). *The true meaning of "duty."* Joint Base McGuire-Dix-Lakehurst. Retrieved June 11, 2022, from https://www.jbmdl.jb.mil/News/Commentaries/Display/Article/246936/the-true-meaning-of-duty/

Ballenger, J. C., Best, S. R., Metzler, T. J., Wasserman, D. H., Mohr, D. C., Liberman, A., Delucchi, K. L., Weiss, D. J., Fagan, J., Waldrop, A. E., & Marmar, C. R. (2011). Patterns and predictors of alcohol use in male and female urban police officers. *American Journal on Addictions, 20*(1), 21–29. https://doi.org/10.1111/j.1521-0391.2010.00092.x

Beks, T. A. (2016). Walking on eggshells: The lived experience of partners of veterans with PTSD. *The Qualitative Report, 21*(4), 645–660. https://doi.org/10.46743/2160-3715/2016.2269

Cochran, S. V., & Rabinowitz, F. E. (1999). *Men and depression: Clinical and empirical perspectives*. Academic Press: San Diego.

Davis, J. P., Prindle, J. P., Saba, S., Lee, D. S., Leightley, D., Tran, D. D., Sedano, A., Fitzke, R., Castro, C. A., & Pederson, E. R. (2022). Childhood adversity, combat experiences, and military sexual trauma: A test and extension of the stress sensitization hypothesis. *Psychological Medicine, April*(20), 1–9. https://doi.org/10.1017/S0033291722000733

Delehanty, C., Mewhirty, J., Welch, R., & Wilks, J. (2017). Militarization and police violence: The case of the 1033 program. *Research & Politics, 4*(2), 1–7. https://doi.org/10.1177/2053168017712885

Eastwood, C. (1986). *Heartbreak ridge*. Warner Bros.

Elbogen, E. B., Johnson, S. C., Wagner, H. R., Sullivan, C., Taft, C. T., & Beckham, J. C. (2014). Violent behaviour and post-traumatic stress disorder in US Iraq and Afghanistan veterans. *British Journal of Psychiatry, 204*(5), 368–375. https://doi.org/10.1192/bjp.bp.113.134627

Escott, T. (2019, October 24). *Mission first, Marines always: Back to basics for leaders*. Marines.mil. Retrieved May 12, 2023, from https://www.marines.mil/News/News-Display/Article/1998053/mission-first-marines-always-back-to-basics-for-leaders/

French, G. (2018, October 30). *4 reasons why military veterans make great cops*. Police1.Com. Retrieved June 11, 2022, from https://www.police1.com/police-jobs-and-careers/articles/4-reasons-why-military-veterans-make-great-cops-CXnbR6T9Kub4OwdK/

Gonzalez, J. M. R., Bishopp, S. A., Jetelina, K. K., Paddock, E., Gabriel, K. P., & Cannell, M. B. (2019). Does military veteran status and deployment history impact officer involved shootings? A case-control study. *Journal of Public Health (Oxf.), 41*(3), e245–e252. https://doi.org/10.1093/pubmed/fdy151

Groll, D. L., Ricciardelli, R., Carleton, R., Anderson, G., & Cramm, H. (2020). A Cross-Sectional study of the relationship between previous military experience and mental health disorders in currently serving public safety personnel in Canada. *Canadian Journal of Psychiatry, 65*(5). https://doi.org/10.1177/0706743719895341

Haddock, C. K., Jitnarin, N., Caetano, R., Jahnke, S. A., Hollerbach, B. S., Kaipust, C. M., & Poston, W. S. C. (2022). Norms about alcohol use among US firefighters. *Safety and Health at Work, 13*(4), 387–393. https://doi.org/10.1016/j.shaw.2022.08.008

Jakupcak, M., Conybeare, D., Phelps, L., Hunt, S., Holmes, H. A., Felker, B., Klevens, M., & McFall, M. E. (2007). Anger, hostility, and aggression among Iraq and Afghanistan war veterans reporting PTSD and subthreshold PTSD. *Journal of Traumatic Stress, 20*(6), 945–954. https://doi.org/10.1002/jts.20258

Kaplan, D. A. (2019, July 8). *Reducing military mental health stigma to improve treatment engagement guidance for clinicians*. Health.Mil.Com. Retrieved June 17, 2022, from https://health.mil/Military-Health-Topics/Centers-of-Excellence/Psychological-Health-Center-of-Excellence/Clinicians-Corner-Blog/Reducing-Military-Mental-Health-Stigma-to-Improve-Treatment-Engagement-Guidance-for-Clinicians#:~:text=Mental%20health%20stigma%20in%20the,seeking%20care%2C%20including%20career%20harm

Katpitulik, E., & MacDonald, J. (2019). *The program: Lessons from elite military units for creating and sustaining high performing leaders and teams*. Wiley.

Kindy, K. (2015, December 10). Creating guardians, calming warriors. *Washington Post*. Retrieved June 18, 2022, from https://www.washingtonpost.com/sf/investigative/2015/12/10/new-style-of-police-training-aims-to-produce-guardians-not-warriors/

Kulka, R., Schlenger, W. E., Fairbank, J. A., Marmar, C. R., & Weiss, D. D. (1988). *National Vietnam veterans readjustment study (NVVRS): Description, current status, and initial PTSD prevalence estimates*. Veterans Administration.

Larson, M. J., Wooten, N. R., Adams, R., Sayko, R. S., & Merrick, E. L. (2012). Military combat deployments and substance use: Review and future directions. *Journal of Social Work Practice in the Addictions, 12*(1). https://doi.org/10.1080/1533256X.2012.647586

Lawn, S., Waddell, E., Rikkers, W., Roberts, L., Beks, T., Lawrence, D., Rioseco, P., Sharp, T., Wadham, B., Daraganova, G., & van Hooff, M. (2022). Families' experiences of supporting Australian veterans and emergency service first responders (ESFRs) to seek help for mental health problems. *Health and Social Care in the Community*. https://doi.org/10.1111/hsc.13856

LeardMann, C. A., Powell, T. M., Smith, T. C., Bell, M. R., Smith, B., Boyko, E. J., Hooper, T. I., Gackstetter, G. D., Ghamsary, M., & Hoge, C. W. (2013). Risk factors associated with suicide in current and former US military personnel. *JAMA, 310*(5), 496–506. https://doi.org/10.1001/jama.2013.65164

Lewis, G. B., & Pathak, R. (2014). The employment of veterans in state and local government service. *Public Works Management & Policy, 46*(2). https://doi.org/10.1177/0160323X14537835

Marmar, C. R., Schlenger, W. E., Henn-Haase, C., Qian, M., Purchia, E., Liu, L., Corry, N. H., Williams, C. S., Ho, C., Horesh, D., Karstoft, K., Shalev, A. Y., & Kulka, R. G. (2015). Course of posttraumatic stress disorder 40 years after the Vietnam war. *JAMA Psychiatry, 72*(9), 875. https://doi.org/10.1001/jamapsychiatry.2015.0803

McLaughlin, K. A., Conron, K. J., Koenen, K. C., & Gilman, S. E. (2010). Childhood adversity, adult stressful life events, and risk of past-year psychiatric disorder: A test of the stress sensitization hypothesis in a population-based sample of adults. *Psychological Medicine, 40*(10), 1647–1658. https://doi.org/10.1017/S0033291709992121

Milzarski, E. (2020, April 29). *5 reasons why veterans are perfectly suited to become firefighters*. Wearethemighty.Com. Retrieved June 11, 2022, from https://www.wearethemighty.com/veterans/veterans-make-great-firefighters/

Mitchell, J. T., & Everly, G. S. (1996). *Critical incident stress debriefing: An operations manual for the prevention of traumatic stress among emergency servicers and disaster workers*. Chevron Publishing Corporation.

Nasveld, P., Cotea, C., Pullman, S., & Pietrzak, E. (2012). Effects of deployment on mental health in modern military forces: A review of longitudinal studies. *Journal of Military and Veterans Health, 20*(3).

Nevarez, M. D., Yee, H. M., & Waldinger, R. J. (2017). Friendship in war: Camaraderie and prevention of posttraumatic stress disorder prevention: Friendship in war. *Journal of Traumatic Stress, 30*(1), 512–520. https://doi.org/10.1002/jts.22224

Petr, B. (2016). Stress, kindling and PTSD: Typical symptoms of temporal lobe epilepsy and antiepileptic medication. In C. Martin, V. Preedy, & V. Patel (Eds.), *Comprehensive guide to post-traumatic stress disorder* (pp. 181–191). Springer. https://doi.org/10.1007/978-3-319-08359-9_94

President's Task Force. (2015). *21st century policing*. US Dept. of Justice.

Rand Corporation, Sims, C. S., Trail, T. E., Chen, E. K., Meza, E., Roshan, P., & Lachman, B. E. (2018). *Assessing the needs of soldiers and their families at the garrison level*. Rand Corporation. https://rand.org/pubs/research_reports/RR2148.html

Richardson, L. K., Frueh, B. C., & Acierno, R. (2010). Prevalence estimates of Combat-Related PTSD: A critical review. *Australian New Zealand Journal of Psychiatry, 44*(1), 4–19. https://doi.org/10.3109/00048670903393597

Ruderman Foundation. (2022, June). *The Ruderman white paper update on mental health and suicide of first responders*. Ruderman Family Foundation.

Sachs-Ericsson, N., Joiner, T. E., Cougle, J. R., Stanley, I. H., & Shefler, J. L. (2016). Combat exposure in early adulthood interacts with recent stressors to predict PTSD in aging male veterans. *The Gerontologist, 56*(1), 82–91. https://doi.org/10.1093/geront/gnv036

SAMHSA. (2018, May). *First responders: Behavioral health concerns, emergency response, and trauma*.

Schafer, K., Sutter, R. C., & Gibbons, S. (2015). Characteristics of individuals and employment among first responders. *ResearchGate*. Retrieved May 10, 2023, from https://www.researchgate.net/profile/Ryan_Sutter/publication/281293262_Characteristics_of_Individuals_and_Employment_Among_First_Responders/links/55e07a8008aecb1a7cc45313.pdf

Schnittker, J. (2018). Scars: The long-term effects of combat exposure on health. *Socius: Sociological Research for a Dynamic World, 4*. https://doi.org/10.1177/2378023118813017

Schnurr, P. P. (n.d.). *Epidemiology and impact of PTSD*. https://www.ptsd.va.gov/. https://www.ptsd.va.gov/professional/treat/essentials/epidemiology.asp

Seal, K. H., Metzler, T. J., Gima, K. S., Berenthal, D., Maguen, S., & Marmar, C. R. (2009). Trends and risk factors for mental health diagnoses among Iraq and Afghanistan veterans using department of veterans affairs health care, 2002–2008. *American Journal of Public Health, 99*, 1651–1658. https://doi.org/10.2105/AJPH.2008.150284

Seal, K. H., Cohen, G., Waldrop, A., Cohen, B. E., Maguen, S., & Ren, L. (2011). Substance use disorders in Iraq and Afghanistan veterans in VA healthcare, 2001–2010: Implications for screening, diagnosis and treatment. *Drug and Alcohol Dependence, 116*(1–3), 93–101. https://doi.org/10.1016/j.drugalcdep.2010.11.027

Suitt, III, T. H. (2021, June). *High suicide rates among United States service members and veterans of the post9/11 wars*. Watson Institute, Brown University.

Taylor, M. G., Ureña, S., & Kail, B. L. (2016). Service-related exposures and physical health trajectories among aging veteran men. *Gerontologist, 56*(1), 92–103.

U.S. Army Training and Doctrine Command. (2019, August). *Enlisted initial entry training policies and administration* (No. 350–6). U.S. Army.

U.S. Dept. of Veteran Affairs. (n.d.). *About VHA*. VA.Gov. Retrieved June 19, 2022, from https://www.va.gov/health/aboutvha.asp#:~:text=VA%2C%20the%20nation's%20largest%20health,complexity%20(VHA%20outpatient%20clinics)

University of Phoenix. (2019, September 16). *University of Phoenix survey finds more than half of first responders feel there are job repercussions for seeking professional mental health counseling* [Press release]. https://www.phoenix.edu/media-center/press-release/university-of-phoenix-survey-finds-more-than-half-of-first-responders-feel-there-are-job-repercussions-for-seeking-professional-mental-health-counseling.html

van Brocklin, V. (2019, May 7). *Warriors vs. Guardians: A seismic shift in policing or just semantics?* Police1.Com. Retrieved June 17, 2022, from https://www.police1.com/21st-century-policing-task-force/articles/warriors-vs-guardians-a-seismic-shift-in-policing-or-just-semantics-EXBkY2pEWCHi6Mni/

Weichselbaum, S., Schwartzapel, B., & Meagher, T. (2017, March 30). *When warriors put on the badge*. The Marshall Project. Retrieved May 6, 2022, from https://www.themarshallproject.org/2017/03/30/when-warriors-put-on-the-badge

Wolfe, T. (2012). *Out of uniform: Your guide to a successful military-to-civilian career transition*. Potomac Books.

Legal and Legislative Issues in Public Safety Contexts

Leonard N. Chan and Caitlin N. Dryden

Law enforcement officers, firefighters, emergency medical services providers, and dispatchers routinely face high stress environments when responding to emergencies, disasters, pandemics, and other crises. The weight of accumulated day-to-day stress impacts a first responder professionally and personally as each shift, call, and response brings uncertainty. For these reasons, prior to COVID-19, first responders were more likely to die by suicide than in the line of duty (Heyman et al., 2018). The perceived stigma around mental health issues in these professions leads to silence that exacerbates the effects of post-traumatic stress such as hopelessness, anxiety, depression, and suicidal ideation (Tiesman et al., 2021). Unfortunately, legal realities have not always matched human realities; while the problem prevails, solutions and support are lacking. The growing political will to develop and implement public policy demonstrates a recognition that treating mental health injuries in first responders not only will strengthen the first responder as a person, but also strengthen the profession and broader community.

First Responder Vulnerability

First responders encounter trauma far more frequently than the general population. Trauma is not limited to mass casualty incidents such as natural disasters or active shooter events, but may also include witnessing suicide attempts, responding to

L. N. Chan (✉)
Houston Fire Department, Houston, TX, USA
e-mail: Leonard.Chan@houstontx.gov

C. N. Dryden
Villari, Lentz & Lynam, LLC, Philadelphia, PA, USA
e-mail: cdryden@vll-law.com

M. L. Bourke et al. (eds.), *First Responder Mental Health*,
https://doi.org/10.1007/978-3-031-38149-2_27

motor vehicle fatalities, and operating under the general day-to-day stress of the job. The cumulative impact of the constant exposure to death and destruction has the substantial potential to chip away at the mental health of first responders.

Comprehensive national data on first responder mental health remains elusive because there is currently no federal government mandate that requires reporting. Instead, first responders or the families of first responders have to voluntarily identify themselves (Kohr, 2019). The anguish first responders endure is often hidden from the public. This leads to a lack of awareness and action to prevent and mitigate mental health issues (Heyman et al., 2018).

To fully understand the scope of mental injures, and to build safe and effective programs for the prevention, mitigation, and treatment of those injuries, increased investment in comprehensive data collection and research is paramount. Professional associations such as the National Fire Protection Association (NFPA), International Association of Fire Chiefs (IAFC), International Association of Fire Fighters (IAFF), International Association of Chiefs of Police (IACP), and International Union of Police Associations (IUPA) recognize the importance of these issues through advocacy efforts, but federal and state governments bear responsibilities in establishing the legal frameworks and appropriating the necessary funds.

Current Legal and Legislative Framework

Federal Programs

Recognizing the issue of mental health–related risks to first responders, the federal government funds an array of programs in an attempt to identify, prevent, or mitigate these issues. However, these initiatives are typically piecemeal and uncoordinated. With COVID-19 came new legislation in the form of the American Rescue Plan Act of 2021, which has helped increase broad-level collaboration. The type of first responder determines which executive department or program has responsibility in providing support: The U.S. Department of Justice, U.S. Department of Homeland Security, U.S. Department of Health and Human Services, or general public programming bear most of the responsibility (Duff et al., 2020).

Law Enforcement Officers

The U.S. Department of Justice serves as the primary federal agency that administers mental health programs for law enforcement officers. Programs under its jurisdiction include the Law Enforcement Mental Health and Wellness Act (LEMHWA), Edward Byrne Memorial Justice Assistance Grant (JAG) Program, Preventing Violence Against Law Enforcement and Ensuring Officer Resilience and Survivability (VALOR) Initiative, and National Officer Safety Initiative.

Law Enforcement Mental Health and Wellness Act (LEMHWA) Passed unanimously in December 2017, LEMHWA charges the Office of Community Oriented Policing Services to address mental health issues in the law enforcement profession. One component of LEMHWA includes distributing grants without any match requirements "to improve the delivery of and access to mental health and wellness services [...] through the implementation of peer support, training, family resources, suicide prevention, and other promising practices for wellness programs" (The Office of Community Oriented Policing Services, 2022). Eligible recipients include state, tribal, and local law enforcement agencies. The LEMHWA program also includes a training and technical assistance program, which is available to public, private, and nonprofit entities.

Edward Byrne Memorial Justice Assistance Grant (JAG) Program The Edward Byrne Memorial JAG Program is the leading source of federal justice funding to state, tribal, and local law enforcement agencies. The Bureau for Justice Assistance (BJA) for each state determines the minimum base allocation by evaluating state population and violent crime statistics. The JAG funds may support a wide range of law enforcement functions including "mental health programs and related law enforcement and corrections programs such as behavioral programs and crisis intervention teams" (Bureau of Justice Assistance, 2022a).

Preventing Violence Against Law Enforcement and Ensuring Officer Resilience and Survivability (VALOR) Initiative The VALOR Initiative, also administered by the BJA, intends "to improve the immediate and long-term safety, wellness, and resilience of law enforcement officers" through professional education, conducting research, developing references, and establishing partnerships (Bureau of Justice Assistance, 2022b). These efforts are inclusive of mental and behavioral health. Through the Field-Driven Officer Safety and Wellness Program, law enforcement officers have the opportunity to obtain training related to survivor's guilt and post-traumatic stress. The Law Enforcement Agency and Resilience Training Program assists law enforcement officers in dealing with day-to-day challenges and stressors as well as larger critical incidents. Other programs supported by the VALOR Initiative include the National Suicide Awareness for Law Enforcement Officers Program and National Consortium Preventing Law Enforcement Suicide. The latter develops informational material that illustrates how the cumulative exposure to traumatic events may lead to post-traumatic stress symptoms, substance misuse, depression, and suicide ideation (IACP, 2022).

National Officer Safety Initiative Issued in February 2017, the executive order on Preventing Violence Against Federal, State, Tribal, and Local Law Enforcement Officers led to the National Officer Safety Initiative by the BJA. The executive order focuses developing strategies on deterring intentional attacks against law enforcement officers, but also directs federal agencies to evaluate grant programs that protect law enforcement officers (Executive Order No. 13774, 2017). Suicide prevention grants fall under this umbrella. The National Officer Safety Initiative serves as complementary source of support for the National Consortium Preventing Law Enforcement Suicide mentioned above.

Firefighters

Multiple agencies share responsibility in supporting the fire service at the federal level. Embedded within the Federal Emergency Management Agency (FEMA), the United States Fire Administration (USFA) provides policy direction and training resources. The USFA promotes resources from partner organizations on its website including the 2021 update to the IAFCs' Volunteer and Combination Officers Section's *Yellow Ribbon Report on Behavioral Health and Wellness* (USFA, 2021). Since 1998, the National Institute for Occupational Safety and Health (NIOSH) has addressed work-related firefighter deaths by conducting independent investigations and issuing recommendations. NIOSH, however, does not have jurisdiction to enforce compliance with safety and health standards nor determine fault or blame for deaths and injuries (United States Department of Health and Human Services, 2021). As direct employers of firefighters, the United States Department of Agriculture's National Forest Service (NFS) and the United States Department of Interior's National Park Service have developed programs to address mental health issues within their respective workforce.

National Fire Incident Reporting System (NFIRS) The USFA relies on NFIRS to meet its congressional obligation to select, analyze, and disseminate information related to the occupational hazards faced by firefighters that may lead to death or injuries (15 United States Code, sec. 2208). The NFIRS Fire Service Casualty Module intends to capture injury and fatality data of any firefighter on duty, and this is inclusive of emotional and psychological stress (FEMA, 2015). As noted by Dr. Matthew Hinds-Aldrich (2020) in his commentary on NFIRS, the system has not kept pace with the data needs of the fire service potentially because the system may be too burdensome to collect and analyze the appropriate information. This perspective echoes the concerns raised at the 2nd National Fire Service Research Agenda Symposium in 2011 (National Fire Academy, 2011). The lack of quality data and analysis hamstrings the ability of policymakers to describe the depth of the problem, identify effective and meaningful solutions, and justify budgets and programs.

National Fire Academy (NFA) The NFA falls under administrative aegis of the USFA. Although the majority of courses focus on community risk reduction and emergency operations, the NFA offers health and wellness training at no cost to the participants. The onsite Department Wellness Program and online Empowering Responding Wellness courses feature mental health as part of the curriculum (USFA, 2022a, b). In addition, dozens of A-level research papers that have focused on mental health have been produced from participants of the NFA's Executive Fire Officer (EFO) Program (USFA, 2022d).

National Wildfire Coordinating Group (NWCG) Established in 1976, NWCG intends to avoid duplication of effort and increase collaboration in executing each agency's fire management programs. Its roster of over 900 members includes representatives across a dozen federal agencies and professional associations (NWCG, 2022). NWCG's mental health subcommittee meets monthly to address wildland firefighter mental health through an interagency approach. Published mental health newsletters cover topics such as stigma and mental illness, maintaining social connections, and burnout. NWCG has also facilitated stress first aid train-the-trainer courses to first responders (NWCG, 2021).

Assistance to Firefighters Grants (AFG) Congress established FEMA's Assistance to Firefighters Grant (AFG) to support state, tribal, and local fire departments in protecting the health and safety of the public and firefighter personnel (United States Fire Administration, AFG, and SAFER Program Reauthorization Act of 2017, 2018). Eligible activities include wellness and fitness activities that strengthen mental and emotional capabilities to "withstand the demands of all hazardous operations" (Department of Homeland Security, 2021, p. 66). FEMA classifies behavioral health programs as Priority 1 projects. The annual amount available varies based on congressional appropriations.

Emergency Medical Services (EMS) Personnel

Depending on the community served, EMS may operate independently as a separate government agency, nonprofit organization, private for-profit entity, or be embedded into a fire department or hospital system. Responses to emergency medical incidents also tend to require collaboration between multiple entities, which can lead to a fragmented approach at the federal level. The National Highway Traffic Safety Administration (NHTSA)'s Office of EMS serves as one of the lead agencies for EMS and 9-1-1 systems. As part of the Surgeon General's national strategic plan to prevent suicide, the NHTSA Office of EMS has increased its focus on first responder mental health issues. This includes participating in interagency research with Centers of Disease Control and Prevention (CDC)'s National Center for Injury Prevention and Control and NIOSH to investigate first responder suicides (Tiesman et al., 2021). Since the fire service has become inextricably connected to emergency medical services, the USFA has plans underway to build a "true EMS section" as it increases its role in shaping EMS policy and training (USFA, 2022c). Many of the existing support programs for the fire service have also been available to EMS personnel.

General Programs

The federal government offers an assortment of mental health programs open to the public, which first responders may access, as well as channeling grant support to the state, tribal, and local levels. Agencies facilitating these programs include the CDC, Substance Abuse and Mental Health Services Administration (SAMHSA), and National Institutes of Health (NIH).

State Programs

Support Programs

The wealth of programs supporting first responder mental health is countless and cannot be captured in this chapter alone. State governments administer many of the initiatives funded by the federal government described above. The following describes a sample of the programs available, which may be found in multiple states.

Nevada requires agencies that employ first responders to provide training related to the awareness, prevention, mitigation, and training of mental health issues (Nevada Revised Statues, sec. 616C.180, 1993). This requirement was largely in response to the Las Vegas Route 91 Harvest musical festival shooting that killed 60 people and wounded over 400 in October 2017. The Nevada Division of Public and Behavioral Health Office of Suicide Prevention facilitates suicide prevention, mental health first aid, and applied suicide intervention skills training (Nevada Division of Public and Behavioral Health Office of Suicide Prevention, 2021). Services offered by other entities also may be used to meet this requirement.

The Nebraska Department of Health and Human Services has facilitated the training of volunteer peers to provide crisis support for the full spectrum of first responders through the National Critical Incident Stress Management Program. The Nebraska Legislature has allocated funds to reimburse first responders for annual training in this program if not paid by their employer (Nebraska Revised Statute, sec. 48-101.01, 2022). Administrative rules by the Nebraska Department of Health and Human Services ensure that the program maintains the confidentiality of participants (Nebraska Administrative Code, title 176, chapter 1, 2021).

The Texas Sunset Advisory Commission reported that the Texas Commission on Fire Protection (TCFP), the primary regulatory body over the Texas fire service, missed opportunities to identify causal factors and consequent costs of firefighter injuries. As a result in 2009, the 81st Texas Legislature mandated that TCFP develop an annual report on firefighter injuries and workers' compensation data as well as issue recommendations to reduce injuries. The statute also permits TCFP to provide technical assistance in reducing injuries (Texas Government Code, sec. 419.048, 2009). Mental health is considered part of this mandate, but psychological injuries account for less than 0.5% of reported injuries each year. Recommendations also rarely focus on addressing psychological issues. Recognizing the injury report understates the mental health problem, TCFP's Health and Wellness Committee has identified mental health as a priority since summer 2019 (TCFP, 2019).

Some states have more general organizations, such as the Pennsylvania Fire and Emergency Services Institute, which seeks to organize members of fire and emergency service organizations and provide education and support for the general needs of the profession (Pennsylvania Fire & Emergency Services Institute, 2019). Organizations like these advocate legislatively and help provide resources to these communities.

Workers' Compensation

Through workers' compensation, workers and their families are eligible to receive benefits for covered injuries, illnesses, and death arising from their employment, without regard to fault or liability. Workers' compensation systems in each state operate under their "own set of laws, regulations, and legal precedents" as the federal government has set no minimum standards for state systems, nor does it require states to have workers' compensation systems at all (Szymendera, 2020). This has led to substantive divergence in the states on eligibility, benefits, funding, and participation. The treatment of work-related mental injuries is no exception.

Each state recognizes that work-related mental injuries may occur but differs on what conditions must exist for them to be eligible for workers' compensation. States can generally be classified as treating mental injuries in two categories: physical-mental and mental-mental. In states considered physical-mental, a physical injury must be associated with the mental injury. Whereas for states considered mental-mental, a mental injury may qualify without an associated physical injury. Within the latter category, states have specified whether a single or an accumulation of stimuli inflicted the mental injury. Standard employment or disciplinary actions may not be the source of the mental injury for these purposes. This may be determined by statute or case law.

Some legislatures have also made special exceptions for first responders recognizing the increased risk they face in witnessing and encountering traumatic incidents. As of May 2022, the majority of states allow mental-mental cases to be eligible for workers' compensation at least for first responders, though significant barriers still exist to actually receiving these benefits. The trend has been moving toward this direction with a surge of legislation since 2018, which is summarized in a later section. Some states, however, such as Idaho, Nebraska, and West Virginia, have only adopted the expansion of workers' compensation eligibility on a trial basis by including sunset dates, or automatic termination dates, into their legislation. The table below summarizes how each state addresses mental injuries for workers' compensation.

	Never compensable unless there is a physical component[a]	Compensable only when there is sudden stimuli[b]	Compensable when there is unusual stimuli[c]	Compensable regardless of stimuli including accumulation of events[d]
General	Alabama Arkansas Georgia Indiana Kansas Kentucky (may include physical exertion, not just physical injuries) Montana North Dakota Ohio Oklahoma South Dakota	Louisiana Maryland Tennessee Utah Washington (has to be tied to an immediately preceding event)	Alaska Arizona Colorado District of Columbia Illinois Iowa Maine Michigan Mississippi Missouri New Jersey New Mexico New York North Carolina Pennsylvania Rhode Island South Carolina Wisconsin	California Delaware (considers brain as part of the body) Hawaii Massachusetts Minnesota (PTSD only) Oregon
First-Responders Only		Nevada	Connecticut (limited) Florida (limited) Virginia (limited)	Idaho – S Louisiana Minnesota Nebraska – S New Hampshire Texas Vermont West Virginia – S Washington Wyoming

S – Denotes sunset date provisions

[a]Alabama Code, sec. 25-5-1; Arkansas Code, sec. 11-9-13 (2020); Court of Appeals of Georgia (1999); Indiana Code, sec. 22-3-6-1; United States Court of Appeals, 10th Circuit (2003); Kentucky Statutes, sec. 342.0011; Montana Code Annotated, sec. 39-71-119; North Dakota Century Code, ch. 65-01; Ohio Revised Code, sec. 4123.01; 85A Oklahoma Statute, sec. 85A-13 (2014); South Dakota Codified Laws 62-1-1

[b]Louisiana Laws Revised Statutes, sec. 23:1021; Court of Special Appeals of Maryland (1998); Tennessee Code, sec. 50-6-102; Utah Code, sec 34A-2-401; Washington Revised Code, sec. 51.08.100; Nevada Revised Code, sec. 616C.180 (2019)

[c]Alaska Statutes, sec 23.30.010 (2014); Arizona Revised Statutes, sec. 23-1043.01; Colorado Revised Statutes, sec. 8-41-301; District of Columbia Court of Appeals (1998); Illinois Compiled Statues, chapter 820, sec. 305; Michigan Compiled Laws, sec. 418.401; Maine Workers' Compensation Act of 1992 Title 39-A chapt. 5-3A; Mississippi Code Title 71 sec. 71.3.3; Revised Statutes of Missouri, sec. 287.120; New Jersey Revised Statues, sec. 34:15-1; New Mexico Statutes, sec. 52-1-24; Consolidated Laws of New York, ch. 67; North Carolina Statutes, sec. 97.53; Commonwealth Court of Pennsylvania (2017); Rhode Island General Laws, sec. 28-34-2; South Carolina Code of Laws, title 42, ch. 1; Wisconsin Statutes and Annotations, sec. 102.01; Connecticut Statutes, sec. 31-275; Florida Statutes, sec. 440.093; Maine Statutes, title 39-A; Code of Virginia, sec. 65.2-400

[d]California Labor Code, sec. 3208.3; Delaware Code, title 19, sec. 2301; Hawaii Statute, sec. 386-3; L.S.A-R.S. title 23 sec. 1307; Massachusetts General Laws, chapter 143, sec. 1; Minn. Stat. sec. 176.011; Idaho Statutes, title 72, ch. 4; Minnesota Statutes, sec. 176.011; Nebraska Revised Statute, sec. 48-101.01, 2022; New Hampshire Revised Statutes, sec. 281-A:17-c (2017); Oregon Revied Statutes, sec. 656.802 (2022); Texas Labor Code, ch. 504; Vermont Statutes, title 21, ch. 9; West Virginia Code, sec. 23-4-1; Wyoming Statutes, title 27, ch. 1; RCW title 51, chapt. 9, section 142.

Alabama is a state that explicitly places itself in the physical-mental through its legislation. The Code of Alabama defines injuries in workers' compensation explicitly stating, "injury does not include a mental disorder or mental injury that has neither been produced nor been proximately caused by some physical injury to the body" (Alabama Code, sec. 25-5-1). Montana has adopted a similar approach by explicitly declaring that injuries do "not mean a physical or mental condition arising from: (a) emotional or mental stress; or (b) a nonphysical stimulus or activity" (Montana Code Annotated, sec. 39-71-119). The North Dakota Century Code also specifies that injuries eligible for workers' compensation do not include "a mental injury arising from mental stimulus" (North Dakota Century Code, sec. 65-01-02).

The judiciary has affirmed the dismissal of mental-mental injuries for workers' compensation in states such as Kansas. The Kansas Supreme Court decided in *Followill v. Emerson Electric Company* that physical injuries must be the root cause of mental injuries for them to be eligible for workers' compensation as its statute defines injuries as "any lesion or change in physical structure of the body, causing damage or harm thereto" (Kansas Statutes, sec. 44-508). Although acknowledging that other states award workers' compensation for mental-mental injuries, the Kansas Supreme Court determined that the statutes and legal precedent in Kansas have not permitted that, and any changes would have to come from the Kansas Legislature, not the court (*Followill v. Emerson Electric Co.*, 1984).

The Supreme Court of Kentucky had a different perspective despite what could be considered as more restrictive statutory language. The Kentucky Revised Statutes explicitly state that injuries "shall not include a psychological, psychiatric, or stress-related change in the human organism, unless it is a result of a physical injury" (Kansas Revised statues, sec. 342.0011). In *White v. Lexington-Fayette* (2005), the Kentucky Supreme Court opined that physical harm caused by an outside force is not necessary for a mental injury to be eligible for workers' compensation, but rather only physical exertion is needed to qualify (*White v. Lexington-Fayette*, 2005). Delaware adopted an even more unique approach that had the same effect, despite its statute defining injuries as "violence to the physical structure of the body." In *State v. Cephas* (1994), the Delaware Supreme Court ruled that the mind is inclusive of the physical body.

States may also specify by statute conditions in which mental injuries may be considered for workers' compensation. Alaska's statute states that mental injuries caused by mental stress may be considered if "(1) the work stress was extraordinary and unusual in comparison to pressures and tensions experienced by individuals in a comparable work environment; and (2) the work stress was the predominant cause of the mental injury" (Alaska Statue, sec. 23.30.010, 2014). Missouri largely mirrors this language in its revised statutes. States that allow for mental-mental workers' compensation claims in statute still recognize mental injuries resulting from physical injuries (Revised Statute of Missouri, sec. 287.120). For example, Louisiana allows for mental injury claims from "sudden, unexpected, and extraordinary stress" but also for "mental injury caused by physical injuries." Louisiana has separate provisions for first responders (Louisiana Laws Revised Statutes, sec. 23:1021).

The court system has also ruled in favor of supporting the legitimacy of mental-mental claims for workers' compensation in select states where the statute remains silent on the issue. One such state is Iowa, which does not define "personal injuries" in its code (Iowa Code, sec. 85.3, 2016). The Supreme Court of Iowa ruled in *Dunlavey v. Economy Fire and Casualty Co.* (1995) that "personal injuries" are inclusive of "pure mental injuries" and established the conditions for mental injury claims. These conditions include specifying that the workplace stress must be more than the day-to-day mental stresses experienced by others employed in the same or similar jobs. Wisconsin takes this one step further by stating that the stress must be greater than what all employees in the workforce experience, not only within a specified profession (*Swiss Colony, Inc. v. DILHR*, 1976).

Approximately a dozen states have carved out first responders as a separate class for determining eligibility of mental injury-related workers' compensation benefits. Nebraska enacted such legislation as it found that first responders face the high potential of constant, cumulative exposure to horrific events "in their sworn mission to keep the people safe" (Nebraska Revised Statute, sec. 48-101.01, 2022). The statute, however, does require pre-employment mental screening, mental health professional diagnosis, evidence of potentially traumatic events, and completion of resiliency training. Oregon sets its own parameters for presumption for mental injury claims and covers dispatchers along with firefighters, law enforcement officers, correction officers, and emergency medical services providers (Oregon Revised Statutes, sec. 656.802, 2019). Other states such as Vermont and New Hampshire have presumption provisions in place but with fewer conditions (Vt. Stat. Ann., Tit. 21, sec. 601, 2017; New Hampshire Revised Statutes, sec. 281-A:17-c, 2020).

Political Climate

The spotlight on mental health issues in first responders has grown brighter with an increasing volume of legislation being introduced and passed in recent years.

Federal Level

As a component of LEHWA, Congress charged the Department of Justice to publish a report on the evaluating effectiveness of crisis lines for law enforcement officers and the efficacy of annual mental health checks for law enforcement officers, as well as strategizing for the expansion of peer mentoring programs and addressing privacy considerations for these types of programs. Published in March 2019, the report issued a series of 19 recommendations that includes embedding mental health professionals in law enforcement agencies, allowing retirees to access peer support programs, improving privacy protections for officers seeking support, and supporting rigorous research evaluating the efficacy of crisis hotlines (The Office of Community Oriented Policing Services, 2022).

The Congressional Research Service highlighted first responder mental health issues that could be addressed through congressional action in October 2020: (1) Tailoring Mental Health Programming to First Responders and Increasing Access, (2) Addressing Barriers to First Responder Utilization of Mental Health Care, (3) Including a Spectrum of Mental Health Services, (4) Identifying Empirical Support for First Responder Mental Health Interventions, and (5) Coordinating First Responder Mental Health Programs across Agencies (Duff et al., 2020). Congress addressed several of these issues through the American Rescue Plan Act of 2021 by appropriating funds specifically to mental health and substance use disorder research, prevention, training, and treatment for health care professionals and public safety officers (American Rescue Plan Act of 2021, 2021).

Filed in March 2022, Improving Law Enforcement Officer Safety and Wellness Through Data Act includes provisions to further develop reports that analyze the type, frequency, and severity of stress-related responses of law enforcement officers to trauma-inducing incidents with the intent to identify solutions in assessing, monitoring, and improving law enforcement mental health and wellness. As of October 2022, the bill awaits a committee hearing (Improving Law Enforcement Officer Safety and Wellness Through Data Act, 2022).

As a response to the four suicides following the Capitol insurrection on January 6, 2021, Congress passed the bi-partisan Public Safety Officer Support Act of 2022 with only 17 members of House of Representatives in opposition. This legislation, signed into law in August 2022, represents a paradigm shift. By recognizing suicides following traumatic events as line-of-duty deaths for public safety officers including police officers, and emergency medical technicians, families now can seek financial support through the Public Safety Officers' Benefits Program, which was previously limited to disbursing benefits for physical injuries. In addition, officers permanently disabled due to post-traumatic stress disorder have a new avenue to seek disability benefits (Public Safety Officer Support Act of 2022, 2022). As of October 2022, regulations for this program remain in development.

State Level

Significant progress has been made in addressing mental health issues of first responders at the state level, especially in establishing intervention programs and reforming workers' compensation laws. The COVID-19 pandemic and the police reform movement played key roles in catalyzing and accelerating these bi-partisan initiatives.

The Illinois General Assembly passed its state's First Responders Suicide Prevention Act in August 2019. Through this legislation, Illinois establishes the parameters of peer support programs while protecting the confidentiality of those seeking support with exceptions made regarding criminal behavior. The creation of the Illinois First Responders Suicide Task Force also resulted from this legislation. The task force compiled recommendations regarding employee assistance programs, health care plans, public education campaigns, training requirements, and treatment programs, as well as recommendations for ways to eliminate stigma (First Responders Suicide Prevention Act, 2019). The 102nd Illinois General Assembly (2022) implemented some of these recommendations including the creation of an online database of mental health resources for first responders.

The 85th Texas Legislature commissioned the Texas Health and Human Services Commission to convene stakeholders to draft a report on mental health access for first responders, which was completed in December 2018. The report addresses issues that included disparity in services, sufficiency in health insurance policies, first responder certification training, critical incident mental health needs, and effectiveness of the workers' compensation system, among others. The report's 18 recommendations align with the Texas Statewide Behavioral Health Strategic Plan (Texas Health and Human Services Commission, 2018).

In subsequent legislative sessions, the Texas Legislature passed bills implementing some of these recommendations. The 86th Texas Legislature in 2019 passed House Bill 2143, which permits workers' compensation claims for mental injuries to be linked to multiple events rather than a single event despite concerns about cost by local government organizations (Texas Legislature, 2019a). However, House Bills 751 and 1054, which would have standardized peer support training and operations, did not pass because it was too prescriptive and did not appreciate the differences between the different classifications of first responders (Texas Legislature, 2019b, c). The 87th Texas Legislature in 2021 continued to address first responder mental health issues by requiring law enforcement agencies to develop a mental health leave policy for those experiencing traumatic events (Texas Legislature, 2019d).

Like other states, Florida has passed legislation commissioning studies to assess mental health of first responders. Senate Bill 7012 in 2020 resulted in the creation of the First Responders Suicide Deterrence Task Force, which is required to release annual reports from 2021 to 2023. The annual reports assess individual, relationship, community, and societal gaps with recommendations focused on awareness, prevention, intervention, and follow-up and support. The report follows up efforts by the Florida Department of Law Enforcement and Florida Firefighters Safety and Health Collaborative white paper titled *Florida First Responder Mental Health* completed in March 2020 (Florida Department of Children and Families, 2021).

Workers' compensation in Florida previously covered mental injuries only if they were accompanied by a physical injury that required medical treatment. That changed with the passage Senate Bill 376 in spring 2018, which permits workers' compensation for post-traumatic stress disorder for first responders if encountering or witnessing events such as a death of a minor, deaths involving grievous bodily harm, homicides, and suicides (Florida Statutes, sec. 112.1815, 2021). Advocates suggested that the legal recognition of post-traumatic stress disorder lowers the stigma of seeking help while increasing the access for comprehensive treatment and reducing vulnerability to substance use disorders (Gonzales, 2018). Despite concerns regarding the negative fiscal impact on local governments, House Bill 689 passed unanimously in spring 2022. The legislation accounts for the delayed manifestation of symptoms by expanding the filing period for mental injury-related workers' compensation claims (Florida House of Representatives, 2022; Florida Legislature, 2021).

States such as Idaho in 2019, Virginia and Wyoming in 2020, and West Virginia in 2021 also passed legislation substantially expanding the eligibility of mental injuries for workers' compensation claims. These changes only affect first responders as defined by their respective statutes. For example, Wyoming modified the definitions for compensable mental injuries by creating an exception for first responders (Wyoming Statues, sec. 27-14-102). By requiring employers of law enforcement officers and firefighters to establish peer support programs by January 2021, Virginia adopted a proactive route in mitigating the potential increase in costs of workers' compensation claims (Code of Virginia, sec. 65.2-107). Although passing its legislation with overwhelming majorities, Idaho displayed some hesitation in changing its approach on mental injuries by writing a July 2023 sunset date written into Senate Bill 1028 (Idaho Legislature, 2019). West Virginia has similar provisions in place but with a July 2026 sunset date (West Virginia Code, sec. 23-4-1). Other states that already allow workers' compensation claims to cover mental-mental injuries passed presumption legislation that effectively shifts the burden of proof away from first responders to their employers. This includes legislative action in 2021 for Nebraska and New Hampshire (New Hampshire Revised Statutes, sec. 281-A:17-c, 2017; Nebraska Revised Statute, sec. 48-101.01, 2022). Mental health for the general population continues to be a focus of state legislatures, especially during the COVID-19 pandemic, as 14 states have passed legislation in 2021 related to suicide prevention (Severance-Medaris, 2021).

The momentum for the adoption of legislation recognizing the mental injuries for workers' compensation, however, has not been universal. For example, Senate Bill 193 during the 2021 Kansas legislative session proposed to expand the definition of personal injury to include mental injuries suffered from emotional shock or a series of work-related events. Due to its estimated fiscal note, the bill "died" without receiving a committee hearing in Spring 2021 (Kansas Division of the Budget, 2021). In Alabama, House Bill 274, which intended to create a fund to support post-traumatic stress disorder health care costs for first responders, also stalled in committee in 2022 but without a fiscal note even being drafted (Alabama Legislature, 2022).

Tennessee's 112th General Assembly's James "Dustin" Samples Act failed to pass despite bi-partisan support in late April 2022. The official bill summary stated that it would create "the legal presumption that a firefighter diagnosed with post-traumatic stress disorder by a mental health professional incurred the injury in the line of duty" (James "Dustin" Samples Act, 2022). The Tennessee General

Assembly's Fiscal Review Committee projected a $4.63 million cost annually to local governments, which they viewed as an unfunded mandate since current Tennessee workers' compensation statutes did not cover mental-mental injuries (Sher, 2022). The fiscal note, however, did not account for the resulting financial and human costs for not providing the necessary timely interventions for post-traumatic stress disorder. Supporters of the legislation intend to raise the issue once more at the next general assembly.

Recommendations

A complete menu of policy options is available to improve mental health support for first responders. Legislatures and government agencies at the federal and state levels have begun to act. Focus should be placed in the following areas: (1) facilitate data collection and information sharing on first responder mental health; (2) ensure worker's compensation systems address mental injuries; and (3) secure funding for mental health programs.

Facilitate Data Collection and Information Sharing on First Responder Mental Health

The disconnected and disparate nature of information regarding first responder mental health should be resolved. The Congressional Research Service proposes "a central clearinghouse for first responder mental health services, administration and funding from a single agency, or more comprehensive mental health prevention and treatment services that address gaps in care" (Duff et al., 2020). Coordination could also help identify which post-crisis and trauma-based interventions can be deemed safe and effective. Initial steps are underway, especially following the passage of the American Rescue Plan Act of 2021.

Ensure Workers' Compensation Addresses Mental Injuries

Refusing to recognize mental injuries for workers' compensation causes two major issues: (1) perpetuating the stigma surrounding mental health by discounting mental injuries as not legitimate; and (2) delaying treatment, potentially allowing conditions and symptoms to worsen. These issues undermine the argument that expanding the eligibility for workers' compensation benefits would lead to substantial negative fiscal implications. The majority of states have at least recognized that first responders face occupational hazards to their mental health and have acted accordingly.

Additional progress still needs to be made in educating legislators, judges, and communities that mental injuries may result from an accumulation of events rather than a single traumatic incident. In addition, more work is needed in providing financial support to families affected by first responder suicide, which entails improving clarity on what is classified as a line-of-duty death.

Secure Funding for Mental Health Programs

Mental health programs, including those catering to the needs of first responders, received an injection of funding as part of COVID-19 recovery and response legislation. Support for mental health programs, however, should not be a one-time effort. Data collection and research is a continuous endeavor that requires consistent funding. Awareness campaigns that help break the stigma regarding first responder mental health need financial support to be ingrained into the psyche of the profession as well as the public. Mental injuries to first responders do not have overnight cures. Completely shielding first responders from exposure to trauma is not feasible, as such events are inherently part of the occupation. Thus, the need to provide support will remain ever-present.

References

15 United States Code, sec. 2208.

Alabama Code, sec. 25-5-1. http://alisondb.legislature.state.al.us/alison/codeofalabama/1975/coatoc.htm

Alabama Legislature. HB 274. (2022, February). http://alisondb.legislature.state.al.us/ALISON/SearchableInstruments/2022RS/PrintFiles/HB274-int.pdf

Alaska Statutes, sec 23.30.010. (2014). https://www.akleg.gov/basis/statutes.asp#23.30.010

American Rescue Plan Act of 2021. (2021). Pub. L. 117-2, 135 Stat. 4. https://www.congress.gov/117/plaws/publ2/PLAW-117publ2.pdf

Arizona Revised Statutes, sec. 23-1043.01. https://www.azleg.gov/ars/23/01043-01.htm#:~:text=If%20compensation%20is%20payable%20for,A%20or%20B%20are%20met

Arkansas Code, sec. 11-9-13. (2020). https://advance.lexis.com/container?config=00JAA3ZTU0NTIzYy0zZDEyLTRhYmQtYmRmMS1iMWIxNDgxYWMxZTQKAFBvZENhdGFsb2cubRW4ifTiwi5vLw6cI1uX&crid=7c3c160e-cb7b-474b-9827-9df1e79e3071&prid=726dc991-0259-40bf-a4c7-2df825a0a507

Bureau of Justice Assistance. (2022a, February). *Fact sheet: Edward Byrne Memorial Justice Assistance Grant program*, 1. https://bja.ojp.gov/doc/jag-program-fact-sheet.pdf

Bureau of Justice Assistance. (2022b, May 19). *VALOR officer safety and wellness initiative*. https://bja.ojp.gov/program/valor/overview

California Labor Code, sec. 3208.3. https://leginfo.legislature.ca.gov/faces/codesTOCSelected.xhtml?tocCode=LAB&tocTitle=+Labor+Code+-+LAB

Code of Virginia, sec. 65.2-107. https://law.lis.virginia.gov/vacode/65.2-107/

Code of Virginia, sec. 65.2-400. https://law.lis.virginia.gov/vacode/65.2-400/

Colorado Revised Statutes, sec. 8-41-301. https://codes.findlaw.com/co/title-8-labor-and-industry/co-rev-st-sect-8-41-301.html

Commonwealth Court of Pennsylvania. (2017). *Frankiewicz v Workers' Compensation Appeal Board*. 177 A.3d 991. https://casetext.com/case/frankiewicz-v-workers-comp-appeal-bd

Connecticut Statutes, sec. 31-275. https://portal.ct.gov/WCC/Statutes-and-Regulations/Workers-Compensation-Regulations/31-275-1

Consolidated Laws of New York, ch. 67. https://www.nysenate.gov/legislation/laws/WKC

Court of Appeals of Georgia. (1999, September 29). *Columbus Fire Department/Columbus Consolidated Government v. Ledford*. https://caselaw.findlaw.com/ga-court-of-appeals/1434695.html

Court of Special Appeals of Maryland. (1998). *King v. Board of Education*, 123 Md. App. 73, 716 A.2d 1077. https://caselaw.findlaw.com/md-court-of-appeals/1396331.html

Delaware Code, title 19, sec. 2301. https://delcode.delaware.gov/title19/c023/sc01/index.html

Department of Homeland Security. (2021). *Notice of funding opportunity (NOFO): Fiscal year 2021 assistance to firefighters grant (AFG) program*, November 2, 2011, 66. https://www.fema.gov/sites/default/files/documents/fema_fy21-afg-nofo.pdf

District of Columbia Court of Appeals. (1998). *Cora M. Gray v. District of Columbia Department of Employment Services*, No. 95-AA-1359. https://www.dccourts.gov/node/16232

Duff, J. H., Gallagher, J. C., James, N., & Cornell, A. S. (2020, October 1). *Federal efforts to address the mental health of first responders: Resources and issues for Congress*, 3. https://crsreports.congress.gov/product/details?prodcode=R46555

Federal Emergency Management Agency. (2015, January). *National fire incident reporting system: Complete reference guide*. https://www.usfa.fema.gov/downloads/pdf/nfirs/NFIRS_Complete_Reference_Guide_2015.pdf

Florida Department of Children and Families. (2021, July 1). *First Responder Suicide Deterrence Task Force: 2021 annual report*. https://www.myflfamilies.com/FirstResponderResiliency/docs/First%20Responder%20Task%20Force%202021%20Report%20-%20Final%20-%208-4-21.pdf

Florida House of Representatives. (2022). *House of Representatives staff analysis: HB 689*. https://www.myfloridahouse.gov/Sections/Documents/loaddoc.aspx?FileName=h0689d.SAT.DOCX&DocumentType=Analysis&BillNumber=0689&Session=2022

Florida Legislature. Florida Statutes, sec. 112.1815. (2021). *Online Sunshine*. https://m.flsenate.gov/statutes/112.1815.

Florida Statutes, sec. 440.093. http://www.leg.state.fl.us/statutes/index.cfm?App_mode=Display_Statute&URL=0400-0499/0440/Sections/0440.093.html

Gonzales, M. (2018, March 29). Florida law extends benefits for first responders with PTSD. *DrugRehab.com*. https://www.drugrehab.com/2018/03/29/florida-law-expands-ptsd-benefits/

Hawaii Statute, sec. 386-3. https://www.hawaii.edu/uhwo/clear/home/HRS386-1.html#:~:text=%C2%A7386-3

Heyman, M., Dill, J., & Douglas, R. (2018). *The Ruderman white paper on mental health and suicide of first responders*, 7. https://dir.nv.gov/uploadedFiles/dirnvgov/content/WCS/TrainingDocs/First%20Responder%20White%20Paper_Final%20(2).pdf

Hinds-Aldrich, M. (2020, April 20). Now is the time to finally fix NFIRS: Let's make "timely information sharing" the rallying cry for the post-COVID fire service. *Medium*. https://medium.com/@dr._matt/now-is-the-time-to-finally-fix-nfirs-2e6040dbb2cd

Idaho Legislature. (2019). *2019 Legislation: SB 1028*. Idaho Legislature. https://legislature.idaho.gov/sessioninfo/2019/legislation/S1028/

Idaho Statutes, title 72, ch. 4. https://legislature.idaho.gov/statutesrules/idstat/title72/

Illinois Compiled Statues, chapter 820, sec. 305. https://www.ilga.gov/legislation/ilcs/ilcs2.asp?ChapterID=68

Illinois General Assembly. (2019, August). *GENERAL PROVISIONS: (5 ILCS 840/) First Responders Suicide Prevention Act*. Illinois Compiled Statutes. https://www.ilga.gov/legislation/ilcs/ilcs3.asp?ActID=4020&ChapterID=2

Illinois General Assembly. (2022). *Bill status of SB1575*. Illinois General Assembly, August 2021. https://www.ilga.gov/legislation/BillStatus.asp?DocNum=1575&GAID=16&DocTypeID=SB&LegId=134209&SessionID=110

Improving Law Enforcement Officer Safety and Wellness Through Data Act. S. 3981. (2022). *Congress.gov*. https://www.congress.gov/bill/117th-congress/senate-bill/3981/text

Indiana Code, sec. 22-3-6-1. https://iga.in.gov/legislative/laws/2020/ic/titles/022

Iowa Code, sec. 85.3. (2016). https://www.legis.iowa.gov/docs/code/2016/85.pdf

James "Dustin" Samples Act, S.B. 1023, 112th Gen. Assem. (Tenn. 2022). https://wapp.capitol.tn.gov/apps/BillInfo/Default.aspx?BillNumber=SB1023&ga=112

Kansas Division of the Budget. (2021, March 1). *Fiscal note for SB 193 by Senator Holland*. http://www.kslegislature.org/li/s/images/pdf.png

Kansas Statutes, sec. 44-508. https://www.ksrevisor.org/statutes/chapters/ch44/044_005_0008.html#:~:text=44%2D508.,in%20the%20workers%20compensation%20act%3A&text=(b)%20%22Workman%22%20or,or%20apprenticeship%20with%20an%20employer

Kentucky Statutes, sec. 342.0011. https://apps.legislature.ky.gov/law/statutes/chapter.aspx?id=38914

Kohr, D. (2019, January 2). *For third straight year, police suicides outnumbers line-of-duty deaths*. Huffpost. https://www.huffpost.com/entry/for-third-straight-year-police-suicides-outnumber-line-of-duty-deaths_n_5c2d110de4b05c88b70542fa

Louisiana Laws Revised Statutes, sec. 23:1021. https://www.legis.la.gov/legis/Laws_Toc.aspx?folder=97&title=23

Maine Statutes, title 39-A. https://legislature.maine.gov/statutes/39-A/title39-Asec201.html

Massachusetts General Laws, chapter 143, sec. 1. https://malegislature.gov/Laws/GeneralLaws/PartI/TitleXXI/Chapter152/Section1

Michigan Compiled Laws, sec. 418.401. https://www.legislature.mi.gov/(S(0z41nedo0llttglsyfmb4dfu))/mileg.aspx?page=getObject&objectName=mcl-317-1969-4

Minnesota Statutes, sec. 176.011. https://www.revisor.mn.gov/statutes/2011/cite/176.011

Montana Code Annotated, sec. 39-71-119. https://leg.mt.gov/bills/mca/title_0390/chapter_0710/part_0010/section_0190/0390-0710-0010-0190.html

National Fire Academy. (2011, May 20–22). *Report of the 2nd National Fire Service Research Agenda Symposium*, 20. https://www.everyonegoeshome.com/wp-content/uploads/sites/2/2014/03/report2.pdf

National Wildfire Coordinating Group. (2021, December 16). *Mental Health Subcommittee*. National Wildfire Coordinating Group. https://www.nwcg.gov/committees/mental-health-subcommittee

National Wildfire Coordinating Group. (2022). National Wildfire Coordinating Group. https://www.nwcg.gov/

Nebraska Administrative Code, title 176, chapter 1. (2021, September 4). https://www.nebraska.gov/rules-and-regs/regsearch/Rules/Health_and_Human_Services_System/Title-176/Chapter-1.pdf

Nebraska Revised Statute, sec. 48-101.01. (2022). https://nebraskalegislature.gov/laws/statutes.php?statute=48-101.01#

Nevada Division of Public and Behavioral Health Office of Suicide Prevention. (2021). *Training*. Nevada Division of Public and Behavioral Health (DPBH) Office of Suicide Prevention. https://suicideprevention.nv.gov/Training/Training/

Nevada Revised Statues, sec. 616C.180. (2019). https://www.leg.state.nv.us/NRs/NRS-616c.html#NRS616CSec180

New Hampshire Revised Statutes, sec. 281-A:17-c. (2017). http://www.gencourt.state.nh.us/rsa/html/NHTOC/NHTOC-XXIII-281-A.htm

New Jersey Revised Statues, sec. 34:15-1. https://www.nj.gov/labor/workerscompensation/assets/PDFs/Forms/wc_law.pdf

New Mexico Statutes, sec. 52-1-24. https://nmonesource.com/nmos/nmsa/en/item/4394/index.do
North Carolina Statutes, sec. 97.53. https://www.ic.nc.gov/ncic/pages/statute/97-53.htm
North Dakota Century Code, ch. 65-01. https://ndlegis.gov/cencode/t65c01.pdf
Ohio Revised Code, sec. 4123.01. https://codes.ohio.gov/ohio-revised-code/chapter-4123
Oklahoma Statute, sec. 85A-13. (2014). https://oksenate.gov/sites/default/files/2019-12/os85A.pdf
Oregon Revied Statutes, sec. 656.802. (2019). https://oregon.public.law/statutes/ors_656.802
Pennsylvania Fire & Emergency Services Institute. (2019). https://pfesi.org/
Public Safety Officer Support Act of 2022. (2022). https://www.congress.gov/bill/117th-congress/house-bill/6943?q=%7B
Revised Statutes of Missouri, sec. 287.120. https://revisor.mo.gov/main/OneSection.aspx?section=287.120#:~:text=287.120.,requirements%2C%20firefighter%20stress%20not%20affected
Rhode Island General Laws, sec. 28-34-2. http://webserver.rilin.state.ri.us/Statutes/TITLE28/28-34/28-34-2.HTM
Severance-Medaris, C. (2021, April 30). *Legislation related to suicide prevention and NCSL resources*. National Conference of State Legislatures. https://www.ncsl.org/documents/meetings/Suicide-Prevention-Legislative-Resources_April.pdf
Sher, A. (2022, May 5). Despite Cleveland, Tennessee, widow's efforts, firefighter PTSD benefits bill fails in state legislature. *Chattanooga Times Free Press*. https://www.timesfreepress.com/news/local/story/2022/may/05/tennessee-firefighter-ptsd-benefits-bill-fails/568464/
South Carolina Code of Laws, title 42, ch. 1. https://www.scstatehouse.gov/code/title42.php
South Dakota Codified Laws 62-1-1. https://sdlegislature.gov/Statutes/Codified_Laws/2078124
State v. Cephas. Delaware Supreme Court. 637 A.2d 20 (1994). https://law.justia.com/cases/delaware/supreme-court/1994/637-a-2d-20-5.html
Supreme Court of Iowa. (1995). *Dunlavey v. Economy Fire and Casualty Co. 526 N.W.2d 845*. https://law.justia.com/cases/iowa/supreme-court/1995/93-1429-0.html
Supreme Court of Kanas. (1984, January 13). *234 Kan. 791 (1984): Followill v. Emerson Electric Co*. https://law.justia.com/cases/kansas/supreme-court/1984/55-753-1.html
Swiss Colony, Inc. v. DILHR, 72 Wis. 2d 46, 240 N.W.2d 128 (1976). https://law.justia.com/cases/wisconsin/supreme-court/1976/675-1974-4.html
Szymendera, S. D. (2020, February 18). *Workers' compensation: Overview and issues*. Congressional Research Service, 8. https://sgp.fas.org/crs/misc/R44580.pdf
Tennessee Code, sec. 50-6-102. https://law.justia.com/codes/tennessee/2021/title-50/chapter-6/part-1/section-50-6-102-d-1/#
Texas Commission on Fire Protection. (2019, July). *Commission hearing*. https://www.tcfp.texas.gov/Services/GetMp3?filename=%2FMeeting%2FCommission%2FRecording%2Fcomm_2019_0718.mp3
Texas Government Code, sec. 419.048. (2009). https://statutes.capitol.texas.gov/Docs/GV/htm/GV.419.htm
Texas Health and Human Services Commission. (2018, December). *Report on mental health access for first responders*. https://www.hhs.texas.gov/sites/default/files/documents/laws-regulations/reports-presentations/2018/hb1794-mental-health-access-first-responders-dec-2018.pdf
Texas Labor Code, ch. 504. https://statutes.capitol.texas.gov/Docs/LA/htm/LA.504.htm
Texas Legislature. (2019a). *HB 751 86(R)*. Texas Legislature Online. https://capitol.texas.gov/BillLookup/History.aspx?LegSess=86R&Bill=HB751
Texas Legislature. (2019b). In Texas Legislature Online (Ed.), *HB 2404 86(R)*. https://capitol.texas.gov/BillLookup/History.aspx?LegSess=86R&Bill=HB2404
Texas Legislature. (2019c). In Texas Legislature Online (Ed.), *HB 4147 86(R)*. https://capitol.texas.gov/BillLookup/History.aspx?LegSess=86R&Bill=HB4147
Texas Legislature (2019d). "SB 1359 87(R)." Texas Legislature Online. https://capitol.texas.gov/BillLookup/History.aspx?LegSess=87R&Bill=SB1359
The International Association of Chiefs of Police. (2022). *The National Consortium on Preventing Law Enforcement Suicide*. IACP. https://www.theiacp.org/projects/the-national-consortium-on-preventing-law-enforcement-suicide

The Office of Community Oriented Policing Services. (2022). *Law enforcement mental health and wellness act (LEMHWA) program*. https://cops.usdoj.gov/lemhwa

Tiesman, H. M., Elkins, K. L., Brown, M., Marsh, S., & Carson, L. M. (2021, April 6). *Suicides among first responders: A call to action*. Centers for Disease Control and Prevention. https://blogs.cdc.gov/niosh-science-blog/2021/04/06/suicides-first-responders/

Trump, D. J. (2017, February 9). Executive order 13774: Preventing violence against Federal, State, tribal, and local law enforcement officers. *Federal Register*. https://www.federalregister.gov/documents/2017/02/14/2017-03115/preventing-violence-against-federal-state-tribal-and-local-law-enforcement-officers

United States Court of Appeals, 10th Circuit. (2003). *Doebele v. Sprint/United Management Company*, 342 F.3d 1117 (10th Cir.). https://caselaw.findlaw.com/us-10th-circuit/1292845.html

United States Department of Health and Human Services. (2021, September 9). *The National Institute for Occupational Safety and Health (NIOSH): Fire fighter fatality investigation and prevention program*. Centers for Disease Control and Prevention. https://www.cdc.gov/niosh/fire/iafcpgmreview.html

United States Fire Administration. (2021, December 9). *2021 Update to Yellow Ribbon report on behavioral health and wellness is now available*. United States Fire Administration. https://www.usfa.fema.gov/blog/ig-120921.html

United States Fire Administration. (2022a). *Department wellness program*. United States Fire Administration. https://apps.usfa.fema.gov/nfacourses/catalog/details/10572

United States Fire Administration. (2022b). *Empowering responder wellness*. United States Fire Administration. https://apps.usfa.fema.gov/nfacourses/catalog/details/10595

United States Fire Administration. (2022c, January 20). *Interviews with USFA leadership*. United States Fire Administration. https://www.usfa.fema.gov/podcasts/2022-episode-1.html

United States Fire Administration. (2022d). *National Emergency Training Center Library*. https://usfa.bibliovation.com/

United States Fire Administration, AFG, and SAFER Program Reauthorization Act of 2017. (2018). *15 United States Code Chapter 49, §2229*. http://uscode.house.gov/view.xhtml?path=/prelim@title15/chapter49&edition=prelim

Utah Code, sec 34A-2-401. https://le.utah.gov/xcode/Title34A/Chapter2/34A-2.html?v=C34A-2_1800010118000101

Vermont Statutes, title 21, ch. 9. https://legislature.vermont.gov/statutes/title/21

Washington Revised Code, sec. 51.08.100. https://app.leg.wa.gov/rcw/default.aspx?cite=51.08&full=true

West Virginia Code, sec. 23-4-1. https://www.wvlegislature.gov/wvcode/chapterentire.cfm?chap=23&art=4&section=1#

White v. Lexington-Fayette, No. 2004-CA-001457-WC (Ky. Ct. App. May 27, 2005). https://casetext.com/case/white-v-lexington-fayette

Wisconsin Statutes and Annotations, sec. 102.01. https://docs.legis.wisconsin.gov/statutes/statutes/102/01

Wyoming Statutes, title 27. https://wyoleg.gov/statutes/compress/title27.pdf

Index

M. L. Bourke et al. (eds.), *First Responder Mental Health*,
https://doi.org/10.1007/978-3-031-38149-2

www.ingramcontent.com/pod-product-compliance
Lightning Source LLC
Chambersburg PA
CBHW061721100826
49620CB00003B/51
* 9 7 8 3 0 3 1 3 8 1 4 8 5 *